Internal Organs

THIEME Atlas of Anatomy
Third Edition

Latin Nomenclature

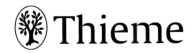

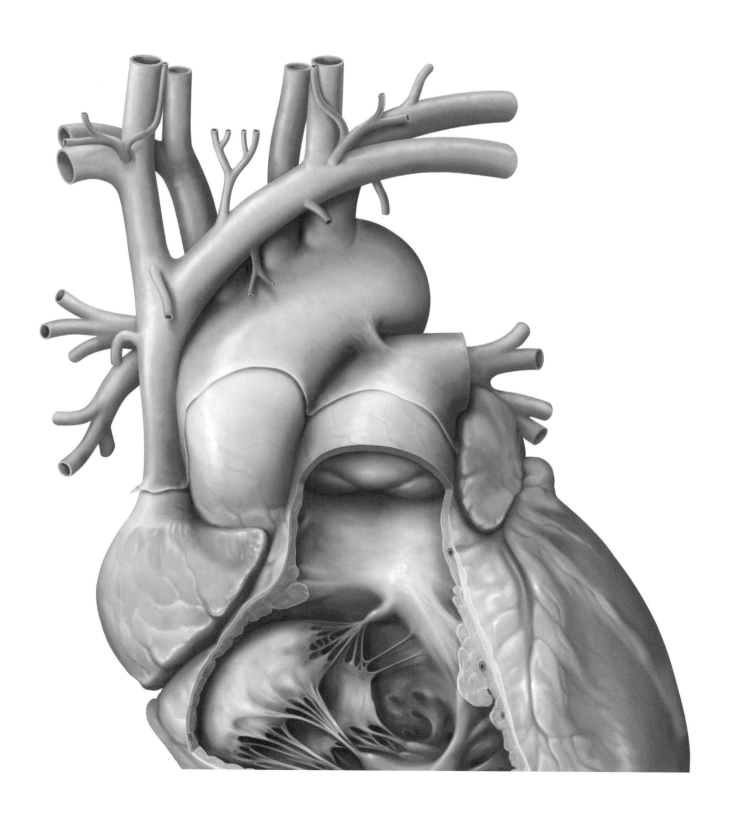

Internal Organs

THIEME Atlas of Anatomy
Third Edition

Latin Nomenclature

Authors

Michael Schuenke, MD, PhD
Institute of Anatomy
Christian Albrechts University, Kiel

Erik Schulte, MD
Institute of Functional and Clinical Anatomy
Johannes Gutenberg University, Mainz

Udo Schumacher, MD
FRCPath, CBiol, FIBiol, DSc
Institute of Anatomy and Experimental
    Morphology
University Medical Center,
    Hamburg-Eppendorf

Illustrations by
Markus Voll
Karl Wesker

Consulting Editor
Wayne A. Cass, PhD
Department of Neuroscience
University of Kentucky College of Medicine
Lexington, Kentucky

**Consulting Editor, Latin
Nomenclature**
Hugo Zeberg, MD
Department of Neuroscience
Karolinska Institute, Stockholm

Thieme
New York • Stuttgart • Delhi • Rio de Janeiro

Translators: Terry Telger, John Grossman, and Judith Tomat

Illustrators: Markus Voll and Karl Wesker

Compositor: DiTech Process Solutions

Library of Congress Cataloging-in-Publication Data is available from the publisher.

Important note: Medicine is an ever-changing science undergoing continual development. Research and clinical experience are continually expanding our knowledge, in particular our knowledge of proper treatment and drug therapy. Insofar as this book mentions any dosage or application, readers may rest assured that the authors, editors, and publishers have made every effort to ensure that such references are in accordance with **the state of knowledge at the time of production of the book.**

Nevertheless, this does not involve, imply, or express any guarantee or responsibility on the part of the publishers in respect to any dosage instructions and forms of applications stated in the book. **Every user is requested to examine carefully** the manufacturers' leaflets accompanying each drug and to check, if necessary in consultation with a physician or specialist, whether the dosage schedules mentioned therein or the contraindications stated by the manufacturers differ from the statements made in the present book. Such examination is particularly important with drugs that are either rarely used or have been newly released on the market. Every dosage schedule or every form of application used is entirely at the user's own risk and responsibility. The authors and publishers request every user to report to the publishers any discrepancies or inaccuracies noticed. If errors in this work are found after publication, errata will be posted at www.thieme.com on the product description page.

Some of the product names, patents, and registered designs referred to in this book are in fact registered trademarks or proprietary names even though specific reference to this fact is not always made in the text. Therefore, the appearance of a name without designation as proprietary is not to be construed as a representation by the publisher that it is in the public domain.

©2021. Thieme. All rights reserved.
Thieme Medical Publishers, Inc.
333 Seventh Avenue, 18th Floor
New York, NY 10001, USA
www.thieme.com
+1 800 782 3488, customerservice@thieme.com

Printed in Germany by Appl   5 4 3 2 1

ISBN 978-1-68420-082-5

Also available as an e-book:
eISBN 978-1-68420-083-2

Foreword

Each of the authors of the single volume *Thieme Atlas of Anatomy* was impressed with the extraordinary detail, accuracy, and beauty of the illustrations that were created for the Thieme three volume series of anatomy atlases. We felt these images were one of the most significant additions to anatomic education in the past 50 years. The effective pedagogical approach of this series, with two-page learning units that combined the outstanding illustrations and captions that emphasized the functional and clinical significance of structures, coupled with the numerous tables summarizing key information, was unique. We also felt that the overall organization of each region, with structures presented first systemically — musculoskeletal, vascular, and nervous — and then topographically, supported classroom learning and active dissection in the laboratory.

This series combines the best of a clinically oriented text and an atlas. Its detail and pedagogical presentation make it a complete support for class and laboratory instruction and a reference for life in all the medical, dental, and allied health fields. Each of the volumes — *General Anatomy and Musculoskeletal System, Internal Organs,* and *Head, Neck, and Neuroanatomy* — can also be used as a stand-alone text/atlas for an in-depth study of systems often involved in the allied health/medical specialty fields.

We were delighted when Thieme asked us to work with them to create a single-volume atlas from this groundbreaking series, and we owe a great debt to the authors and illustrators of this series inasmuch as their materials and vision formed the general framework for the single volume *Thieme Atlas of Anatomy*.

We thank the authors and illustrators for this very special contribution to the teaching of anatomy and recommend it for thorough mastery of anatomy and its clinically functional importance in all fields of health care-related specialties.

Lawrence M. Ross, Brian R. MacPherson, and Anne M. Gilroy

A Note on the Use of Latin Terminology

To introduce the Latin nomenclature into an English-language text-book is a delicate task, particularly because many Latin loanwords have passed into general use. Some loanwords are so common that fluency of the text would be disturbed if they were to be translated back into Latin. These Latin loanwords have typically undergone several adaptations before becoming part of the English language. A term such as *sympathetic trunk* (lat. *truncus sympaticus*) has undergone morphological adaptation (through the loss of masculine suffix -us), orthographical adaptation (through the substitution of a "Germanic" k for a Latin c), and phonological adaptation (th and e instead of t and i). In addition, the word order has been reversed. The Latin term *sympaticus* is in fact borrowed from the late Greek word *sympathetikos* (from sympathes "having a fellow feeling, affected by like feelings"), thereby illustrating that words move between languages when cultures meet. Other anatomical terms are so colloquial (e.g. *hand*), that a Latin word (e.g. *manus*) would be inappropriate to use at all occasions. Clearly, the text would become unreadable if a strict translation of all English terms into Latin were imposed.

As a result, Latin has been used as long as it does not disrupt the flow of the text and whenever possible in figures and tables. In some cases, dual terminology has been used, with either the English or Latin word in parentheses. As much as possible, the terminology of *Terminolgia Anatomica* (1998) has been followed.

Hugo Zeberg

Preface of the Authors and Illustrators

When Thieme started planning the first edition of this atlas, they sought the opinions of students and instructors alike in both the United States and Europe on what constituted an "ideal" atlas of anatomy — ideal to learn from, to master extensive amounts of information while on a busy class schedule, and, in the process, to acquire sound, up-to-date knowledge. The result of our work in response to what Thieme had learned is this atlas. The *Thieme Atlas of Anatomy*, unlike most other atlases, is a comprehensive educational tool that combines illustrations with explanatory text and summary tables, introducing clinical applications throughout, and presenting anatomic concepts in a step-by-step sequence that includes system-by-system and topographical views.

For the first edition we had hoped that our *Atlas of Anatomy* would help the medical student to understand the anatomical basis of clinical medicine. This indeed was accepted by the students all over the world and soon a second edition had to come on the market in Germany, which was extensively extended and revised. More and more information had been added, including spreads on important foundational information on the common imaging planes for plain film, MRI, and CT scans, the structure of skeletal muscle fibers, the structure and chemical composition of hyaline cartilage, and the regeneration of peripheral nerves, bone marrow, and paraganglia, as well as new graphical summaries in neuroanatomy. Hence the fifth German edition looks ever more distinctly different from the first one. Of course, we have also checked, corrected, and updated all of the information in this atlas.

We are grateful to the American branch of Thieme that they have made this third English edition possible. We hope that this updated version will serve the medical students and practitioners of medicine alike in helping them to understand human morphology which is indispensable for diagnosis and therapy.

Michael Schünke, Erik Schulte, Udo Schumacher,
Markus Voll, and Karl Wesker

Acknowledgments

First we wish to thank our families. This atlas is dedicated to them.

Since the publication of the first volume of the *Thieme Atlas of Anatomy* in 2006, we have received numerous suggestions for refinements and additions. We would like to take this opportunity to express our sincere thanks to all those who through the years have helped us to improve the *Thieme Atlas of Anatomy* in one way or another. Specifically, this includes Kirsten Hattermann, Ph.D.; Runhild Lucius, D.D.S.; Prof. Renate Lüllmann-Rauch, M.D.; Prof. Jobst Sievers, M.D.; Ali Therany, D.D.S.; Prof. Thilo Wedel, M.D. (all at the Anatomic Institute of Christian Albrecht University of Kiel); as well as Christian Friedrichs, D.D.S. (Practice for Tooth Preservation and Endodontics, Kiel); Prof. Reinhart Gossrau, M.D. (Charité Berlin, Institute of Anatomy); Prof. Paul Peter Lunkenheimer, M.D. (Westphalian Wilhelm University Münster); Thomas Müller, M.D., associate professor (Institute of Functional and Clinical Anatomy of the Johannes Gutenberg University of Mainz); Kai-Hinrich Olms, M.D., Foot Surgery, Bad Schwartau; Daniel Paech, M.S. physics, medical student (Department of Neuroradiology of the University Medical Center, Heidelberg); Thilo Schwalenberg, M.D., supervising physician (Urologic Clinic of the University Medical Center, Leipzig); Prof. emeritus Katharina Spanel-Borowski, M.D. (University of Leipzig); Prof. Christoph Viebahn, M.D. (Georg August University of Göttingen). For their extensive proofreading we thank Gabriele Schünke, M.S. biology; Jakob Fay, M.D.; as well as medical students Claudia Dücker, Simin Rassouli, Heike Teichmann, Susanne Tippmann, and dental student Sylvia Zilles; also, Julia Jörns-Kuhnke, M.D., especially for her assistance with the figure labels.

We extend special thanks to Stephanie Gay and Bert Sender, who prepared the layouts. Their ability to arrange the text and illustrations on facing pages for maximum clarity has contributed greatly to the quality of the atlas.

We particularly acknowledge the efforts of those who handled this project on the publishing side:

Jürgen Lüthje, M.D., Ph.D., executive editor at Thieme Medical Publishers, has "made the impossible possible." He not only reconciled the wishes of the authors and artists with the demands of reality but also managed to keep a team of five people working together for years on a project whose goal was known to us from the beginning but whose full dimensions we only came to appreciate over time. He is deserving of our most sincere and heartfelt thanks once more this year, in which Jürgen Lüthje, M.D., Ph.D., is retiring. We welcome his successor Dr. Jochen Neuberger, who has shown great initiative is taking over the *Thieme Atlas of Anatomy* and will continue to lead and develop the existing team.

Sabine Bartl, developmental editor, became a touchstone for the authors in the best sense of the word. She was able to determine whether a beginning student, and thus one who is not (yet) a professional, could clearly appreciate the logic of the presentation. The authors are indebted to her.

We are grateful to Antje Bühl, who was there from the beginning as project assistant, working "behind the scenes" on numerous tasks such as repeated proofreading and helping to arrange the figure labels.

We owe a great debt of thanks to Martin Spencker, managing director of Educational Publications at Thieme, especially to his ability to make quick and unconventional decisions when dealing with problems and uncertainties. His openness to all the concerns of the authors and artists established conditions for a cooperative partnership.

We are also indebted to Yvonne Strassburg, Michael Zepf, and Laura Diemand who saw to it that the *Thieme Atlas of Anatomy* was printed and bound on schedule, and that the project benefited from the best practical expertise throughout the entire process of publication. We also thank Susanne Tochtermann-Wenzel and Anja Jahn for their assistance with technical issues involving every aspect of the illustrations; Julia Fersch who ensured that the *Thieme Atlas of Anatomy* is also accessible via eRef; Almut Leopold for the exceptional index; Marie-Luise Kürschner and Nina Jentschke for the appealing cover design; as well as Dr. Thomas Krimmer, Liesa Arendt, Birgit Carlsen, Stephanie Eilmann, and Anne Döbler, representing all those now and previously involved in the marketing, sale, and promotion of the *Thieme Atlas of Anatomy*.

The authors, October 2019

I thank my wife, Valerie, and son, Robert, for their love, support and understanding. Nothing means more to me than the two of you.

As consulting editor I was asked to review the English translation of *Thieme Atlas of Anatomy: Internal Organs*, third edition. My work involved reviewing and editing the translation and nomenclature conversion of the German text to currently used English terms. In addition, some minor changes in presentation were made to reflect commonly accepted approaches in North American educational programs. This task was facilitated by the clear organization of the original text and the exceptional work of the translators. Throughout this process I have tried to remain faithful to the intentions and insights of the authors and illustrators, whom I thank for this outstanding revision.

I would also like to thank the entire team at Thieme Medical Publishers who worked on this edition. In particular I would like to give special thanks to Delia DeTurris, Executive Editor, for inviting me to work on this atlas and for her continued support, and Torsten Scheihagen, Managing Editor, for his support and help throughout the process of completing this atlas. I also thank Brian R. MacPherson, Ph.D., Professor of Neuroscience at the University of Kentucky, for his support.

Wayne A. Cass

It has been a great honor to act as a consulting editor, with responsibility for the Latin nomenclature, for *Thieme Atlas of Anatomy: Internal Organs*, Third Edition. There were several people from whom I received a great deal of assistance and guidance, and must express my gratitude towards. Regarding the discussion of nomenclature, I would wish to thank my mentor Prof. Peter Århem, Ph.D., my father Lennart Zeberg, M.D., and Prof. Jonas Broman, Ph.D. In addition, I would also like to express my gratitude to Prof. Björn Meister, M.D., Ph.D., for putting forward my name for this task.

Moreover, I am deeply grateful to the staff at Thieme Medical Publishers that I have been in close contact with, in particular, the editorial director Anne Sydor, Ph.D., managing editor Judith Tomat, editorial assistant Huvie Weinreich, and marketing agent David Towle.

I would also like to acknowledge the Federative International Programme for Anatomical Terminology (FIPAT) for their work towards a standard nomenclature in the field of anatomy.

In addition, I would like to express my gratitude to my talented assistant teachers — C. Stening-Soppola, D.F. Åström, A. Javanmardi, E.N. Sögutlu, A. Sotoodeh, N. Aziz, A.-M. Al-Khabbaz, K. Ma, and T. Engström — for performing an initial review of the Latin nomenclature.

Hugo Zeberg

The people behind the *Thieme Atlas of Anatomy*

A work such as the *Thieme Atlas of Anatomy* can only arise when the people involved in the project work hand in hand. The integrated educational and artistic work you now hold in your hands is the product of an intensive discourse between anatomy professors Michael Schünke, Erik Schulte, and Udo Schumacher and anatomic illustrators Markus Voll and Karl Wesker.

Creating learning units that comprehensively treat a topic on a two-page spread is a challenge in itself. The authors must carefully select the content, assemble it, and add explanatory legends. Yet how this content is presented in the atlas, how appealing and memorable it is, depends largely on the illustrations. And the *Thieme Atlas of Anatomy* now includes a good 5000 of them. In creating them, Markus Voll and

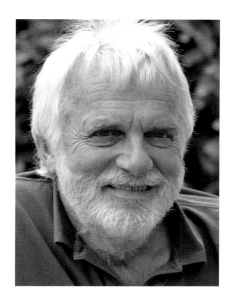 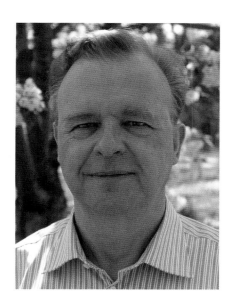 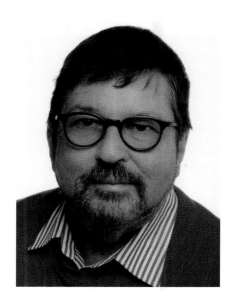

Michael Scheunke, MD, PhD, professor

Institute of Anatomy of the University of Kiel, studied biology and medicine in Tübingen and Kiel, extensive teaching of medical students and physical therapists, author and translator of other textbooks.

Erik Schulte, MD, professor

Institute of Functional and Clinical Anatomy of the Johannes Gutenberg University of Mainz, studied medicine in Freiburg, extensive teaching of medical students, award for excellence in teaching in Mainz.

Udo Schumacher, MD, professor

Institute of Anatomy of the University of Hamburg; studied medicine in Kiel with one year of study at the Wistar Institute of Anatomy and Biology in Philadelphia; extensive teaching of medical students, physical therapists, and residents (FRCS). Spent several years in Southampton and gained experience in integrated interdisciplinary instruction.

Karl Wesker drew on many years of experience in anatomic illustration, visited anatomic collections, studied specimens, and immersed themselves in old and new works of anatomy. This was the foundation on which the *Thieme Atlas of Anatomy* arose.

It guides the reader through anatomy step by step, revealing what a crucial role anatomy will later play in medical practice. This was a particularly important consideration for the authors. Whether performing bowel surgery for a tumor, puncturing the tympanic membrane in a middle ear infection, or examining a pregnant patient, no physician lacking knowledge of anatomy is a good physician. Even the *Thieme Atlas of Anatomy* cannot spare you the effort of learning, yet the authors and illustrators can assure you that it will make it a lot more pleasant.

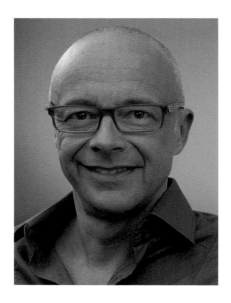

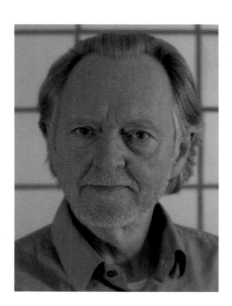

Markus Voll

Freelance illustrator and graphic artist in Munich, trained as an artist at the Blocherer School of Design in Munich, studied medicine at the University of Munich. He has worked as a scientific illustrator on numerous book projects for 25 years.

Karl Wesker

Freelance painter and graphic artist in Berlin. Apprenticeship as a plate etcher and lithographer, studied visual communication at the University of Applied Sciences in Münster and at the Berlin University of the Arts and art science at the Technical University of Berlin. For over 30 years he has been active as a freelance painter and graphic artist, including book projects in anatomy.

Contents

A Structure and Development of Organ Systems

B Thorax

C Abdomen and Pelvis

D Neurovascular Supply to the Organs

E Organ Fact Sheets

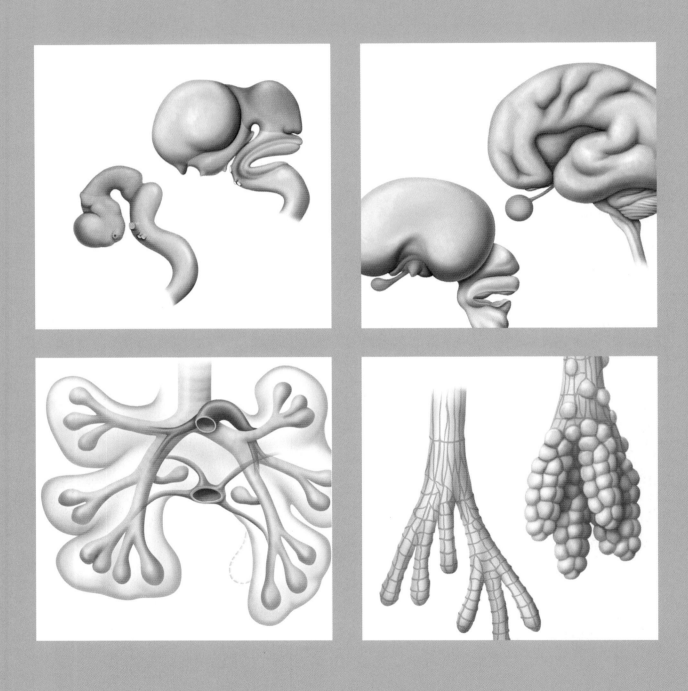

A Structure and Development of Organ Systems

1.1   Definitions, Overview, and Evolution of Body Cavities

Definitions

The human body, similar to all higher organisms, is organized into a hierarchy of different levels:

- A **cell** is the smallest unit of life, that in principle can survive on its own.

- A **tissue** consists primarily of cells from the same origin, and the extracellular matrix they form. A tissue is an ensemble of cells, organized to do a specific job.

- An **organ** is a structural unit composed of different tissues. Thus, it combines the functions of the various tissue components.

- An **organ system** is made up of organs that function together to perform a specific function. For example, the digestive organs make up the *digestive system*. For the most part, the individual organs are related to each other morphologically.

- An **organism** is composed of several organ systems.

A Overview of the internal organs of the human body

Anterior view of the human body, displaying the internal organs. For clarity, the nervous system and most of the intestinum tenue and endocrine organs are not shown.

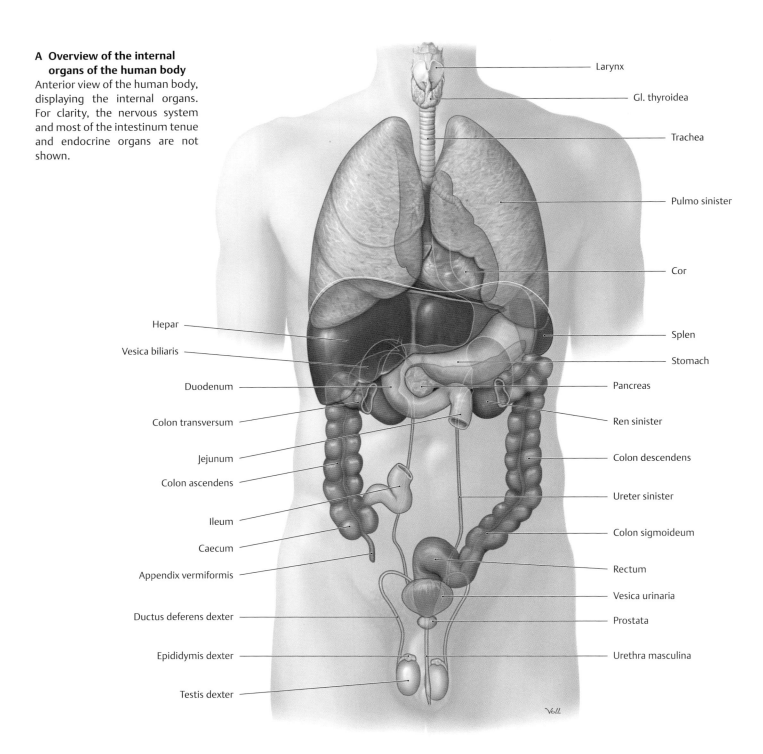

Larynx
Gl. thyroidea
Trachea
Pulmo sinister
Cor
Splen
Stomach
Pancreas
Ren sinister
Colon descendens
Ureter sinister
Colon sigmoideum
Rectum
Vesica urinaria
Prostata
Urethra masculina

Hepar
Vesica biliaris
Duodenum
Colon transversum
Jejunum
Colon ascendens
Ileum
Caecum
Appendix vermiformis
Ductus deferens dexter
Epididymis dexter
Testis dexter

Voll

B Overview of organ systems

Since, by definition, every structural unit composed of different tissues is referred to as an organ (according to this definition, every muscle is an organ), the term is commonly used for structures in the cranium, neck, and body cavities. The organs situated inside the body cavities are referred to as internal organs or viscera. This atlas is a study aid for learning gross anatomy. Thus, the individual organs are discussed with respect to their topography. However, since groups of individual organs form morphological and functional systems, which due to evolutionary processes don't conform to topographical anatomy, those organ systems along with their embryology will be discussed first. This overview will aid in understanding the location, shape and function of the internal organs in the developing organism.

Note: Peripheral nerves, bone marrow, and blood are usually not referred to as "organs." For the sake of completeness, they will also be discussed since they are part of whole organ systems.

* Organs that are highlighted in italics are located in the neck or cranium and thus will not be discussed here.

System	Organs*
Systema digestorium	*Cavitas oris with dentes and gll. salivariae, pharynx, oesophagus,* stomach (gaster), intestinum tenue, intestinum crassum, rectum, pancreas, liver (hepar), and vesica fellea
Systema respiratorium	*Cavitas nasi and sinus paranasales, larynx, trachea,* pulmones
Systema urinarium	Kidneys (renes), ureteres, vesica urinaria, urethra
Systema genitale	♀ Uterus, tubae uterinae (salpinges), ovarium, vagina, gll. vestibulares majores
	♂ Testes, epididymis, ductus deferens, vesiculae seminales, prostata, gl. bulbourethralis
Systema cardiovasculare	Heart (cor), vessels, blood, and *medulla ossium rubra*
Systema lymphoideum	*Medulla ossium, tonsillae,* thymus, splen, nodi lymphoidei, ductus thoracicus
Systema endocrinum	*Gl. thyroidea, gll. parathyroideae,* gll. suprarenales (adrenal), paraganglia, pancreas (islet cells), ovaria, testes, *hypophysis, hypothalamus*
Systema nervosum	*Encephalon, medulla spinalis,* systema nervosum periphericum (with *somatic* and autonomic components)

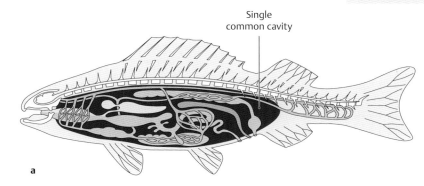

Single common cavity

a

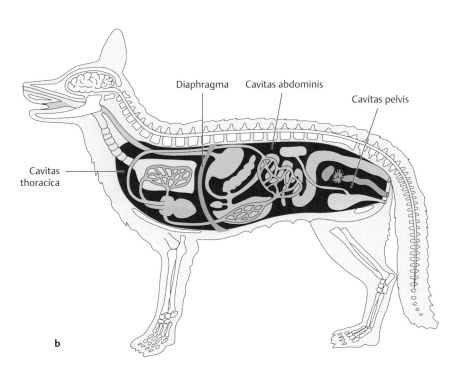

Diaphragma   Cavitas abdominis

Cavitas pelvis

Cavitas thoracica

b

C Evolution of body cavities

While in fish **(a)** all internal organs are situated in a single common body cavity, in mammals **(b)**, the diaphragma separates the cavitas thoracica from the cavitas abdominis. Due to shared evolutionary history, the structures of these two body cavities are basically identical. The different anatomical terms used for similar structures (e.g., pleura – peritoneum) are functionally meaningless. In mammals, there is no physical structure that separates the cavitas abdominis from the cavitas pelvis. They form a continuous space that in terms of its topographical anatomy is divided only by the superior border of the bony pelvis. The anatomical unit of the cavitates abdominis and pelvis is of clinical significance as there are no anatomical barriers to restrict the spread of inflammation or tumors between these two compartments. The diaphragma acts as a barrier to stop tumors or inflammation from spreading from the cavitas abdominis to the cavitas thoracica and vice versa.

3

1.2 Organogenesis and the Development of Body Cavities

A Differentiation of the germ layers (after Christ and Wachtler)

After the formation of the trilaminar discus embryonicus at the end of the third week (see **B**) the primordia (precursor cells destined to become a specific tissue or organ) of the different tissues and organs are arranged according to the body plan. In the subsequent embryonic period (weeks 4 to 8), the three germ layers (ectoderma, mesoderma, and endoderma) give rise to all major external and internal organs (organogenesis). At the same time, the trilaminar discus embryonicus begins to fold, resulting in major changes in body form and internal structure. By the end of the embryonic stage, the major features of the body are recognizable and the organs have moved into their eventual position within and outside of the body cavities.

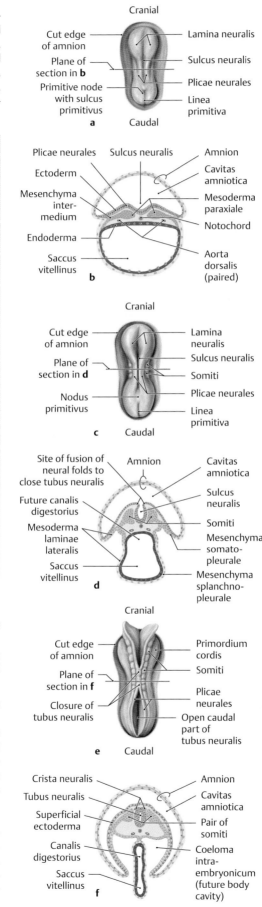

Ectoderma	Tubus neuralis		Encephalon, retina, medulla spinalis
	Crista neuralis	Crista neuralis cranialis	Ganglia sensoria and parasympathica, pars enterica systematis nervosi, thyrocyti C, textus muscularis levis, pigment cells, glomus caroticum, bone, cartilage, connective tissue, dentinum and cementum of the teeth, dermis, and tela subcutanea of the head
		Crista neuralis truncalis	Ganglia sensoria and autonomica, gliocyti peripherici, medulla suprarenalis, melanocyti, intramural plexuses
	Surface ectoderma	Ectodermal placodesae	Adenohypophysis, ganglia sensoria nervorum cranialium, epithelium olfactorium, auris interna, lens
			Enamelum of the teeth, epithelium cavitatis oris, gll. salivariae, cavitates nasi, sinus paranasales, lacrimal passages, porus acusticus externus, epidermis, hair, nails, cutaneous glands
Mesoderma	Axial	Notochorda, prechordal mesoderma	Musculi externi bulbi oculi
	Paraxiale		Columna vertebralis, costae, textus muscularis striatus, connective tissue, dermis and subcutis of the back and part of the head, smooth muscle, blood vessels
	Mesenchyma intermedium		Renes (kidneys), gonada, renal and genital excretory ducts
	Mesoderma laminae lateralis	Visceral (mesenchyma splanchnopleurale)	Cor (heart), vasa sanguinea, textus muscularis levis, bowel wall, blood, cortex suprarenalis, tunica serosa pleurae visceralis
		Parietal (mesenchyma somatopleurale)	Sternum, limbs (cartilage, bones, and ligaments), dermis and tela subcutanea of the anterolateral body wall, textus muscularis levis, connective tissue, tunica serosa pleurae parietalis
Endoderma			Epithelium of the bowel, respiratory tract, digestive glands, gll. pharyngeales, tuba auditiva, cavitas tympani, vesica urinaria, thymus, gll. parathyroideae, gl. thyroidea

B Neurulation and Somitus Formation (after Sadler)

a, **c**, and **e** Dorsal views of the discus embryonicus after removal of the amnion;

b, **d**, and **f** Schematic cross-sections of the corresponding stages at the planes of section as marked in **a**, **c**, and **e**; Age is in postovulatory days.

During neurulation (formation of the tubus neuralis from the lamina neuralis), the neurectoderma differentiates from the surface ectoderma, due to inductive influences from the notochorda, and the tubus neuralis and crista neuralis cells move inside the embryo.

a and **b** Discus embryonicus at 19 days: The sulcus neuralis is developing in the area of the lamina neuralis.

c and **d** Discus embryonicus at 20 days: In the mesoderma paraxiale, flanking both sides of the sulcus neuralis and notochorda, the first somiti have formed (they contain cellular material assigned to form the columna vertebralis, muscles, and subcutaneous tissue). Immediately lateral to the mesoderma paraxiale is the mesenchyma intermedium, and lateral to that is the mesoderma laminae lateralis. The sulcus neuralis is beginning to close to form the tubus neuralis and the embryo begins to fold.

e and **f** Discus embryonicus at 22 days: Eight pairs of somiti are seen flanking the partially closed tubus neuralis which is sinking below the ectoderma. In the mesoderma laminae lateralis, the coeloma intraembryonicum, or future body cavity, arises. It will later develop both a parietal and a visceral layer (somatopleure and splanchnopleure). On the side facing the coeloma, a mesothelial lining develops from the somato- and splanchnopleure. It later forms the tunicae serosae lining the cavitates pericardiaca, pleurales, and peritonealis. The tubus neuralis migrates deeper into the mesoderma, and the somiti differentiate into sclerotomus, myotomus, and dermatome.

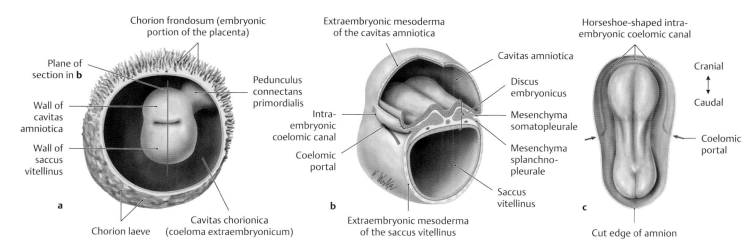

Chorion frondosum (embryonic portion of the placenta)

Plane of section in **b**

Wall of cavitas amniotica

Wall of saccus vitellinus

Pedunculus connectans primordialis

Intra-embryonic coelomic canal

Coelomic portal

a

Chorion laeve

Cavitas chorionica (coeloma extraembryonicum)

Extraembryonic mesoderma of the cavitas amniotica

Cavitas amniotica

Discus embryonicus

Mesenchyma somatopleurale

Mesenchyma splanchno-pleurale

Saccus vitellinus

b

Extraembryonic mesoderma of the saccus vitellinus

Horseshoe-shaped intra-embryonic coelomic canal

Cranial

Caudal

Coelomic portal

c

Cut edge of amnion

C Formation of the coeloma intraembryonicum (after Waldeyer)
a View into the chorionic cavity (coeloma extraembryonicum); **b** Cut through the cavitas amniotica, discus embryonicus and saccus vitellinus (the cavitas chorionica has been removed); **c** View of the discus embryonicus (the intraembryonic coelomic canal has been highlighted in red). The eventual definitive serous cavities (cavitates pericardiaca, pleuralis, and peritonealis) arise from the coeloma intraembryonicum which begins to form in week 4 when intercellular clefts (not shown) appear in the mesoderma laminae lateralis (see **B**). The coeloma intraembryonicum divides the mesoderma laminae lateralis into parietal and visceral layers (*mesenchymata somatopleurale* and *splanchnopleurale*). At the edges of the discus embryonicus, the mesenchyma somatopleurale adjacent to the surface ectoderm is continuous with the extraembryonic mesoderm of the amnion. The mesenchyma splanchnopleurale

adjacent to the endoderma is continuous with the extraembryonic mesoderm of the saccus vitellinus. Thus, the coeloma intraembryonicum surrounds the opening of the saccus vitellinus like a ring (the *coelomic ring*). In the cranial part of the embryo, the coelomic ring closes off from the coeloma extraembryonicum (cavitas chorionica) and forms a horseshoe shaped intraembryonic *coelomic canal*, which is visible when viewed from above. The caudal coelomata intra and extraembryonicum (see **D**) continue to communicate with one another through the *coelomic portals*. Later, as a result of embryonic folding, the caudal coelomata intra- and extraembryonicum become separated from each other. During the course of embryonic development, the coeloma intraembryonicum compartmentalizes with the cavitas pericardiaca arising from the unpaired cranial part of the coeloma and the paired cavitates pleuralis and peritonealis arising from the lateral limbs of the coelom.

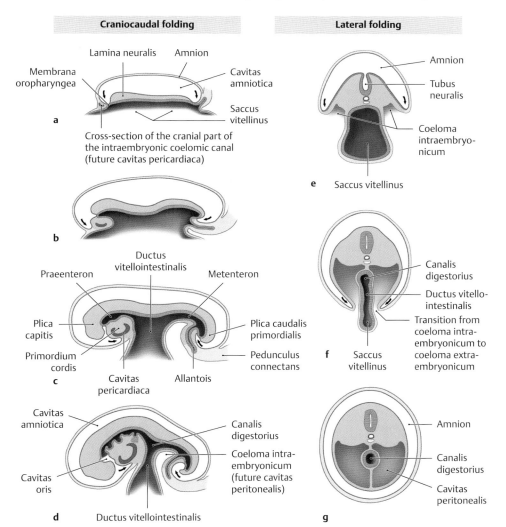

Craniocaudal folding

Lamina neuralis   Amnion

Membrana oropharyngea

Cavitas amniotica

Saccus vitellinus

a

Cross-section of the cranial part of the intraembryonic coelomic canal (future cavitas pericardiaca)

b

Ductus vitellointestinalis

Praeenteron

Metenteron

Plica capitis

Primordium cordis

Cavitas pericardiaca

Allantois

Plica caudalis primordialis

Pedunculus connectans

c

Cavitas amniotica

Canalis digestorius

Coeloma intra-embryonicum (future cavitas peritonealis)

Cavitas oris

d

Ductus vitellointestinalis

Lateral folding

Amnion

Tubus neuralis

Coeloma intraembryonicum

e   Saccus vitellinus

Canalis digestorius

Ductus vitello-intestinalis

Transition from coeloma intra-embryonicum to coeloma extra-embryonicum

f   Saccus vitellinus

Amnion

Canalis digestorius

Cavitas peritonealis

g

D Embryonic folding
a–d Midsagittal sections; **e–g** Frontal sections at the level of the saccus vitellinus.
During folding the embryo is rapidly growing and it rises up from the surface of the original discus. The lamina neuralis grows rapidly and extends in both the cranial and caudal directions. As a result, the embryo curves upon itself (**a–d**). The formation of somiti causes a lateral expansion (lateral folding) of the embryo in the area above the saccus vitellinus (**e–g**). As a result, the intraembryonic coelomic canal shifts ventrally. Due to cranial folding (head fold), the cranial portion of the coeloma intraembryonicum moves ventral to the praeenteron and broadens into the cavitas pericardiaca. The folding of the caudal tail moves the pedunculus connectans (the future funiculus umbilicalis) and the allantois to the ventral aspect of the embryo. While lateral folding occurs, the coeloma intraembryonicum progressively separates from the coelom extraembryonicum. These processes result in the junction between embryonic endoderma (primitive canalis digestorius) and saccus vitellinus (future pedunculus sacci vitellini) becoming increasingly narrow. At the same time, the left and right caudal parts of the coeloma intraembryonicum merge with one another forming a single large cavitas coelomica, which is the future cavitas peritonealis (for position of cavitates pleurales see p. 6).

5

1.3 Compartmentalizatioan of the Coeloma Intraembryonicum

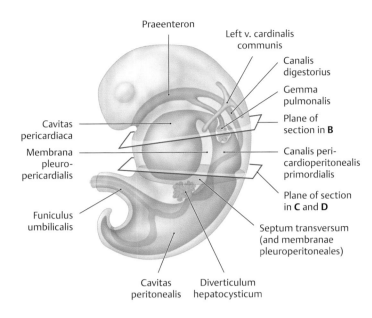

Praeenteron
Left v. cardinalis communis
Canalis digestorius
Gemma pulmonalis
Plane of section in **B**
Cavitas pericardiaca
Membrana pleuro-pericardialis
Canalis peri-cardioperitonealis primordialis
Plane of section in **C** and **D**
Funiculus umbilicalis
Septum transversum (and membranae pleuroperitoneales)
Cavitas peritonealis
Diverticulum hepatocysticum

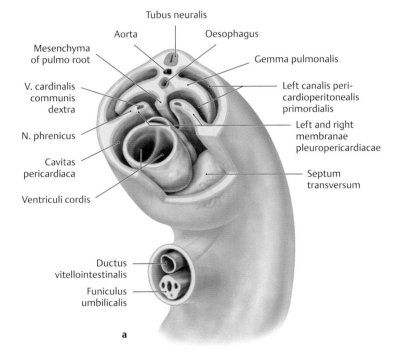

Tubus neuralis
Aorta
Oesophagus
Mesenchyma of pulmo root
Gemma pulmonalis
V. cardinalis communis dextra
Left canalis peri-cardioperitonealis primordialis
N. phrenicus
Left and right membranae pleuropericardiacae
Cavitas pericardiaca
Septum transversum
Ventriculi cordis
Ductus vitellointestinalis
Funiculus umbilicalis

a

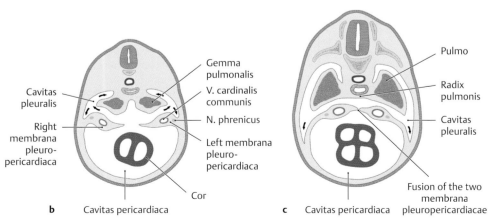

Cavitas pleuralis
Gemma pulmonalis
V. cardinalis communis
N. phrenicus
Right membrana pleuro-pericardiaca
Left membrana pleuro-pericardiaca
Cor
b Cavitas pericardiaca

Pulmo
Radix pulmonis
Cavitas pleuralis
Fusion of the two membrana pleuropericardiacae
c Cavitas pericardiaca

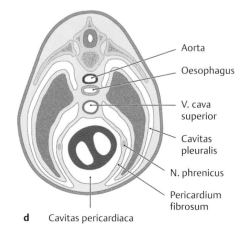

Aorta
Oesophagus
V. cava superior
Cavitas pleuralis
N. phrenicus
Pericardium fibrosum
d Cavitas pericardiaca

A Overview of the compartmentalization of the coeloma intraembryonicum (after Drews)

Embryo at 4 weeks (viewed from left side).

Due to cranial folding, the cranial portion of the coeloma intraembryonicum moves ventral to the praeenteron and broadens into the cavitas pericardiaca. The cavitas pericardiaca flanking the canalis digestorius (gut tube) communicates with the caudally located cavitas peritonealis through the canales pericardioperitoneales primordiales. The still unfolded parts of the future cavitas peritonealis initially open laterally into the cavitas chorionica. The gemmae pulmonales, which push from the canalis digestorius into the canales pericardioperitoneales, grow into the future paired cavitates pleurales. Through the formation of partitions, the pleural cavities separate from both the cavitas pericardiaca (membranae or plicae pleuropericardiacae) and the cavitas peritonealis (septum transversum and membranae or plicae pleuroperitoneales) (see **B**). In the frontal plane the plicae pleuropericardiacae originate on the craniolateral side of the two canales pericardioperitoneales primordiales in the area surrounding the vv. cardinales communes. They fuse with the mesoderma located ventral to the canalis digestorius (the future oesophagus). The plicae pleuroperitoneales develop in the caudolateral wall of the canales pericardioperitoneales and, together with the mesooesophagum dorsale and the septum transversum, form the future diaphragma (see **D**).

B Separation of the cavitas pericardiaca from the cavitates pleurales (after Sadler)

Embryo at 5 weeks. Frontal section at the level of the future cavitas pericardiaca; for plane of section see **A**.

In the 5th week, at the junction between the unpaired cavitas pericardiaca and the two canales pericardioperitoneales, two thin mesoderm folds (plicae pleuropericardiacae), coming from the lateral direction, grow toward one another. They contain the trunks of the vv. cardinales communes and the nn. phrenici. The cavitates pleurales form as a result of the gemmae pulmonales growing into the canales pleuroperitoneales (see p. 36 development of the pulmones). In the course of further development, the cavitates pleurales further expand and become separate from the cavitas pericardiaca. The separation is complete once both of the plicae pleuropericardiacae have fused with the mesenchyma at the root of the lungs. The anterior vv. cardinales merge to form the v. cava superior; and the two plicae pleuropericardiacae give rise to the future pericardium fibrosum (see p. 14, development of the heart).

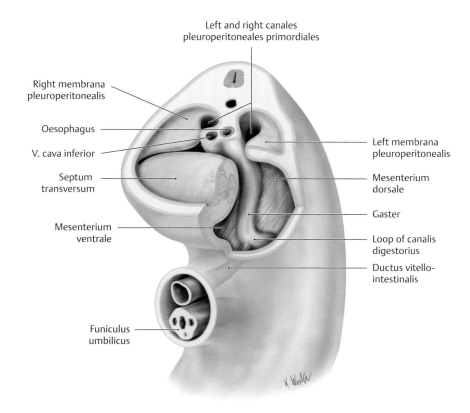

Left and right canales
pleuroperitoneales primordiales

Right membrana
pleuroperitonealis

Oesophagus

V. cava inferior

Septum
transversum

Mesenterium
ventrale

Funiculus
umbilicus

Left membrana
pleuroperitonealis

Mesenterium
dorsale

Gaster

Loop of canalis
digestorius

Ductus vitello-
intestinalis

C Separation of the cavitates pleurales from the cavitas peritonealis

(after Sadler)

After the cavitates pleurales have separated from the cavitas pericardiaca, they are still temporarily connected to the cavitas peritonealis through the canales pericardioperitoneales. They become completely sealed off by the end of the 7th week with the development of the diaphragma, which is formed from several different structures (see **D**). Faulty closure of the canales pericardioperitoneales can lead to a *congenital hernia diaphragmatica* (e.g., Bochdalek hernia) allowing abdominal viscera to enter into the cavitates pleurales.

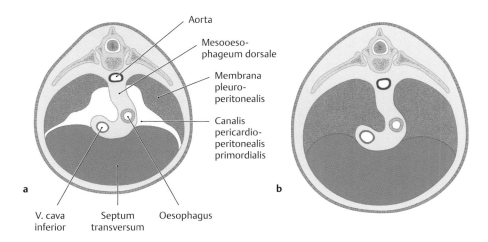

Aorta

Mesooeso-
phageum dorsale

Membrana
pleuro-
peritonealis

Canalis
pericardio-
peritonealis
primordialis

a

V. cava
inferior

Septum
transversum

Oesophagus

b

D Development of the diaphragma

(after Sadler)

The diaphragma is derived from four different structures:

- the septum transversum
- the left and right plicae pleuroperitoneales
- the mesooesophagum dorsale
- body wall musculature

In the 4th week the septum transversum develops as a thick mesenchymal plate in the area between the cavitas pericardiaca and pedunculus sacci vitellini. In the 6th week, the septum transversum moves caudally (**a**). The hepar (liver) forms in the ventral mesenterium directly below it. During further development, the septum transversum fuses with both of the plicae pleuroperitoneales and forms the future *centrum tendineum* (**b**). The mesooesophagum dorsale and the adjacent body wall musculature give rise to the muscular part of the diaphragma (**c**).

Note: The nn. phrenici (C3, C4, and C5), located in the plicae pleuropericardiacae directly next to the trunks of the vv. cardinales communes, provide motor innervation to the diaphragma. The textus muscularis striatus of the diaphragm (from somiti), as well as the septum transversum, are originally from cervical regions. This explains why the nerve supply to the diaphragma (the nn. phrenici) comes from cervical medulla spinalis levels.

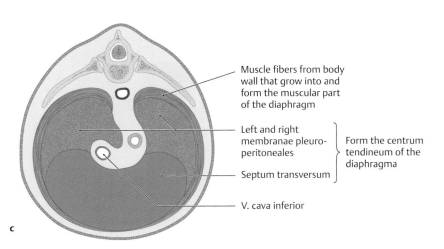

Muscle fibers from body
wall that grow into and
form the muscular part
of the diaphragm

Left and right
membranae pleuro-
peritoneales

Septum transversum

Form the centrum
tendineum of the
diaphragma

V. cava inferior

c

1.4 Organization and Architecture of Body Cavities

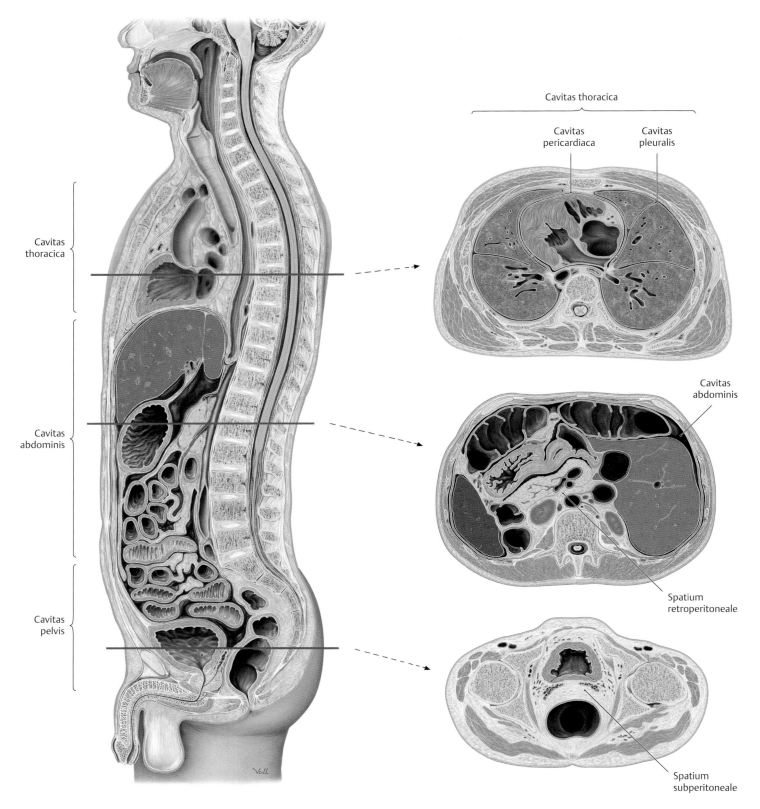

A Organization of the body cavities
Midsagittal section, viewed from the left side. Three large body cavities can be identified. From from the top down they are as follows

- Cavitas thoracica
- Cavitas abdominis
- Cavitas pelvis

These body cavities are completely surrounded by parts of the body wall. The majority of the walls consists of muscle and connective tissue. In addition, the thorax is surrounded by costae, and the pelvis by the ossa coxae. At its upper end, the connective tissue space of the cavitas thoracica is continuous with the connective tissue space of the neck. The diaphragma pelvis muscles close off the apertura pelvis inferior. Depending on their location in one of the three cavities, organs are referred to as thoracic, abdominal or pelvic organs (see **C**).

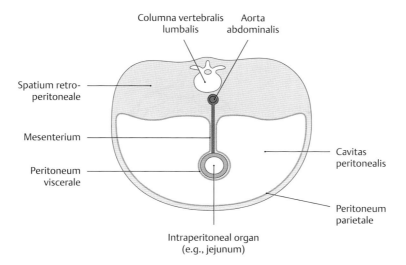

Columna vertebralis lumbalis — Aorta abdominalis

Spatium retro-peritoneale

Mesenterium

Peritoneum viscerale

Cavitas peritonealis

Peritoneum parietale

Intraperitoneal organ (e.g., jejunum)

B Structure of the body cavities

Highly schematic cross-section of a human body; superior view. Every body cavity can be divided into two differently structured spaces:

- A **hollow space**: A smooth, moist epithelial layer, the serous membrane or tunica serosa, lines the inner wall of the cavity and the adjacent outer wall of the organs. The portion of the tunica serosa that covers the organ is called the *lamina visceralis* (viscera refers to internal organ). The portion lining the walls of the cavity is called the *lamina parietalis* (parietal refers to wall). The organs located in the cavity are movable. They are attached to the connective tissue space (see below) by a connective tissue bridge covered by a serous membrane (a mesenterium).
- A **connective tissue space** within which run the pathways leading to and from the organ. Organs situated in these spaces are surrounded by connective tissue and are more or less immovable.

While this general structure applies to all three body cavities, the terms for the individual regions vary (see **C**):

- In the **thorax**, most of the connective tissue is located in the central compartment of the cavitas thoracica, the mediastinum, in which the cavitas pericardiaca (a hollow space lined with a serous membrane) is embedded. The cavitates pleurales are located lateral to the mediastinum.

- In the **abdomen**, the connective tissue is situated behind the cavitas peritonealis in the spatium retroperitoneale (an extraperitoneal space).
- In the **pelvis**, the connective tissue is situated both behind and below the cavitas peritonealis in the spatia retroperitoneale and subperitoneale (spatia extraperitonealia).

Correspondingly, all organs in the thorax, abdomen and pelvis can be organized according to their location in the connective tissue space or in one of the serous-membrane lined cavities (see **C**).
Note: While the partition between the cavitates thoracica and abdominis is clearly defined by the diaphragma, the separation between the cavitates abdominis and pelvis is often only demarcated by bony reference points on the body wall. Thus, the cavitates abdominis and pelvis essentially remain a single cavity, and therefore form a single region where disease processes can spread from one cavity to the other.
A mesenterium is a layer of connective tissue covered by peritoneum. Within it run the organ's neurovascular supply (vasa sanguinea and lymphatica, nervi). With reference to organs, the mesenterium is often identified with the prefix "meso" (e.g., mesocolon transversum).

C Spaces and body cavities and their respective organs in the thorax, abdomen, and pelvis

Body cavity and the organs it contains	Serous cavities and the organs they contain	Serous membrane	Connective tissue spaces and their embedded organs
Cavitas thoracica (thorax) Thoracic organs	• Paired cavitates pleurales with pulmones: *Intrapleural organs* • Cavitas pericardiaca *Intrapericardial organ*	• Pleura visceralis and parietalis • Laminae visceralis and parietal is pericardii serosi	• Mediastinum (middle section of the cavitas thoracica) between the cavitates pleurales as well as behind the unpaired cavitas pericardiaca with the mediastinal organs: oesophagus, trachea, and thymus as well as vessels and nerves: – *Mediastinal organs*
Cavitas abdominis (abdomen) Abdominal organs	• Abdominal cavitas peritonealis with gaster (stomach), parts of the intestina tenue and crassum, splen (spleen), hepar (liver), vesica biliaris, and caecum with appendix vermiformis: *Intraperitoneal organs*	• Peritoneum visceralis and parietale	• Spatium extraperitoneale behind the abdominal cavitas peritonealis (spatium retroperitoneale, retropubicum) with renes, ureteres, pancreas and parts of the duodenum, intestinum crassum, and rectum: – *Extraperitoneal organs*
Cavitas pelvis (pelvis) Pelvic organs	• Pelvic cavitas peritonealis with fundus and corpus uteri, ovaria, tubae uterinae, and upper rectum: *Intraperitoneal organs*	• Peritoneum visceralis and parietale	• Spatia extraperitonealia behind and below the pelvic cavitas peritonealis (spatia retroperitoneale and subperitoneale) with vesica urinaria and adjacent portions of the ureteres, prostata, gll. vesiculosae, cervix uteri, vagina, and parts of the rectum: – *Extraperitoneal organs*

2.1   Overview and Basic Wall Structure

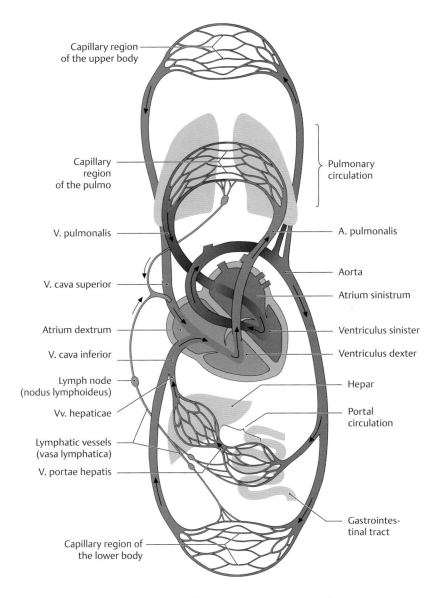

Capillary region of the upper body

Capillary region of the pulmo

Pulmonary circulation

V. pulmonalis

A. pulmonalis

V. cava superior

Aorta

Atrium sinistrum

Atrium dextrum

Ventriculus sinister

V. cava inferior

Ventriculus dexter

Lymph node (nodus lymphoideus)

Hepar

Vv. hepaticae

Portal circulation

Lymphatic vessels (vasa lymphatica)

V. portae hepatis

Gastrointestinal tract

Capillary region of the lower body

A Overview of the cardiovascular system
The **cardiovascular system** is a closed system of vessels through which the blood is transported. This circulation is necessary to supply the organs with oxygen, nutrients, and hormones and to carry carbon dioxide and other metabolic waste products away to the excretory organs. Additionally, cells and proteins of the immune system travel through the bloodstream. Using blood as a transport medium, they "patrol" the body by constantly looking out for pathogens. The blood can also transport heat, so that circulation helps to regulate body temperature. In addition to these functions, the blood also helps to seal off leaks. It contains clotting factors that are activated when vessels gets damaged. The circulation is powered by the cor (heart) which functions as a pressure pump.

The circulatory system can be divided into two main circuits:

- the systemic circulation (high-pressure system, average blood pressure of 100mmHg in the major arteries) and
- the pulmonary circulation (low-pressure system, average blood pressure of 12mmHg; the difference in pressure from the systemic circulation is almost a factor of 10).

Regarding the vessels and pump, both circulatory systems can be divided into four parts:

- arteriae (aa.) and arteriolae: they lead away from the heart and distribute blood to the organs
- capillaries: they connect arterioles to venules and enable the exchange of substances in organs
- venulae and venae (vv.): receive blood from the capillaries and carry it back to the cor
- cor: functions as a circulation pump and transports the blood back to the arteriae

The **lymphatic system** is an additional vascular system that carries fluid away from the organs. It begins with lymphatic capillaries (vasa lymphocapillaria) in the organs and transports lymph back to the venous system.
Note: Whether to refer to a vessel as an artery or vein depends on the direction of blood flow, not on blood oxygen level. Arteriae carry blood away from the heart, and venae carry blood toward the heart. Hence, in the diagram, the a. pulmonaria contains oxygen-low blood (blue), while the v. pulmonaria contains oxygen-rich blood (red).

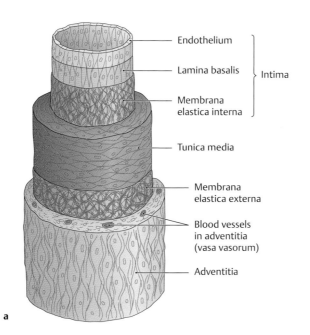

Endothelium ⎱
Lamina basalis ⎰ Intima
Membrana elastica interna ⎰

Tunica media

Membrana elastica externa

Blood vessels in adventitia (vasa vasorum)

Adventitia

a

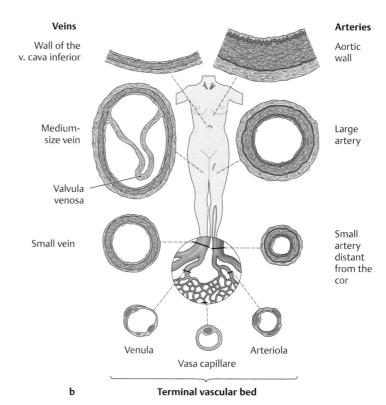

Veins

Wall of the v. cava inferior

Medium-size vein

Valvula venosa

Small vein

Venula

Vasa capillare

Arteries

Aortic wall

Large artery

Small artery distant from the cor

Arteriola

b **Terminal vascular bed**

B Basic wall structure of large blood vessels

a The major blood vessels (arteries and veins) generally consist of three layers:

- The tunica intima (intima): an endothelium consisting of a single layer of squamous epithelial cells, with the cells elongated in the direction of blood flow, and a thin layer of subendothelial connective tissue
- The tunica media (media): consisting of a circular arrangement of smooth muscle cells, and elastic fibers of the internal elastic membrane (which separates the intima from the media) and external elastic membrane (which separates the media from the adventitia)
- The tunica adventitia (adventitia): consisting mainly of loose connective tissue, which integrates the blood vessel into its surroundings and allows for movement of vessels with organ movements. It can contain blood and lymphatic vessels as well as nerves.

b While veins have a similar three-layered structure as arteries, they have fewer and less dense layers of smooth muscle cells, giving the media of veins a looser structure. These structural characteristics are the result of lower venous blood pressure compared to arterial blood pressure. The peripheral veins in limbs contain valves to help direct blood flow back to the cor. The small exchange vessels, the capillaries, have no muscle tissue and consist only of endothelium and basement membrane.

C Blood pressure in different regions of the cardiovascular system

The function and structure of the cardiovascular system are closely interconnected, as higher blood pressure leads to the thickening of blood vessel walls and lower blood pressure allows walls to thin. Thus, knowledge of blood pressures is important when interpreting morphology. In the cor and major arteries closest to the cor, blood pressure fluctuates substantially with each cardiac cycle. While blood pressure in the ventriculus sinister reaches 120 mmHg during systole, during diastole it drops to 0 mmHg. Due to the vessel wall properties of the arteriae close to the heart, blood pressure fluctuations in them during the cardiac cycle are less extreme. Resistance vessels further help regulation so that capillary pressure remains constant. Pressure is lowest in the central veins closest to the heart. Because of their thin walls, they can expand and store blood.

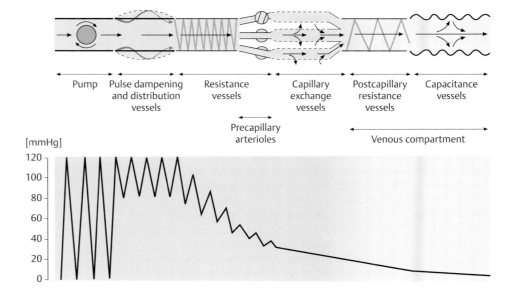

Pump | Pulse dampening and distribution vessels | Resistance vessels | Capillary exchange vessels | Postcapillary resistance vessels | Capacitance vessels

Precapillary arterioles

Venous compartment

[mmHg]
120
100
80
60
40
20
0

Note: The different regions of the vascular system are assigned specific functions, which are described in the illustration above.

2.2 Terminal Vessels and Overview of the Major Blood Vessels

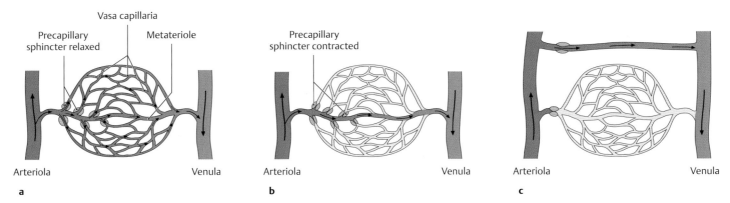

a   b   c

A Terminal vessels

a The primary function of the arteries and veins is to transport blood. Terminal vessels are concerned with the exchange of substances between blood and tissue. This is often called the *microcirculation.* The terminal vascular bed consists of

- Arteriolae
- Capillaries
- Venulae

b It is important to point out that capillary perfusion can vary within organs. Precapillary sphincters, which consist of smooth muscle cells,

help to regulate perfusion in *one* capillary. Terminal vessel perfusion within a specific organ is related to the organ's function and varies from organ to organ.

c Additionally, arteriovenous anastomoses help regulate the circulation in a group of neighboring capillaries that have formed one functional unit. Thus, entire capillary beds can be shut down.
Disruption of the fine regulation of the microcirculation is a major problem when patients go into shock because blood can pool in capillaries.

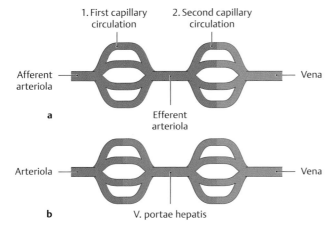

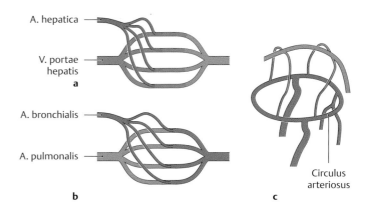

B Vascular relationships

In addition to the above mentioned descriptions of typical organ circulation: artery – capillary – vein, there are additional blood flow patterns in some organs.

a Flow of arterial blood through two serially connected capillary beds: Two serially connected capillary beds are found in the ren (kidney) where arterial blood initially flows through the corpuscula renalia (glomeruli) and then into the capillaries of the medulla renalis.

b Flow through two venous circuits (portal venous system): Venous blood flowing through two serially connected capillary beds is known as a portal venous system. For clarification, the blood in the first capillary bed is colored purple because it is not yet completely deoxygenated. Such a portal venous system exists in the digestive tract, where the v. portae hepatis collects the venous blood from the unpaired abdominal organs (gaster, intestina, splen). From there it flows to the capillaries of the hepar.

C Dual organ circulation

The **hepar (liver)** receives its blood supply from the a. hepatica propria and the v. portae hepatis (**a**). The vessel responsible for suppling oxygenated blood to the liver tissue is the a. hepatica propria. The vessel that contains the blood with the substances to be metabolized in the liver is the v. portae hepatis. The **pulmones** also have a dual arterial supply (**b**). Here, the aa. pulmonariae contain deoxygenated blood and the rr. bronchiales contain oxygenated blood. Another pattern of multiple blood supply can be found in the **encephalon**. Four arteriae form a closed ring (the circulus arteriosus cerebri, circle of Willis) from which other vessels supply the encephalon (**c**). All three forms of blood supply through multiple vessels allow for a certain degree of compensation in case one of the supplying vessels fails.

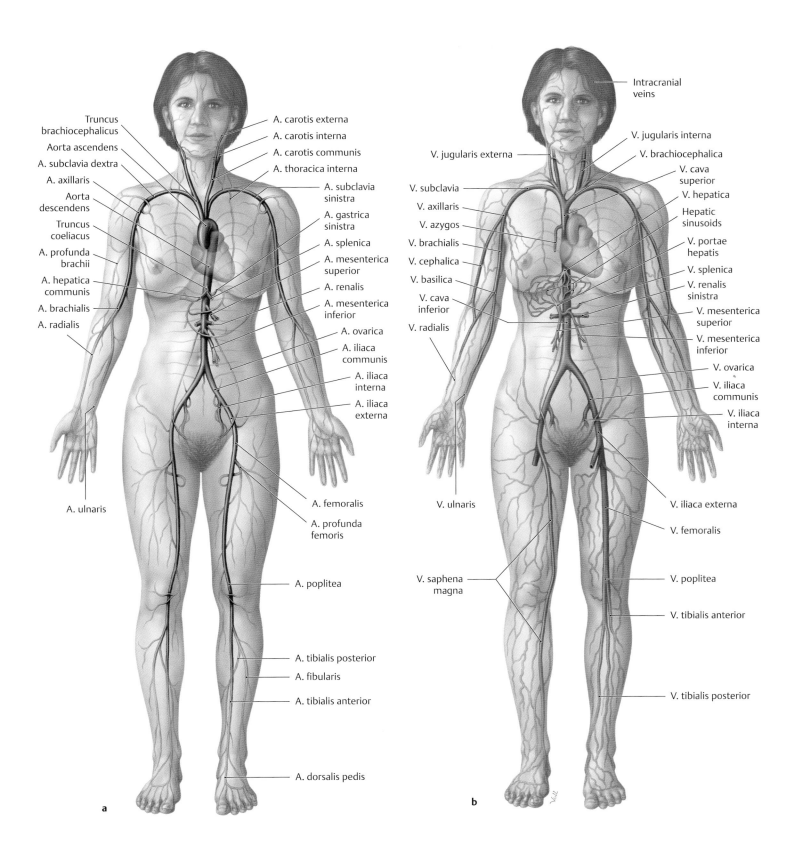

Truncus brachiocephalicus
Aorta ascendens
A. subclavia dextra
A. axillaris
Aorta descendens
Truncus coeliacus
A. profunda brachii
A. hepatica communis
A. brachialis
A. radialis

A. carotis externa
A. carotis interna
A. carotis communis
A. thoracica interna
A. subclavia sinistra
A. gastrica sinistra
A. splenica
A. mesenterica superior
A. renalis
A. mesenterica inferior
A. ovarica
A. iliaca communis
A. iliaca interna
A. iliaca externa

A. ulnaris

A. femoralis
A. profunda femoris

A. poplitea

A. tibialis posterior
A. fibularis
A. tibialis anterior

A. dorsalis pedis

a

Intracranial veins

V. jugularis externa

V. jugularis interna
V. brachiocephalica
V. cava superior
V. hepatica
Hepatic sinusoids
V. portae hepatis
V. splenica
V. renalis sinistra
V. mesenterica superior
V. mesenterica inferior
V. ovarica
V. iliaca communis
V. iliaca interna

V. subclavia
V. axillaris
V. azygos
V. brachialis
V. cephalica
V. basilica
V. cava inferior
V. radialis

V. ulnaris

V. iliaca externa
V. femoralis

V. saphena magna

V. poplitea

V. tibialis anterior

V. tibialis posterior

b

D Major blood vessels

This overview depicts the major arteriae (**a**) and venae (**b**) in the human body. In the following organ descriptions, knowledge of the major vascular trunks is assumed, and the smaller organ-supplying vessels will be discussed with the respective organs.

2.3   Cardiogenic Area, Development of the Heart Tube

Characteristics

In many respects, the cardiovascular system is extraordinary. It is the first system to function in the human embryo; it is already functional by the end of the third week (first contractions of the primitive cor tubulare). Additionally, the cardiac loop (see below) is the body's first asymmetrical structure. Since the human embryo is poorly supplied with yolk, which ensures nutrition by diffusion for a limited time only, it depends on extraembryonic circulation from a very early stage. While the saccus vitellinus circulation appears earlier, it is the placental circulation that ultimately provides nutrients and removes waste over the course of embryonic and fetal development (see **D**).

A Origins of the cardiac tissue (cardiogenic area)

Dorsal view of the discus embryonicus from the cavitas amniotica. During the third week of development (presomite stage), the mesenchyma cardiogenicum, from which the cor develops, forms a horseshoe-shaped area (campus cordis primus) that consists of a thickened layer of mesenchymal cells. It lies anterolateral to the lamina neuralis. At this stage in development, the mesenchyme is still located under the similarly horseshoe-shaped intraembryonic cavitas coelomica. The campus cordis primus is composed of mesenchyma splanchnopleurale (the layer of mesoderma laminae lateralis facing the viscera) and it borders the future cavitas pericardiaca (see **Be**). During craniocaudal and lateral embryonic folding, the campus cordis primus, which originally lies in the anterolateral portion of the discus embryonicus, moves ventrally under the developing praeenteron along with the adjacent coelomic cleft (see **Bc**).

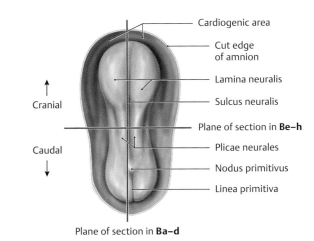

B Formation of the heart

a–d Sagittal sections; **e–h** Cross-sections (21–23 days / 4–12 somites); Lateral (**a–d**) and rostral (**e–h**) views; For location of the respective plane of section see **A**.

As a result of craniocaudal folding (**a–d**) the primordium cordis and the adjacent cavitas pericardiaca rotate 180 degrees and move under the praeenteron (descent of the heart). The lamina praechordalis (the future site of the cavitas oris), which previously was located caudally, is now rostral to the developing cor. The septum transversum (future centrum tendineum of the diaphragma) also moves caudally under the cor and cavitas pericardiaca. During the slightly delayed process of lateral folding (**e–h**) the initially paired primordia cordis fuse to form the unpaired cor tubulare (**h**). During this fusion, endothelial-lined embryonic vessels (endocardial tubes) that developed from angioblasts in the cardiogenic area fuse to form a single cavity in the cor tubulare. After fusing with the opposite side, the adjoining mesenchyma splanchnopleurale thickens and develops into cardiac muscle (myocardium). Between the endocardial and myocardial layers develops a basement membrane-like structure consisting of a gelantinous extracellular matrix (gelatinoreticulum). Thus, the fused embryonic heart tube consists of three layers—from inside to outside: endocardium, gelatinoreticulum, and myocardium. The visceral layer of the pericardium, the epicardium, develops from progenitor cells in the area around the sinus venosus, which then overgrow the myocardium.

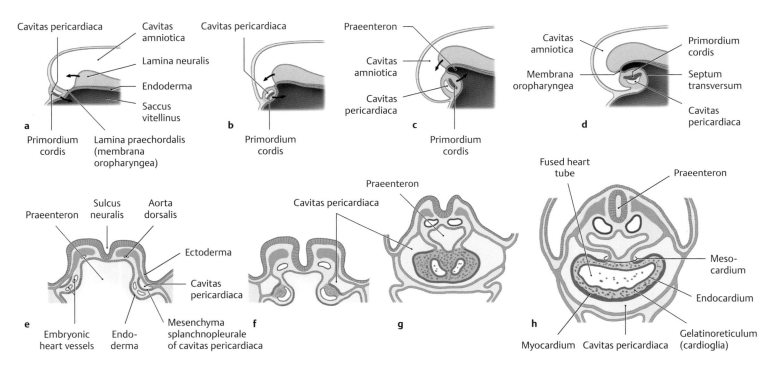

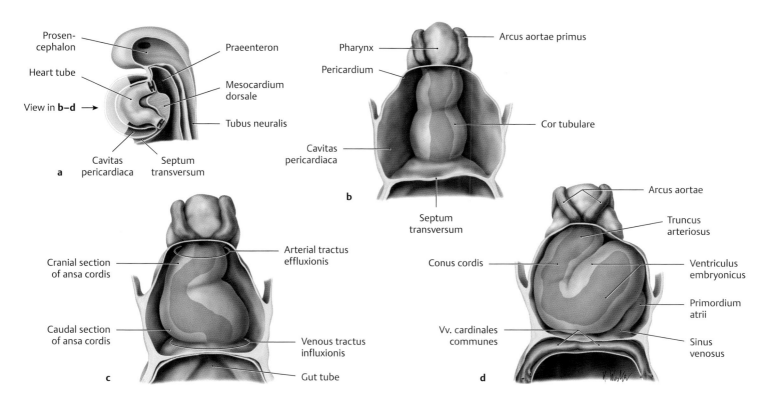

C Formation of the ansa cordis dextra

a Left lateral view; **b–d** Anterior view (with the cavitas pericardiaca opened).

During cranial embryonic folding, the developing cor and cavitas pericardiaca shift in a ventral and caudal direction. With the start of the fourth week, the cor tubulare elongates and curves to form the ansa cordis, which at this stage is attached by a mesocardium dorsale to the posterior wall of the cavitas pericardiaca. Over the course of development, this connection regresses (allowing formation of the sinus transversus pericardii), so that only the tractus influxionis (venosus) and effluxionis (arteriosus) attach the cor tubulare to the pericardium (see **c**). During formation of the ansa cordis, the cranial portion of the cor tubulare shifts ventrocaudally and to the right, while the caudal portion moves dorsocranially and to the left (**d**). Thus, the tractus influxionis lies dorsal and the tractus effluxionis ventral. At the same time, the ansa cordis dextra subdivides into multiple portions as a result of constriction and expansion, forming the following regions:

- truncus arteriosus
- conus cordis
- ventriculus embryonicus
- primordium atrii
- sinus venosus

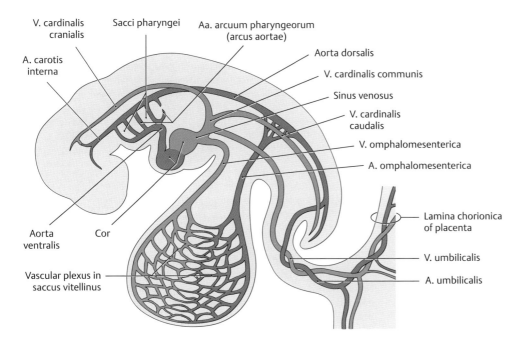

D Early embryonic circulation (after Drews)

Lateral view. The cardiovascular system of a 3 to 4 week old embryo consists of a contractile muscular cor tubulare and three distinct circulatory systems:

- An **intraembryonic systemic circulation** (aorta ascendens and aorta dorsalis, aa. arcuum pharyngeorum and arcus aortae, vv. praecardinales and postcardinales)
- An **extraembryonic vitelline circulation** (aa. and vv. omphalomesentericae)
- A **placental circulation** (aa. and vv. umbilicales).

Deoxygenated blood in the six major venous trunks (two vv. vitellinae or omphalomentericae, two vv. umbilicales, and two vv. cardinales communes) flows into a common, venous cavity close to the heart called the sinus venosus. It then flows through the cor tubularis and out the aortae dorsales pares to enter the systemic circulation, saccus vitellinus or placenta (for development of the sinus venosus see p. 17).

15

2.4 Development of the Inner Chambers of the Heart and Fate of the Sinus Venosus

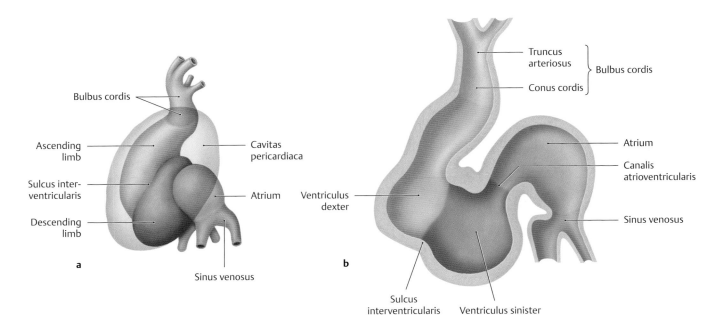

A The ansa cordis and the parts of the cor that develop from it

a Ansa cordis, left lateral view; **b** Sagittal section of the ansa cordis.
By the end of the 3rd or beginning of the 4th week, the precursors of the definitive parts of the cor are clearly visible:

- The bulbus cordis (truncus arteriosus and conus cordis) differentiates into the smooth-walled tractus effluxionis of the ventriculi sinister and dexter as well as the proximal portion of the aorta ascendens and truncus pulmonalis.
- The ascending limb of the ansa cordis forms the ventriculus dexter.

- The descending limb of the ansa cordis forms the ventriculus sinister.
- The sulcus interventricularis marks the boundary between the definitive ventriculi sinister and dexter.
- The future valvae atrioventriculares will form at the level of the canalis atrioventricularis.

Between the 27th and 37th day of development, a complex series of steps occurs in the ansa cordis to form septa in the atrium, ventriculus and tractus effluxionis (see p. 18) to divide the cor into right and left sides.

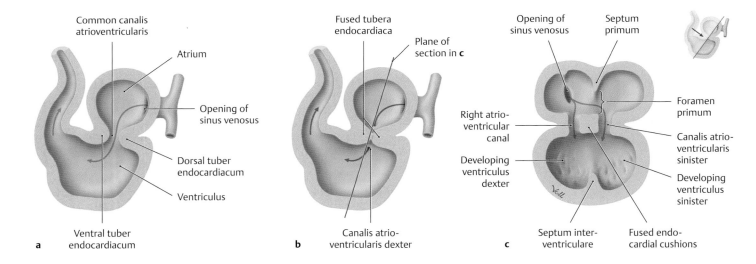

B Formation of the tubera endocardiaca and development of the cor's internal chambers

a and **b** Sagittal section of the ansa cordis; **c** Anterior view at the level of the tubera endocardiaca (for plane of section see **b**).
During the 4th week, the cor tubulare narrows at the junction of the atrium, ventriculus and canalis atrioventricularis (AV canal). This narrowing is a result of the formation of dorsal and ventral tubera

endocardiaca. These are thickened areas of mesenchyma that develop in the region of the gelatinoreticulum. The tubera fuse, and with continued development divide the AV canal into right and left sides (right and left canales atrioventriculares). Later, the fused tubera endocardiaca give rise to the valvae atrioventriculares (valvae tricuspidalis and mitralis), which separate the atria from the ventriculi. Simultaneously, the atrium begins to separate into two chambers (see p.18).

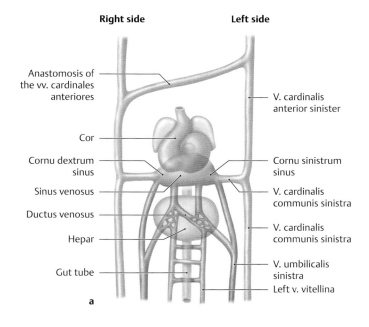

Right side | Left side

- Anastomosis of the vv. cardinales anteriores
- V. cardinalis anterior sinister
- Cor
- Cornu dextrum sinus
- Cornu sinistrum sinus
- Sinus venosus
- V. cardinalis communis sinistra
- Ductus venosus
- V. cardinalis communis sinistra
- Hepar
- Gut tube
- V. umbilicalis sinistra
- Left v. vitellina

a

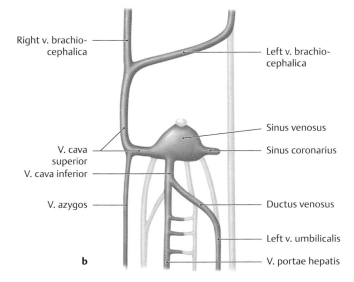

- Right v. brachiocephalica
- Left v. brachiocephalica
- Sinus venosus
- V. cava superior
- Sinus coronarius
- V. cava inferior
- V. azygos
- Ductus venosus
- Left v. umbilicalis
- V. portae hepatis

b

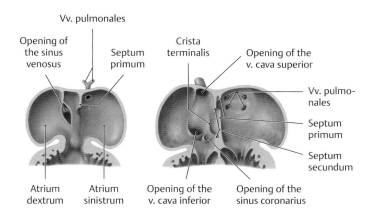

- Vv. pulmonales
- Opening of the sinus venosus
- Septum primum
- Crista terminalis
- Opening of the v. cava superior
- Vv. pulmonales
- Septum primum
- Septum secundum
- Atrium dextrum
- Atrium sinistrum
- Opening of the v. cava inferior
- Opening of the sinus coronarius

D Transformation of the atria

The separation of the common atrium into atria sinistrum and dextrum begins in the 5th week with the formation of the septum primum (see p. 18). Around the same time the chambers of the atria enlarge by incorporating venous wall tissue. On the right side, parts of the cornu dextrum sinus are incorporated into the atrial wall. On the left side, a large part of the atrium sinistrum develops by incorporating the primitive vv. pulmonales. The origins of the parts of the atria are still detectable in the mature heart:

- The partes leves atriorum developed from venous wall tissue (sinus venosus, vv. pulmonales)
- The partes trabeculatae atriorum (mainly the auriculae sinistra and dextra) developed from the former common atrium

In the atrium dextrum, the border between the partes levis and trabeculata is demarcated by a vertical ridge, the crista terminalis. Its cranial portion is the former valva venosa dextra; its caudal portion is the valvulae venae cavae inferioris and sinus coronarii.

E Transformation of the sinus venosus and veins opening into it by the end of the 4th week (see also Cb)

Sinus venosus and veins opening into it through the 4th week	Structures that remain on the right side of the body after the 4th week	Structures that remain on the left side of the body after the 4th week
Cornua dextrum and sinistrum sinus	Pars levis atrii dextri	Sinus coronarius
Vv. cardinales communes dextra and sinistra	Right vein develops into part of the v. cava superior	Left vein becomes part of the sinus coronarius
Vv. praecardinales dextra and sinistra	Right vein also develops into part of the v. cava superior	Left vein regresses
Right and left posterior cardinal veins	Right vein develops into the v. azygos	Left vein regresses
Vv. umbilicales dextra and sinistra	Right vein regresses	Left distal portion remains until birth
Vv. vitellinae dextra and sinistra	• Proximal portion of the right vein develops into part of the v. cava inferior • Distal portion of the right vein develops into the v. portae hepatis	Left vein regresses

C Fate of the sinus venosus and the veins opening into it

a 4th week; **b** 3rd month; ventral view.

By the beginning of the 4th week, the sinus venosus is a separate part of the heart at the opening of the venous tractus influxionis. It opens into the still undivided atrium. Three large paired veins open into each side of the atrium through the cornua sinistrum and dextrum of the sinus venosus. These are the vv. vitellinae, vv. umbilicales, and vv. cardinales communes. Through two *left-right circuits* (see below), the tractus influxionis increasingly shifts to the right side of the body. On the left side, the majority of these veins disappear (see **E**):

1. **Left-right circuit:** Blood flowing from the placenta passes through the v. umbilicalis sinistra and ductus venosus and enters the hepar on the right side. From there it passes through the proximal portion of the right *v. vitellina* (future v. cava inferior) and then to the cornu dextrum sinus.
2. **Left-right circuit:** Both of the vv. praecardinales become connected by an anastomosis. Blood flowing through the systemic circulation enters the cornu dextrum sinus through the right *v. cardinalis communis* (future v. cava superior). The cornu dextrum sinus enlarges and is gradually incorporated into the right atrial wall (**b**). The *cornu sinistrum sinus*, however, increasingly regresses and forms the sinus coronarius.

17

2.5 Cardiac Septation (Formation of Septa Interatriale, Interventriculare, and Aorticopulmonale)

Development of cardiac septa—the basics

Cardiac septation begins at the end of the 4th week and is completed over the next three weeks. Over this period, the embryo grows in length from 5 mm to 17 mm. As a result of the development of the various cardiac septa, the cor tubulare separates into two sides with a circuit for the left heart and another for the right heart. The two circuits are completely separated from one another at the time of birth with the closure of the foramen ovale (see p. 20). This closure is due in part to increased blood flow to the infant's lungs and the resulting decrease in pressure in the right heart circuit.

Note: Septation defects play a key role in many heart malformations (eg. atrial and ventricular septal defects, transposition of large vessels, tetralogy of Fallot, see p. 21). The incidence rate of heart malformations among newborns is 7.5/1000 making them the most frequent congenital diseases. In Germany, 6000 children are born with a heart defect every year.

A Atrial septation (formation of the atrial septum)

a, c, e, g, i, k Frontal sections, ventral view; **b, d, f, h, j** Sagittal section, viewed from the right side.

Septum primum and foramen secundum: After the 4th week the common atrium gradually gets divided into two chambers. From the roof of the still undivided atrium, the crescent-shaped *septum primum* grows and extends toward the already fused tubera endocardiaca of the canalis atrioventricularis (**a** and **b**). Between the margin of the septum and the tuber endocardiacum remains an opening, the *foramen primum*. It becomes progressively smaller and finally disappears as the septum primum continues to grow. At the same time, perforations produced by apoptosis appear in the central part of the septum primum. The perforations coalesce to form a new, large opening between the two atria, the *foramen secundum* (**c** and **d**). From now until birth, this new opening ensures continuous flow of oxygenated blood from the atrium dextrum to the atrium sinistrum.

Septum secundum and foramen ovale: By the end of the 5th week, a second crescent-shaped septum called the septum secundum grows from the ventrocranial wall of the atrium dextrum toward the fused tubera endocardiaca (**g** and **h**). The *septum secundum* does not completely reach the tubera endocardiaca and an opening, the *foramen ovale*, remains in the septum. The extending septum secundum progressively overgrows the *foramen secundum* in the *septum primum* (**i** and **j**). However, blood can continue to flow from the atrium dextrum to the atrium sinistrum due to differing blood pressures in the two sides. Before birth, pressure in the atrium dextrum is higher than in the atrium sinistrum and blood entering the atrium dextrum from the v. cava inferior passes into the atrium sinistrum. This is because the blood pressure is sufficient to push the septum primum aside and open it like a door. In this way, blood can pass through the foramen ovale, into the gap between the septum secundum and septum primum, and through the foramen secundum to enter the atrium sinistrum (**i** and **j**).

Closure of the foramen ovale and the definitive separation of the atria: Due to changes in the pulmonary circulation at birth, blood pressure in the atrium sinistrum increases. As a result, the septum primum is pushed against the septum secundum. The foramen ovale closes and the two atria are separate from one another (**k**). The septum primum forms the future fossa ovalis, and the free edge of the septum secundum develops into the limbus (border) of the fossa ovalis. Once these two septa fuse the foramen ovale remains permanently closed.

Note: Failure of the septa to fuse results in the foramen ovale remaining open (patent foramen ovale [PFO]). However, this is of little significance due to the pressure differences in the atria (see p. 21). The higher pressure in the atrium sinistrum pushes the septum primum firmly against the septum secundum.

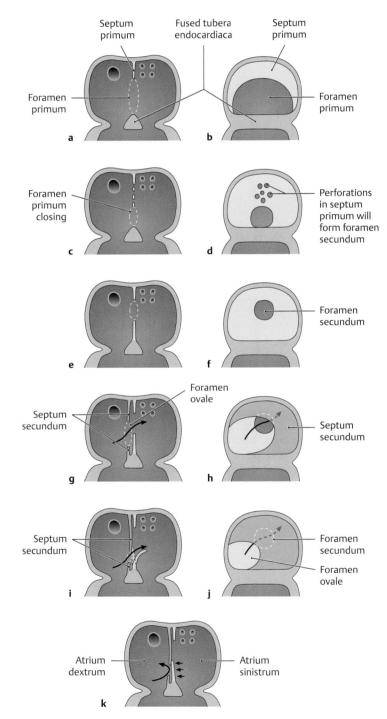

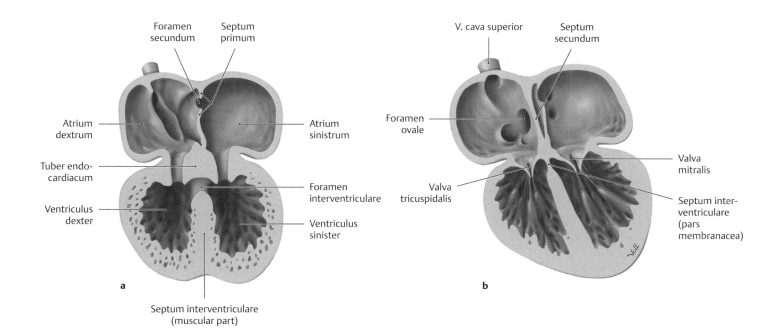

a

Foramen secundum
Septum primum
Atrium dextrum
Atrium sinistrum
Tuber endo-cardiacum
Ventriculus dexter
Foramen interventriculare
Ventriculus sinister
Septum interventriculare (muscular part)

b

V. cava superior
Septum secundum
Foramen ovale
Valva tricuspidalis
Valva mitralis
Septum inter-ventriculare (pars membranacea)

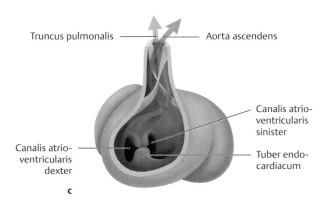

c

Truncus pulmonalis
Aorta ascendens
Canalis atrio-ventricularis sinister
Canalis atrio-ventricularis dexter
Tuber endo-cardiacum

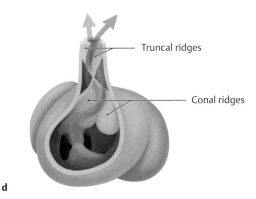

d

Truncal ridges
Conal ridges

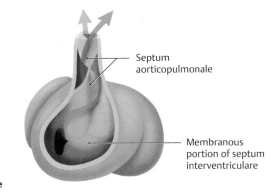

e

Septum aorticopulmonale
Membranous portion of septum interventriculare

B Septation of the ventriculi and the tractus effluxionis (formation of the septa interventriculare and aorticopulmonale)
(after Sadler)

Ventricular septation also begins by the end of the 4th week with the formation of a myocardial wall between the ascending and descending limbs of the ansa cordis.

Ventricular septation (a and b): A crescent-shaped muscular ridge called the pars muscularis of the *septum interventriculare* develops from the wall of the ventriculus and projects into the ventricular lumen. With continued development, its two limbs fuse with the tubera endocardi-aca of the canalis atrioventricularis (however, the bottom of the crescent-shaped ridge does not fuse with the tubera). The remaining opening between the two ventriculi is called the *foramen interventriculare*. In the 7th week, it is completely closed by the *pars membranacea* of the septum interventriculare, which comes from the tubera endocardiaca and the proximal end of the conal ridges (see below).

Outflow tract septation (c–e): While the septum interventriculare forms, the common tractus effluxionis of both ventriculi (bulbus cordis) begins to differentiate into the aorta ascendens and *truncus pulmonalis*. This is the result of the formation of two opposite longitudinal ridges in the lower (conus cordis) and upper (truncus arteriosus) parts of the tractus effluxionis. These conal and truncal ridges develop through increased proliferation of mesenchyma. Their progenitor cells migrated from cranial crista neuralis cells in the arcus pharyngei.

Note: Crista neuralis cells give rise to most of the peripheral nervous system, but also contribute to cardiovascular development. Thus, cranial crista neuralis cells are of central importance for the normal development of the cardiac tractus effluxionis.

Over the course of septum formation, the conal and truncal ridges complete a rotation of 180 degrees. This pattern of fusion leads to the formation of the spiral-shaped *septum aorticopulmonale*, which separates the common tractus effluxionis of the two ventriculi.

Heart valve formation: Formation of the valvae aortae and trunci pulmonalis is related to formation of the *septum aorticopulmonalis*. The valves develop from three subendocardial ridges (tubera endocardiaca) located at the junction of the conus cordis and truncus arteriosus (thus at the root of the aorta and truncus pulmonalis).

19

2.6 Pre- and Postnatal Circulation and Common Congenital Heart Defects

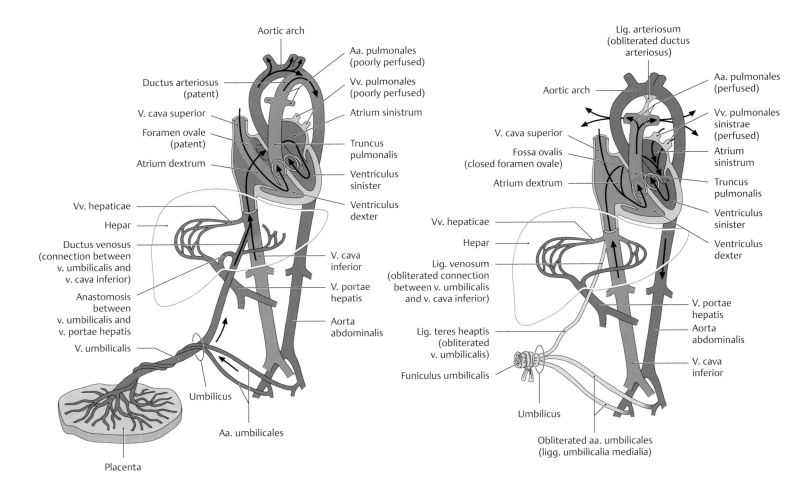

A Prenatal circulation (after Fritsch and Kühnel)
The prenatal circulation is characterized by the following:

- Very little pulmonary blood flow
- Gas exchange in the placenta
- Delivery of oxygen and nutrients to the fetus through the placenta
- A right-to-left shunt in the heart

The fetal **lungs** have not yet expanded, are not aerated and have minimal blood flow. Consequently exchange of O_2 and CO_2 takes place outside the fetus in the placenta. Oxygenated and nutrient-rich fetal blood from the placenta passes to the fetus through the unpaired v. umbilicalis. Near the liver, the v. umbilicalis empties into the v. cava inferior through the ductus venosus (a venovenous anastomosis). There, oxygen-rich blood (from the v. umbilicalis) mixes with oxygen-poor blood (from the v. cava inferior). At the same time, the v. umbilicalis passes nutrient-rich blood, via another venous anastomosis, to the v. portae hepatis which transports it to the hepar for metabolic processing.

Blood flow in the **cor** is characterized by a right-to-left shunt. Blood from both vv. cavae flows into the atrium dextra. Blood from the v. cava inferior passes into the atrium sinistra through the foramen ovale (see p. 18). Most of the blood from the v. cava superior passes through the atrium dextrum to the ventriculus dexter and then enters the truncus pulmonalis. However, it does not enter the unexpanded fetal lungs but passes via the ductus arteriosus (an arterioarterial anastomosis) into the aorta and then to peripheral fetal vessels. Blood returns to the placenta through the paired aa. umbilicales (branches of the aa. iliacae internae). Since the pulmonary circulation is greatly reduced, very little blood is returned to the atrium sinistrum through the vv. pulmonales.

B Postnatal circulation (after Fritsch and Kühnel)
At birth, gas exchange and blood flow undergo a radical change. The postnatal circulation is characterized by the following:

- Loss of the placental circulation
- Pulmonary respiration with pulmonary gas exchange
- Functional occlusion of the right-to-left shunt and all fetal anastomoses

When respiration begins, the lungs are expanded, aerated and become responsible for gas exchange. Vascular resistance in the expanded lungs drops abruptly. The sudden drop in blood pressure in the atrium dextrum (pressure in the atrium sinistrum is now higher than in the atrium dextrum) causes the foramen ovale to close (see p. 18). Contraction of vascular smooth muscle in the ductus arteriosus functionally closes that anastomosis. Later it closes completely by scarring and forms the lig. arteriosum. The ventriculus dexter pumps blood through the aa. pulmonales into the expanded lungs. Blood from the ventriculus sinister is distributed through the aorta to all body regions and returns to the atrium dextrum through the vv. cavae superior and inferior. Both sides of the heart are now hemodynamically separate. The v. umbilicalis is no longer perfused and the ductus venosus connecting it to the v. cava inferior occludes and eventually scars to form the lig. venosum. The v. umbilicalis also becomes occluded and fibrous over its entire length, forming the lig. teres hepatis. The proximal portions of the aa. umbilicales remain patent, while the distal portions become occluded and form the lig. umbilicale mediale on each side.

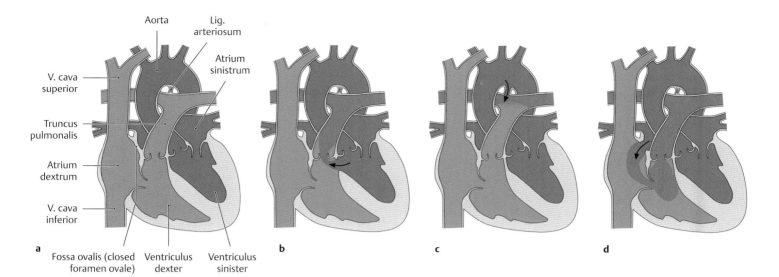

Aorta Lig. arteriosum

Atrium sinistrum

V. cava superior

Truncus pulmonalis

Atrium dextrum

V. cava inferior

a   b   c   d

Fossa ovalis (closed foramen ovale)   Ventriculus dexter   Ventriculus sinister

C Congenital heart defects

Heart defects are the most common birth defects (incidence in live-born infants is 7.5/1000). The factors are usually genetic (trisomy 21) or exogenous (e.g., virus infections/rubella, alcohol, medications, cytostatics, ionizing radiation).

Note: The cor is most sensitive to teratogen exposure between the 4th and 7th weeks, a time period in which a woman may not know yet that she is pregnant.

Thanks to enormous progress in diagnosis and therapy, more than 85% of children born today with congenital heart disease survive and reach adult age. Among the most common congenital heart defects are *acyanotic heart defects* (cyanosis: bluish discoloration of the skin/mucosae due to low oxygen saturation). They are ventricular septal defects (31%), atrial septal defects (10%) and patent ductus arteriosus (9%), in which a non-physiological connection exists between the left and right sides of the heart. Since blood always flows from high pressure to low pressure, and the left side of the heart has the higher pressure in postnatal circulation, the heart abnormalities described are characterized by an initial left-to-right shunt. The shunt leads to higher pressure in the right side of the heart. In response to the increased pressure, the walls of the ventriculus dexter and aa. pulmonales thicken which results in continuously increasing resistance and pressure in the pulmonary circulation (pulmonary hypertension). Over time the pressure in the pulmonary circulation becomes higher than the pressure in the systemic circulation, which leads to a shunt reversal (now right-to-left shunt [Eisenmenger reaction]) and decompensated right-sided failure. As less blood flows through the aa. pulmonales, the oxygen saturation decreases leading secondarily to cyanosis. During childhood, acyanotic heart defects are usually well tolerated and become symptomatic only later in life. If a patent ductus arteriosus is surgically closed (e.g., using an endoscopic catheter) before complications occur, life expectancy is normal.

a **Normal postnatal heart:** The foramen ovale closes, the ductus arteriosus atrophies, and systemic and pulmonary circulation are completely separated.

b **Ventricular septal defect (VSD):** VSDs are usually located in the pars membranacea of the septum interventriculare and arise from failure of fusion of the pars muscularis of the septum interventriculare with the proximal septum aorticopulmonale. As a result, the foramen interventriculare remains open, and with each contraction blood from the ventriculus sinister enters the ventriculus dexter. Ventricular septal defects are frequently associated with an asymmetric septation of the outflow tract such as a narrowed truncus pulmonalis

(stenosis), an "overriding" aorta on the ventricular septum, and right ventricular hypertrophy caused by the pulmonary stenosis (*tetralogy of Fallot*, the most common cyanotic heart defect. An infant's mucous membranes, lips, and fingers have a bluish color because too little blood is pumped through the pulmonary circulation for adequate oxygenation).

c **Patent ductus arteriosus (PDA):** frequently occurs in premature infants (75% will spontaneously close within one week). Symptoms are the result of increased backflow of aortic blood into the truncus pulmonalis, which leads to volume overload on the pulmonary circulation (see above). If the ductus arteriosus is closed (e.g., using an endoscopic catheter), life expectancy is normal.

d **Atrial septal defects (ASD):** depending on location, these defects are subdivided into three types: primum atrial septal defects (ASD I), secundum atrial septal defects (ASD II) and sinus venosus atrial septal defects (SV). The most common type is the secundum atrial septal defect (75% of all cases), characterized by the excessive resorption of septum primum tissue at the site of the foramen ovale (foramen secundum is too large) or inadequate growth of the septum secundum (foramen secundum is not sufficiently covered, see p. 18). As a result, in postnatal circulation, blood flows from the atrium sinistrum to the atrium dextrum which, depending on the shunt volume, leads to volume overload in the pulmonary circulation. Significant symptoms can occur later in life once the shunt has reached a certain size. Thus, ASD II defects are corrected even though patients have not yet shown symptoms. Closure of secundum atrial septal defects is generally performed by using an interventional approach with a stent and a self-expanding double-umbrella device made of a nickel titanium alloy.

Note: Failure of the septum primum to fuse with the septum secundum after birth leads to an anatomically open (through which a probe could be passed) foramen ovale ("probe" patent foramen ovale [PFO]). Due to the valve mechanisms and the existing pressure differences, it is clinically insignificant (see p. 18) and thus is not a true heart defect but rather a normal variant (almost 30% of adults are affected). Pathological conditions, (e.g., resulting from an acute hemodynamically relevant pulmonary embolism) can lead to the formation of a right-to-left shunt. As a result, blood clots (thrombi), which are usually filtered out in the lungs, can enter the systemic circulation causing an ischemic stroke (a paradoxical or crossed embolism). Even smaller clots can be potentially life-threatening. Even routine activities (lifting heavy loads, coughing, etc.) can lead to quick changes in intrathoracic pressures so that a PFO can temporarily cause a right-to-left shunt.

3.1 Blood: Components

A Composition of blood

Blood is a unique tissue in that it is liquid. Yet like every other tissue it consists of an extracellular matrix (plasma) and cellular components (red and white blood cells as well as platelets). A transport and communication organ, it is contained within a closed vascular system that interconnects all organ systems. Its functions are accordingly diverse: transport of gases and substances, protection, thermoregulation, regulation of pH value, and coagulation. Coagulation prevents all of the blood from draining out of the cardiovascular system when its walls have been damaged. A protein-containing fluid (plasma) accounts for 50–63% of the blood volume; 37–50% is blood cells. The ratio of the volume of red blood cells to the total volume of blood is referred to as hematocrit. **Plasma** is obtained by centrifuging whole blood which has been prevented from coagulating by the addition of a substance such as heparin. **Serum** is obtained by initially allowing the blood to coagulate and then centrifuging it. Serum is thus plasma minus clotting factors. About 90% of plasma consists of water; the rest includes proteins, electrolytes, and low-molecular-weight substances of metabolism and metabolic regulation (hormones). Most plasma proteins are synthesized by the liver. Accounting for a full 99% of the hematocrit, the vast majority of **blood cells** (see p. 24) are the non-nucleated red blood cells. Their cytoplasm is filled with hemoglobin, which serves to transport oxygen and buffer the blood. The white blood cells have a protective function; the platelets promote blood coagulation. All blood cells come from stem cells of the red bone marrow (see p. 27) where they are constantly produced.

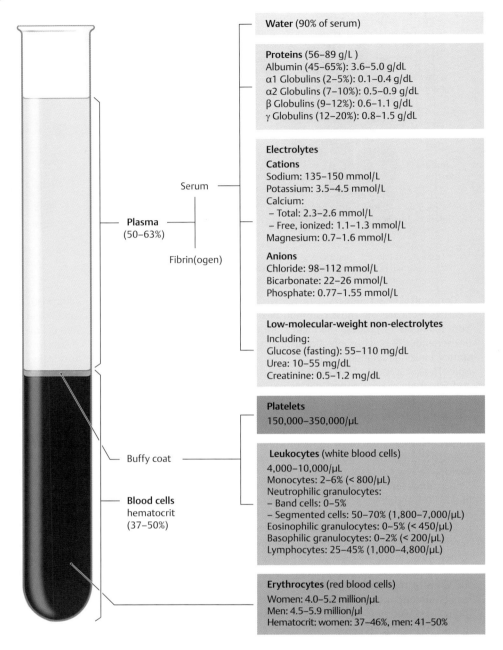

Water (90% of serum)

Proteins (56–89 g/L)
Albumin (45–65%): 3.6–5.0 g/dL
α1 Globulins (2–5%): 0.1–0.4 g/dL
α2 Globulins (7–10%): 0.5–0.9 g/dL
β Globulins (9–12%): 0.6–1.1 g/dL
γ Globulins (12–20%): 0.8–1.5 g/dL

Electrolytes
Cations
Sodium: 135–150 mmol/L
Potassium: 3.5–4.5 mmol/L
Calcium:
– Total: 2.3–2.6 mmol/L
– Free, ionized: 1.1–1.3 mmol/L
Magnesium: 0.7–1.6 mmol/L

Anions
Chloride: 98–112 mmol/L
Bicarbonate: 22–26 mmol/L
Phosphate: 0.77–1.55 mmol/L

Low-molecular-weight non-electrolytes
Including:
Glucose (fasting): 55–110 mg/dL
Urea: 10–55 mg/dL
Creatinine: 0.5–1.2 mg/dL

Platelets
150,000–350,000/μL

Leukocytes (white blood cells)
4,000–10,000/μL
Monocytes: 2–6% (< 800/μL)
Neutrophilic granulocytes:
– Band cells: 0–5%
– Segmented cells: 50–70% (1,800–7,000/μL)
Eosinophilic granulocytes: 0–5% (< 450/μL)
Basophilic granulocytes: 0–2% (< 200/μL)
Lymphocytes: 25–45% (1,000–4,800/μL)

Erythrocytes (red blood cells)
Women: 4.0–5.2 million/μL
Men: 4.5–5.9 million/μl
Hematocrit: women: 37–46%, men: 41–50%

Serum

Plasma (50–63%)

Fibrin(ogen)

Buffy coat

Blood cells hematocrit (37–50%)

B Phases of blood formation during development

Blood is required before birth even prior to the development of red bone marrow. As a result, blood is initially formed elsewhere: in the yolk sac (insular), in the liver (hepatic), in the spleen (splenic), and finally in the secondary bone marrow (medullary). Malignant systemic diseases of the blood and the immune system "remember" these sites that provide favorable conditions for growth, and certain forms of these diseases then colonize the liver and spleen.

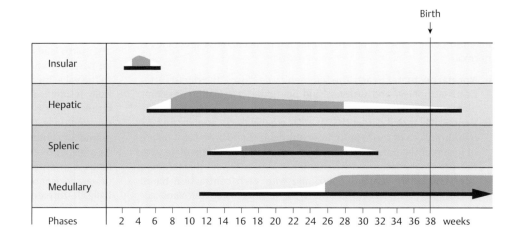

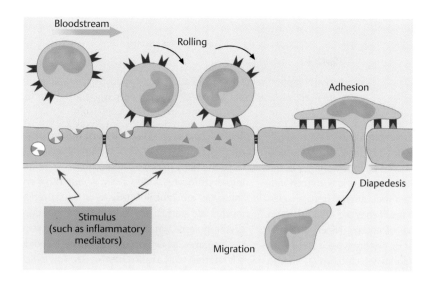

C Blood as a transport medium for blood cells

(modified from Lüllmann-Rauch, Thieme; 2012) White blood cells circulate through the blood and as a result are distributed throughout the body. They constantly migrate out of the blood stream and into the connective tissue of the organs where they attack bacteria or cancer cells. Migration (diapedesis) occurs via the leukocyte adhesion cascade. Upon receiving a stimulus, endothelial cells express cell adhesion molecules on their luminal surface. These molecules either come to the surface immediately through vesicles in the cytoplasm or they are synthesized in response. Ligands on the cell membrane of the leukocytes bind to these molecules. This binding (keying) causes the leukocytes to roll along the endothelium. Sometimes they come to a stop and sometimes they disconnect and rejoin the bloodstream. When they stop, the endothelial cells reduce their intercellular cohesion to allow the leukocytes to pass through the gap between them.

D Innate and adaptive immunity

As the blood has access to all organs, it plays an important role in the immune system in defending against infections and malignant cells. The immune system and the blood are thus tightly integrated. The innate immune system responds immediately to an appropriate stimulus and is nonspecific as it must respond to many possible attacks. Cellular components (cells are transported by the blood) and humoral components are differentiated. Humoral ("liquid") components include complement and cytokines in the blood. Adaptive immunity is specific and is directed toward a specific noxious agent such as a certain virus. The adaptive immune system includes T and B cells, which also circulate in the blood. T cells kill cancer cells or cells infected by viruses by direct contact (cellular immunity); B cells secrete various classes of antibodies (humoral immunity).

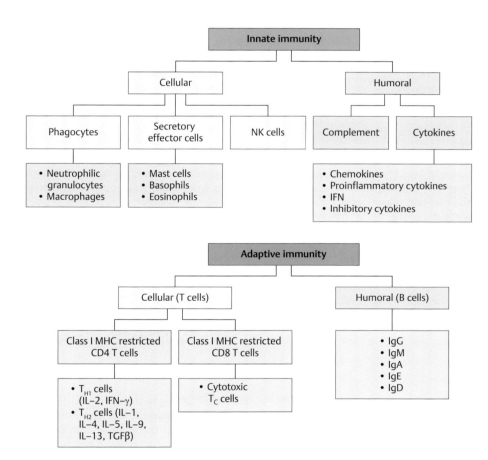

E Lifespan facts of certain blood cells

Type of cell	Retention time in blood	Lifetime in interstitium	Creation of new cells in bone marrow
Erythrocyte	120 days	—	About 8 days
Platelet	10 days unless consumed earlier	—	About 8 days
Neutrophilic granulocyte	< 1 day	1–2 days	About 8 days
Monocyte	About 1–3 days	Months (as a macrophage)	About 8 days

3.2   Blood: Cells

This unit discusses the cells of the blood that can be morphologically distinguished in a normal blood smear. The classic blood smear is colored with Pappenheim stain. Red and white blood cells as well as platelets are readily identifiable. See p. 22 for their normal values in blood.

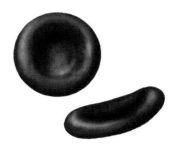

A Red blood cells (erythrocytes)
Erythrocytes (approx. 5 million/µL) are large, biconcave cells measuring about 7.5 µm in diameter. In mammals they contain no nucleus or cytoplasmic organelles. Their lack of organelles and their specially reinforced cell membrane allow erythrocytes to adapt particularly well to different flow characteristics in blood so that they can even squeeze through narrow capillaries. This adaptability allows them to survive in the blood about 120 days. After this, erythrocytes are eliminated by macrophages in the liver and spleen. Because they lack mitochondria, they must obtain their energy from anaerobic glycolysis. As a result they are dependent on glucose as a source of energy. Ninety-five percent of the interior of erythrocytes is filled with the protein hemoglobin, which binds O_2 and, to a lesser extent, CO_2. Erythrocytes are created in a series of morphologically distinct stages from a precursor cell containing a nucleus (see page 27). Reticulocytes represent the stage immediately preceding mature erythrocytes. They can be demonstrated with Cresyl violet stain. This stain binds to the RNA of the rough endoplasmic reticulum of erythrocytes, whose precursor cells ejected their nuclei 1–2 days previously and still contain residual traces of the endoplasmic reticulum. About 2.5 million reticulocytes leave the bone marrow per second. They mature into erythrocytes within a day. About 1% of erythrocytes are reticulocytes. As a result, reticulocytes are particularly suitable for monitoring erythropoiesis. When the number of reticulocytes increases, as can occur after acute bleeding, it is referred to as a reticulocyte crisis. This indicates that the bone marrow has responded to the blood loss by increasing the production of new erythrocytes. Here, the term crisis is used in a positive sense to indicate the regenerative output of the bone marrow.

Note: As the average diameter of erythrocytes is a reliably constant 7.5 µm, it can be used in histologic sections as an intrinsic scale for the size of a histologic structure.

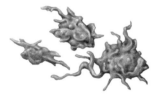

B Platelets (thrombocytes)
Platelets (about 250,000/µL) are non-nucleated fragments of megakaryocytes, multinuclear giant cells that reside in the bone marrow. They survive in blood for about 10 days after which they are phagocytized by macrophages in the liver and spleen, so new cells must be generated constantly. In flowing blood they assume the shape of a biconcave disk measuring 2.5 µm in diameter. Platelets are an essential component of blood coagulation. Increases, decreases, and anomalies of platelets can be diagnosed in blood smears. Below 30,000/µL fine capillary hemorrhaging known as petechial bleeding occurs. Below 10,000/µL life-threatening bleeding occurs. A change in the platelet count is a sensitive indicator of bone marrow function. A decreased platelet count can be an early indicator of worsening bone marrow function. Conversely, an increased platelet count can be an early indicator of increased bone marrow function.

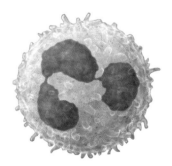

C Neutrophilic granulocytes
Neutrophils (the commonly used short form of neutrophilic granulocytes) represent the largest share of leukocytes in blood (4,000–10,000/µL), accounting for about 60%. A neutrophil measures 10–12 µm in diameter and remains in the blood for less than a day. It is characterized by a cell nucleus consisting of 3–4 segments connected to one another by narrow nucleic bridges. As a result it is also referred to as polymorphonuclear. Granulocytes take their respective name from how their granules stain with Pappenheim dye. The term neutrophilic comes from the fact that their cytoplasmic granules (< 1 µm) don't stain well with either basophilic dyes or eosinophilic dyes. They are therefore neutral.

Neutrophils belong to the nonspecific immune system and phagocytize bacteria (microphages) in particular. Therefore, a large share of their granules are lysosomes in which phagocytized bacteria are broken down. Neutrophils are generated in the bone marrow and are released from there into the peripheral bloodstream when acutely needed (as is the case in bacterial infection). In such cases, a blood smear will reveal increased numbers of neutrophil precursors ("juvenile" cells) with unsegmented or less clearly segmented nuclei. Thus, a reactive increase in neutrophils in a blood smear can suggest a bacterial infection.

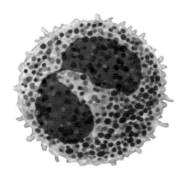

D Eosinophilic granulocytes

Eosinophils (12 μm in diameter) have a bilobed nucleus. They contain eosinophilic granules measuring 1.5 μm which represent modified lysosomes that release their contents to the extracellular matrix in degranulation. The anionic dye eosin binds to the cationic proteins in the granules (such as major basic protein, and eosinophil cationic protein). Eosinophils defend against worms in particular (small eosinophils cannot completely phagocytize large multicellular parasites), which is why their blood count is increased in parasitic diseases. They frequently migrate from the blood into the mucosa of the gastrointestinal tract and lungs. Their numbers are also increased in allergic disorders.

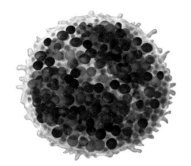

E Basophilic granulocytes

The lobulated nucleus of basophils is often undetectable as it is obscured by granules, which measure 1 μm and stain intensely bluish-violet. The polyanionic heparin contained in the granules takes up cationic dyes (methylene blue, azure). The granules also contain histamine, which is released in an allergic reaction. Although basophils resemble mast cells in their morphology and function, the two are separate types of cells that arise from different stem cells and they do not merge with each other.

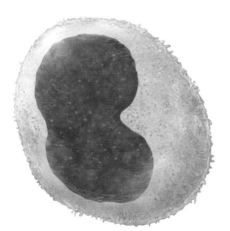

F Monocytes

Measuring 20–40 μm in diameter, monocytes are the largest cells in the blood. They exhibit a pale grayish blue cytoplasm and an indented bean-shaped nucleus that also can assume other shapes. This means that monocytes are the most variable type of cell in a blood smear. Small, barely discernible azure granules may be found in the cytoplasm, especially in the indentation of the nucleus. These represent lysosomes. Monocytes leave the bloodstream after about a day and migrate into the connective tissue of the organs, where they differentiate into macrophages. Macrophages are monocytes that have become resident and in which a number of differentiation processes occur. The number of lysosomes in particular increases greatly. The mononuclear phagocytic system (MPS) is a generic term introduced by van Furth which includes all of these cells.

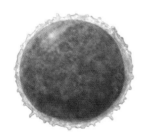

G Lymphocytes

Lymphocytes are characterized by a round nucleus rich in heterochromatin. In small lymphocytes (4–7 μm in diameter), the nucleus is surrounded by a narrow ring of cytoplasm; in medium-sized lymphocytes (up to 15 μm) this ring is wider and can contain granules (see **H**). Lymphocytes are part of the adaptive or specific immune system and occur in two main forms, B lymphocytes and T lymphocytes, which are indistinguishable in a blood smear. They are analyzed with the aid of monoclonal antibodies in flow cytometry (important in AIDS patients). B lymphocytes ultimately differentiate into plasma cells that produce antibodies; T lymphocytes aid in providing specific cell-mediated immunity. Lymphocytes only use the bloodstream for a short time (approximately 1 hour) as a transport medium to enter the lymphatic organs and the interstitium of other organs. Lymphocytes have a similar appearance to monocytes, which is why the two are often grouped together as mononuclear cells. These are distinguished from the granulocytes (polymorphonuclear cells). Reactively increased numbers of lymphocytes in the blood occur often in viral disorders.

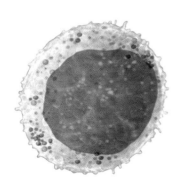

H Azurophilic granulated lymphocytes

Azurophilic granulated lymphocytes are a special form of large lymphocyte distinguishable by their large ring of cytoplasm and their azurophilic granules (large granular lymphocytes or LGL). They represent the natural killer cells (NK cells) that form part of the nonspecific immune system. They react immediately upon contact with virus-infected cells or bloodborne cancer cells and usually destroy these target cells after direct contact.

3.3 Blood: Bone Marrow

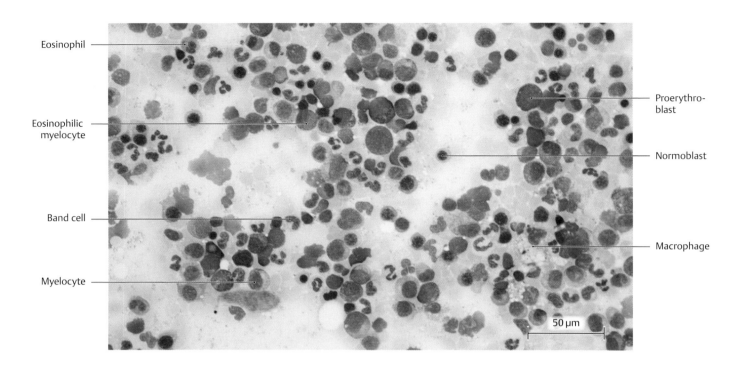

A Bone marrow cytology

Normal medulla ossium contains a bewildering variety of cells. The reason for this is that starting from a single pluripotent stem cell, erythropoiesis, granulopoiesis, and lymphopoiesis all occur simultaneously and produce several different morphologically distinct intermediate stages. A few of the cell types that occur are shown here (see **D** for the classification of cell types in the various lines). In bone marrow cytology, the cells of hematopoiesis from the aspirate are spread out on a slide and are viewed as a single layer of spread out cells. Because the cells are spread out in a single layer in their entirety, cellular details are far more readily discernible than in bone marrow histology where cells may be only partially sectioned because of their size. (Specimen provided by Prof. Hans-Peter Horny, Munich)

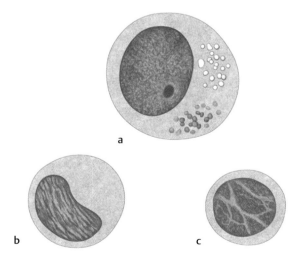

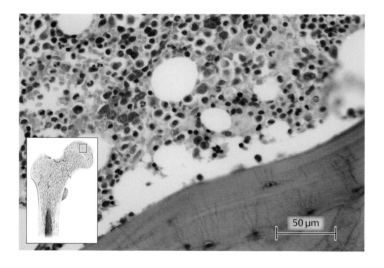

B Cytologic evaluation criteria for bone marrow aspirates (after Haferlach et al. Thieme; 2012)

The various different chromatin structures allow us to identify different cell types: **a** myeloblast through promyelocyte; **b** myeloblast through band cell; **c** lymphocyte; clumped chromatin structure. Aside from the structure of the chromatin in the cell nucleus, the structure of the cytoplasm and its granules are evaluated. When granules are present, their affinity for dye allows their classification within a certain series of cells, such neutrophils (granules that do not easily stain) or eosinophils (red stained granules).

C Bone marrow histology

To obtain a histologic specimen, one removes a section of red bone marrow from the femur (in living patients via a biopsy of the posterior superior iliac spine). The cells of the red marrow fill the spaces between the trabeculae. In contrast to bone marrow cytology, histology allows local classification of the cells of hematopoiesis among themselves and with respect to the trabeculae of the bone marrow. This precise classification can be helpful in certain lines of inquiry.
(Specimen provided by Prof. Hans-Peter Horny, Munich)

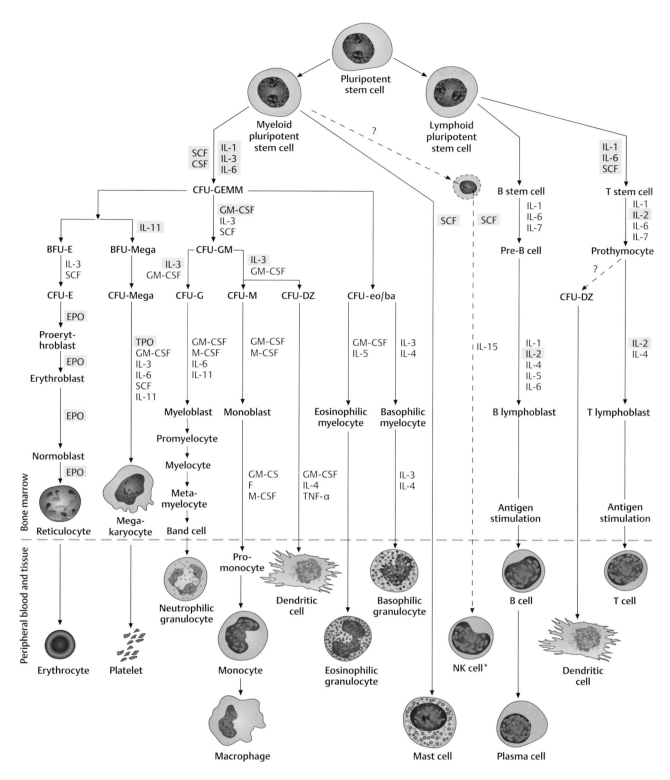

D Hematopoiesis

The yellow highlighted growth factors are the most important hematopoietic growth factors for cell differentiation.

All cells in the blood are descended from the pluripotent stem cell. It gives rise to two other cells also referred to as pluripotent stem cells: the lymphoid (right) and the myeloid (left). The various stem cell populations are morphologically indistinguishable from one another. The stem cells that descend from the two pluripotent stem cells are determined; they are stem cells only for the cell populations that follow them. The hematopoietic system requires such a complex hierarchy of stem cells because cells of the most widely varied functions and lifetimes (an erythrocyte that lives 120 days, a neutrophil that lives only a few

days) must be constantly produced at a single location (bone marrow). Additionally, increased numbers of erythrocytes must be produced when there has been blood loss, and increased numbers of neutrophils in a bacterial infection. This means the system needs a high degree of flexibility in order to produce cells that function differently and have different lifetimes. The various stem cell populations ensure this flexibility. The morphology of the various normal cells of hematopoiesis is used as the basis for classifying leukemic cells (malignant degenerative cells), for example promyelocytic leukemia or erythroleukemia. This hierarchical scheme of a stem-cell-containing tissue was then applied to other types of tumors, including solid ones (concept of the malignant stem cell).

* The exact classification of the natural killer cells with respect to stem cells has not yet been fully clarified.

4.1   Overview of the Lymphatic System

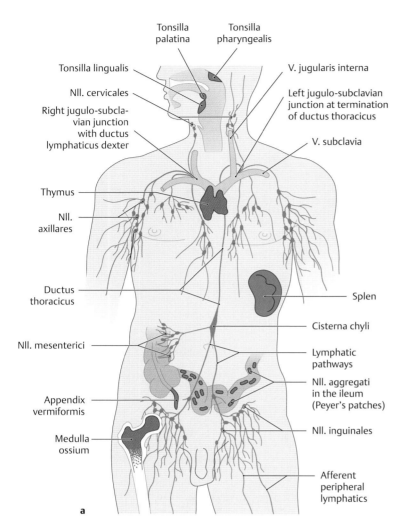

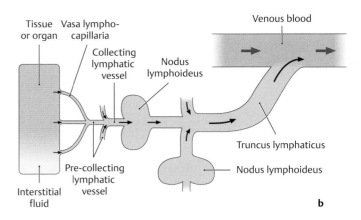

A Lymphatic organs and vessels

The lymphatic system, which is widely distributed throughout most of the body, consists of lymphatic organs and vessels. It has three main functions:

- Immunological defense (lymphatic organs and vessels). The main function of the immune response is to distinguish "self" from "non-self" (or foreign) substances (such as pathogens, or transplanted tissues) and destroy the "nonself" substances.
- Transport of interstitial fluid to venous blood (vasa lymphatica)
- Removal of lipids from the intestinum tenue while bypassing the hepatic portal system. This allows triglycerides to avoid hepatic metabolism and to be transported directly to organs that can utilize them.

a Lymphatic organs: All lymphatic organs have a stroma that is populated by lymphocytes that originated in medulla ossium (bone marrow). They are directly or indirectly responsible for eliminating antigens (immune response). Antigens are molecules (proteins, carbohydrates, lipids), which the immune system recognizes as foreign and mounts a defense against.

There are two types of *lymphocytes,* which can be further subdivided. (For more details see immunology textbooks.)

- B lymphocytes ("B" stands for bone marrow, where the cells are produced) differentiate into plasma cells, which produce antibodies. Antibodies are essential components of the *humoral immune response*. Humoral immunity refers to antibodies dissolved in blood and interstitial fluid that bind to antigens. Thus, the plasma cells are not directly involved in the immune response.
- T lymphocytes ("T" stands for thymus, where the cells mature) attack and destroy foreign substances (e.g., virus-infected cells) on direct contact (*cellular immune response*).

There are both primary lymphatic organs (*organa lymphoidea primaria,* red organs in **a**) and secondary lymphatic organs *(organa lymphoidea secundaria,* green organs in **a**):

- In the primary lymphatic organs, lymphocytes derived from stem cells mature and become immunocompetent cells (meaning they are capable of distinguishing between self and nonself substances).
- From these primary lymphatic organs, lymphocytes migrate to the secondary lymphatic organs where they continue to proliferate and mature. They are then able to fulfill their specific roles in the immune response. Lymphocytes can leave an organ and enter the bloodstream.

The structure and function of the individual lymphatic organs will be discussed in the respective organ chapters.

b Lymphatic vessels: Lymphatic vessels (green in **a**) are part of a tubular system that is distributed to all parts of the body (except for the CNS and medulla renalis). The vessels are responsible for absorbing fluid from the interstitial spaces (it is now called lymph) and transporting it to the venous blood. Lymphatic vessels start out as tiny, thin-walled capillaries (lymphatic capillaries), which drain into larger pre-collecting and collecting vessels (**b**). These eventually coalesce into trunci lymphatici. These trunks join to form two larger ducts that end at each of the two venous angles (the junction of the v. jugularis interna and v. subclavia) (see p. 30). Nodi lymphoidei are incorporated into the system of peripheral lymphatic vessels. Lymphatic vessels converge in the nodi lymphoidei, where the lymph is filtered and checked for pathogens as it passes through.

B Overview of the lymphatic pathways

Lymphatic pathways play a clinically significant role in the classification of tumors and their cells that metastasize to lymphatic nodes (nodi lymphoidei). Since lymphatic node metastases are sometimes discovered before the primary tumor, the organ where the cancer initiated can be determined from the affected lymph nodes. Thus it is crucial to know the lymphatic pathways of organs and regions. The classification of lymph vessels and the nodi lymphoidei associated with them is illustrated below. If one follows the pathway the lymph travels from the site of origin until it flows into the venous blood stream, the basic classification becomes apparent:

- Lymph is formed by ultrafiltration from capillary vessels (vasa capillaria) in the connective tissue (**C**).
- There is a superficial and deep lymphatic network (**D**).
- 5 major trunci lymphatici drain lymph from all areas of the body (see p. 30).
- The nodi lymphoidei incorporated into the lymphatic system can be classified according to their location (see p. 31).

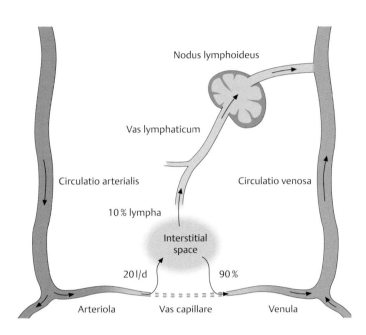

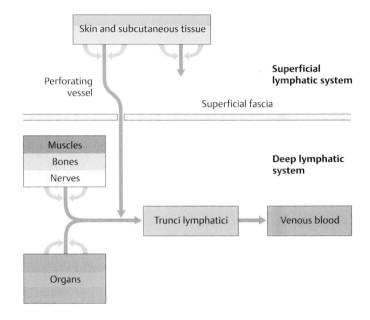

C Lymph formation

Lymph forms as a clear fluid in the capillaries by blood ultrafiltration. Blood passes through capillaries from the arterial to the venous side of the circulatory system. The internal capillary blood pressure is greater than the colloid osmotic pressure in the capillary. As a result, 10% of the fluid from the capillaries remains as interstitial fluid in the interstitial space. This 1.8–2 liters of interstitial fluid (over 24 hours) that is not returned to the blood capillaries is absorbed by lymph capillaries (see **Ab**), and then collected into larger lymphatic vessels and trunks before it drains into venous blood. Eventually all the lymph in the body drains into two trunci lymphatici (ductus thoracicus et ductus lymphaticus dexter, which drain into the anguli venosi sinister et dexter, respectively, at the junction of the neck and thorax [see page 28, Fig. **Aa**]). The lymphatic vessels direct lymph through lymph nodes, and the nodes check the lymph for germs and toxins. In cases of purulent inflammation caused by bacteria, reddened superficial lymphatic pathways are visible, which in layman terms is referred to as "blood poisoning."

Note: After a fat-rich meal, lymph from the small intestine is rich in emulsified lipoprotein particles (chylomicrons) and thus has a milky appearance. Lymph flowing from the small intestine is called chyle and the lymph vessels of the small intestine are sometimes referred to as chyle vessels.

D Superficial and deep lymphatic systems

There are both superficial and deep lymphatic systems.

- The superficial lymphatic system is located in and above the superficial fascia and collects lymph from the cutis (skin) and tela subcutanea (subcutaneus tissue).
- The deep lymphatic system lies underneath the superficial fascia and collects lymph from the organs, muscles, bones, and nerves.

Only the deep lymphatic system has direct contact with the major trunci lymphatici (see p. 30). The superficial lymphatic system transports lymph to the deep vasa lymphatica through perforating vessels (which penetrate the superficial fascia). The connection between superficial and deep vasa lymphatica is very pronounced in three spots:

- the sides of the neck
- the armpit
- the groin

Nodi lymphoidei are also particularly numerous in these sites, where they can be readily palpated during clinical examinations.

4.2 Lymphatic Drainage Pathways

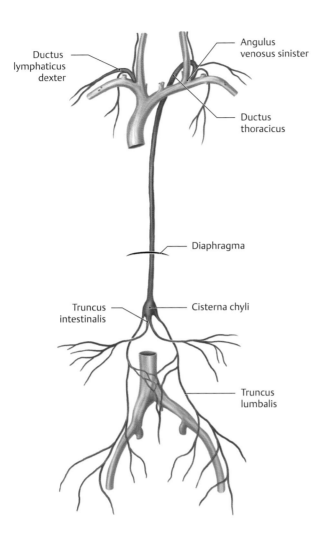

A The major trunci lymphatici

There are 5 major trunci lymphatici, most of them paired, which drain lymph from the various regions of the body. Table **B** lists all the trunci and the regions they drain. Generally, all trunci drain into either theducts thoracicus or the *ductus lymphaticus dexter*, both of which empty into the venous system. The 3 major lymphatic trunks for the abdomen, pelvis, and lower limbs (the truncus intestinalis and the two trunci lumbales) merge just beneath the diaphragma into a dilated collecting sac, the *cisterna chyli*. The ductus thoracicus originates from the cisterna chyli, traverses the diaphragma through the hiatus aorticus, ascends through the cavitas thoracica and eventually drains into the left venous angle. On its way it usually receives the left truncus bronchomediastinalis as well as the left truncus jugularis and left truncus subclavius. However, all these trunks may empty separately into the venous system.

The right truncus bronchomediastinalis, right truncus jugularis, and right truncus subclavius merge to form the very short ductus lymphaticus dexter. The ductus lymphaticus dexter drains into the right venous angle.

Note: Except for the truncus intestinalis, all lymphatic trunks are paired, corresponding with the organization of the body regions they drain. The truncus intestinalis drains the unpaired abdominal viscera (see **B**). Although it is unpaired, it can often be divided into multiple (not individually named) sub-trunks, which in the nomenclature are collectively referred to as trunci intestinales–plural.

B Organization of the trunci lymphatici and the regions they drain
Summary of the lymphatic trunks and the body regions they drain.

Truncus lymphaticus	Drainage area
Head, neck, and upper limbs	
• Left and right trunci jugulares • Left and right trunci subclavii	• Left and right sides of the head and neck • Left and right upper limbs
Thorax	
• Left and right trunci bronchomediastinales	• Organs, internal structures, and walls of the left and right thorax

The trunks located on the right side merge to form the ductus lymphaticus dexter. The trunks located on the left side drain into the ductus thoracicus (see below).

Abdomen, pelvis, and lower limbs	

The ductus thoracicus collects most of the lymph circulating throughout the body. The duct is formed by the convergence of

• The truncus intestinalis	• Unpaired abdominal viscera (digestive tract and splen)
• The left and right trunci lumbales	• Paired abdominal viscera (renes, gll. suprarenales) • All pelvic viscera • Left and right abdominal walls • Left and right pelvic walls • Left and right lower limbs

The ductus thoracicus drains all lymph from areas below the diaphragma and from the left side of the body above the diaphragma. The ductus lymphaticus dexter only drains the lymph from the right side of the body above the diaphragma. Accordingly, it is possible to divide the body into 4 lymphatic drainage quadrants (see **C**).

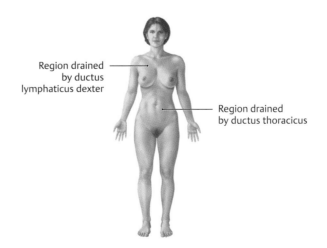

C Organization of the body into lymphatic drainage quadrants
The lymphatic drainage of the body is not symmetrical. Rather, it is organized by quadrants. The ductus lymphaticus dexter drains the right upper quadrant, and the ductus thoracicus drains the other three quadrants.

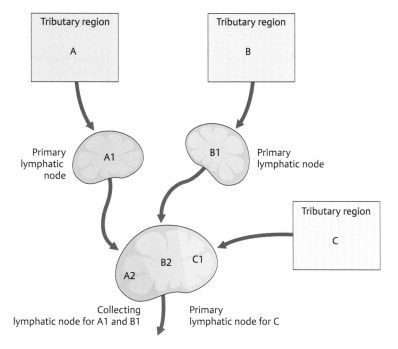

D Classification of lymph nodes (modified after Földi)
Groups of lymph nodes can be classified in different ways. One classification is based on the direction of lymph flow, and another is based on their location relative to the internal organs.

Classification based on direction of lymph flow: If lymph is classified based on the direction it flows (from peripheral tissue to the venous system), it usually passes through several serially connected groups of lymph nodes. These nodes are referred to as primary, secondary, and tertiary lymph nodes:

- Primary lymph nodes (nodi lymphoidei regionales) take up lymph directly from a circumscribed area of the body (organ; limb; part of trunk). The area that passes its lymph to a particular group of primary lymph nodes (blue or green node, A1 or B1) is called the tributary region of the specific group of nodes (in the figure labeled A–C).

- Once the lymph leaves the primary lymph nodes, it can be passed to subsequent (secondary or tertiary) lymph nodes. Since secondary lymph nodes often collect lymph from multiple groups of primary lymph nodes, they are also referred to as collecting lymph nodes (in the figure marked as a multicolored node).

Note: A group of primary lymph nodes for one tributary region can, at the same time, be the secondary or collecting lymph nodes for another region. Thus, the three-colored nodus lymphoideus is a primary node for tributary region C (yellow), while at the same time it is also a collecting node for primary nodes A1 and B1 (blue and green).

Classification based on location relative to the internal organs: Lymph nodes in the abdomen and pelvis are classified as nodi lymphoidei *parietales* or nodi lymphoidei *viscerales* depending on their relationship to major vessels and organs:

- Nodi lymphoidei parietales of the abdomen and pelvis are located either directly adjacent to the major vessels (aorta abdominalis, v. cava inferior cava or iliac vessels) or close to the abdominal wall.
- Nodi lymphoidei viscerales of the abdomen are related to the unpaired abdominal viscera, which are supplied by the three major unpaired arterial trunks. Groups of nodi lymphoidei viscerales are also located next to the organs in the pelvis. These lymph nodes pass their lymph primarily to the (parietal) nodi lymphoidei iliaci, which would then be considered as collecting nodi lymphoidei for the visceral group.

Lymphatic node group	Parietal group	Visceral group
Abdominal	• Nodi lymphoidei lumbales sinistri, dextri, and intermedii • Nodi lymphoidei epigastrici inferiores • Nodi lymphoidei phrenici inferiores	• Named after organ (see p. 222)
Pelvic	• Nodi lymphoidei iliaci interni, externi, and communes	• Named after organ (see p. 223)

E Embryonic development of lymphatic organs and lymphatic vessels
The lymphatic organs and lymphatic vessels (organa lymphoidea and vasa lymphatica) are derived mostly from mesoderma.
Note: Growth and development of the thymus are not complete until after birth. While the other organs develop in the given time frame, they mature in function only around the time of birth (when the immune cells can make the immunologically important distinction between "self" and "nonself").

Lymphatic structure	Time frame	Developmental process
Vasa lymphatica	Approx. weeks 5–9	Endothelial buds of the vv. cardinales form sac-like, enlarged vessels, which are connected to a lymphatic plexus close to the dorsal body wall. The major ducts develop from this plexus.
Tonsillae	Approx. weeks 12–16	Epithelial invagination of the 2nd saccus pharyngeus
Splen	Approx. weeks 5–24	Proliferation of mesenchymal cells in the mesogastrium dorsale. As part of gaster rotation, the splen moves to the left upper quadrant.
Thymus	Approx. weeks 4–16	Epithelial invagination of the ventral endoderma and ectoderma in the 3rd saccus pharyngeus

5.1   Overview of the Respiratory System

Introduction and overview

The respiratory organs are the site of gas exchange between the organism and the atmosphere (external respiration vs. internal respiration = cellular respiration). Additionally, respiratory organs contribute to voice production.

Inhaled air reaches the alveoli pulmonales through a network of finely branched tubes (the trachea, bronchi and bronchioli). *Gas exchange* takes place in the alveoli. In the air passages, incoming air is warmed, moistened and filtered. Blood is transported to the lungs (pulmones) through a similarly finely branched network, the aa. pulmonales and their branches. *Carbon dioxide*, an end product of cellular metabolism,

is carried with the blood to the lungs. During respiration, *oxygen is* absorbed from the air, and then binds with hemoglobin. At the same time, carbon dioxide is excreted. Carbon dioxide in the blood is a component of the bicarbonate buffering system. Thus, respiration influences the body's acid-base balance by releasing CO_2. The gas exchange between air and blood occurs by diffusion, driven by the differences in partial pressure of the two gases (the difference in the pressure of the gas between the blood and air). Blood does not come into direct contact with the air; they are separated by the blood-air barrier. From the lungs, blood is pumped through the vv. pulmonales back to the heart, and from there it reenters the systemic circulation.

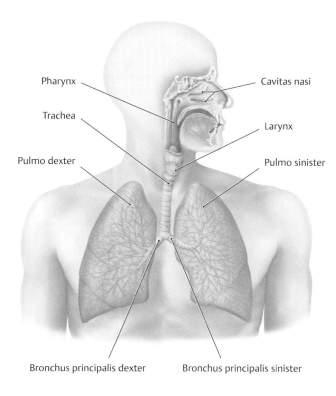

A Structure of the air passages

The respiratory system is divided into an upper and lower respiratory tract:

- **The upper air passages include**
  - the external nose and cavitas nasi,
  - the sinus paranasales,
  - the pharynx (only the upper portion, the pars nasalis pharyngis, is exclusively a part of the respiratory tract; in the middle portion of the pharynx the respiratory and digestive tracts cross each other).
- **The lower air passages include**
  - the larynx, which serves to temporarily close the air passages during swallowing, and also contributes to voice production;
  - the trachea, which divides into the two bronchi principales;
  - the two bronchi principales, which then progressively subdivide;
  - the alveoli, located at the end of the network of progressively narrowing tubes. They are the site of gas exchange.

The histology of the different parts of the respiratory tract will be further discussed in the organ chapters.

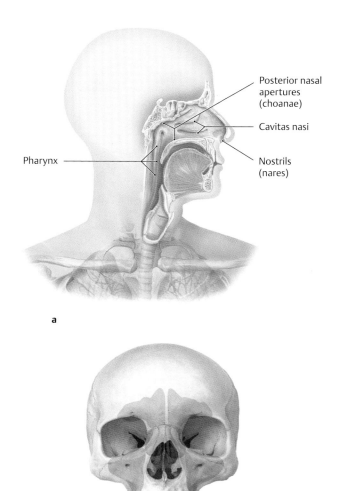

B Upper air passages: Nose, cavitas nasi, and pharynx

a Main cavitas nasi and pharynx viewed from the right side with the head turned left; **b** Bony skull, anterior view of the sinus paranasales.

Air is inhaled through the nostrils (nares) into the cavitas nasi. It then passes through the posterior aperture of the nose (choana) into the pharynx, and then to the larynx. Narrow openings connect the sinus paranasales to the main cavitas nasi.

Note: In addition to conducting air, the main cavitas nasi is also involved in odor perception.

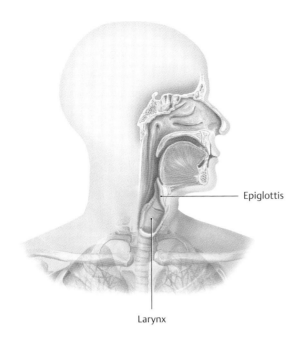

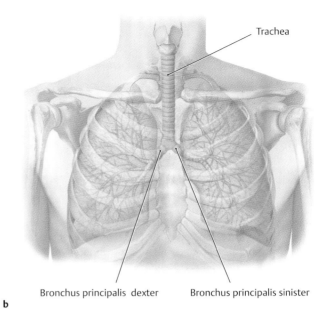

a — Larynx — Epiglottis

b — Trachea — Bronchus principalis dexter — Bronchus principalis sinister

C Lower air passages: Larynx and trachea

a Larynx viewed from the right side; **b** Anterior view of the trachea. The larynx marks the entrance to the lower air passages. The epiglottis, which is part of the larynx, can temporarily close the entrance to the airways during swallowing. This helps to prevent food from entering the lower respiratory passageways (which could lead to choking). Additionally, the larynx contributes to voice production. The trachea is the continuation of the larynx. It is located in the neck and thorax and divides into the two bronchi principales, which carry air to each lung. Cartilage is an important structural component of the larynx and trachea.

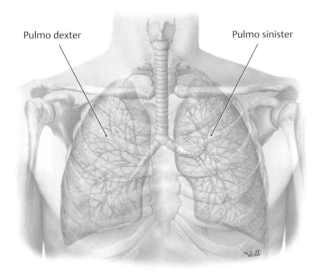

Pulmo dexter — Pulmo sinister

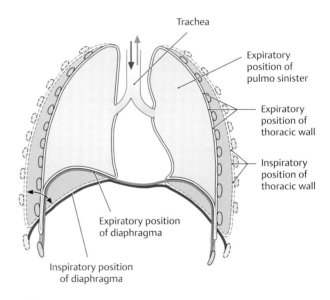

Trachea — Expiratory position of pulmo sinister — Expiratory position of thoracic wall — Inspiratory position of thoracic wall — Expiratory position of diaphragma — Inspiratory position of diaphragma

D Lower air passages: Arbor bronchialis and lungs

Anterior view of the arbor bronchialis and pulmones. On the right side, the two bronchi principales divide into three bronchi lobares, and on the left side into two bronchi lobares. They further subdivide over several more steps with the final bronchioli respiratorii ending in alveoli, where gas exchange takes place. The arbor bronchialis provides the structural framework of the lungs. Each pulmo is located in a separate cavitas pleuralis, which is lined by a pleural membrane (pleura). The function of the arbor bronchialis is to conduct air to and from the lungs.

E Breathing mechanics

Anterior view of the lungs (schematic frontal section). The rhythmic activity of the respiratory muscles causes the cavitas thoracica to expand (upward, downward, and laterally) and contract. The change in thoracic volume also causes the lungs to rhythmically expand, and then retract due to their elasticity. Thus, the bony and muscular structures of the thoracic wall and diaphragma, which surround the lungs, function like a pair of bellows.

33

5.2 Development of the Larynx, Trachea, and Lungs

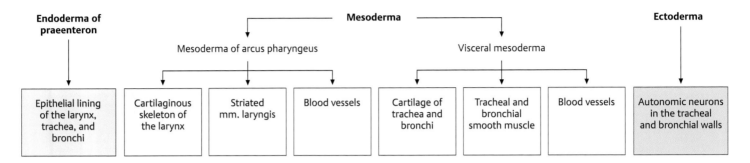

A Development of the respiratory tract from the three germ layers
All three germ layers are involved in the embryonic development of the larynx, trachea, and arbor bronchialis. A protrusion from the praenteron in the area around the oesophagus gives rise to the trachea and arbor bronchialis. While the cartilage, muscle, vessels, and nerves of the larynx are mostly derived from the 4th—6th arcus pharyngei, the laryngeal epithelium is derived from the praenteron.

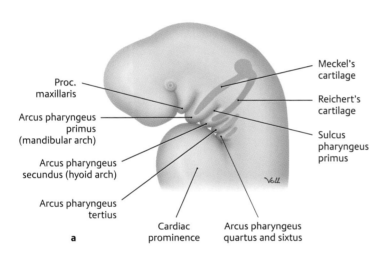

a

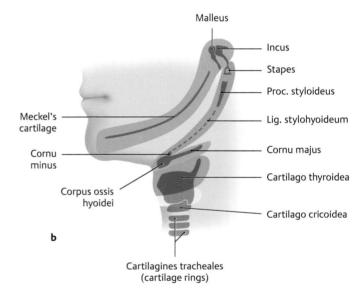

b

B Embryonic development of the larynx (after Sadler)
a Embryo, viewed from the left side; **b** Location of structures derived from the cartilaginous elements of the arcus pharyngei, viewed from the left side; **c** Dorsal view of the arcus pharyngei in an embryo at 6 weeks, frontal section.

In **a**, the embryonic arcus pharyngei are visible. The viscerocranium is derived from arcus pharyngei 1 and 2. Arcus 3 gives rise to most of the os hyoideum. The cartilaginous skeleton of the larynx and the mm. laryngis are from arcus 4 and 6. Corresponding to their embryonic origin, the striated mm. laryngis are innervated by a cranial nerve (the n. vagus).

Note: The laryngeal epithelium is derived from praenteron endoderma, like that of the trachea and bronchi, and not from the arcus pharyngei. The dorsal view of the arcus pharyngei of an embryo at 6 weeks (**c**) shows the developing aditus laryngis adjacent to arcus pharyngei 4 and 6. This is where the passageways for food and air divide and continue in the caudal direction as two separate systems (see **C**).

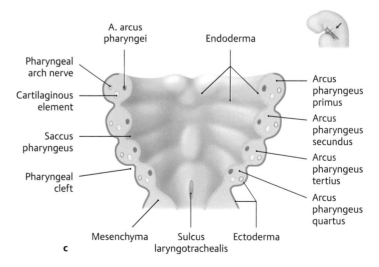

c

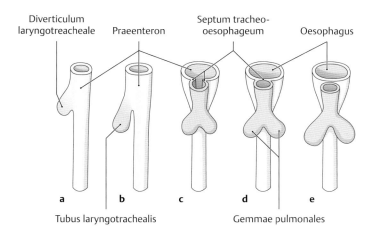

Diverticulum laryngotreacheale — Praeenteron — Septum tracheo-oesophageum — Oesophagus

a **b** **c** **d** **e**

Tubus laryngotrachealis — Gemmae pulmonales

C Development of the trachea and lungs: Tubus laryngotrachealis and gemmae pulmonales

Praeenteron viewed from the left side (**a** and **b**) and ventral view (**c**–**e**). The *diverticulum laryngotracheale* develops as a protrusion on the ventral aspect of the praeenteron towards the end of the 4th week of embryonic development (**a**). It later elongates into the tubus laryngotrachealis (**b**). This tube is initially open to the praeenteron. However, the septum tracheooesophageum, which develops from two lateral folds, soon separates the tubus laryngotrachealis almost completely from the praeenteron. This divides the praeenteron in a ventrodorsal direction into two portions (**d**):

- the developing respiratory tract, located ventral to the septum; and
- the developing oesophagus, located dorsal to the septum (for the location of the praeenteron see p. 40).

Only the cranial end of the tubus laryngotrachealis — the area around the future aditus laryngis — is in open communication with the praeenteron (see **b**). At the caudal end of the tube, a smaller left and a larger right gemma pulmonalis forms (**d**). The gemmae pulmonales are the primordia for the two lungs, and they continue to grow downward while at the same time expanding laterally (**e**). The right gemma pulmonalis gives rise to the bronchus principalis dexter and the left gemma pulmonalis to the bronchus principalis sinister.

D Development of the trachea and lungs: The arbor bronchialis

Arbor bronchialis at 5 (**a**), 6 (**b**), and 8 (**c**) weeks, ventral view; Detail of fully developed arbor bronchialis (**d**).

The gemmae pulmonales initially form the bronchi principales dexter and sinister. These give rise to three bronchi lobares on the right side and two on the left side, corresponding to the lobi of the lungs. These future bronchi lobares further elongate and subdivide into bronchi segmentales that supply the segments of the lung (10 segments in the pulmo dexter and usually only 9 in the pulmo sinister). Further subdivisions lead to bronchi intrasegmentales, which decrease in size, and finally to the bronchioli terminales (**d**). The tubus laryngotrachealis undergoes about 23 dichotomous divisions, beginning with the gemma pulmonalis. The first 17 divisions take place before birth and lead to the formation of simple alveoli, mainly in the form of sacculi alveolares (see p. 37). The remaining 6 divisions take place after birth, resulting in dramatically enlarged pulmones due to the high number of newly formed mature alveoli. The maturation of the lungs begins in their cranial segments and ends in their caudal segments 8 to 10 years after birth.

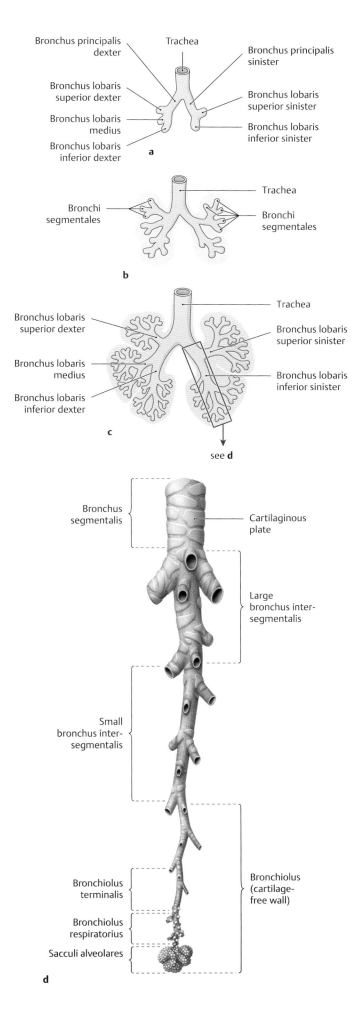

Bronchus principalis dexter — Trachea — Bronchus principalis sinister

Bronchus lobaris superior dexter — Bronchus lobaris superior sinister

Bronchus lobaris medius — Bronchus lobaris inferior sinister

Bronchus lobaris inferior dexter

a

Bronchi segmentales — Trachea — Bronchi segmentales

b

Bronchus lobaris superior dexter — Trachea — Bronchus lobaris superior sinister

Bronchus lobaris medius — Bronchus lobaris inferior sinister

Bronchus lobaris inferior dexter

c

see **d**

Bronchus segmentalis — Cartilaginous plate

Large bronchus inter-segmentalis

Small bronchus inter-segmentalis

Bronchiolus terminalis — Bronchiolus (cartilage-free wall)

Bronchiolus respiratorius

Sacculi alveolares

d

5.3 Lung Development and Maturation

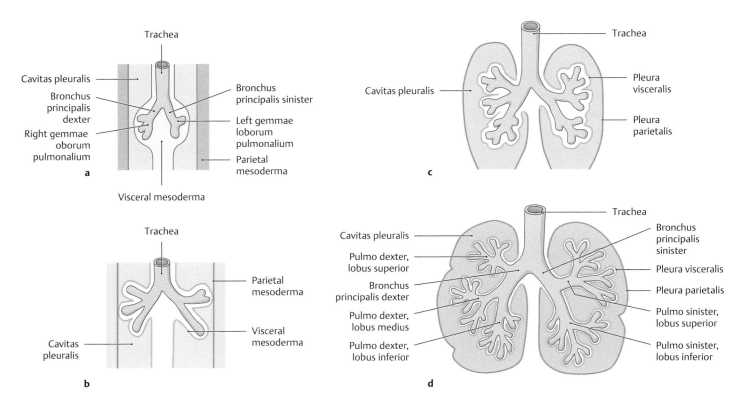

A Development of the trachea and lungs: The cavitates pleurales
Schematic view of the cavitates pleurales at 5 (**a**) and 6 (**b**) weeks; Ventral view of arbor bronchialis.
As part of the branching described above, the arbor bronchialis grows laterally and caudally toward the cavitas abdominis expanding against the visceral mesoderma (**a**) until it almost touches the parietal mesoderma (**b**). The pleura visceralis develops from the visceral mesoderma near the gemmae pulmonales, and the pleura parietalis, which lines the inside of the body cavity, develops from the parietal mesoderma. Thus, the expanding lung tissue, covered by pleura visceralis, progressively fills up the pleura parietalis lined body cavity (**c** and **d**). Due to its channel-like appearance, the still undivided cavity is referred to as the canalis pericardioperitonealis primordialis since it connects the cavitas pericardiaca primordialis (above) with the cavitas peritonealis (below). Two folds, the membranae pleuropericardiacae, grow medially and fuse with each other and connect with the central compartment of the cavitas thoracica (the future mediastinum, see p. 71) thus separating the now paired cavitates pleurales from the cavitas pericardiaca which contains the cor (see p. 6). The septum transversum (the future diaphragma, not shown) separates the cavitates pleurales from the cavitas abdominis, resulting in the complete partitioning of the initially single body cavity.

B Overview of the phases of lung development
The development of the lungs can be roughly divided into four phases: tempora pseudoglandulare pulmonis, canaliculare, sacculare, and alve-

olare. The first three stages end before or at birth (see **C**).
Note: The phases can overlap.

Phase of development	Before birth (weeks of development)	Developmental stages
• Tempus pseudoglandulare pulmonis	5–17	Division of the arbor bronchialis up to the bronchioli terminales. Bronchioli respiratorii and alveoli have not yet formed.
• Tempus canaliculare	16–25	Division of the bronchioli terminales into bronchioli respiratorii, which subdivide into ductuli alveolares with alveoli.
• Tempus sacculare (tempus sacci terminalis)	24 until birth	Primitive alveoli form and are in contact with capillaries. Epithelial cells begin to differentiate into specialized pneumocyti typi I and II. Pulmones are capable of a limited degree of respiration.
	After birth	
• Tempus alveolare	Around birth until 8 to 10 years after birth	Large increase in the number of alveoli as a result of further divisions. Differentiation of mature alveoli and formation of the blood-air barrier.

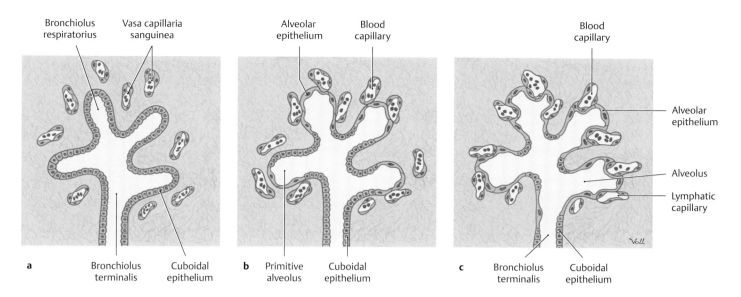

a — Bronchiolus respiratorius | Vasa capillaria sanguinea | Bronchiolus terminalis | Cuboidal epithelium

b — Alveolar epithelium | Blood capillary | Primitive alveolus | Cuboidal epithelium

c — Blood capillary | Alveolar epithelium | Alveolus | Lymphatic capillary | Bronchiolus terminalis | Cuboidal epithelium

C Development of the lungs: Alveolar formation and lung maturation

Alveolar development occurs simultaneously with the previously mentioned stages in lung development (see **B**). From the formation of the gemmae pulmonales around the 5th week to the formation of the bronchioli terminales around the 17th week, the primitive pulmones resemble an endocrine gland (thus, the *tempus pseudoglandulare pulmonis*, see **B**). The alveoli are still unexpanded and resemble an acinous gland with an exit duct. During the subsequent *tempus canaliculare*, the arbor bronchialis subdivides repeatedly into progressively smaller branches, with the bronchioli respiratorii being the smallest bronchi that exhibit alveolar precursors. Cuboidal epithelial cells of the bronchioli respiratorii proliferate to form flat alveolar epithelial cells, which make contact with the capillaries (**b**; morphological correlate to the blood-air barrier). This process results in the formation of *primitive alveoli* (**b**). By the end of the 7th month, sufficient numbers of alveoli guarantee that a premature infant is capable of breathing on its own. In the last two months before birth (*tempus sacci terminalis*), the lungs enlarge as a result of continuous branching of the arbor bronchialis and an increasing number of bronchioli respiratorii and alveoli. The first sacci alveolares form (see **D**, p. 35), and blood capillaries protrude into the alveolar spaces (**c**). In the alveoli, the epithelium further differentiates into pneumocyti typi I and typi II (see p. 155). The pneumocyti typi II produce surfactantum pulmonale, a phospholipid, that reduces surface tension in alveoli, thus enabling the lungs to expand with the newborn's first breath. At the time of birth, only 15–20% of the eventual number of alveoli have formed! There are around 300 million alveoli in a mature lung. The remaining 80–85% develop over the next 8–10 years as the lungs continuously produce new alveoli through differentiation (the *tempus alveolare*).

Note: Fetal lungs contain fluid (amniotic fluid and bronchial secretions). When the newborn takes its first breath, air replaces this fluid. The expansion of the lungs is the result of air replacing lung fluid, not enlargement or distension of the lungs. Surfactantum alveolare lowers the surface tension to such a degree that the ventilated alveoli can expand and remain open. Congenital absence of surfactantum leads to *respiratory distress syndrome* (RDS), which is life threatening. In cases of RDS, surfactantum is administered therapeutically by direct intrapulmonary application. Despite these measures, lung development and maturation is still a critical phase in embryonic development: Failure of the lungs to develop properly is among the most common causes of death in newborns.

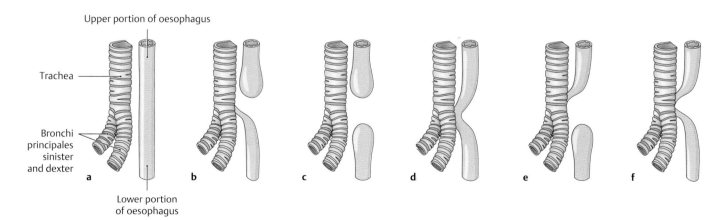

Upper portion of oesophagus

Trachea

Bronchi principales sinister and dexter

a | b | c | d | e | f

Lower portion of oesophagus

D Development of the trachea and lungs: Abnormalities

a Normal case; **b–f** Abnormalities.

Abnormalities in the development of the trachea, including irregular separation from the praeenteron, lead to various malformations that may or may not involve communications between the trachea and oesophagus. Often, the upper portion of the oesophagus ends blindly (**b** and **c**). This requires immediate corrective surgery because the infant is unable to ingest milk into its stomach. If the oesophagus remains in communication with the trachea it is called a tracheoesophageal fistula. There are several types (**b, d–f**), and they can lead to aspiration ("breathing in") of milk resulting in constant inflammation of the trachea and lungs (the infant coughs after drinking milk). Tracheoesophageal fistulas must be surgically corrected.

6.1 Overview of the Digestive System

Introduction

Function, localization, and terms: The digestive organs break down ingested solids and fluids, absorbs their nutrients, and excrete the remaining substances that the body can't use (*digestion*). The organs form a continuous tube from the head to the pelvis minor, and thus traverse the body cavities in the thorax, abdomen, and pelvis. The entire system is also referred to as the *"digestive apparatus,"* and the portions that are contained in the body cavities are called the *"gastrointestinal tract."* In addition to the usual terms of location and direction, the terms "oral and "aboral" are used when discussing the digestive system. They refer to direction along the longitudinal axis of the tract: *"oral"* = "toward the mouth" (os = mouth), *"aboral"* = "away from the mouth."

Structure of the digestive apparatus and processing of food: The digestive system is made up of a continuous series of tube-like organs that transports a bolus of food in an oral to aboral direction. In the first portion of this tube system (cavitas oris to gaster), food is broken up into small pieces. The next, and longest, portion (intestinum tenue to colon) is responsible for absorption of nutrients and water. The terminal portion (rectum and canalis analis) is responsible for temporary storage and controlled excretion (defecation) of feces. In the digestive system:

- Solid food is broken up, mixed with water and converted into a bolus (chyme). Enzymes in the gaster (stomach) and intestinum tenue digest the food into absorbable components. Most of the nutrients are absorbed through the epithelial cells lining the intestinum tenue and into vasa capillaria. They are then transported by the v. portae hepatis to the hepar (liver) where they are further metabolized. Fats, however, are absorbed directly into vasa lymphatica, and they bypass the portal venous system and hepatic metabolism.
- Water is mostly absorbed by the intestinal wall and into vasa capillaria or lymph ocapillaria. As part of the regulation of the osmotic pressure of blood, the renes (kidneys) also control water excretion and resorption (see urinary organs, p. 50).

Additional factors that aid digestion: The gaster and portions of the intestinal tract are in constant motion in order to churn the bolus and propel it along the digestive tract. The movement of the bolus in the aboral direction toward the rectum is called peristalsis. The pars enterica systematis nervosi, which is the gastrointestinal tract's intrinsic nervous system, controls peristalsis. Glandulae, which are either attached to the tube system or located directly in the system's walls, secrete hydrochloric acid, enzymes, and other substances that mix with the bolus and water to aid digestion. Parts of the lymphatic system (tonsillae and lymph follicles in the intestinal wall) are also located in the gastrointestinal tract and play an important role in the body's immune system.

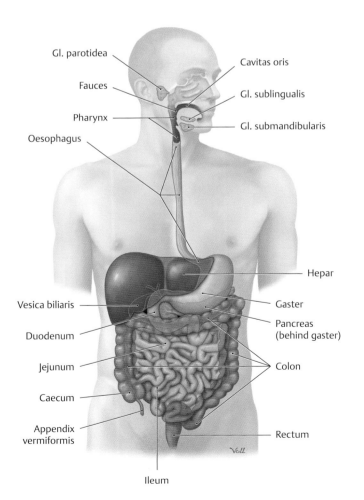

Gl. parotidea
Cavitas oris
Fauces
Gl. sublingualis
Pharynx
Gl. submandibularis
Oesophagus
Hepar
Vesica biliaris
Gaster
Duodenum
Pancreas (behind gaster)
Jejunum
Colon
Caecum
Appendix vermiformis
Rectum
Ileum

A Regional organization of the digestive organs

Digestive organs and associated structures are are located in the following regions:

In the **head** and **upper part of the neck:**
- Cavitas oris with fauces at the transition between mouth and pharynx

In the **middle** and **lower part of the neck**, and in the **thorax:**
- Partes oralis and laryngea pharyngis
- Oesophagus with partes cervicalis and thoracica

In the **abdomen:**
- Pars abdominalis of oesophagus
- Gaster
- Intestinum tenue with duodenum, jejunum, and ileum
- Intestinum crassum with caecum, appendix vermiformis, and colon (ascendens, transversum, descendens, and sigmoideum).

In the **pelvis:**
- Intestinum crassum with rectum and canalis analis.

Glandulae involved in digestion and their locations:
- Gll. salivariae (submandibularis, sublingualis, and parotidea as well as gll. salivariae minores in the cavitas oris)
- Pancreas in the abdomen
- Hepar with vesica biliaris in the abdomen

Numerous small gll. are present in the walls of the digestive organs from the oesophagus to the rectum.

B Cavitas oris, fauces, pharynx, oesophagus, and gaster

In the **cavitas oris** the dentes (teeth), lingua (tongue), and gll. salivariae chop food into small pieces and moisten it with saliva. The three paired gll. salivariae majores, sublingualis, submandibularis, and parotidea, secrete saliva into the cavitas oris through their ducts.

Fauces and pharynx: The cavitas oris connects to the pharynx through the fauces. The pharynx, which is also a part of the respiratory system, is divided into three sections. The lower portion of the pharynx , the pars laryngea pharyngis, connects to the oesophagus. In some textbooks, the entire pharynx is considered part of the neck.

Oesophagus and gaster: The pharynx is continuous with the oesophagus, which traverses the thorax and diaphragma and ends in the gaster. The function of the oesophagus is to transport fluids and food to the gaster, where the food bolus is further broken down by the gaster's churning. The bolus is mixed with acids to help denature proteins, and enzymatically digested. Over time the bolus is parceled out into the intestinum tenue through the ostium pyloricum.

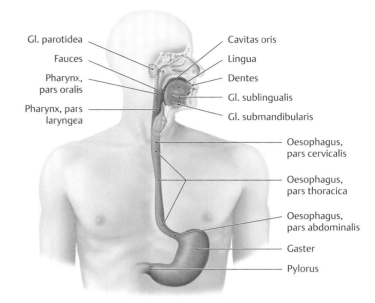

C Intestinum tenue, intestinum crassum, and abdominal glandulae (hepar, vesica biliaris, and pancreas)

Intestina tenue and crassum: The upper portion of the intestinum tenue, the *duodenum*, is a C-shaped structure located behind and beneath the hepar. The subsequent parts of the intestinum tenue, the *jejunum* and *ileum*, are difficult to distinguish from one another. Their multiple loops are located behind the anterior abdominal wall and are surrounded by the intestinum crassum. While nutrients are absorbed along the entire length of the *intestinum tenue*, the *intestinum crassum* absorbs primarily water and electrolytes. Stool is evacuated from the rectum.

The **hepar** is located in the right upper quadrant of the abdomen (**a**). The hepar metabolizes the nutrients and other compounds that are brought to it from the intestinum crassum through the venous portal system (see p. 13). The hepar produces bile, which it delivers to the duodenum via the ductus choledochus. Bile, which emulsifies fats to ease their absorption, is stored in the vesica biliaris located beneath the hepar. The **pancreas** (**b**) is located in the craniodorsal part of the abdomen close to the duodenum and consists of two glands:

- An exocrine gland, which discharges a watery, enzyme-rich secretion into the duodenum through the ductus pancreaticus. These enzymes aid in the digestion of substrates.
- An endocrine gland (the insulae pancreaticae), which produce several compounds including the hormones insulin and glucagon which regulate blood sugar levels.

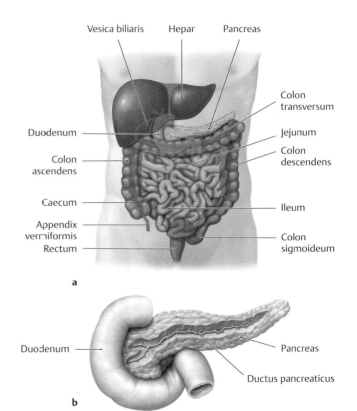

a

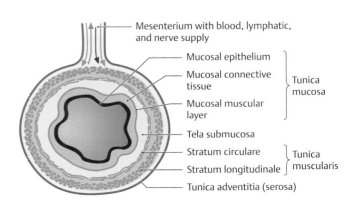

b

D Schematic cross-section illustrating the histology of the gastrointestinal tract

All segments of the gastrointestinal tract are divided into four layers:

- Tunica mucosa: an epithelial layer surrounding the lumen.
- Tela submucosa: a layer of connective tissue surrounding the tunica mucosa; contains vasa sanguinea and lymphatica and nn. autonomici.
- Tunica muscularis: the layer surrounding the tela submucosa; consists of an inner stratum circulare and an outer stratum longitudinale of smooth muscle.
- Tunica adventitia or tunica serosa (depending on its location in the gastrointestinal tract): the outermost layer that attaches the gastrointestinal tract to its surroundings.

39

6.2   Development and Differentiation of the Gastrointestinal Tract

Introduction

The digestive organs are located in the head, neck, and major body cavities. Their complex development influences the structure of the body cavities, and thus their development will be discussed in relation to that of the body cavities. When development is complete there is a continuous tube extending from the cavitas oris ("entrance") to the anus ("exit"). The hepar and vesica biliaris, and the pancreas, discharge their secretions into this tube in the abdomen.

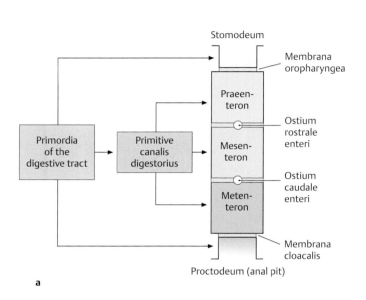

a

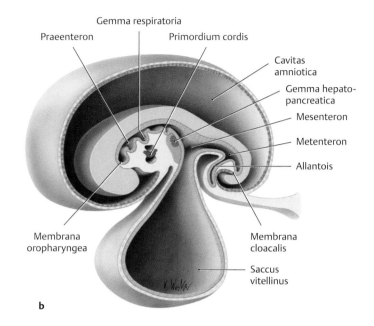

b

A Development of the gastrointestinal tract: Overview (after Sadler)

a Overview; **b** Midsagittal section of an embryo at the beginning of the 5th week.

The primitive canalis digestorius is derived from the dorsal part of the saccus vitellinus, which is incorporated into the body of the embryo. The formation of two intestinal portals divides the primitive canalis digestorius into three sections:

- The cranially located *praeenteron*
- The *mesenteron* (the longest portion of the gut)
- The caudally located *metenteron*

Cranially and caudally the primitive canalis digestorius ends blindly. The cranial end of the praeenteron is closed by the *membrana oropharyngea*

and the caudal end of the metenteron by the *membrana cloacalis*. The two membranes lie in contact with two ectodermal depressions. The depression at the cranial end is called the *stomodeum* and at the caudal end it is called the *proctodeum*. At first, the initially very short mesenteron is in direct communication with the saccus vitellinus along its entire length. During embryonic folding additional portions of the saccus vitellinusbecome incorporated into the developing mesenteron. The mesencephalon is a continuation of the praeenteron at the *ostium rostrale enteri*, and the metenteron is a continuation of the mesenteron at the *ostium caudale enteri*. The metenteron is connected to the allantois, which is an outpouching of the caudal wall of the saccus vitellinus in the early embryo (see **b**).

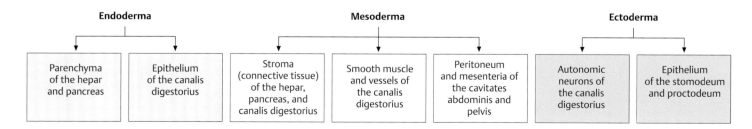

Endoderma		Mesoderma			Ectoderma	
Parenchyma of the hepar and pancreas	Epithelium of the canalis digestorius	Stroma (connective tissue) of the hepar, pancreas, and canalis digestorius	Smooth muscle and vessels of the canalis digestorius	Peritoneum and mesenteria of the cavitates abdominis and pelvis	Autonomic neurons of the canalis digestorius	Epithelium of the stomodeum and proctodeum

B Development of the gastrointestinal tract from the three germ layers

The organs of the gastrointestinal tract are derived from the three germ layers.

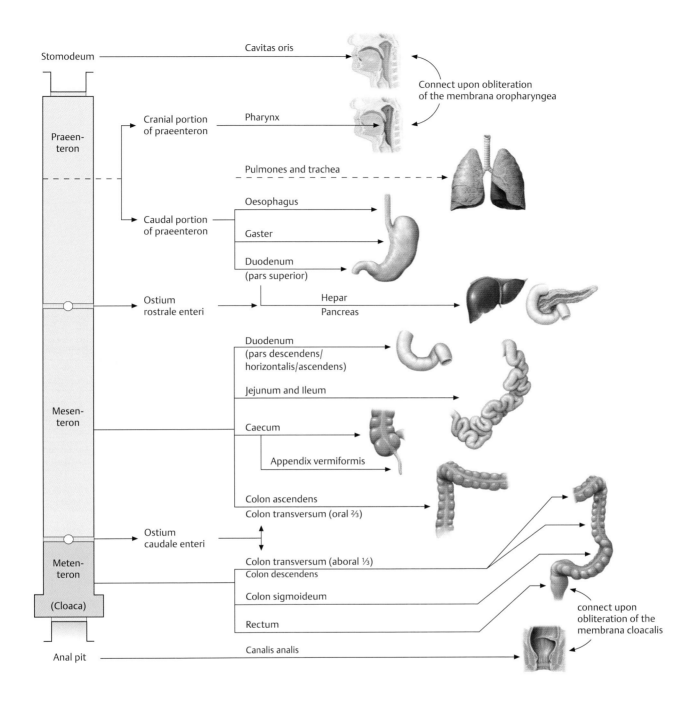

C Differentiation of the gastrointestinal tract

The primitive canalis digestorius gives rise to all parts of the digestive tract. The epithelium of the gut tube is derived from *endoderma* (see **B**). The membrana oropharyngea and membrana cloacalis, which are lined on the outside with ectoderma, break down later in development to allow the canalis digestorius open access to the external environment (see p. 47).

- The **praeenteron** divides into a *cranial portion*, which gives rise to the pharynx, and a *caudal portion*, which gives rise to the oesophagus, gaster and the pars superior of the duodenum (see p. 42). The diverticulum laryngotracheale, which will develop into the trachea and lungs, marks the boundary between the two portions of the praeenteron (see p. 35).
- The **mesenteron** gives rise to the remainder of the intestinum tenue as well as the colon ascendens and oral ⅔ of the colon transversum.
- The **metenteron** gives rise to the remainder of the colon and the rectum. The expanded caudal end of the metenteron is called the *cloaca*. Both the rectum and part of the urogenital system develop from the cloaca.

The **ostium rostrale enteri** marks the border between the praeenteron and mesenteron. It is located along the duodenum and it gives rise to the hepar, vesica biliaris and pancreas. The junction between the mesenteron and metenteron is called the **ostium caudale enteri** and it lies between the oral ⅔ and aboral ⅓ of the colon transversum. This region, also referred to as the Cannon-Boehm-point, plays a significant role in the arrangement of the colon's autonomic innervation. The **stomodeum** develops into the cavitas oris and the **proctodeum** gives rise to the canalis analis. The epithelial lining of both structures is derived from ectoderm and is continuous with the outer lining of the membranae oropharyngealis and cloacalis. At these two sites, the endodermal and ectodermal epithelium are adjacent to each other. The obliteration of the membranae oropharyngealis and cloacalis results in the primitive canalis digestorius becoming open to the embryo's external environment.

6.3 Mesenteria and Primordia of the Digestive Organs in the Caudal Praeenteron Region; Stomach Rotation

Introduction

Two processes are crucial for the embryological development of the digestive organs:

- The rotation of the gaster in the *caudal foregut* (see p. 44)
- The rotation of the intestinal loop (the loop-shaped fetal canalis digestorius, see p. 46) in the *midgut and hindgut*.

A Mesenteries of the canalis digestorius in the embryo (overview)

The oesophagus, gaster, and pars superior of the duodenum originate from the caudal portion of the praeenteron. Like all organs of the digestive system in the abdomen and pelvis, they have a mesenterium dorsale (a passageway extending from the posterior wall of the cavitas peritonealis to the posterior wall of the organ). In the area surrounding the gaster and the pars superior of duodenum, there is also a mesenterium ventrale. It arises from the anterior wall of the cavitas peritonealis and attaches to the anterior wall of the organs. The v. umbilicalis carries oxygenated blood from the placenta to the liver and v. cava inferior of the embryo through this mesenterium ventrale. Due to this additional mesenterium, the cavitas peritonealis at the level of the gaster and duodenum is divided into a left and a right half (see p. 44).

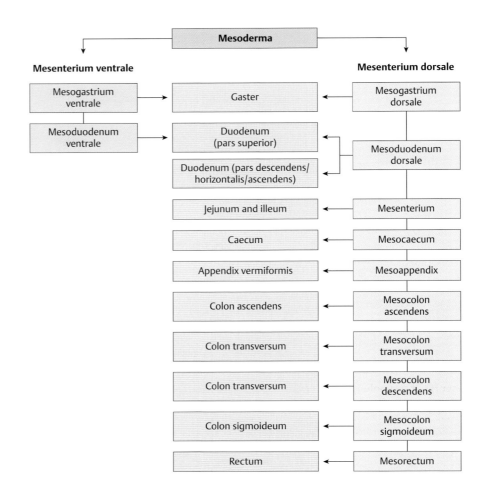

B Mesenteries of the caudal praeenteron in the embryo

The following organs arise from the duodenal epithelium and grow into the mesentera of the duodenum and gaster (see **A**):

- The ductus hepaticus and biliaris grow into the area between meso*duodenum* ventrale and meso*gastrium* ventrale.
- The gemma pancreatica ventralis and gemma pancreatica dorsalis grow into the mesoduodenum *ventrale* and mesoduodenum *dorsale*, respectively.

In the 5th week, the splen, a lymphatic organ (not a digestive organ), migrates from mesenchyma in the spatium retroperitoneale located dorsal to the cavitas peritonealis, to the mesogastrium dorsale. Thus, both the splen and gemma pancreatica dorsalis are located in the mesenterium dorsale. During stomach rotation (see **D**), the mesenteria shift along with the organs they contain (see p. 44). The terminology for the mesenteria in the mature organism is indicated in **E**.

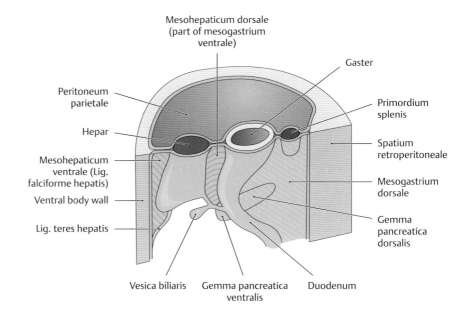

C Fusion of the gemmae pancreaticae dorsalis and ventralis
(after Sadler)

Schematic view of the caudal praeenteron from the left side. The two gemmae pancreaticae form as outgrowths from the duodenal epithelium (**a**) into the mesenteria ventrale and dorsale (see **B**). The gemma pancreatica ventralis develops in close association with the bile ducts. It migrates with the developing bile ducts around the right side of the duodenum toward the gemma pancreatica dorsalis (**b**) (for the effect of stomach rotation on the gemma pancreatica ventralis see p. 44). Both gemmae pancreaticae fuse and their ducts anastomose, forming the ductus pancreaticus, and, when present, a ductus pancreaticus accessorius.

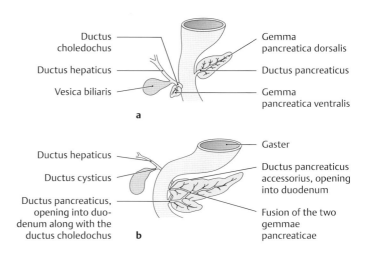
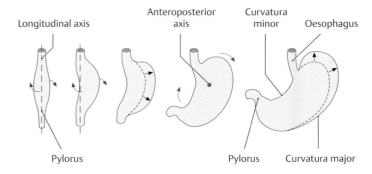

D Stomach rotation
Ventral view. At the beginning of the 5th week, the gaster rotates clockwise 90 degrees around its longitudinal axis (see arrows). At the same time, it grows wider with the left wall (original dorsal wall) growing faster than the right wall (original ventral wall). This differential growth forms the curvaturae major and minus. The entire gaster also rotates clockwise around an anteroposterior axis and now sits obliquely in the abdomen. The curvatura major now points to the left and downward, and the curvatura minor points to the right and upward. The mesenteria of the stomach are also affected by the asymmetrical growth and rotation of the stomach: the mesogastrium ventrale shifts to the right and upward, and the mesogastrium dorsale shifts to the left and downward.

E Mesentery terminology in the caudal praeenteron: Comparison of embryonic and mature organisms
As a result of the rapid growth of the hepar and splen in the embryo, both mesenteria of the stomach, the mesogastria dorsale and ventrale, are further subdivided into a mesohepaticum ventrale and dorsale and a mesosplenicum ventrale and dorsale. In the mature organism, these mesenteria are referred to as omenta and ligaments.

Term in the embryonic organism	Term in the mature organism
Mesogastrium ventrale with subsections	
• Mesohepaticum dorsale ("in the back of the hepar")	• Omentum minus; connection from hepar to curvatura minor of the gaster and pars superior of duodenum; divided into – lig. hepatogastricum (hepar to gaster) with flaccid and hard portions – lig. hepatoduodenale (hepar to duodenum)
• Mesohepaticum ventrale ("at the front of the hepar")	• Connection between liver and anterior trunk wall; divided into – lig. falciforme – lig. teres hepatis (contains the obliterated v. umbilicalis)
Mesogastrium dorsale with subsections • *At the level of the primordium splenis* – mesosplenicum ventrale ("at the front of the splen") – dorsal mesosplenicum ("in the back of the splen")	• Part of omentum majus as well as other ligaments: – lig. gastrosplenicum (part of omentum majus, gaster to splen) – lig. phrenicosplenicum (diaphragma to splen) – lig. splenorenale (splen to ren and posterior wall of cavitas peritonealis)
• *Above the primordium splenis* (no anatomical terms for the embryonic organism)	– lig. gastrophrenicum (part of omentum majus, gaster to diaphragma)
• *Below the primordium splenis* (no anatomical terms for the embryonic organism)	– lig. gastrocolicum (part of omentum majus, gaster to colon transversum) – lig. phrenicocolicum (posterior wall of cavitas peritonealis to flexura coli sinister)

Note: In the mature organism, all structures arising from the mesogastrium dorsale are often referred to as omentum majus.

6.4 Stomach Rotation and Organ Location in the Caudal Praeenteron Region; Formation of the Bursa Omentalis

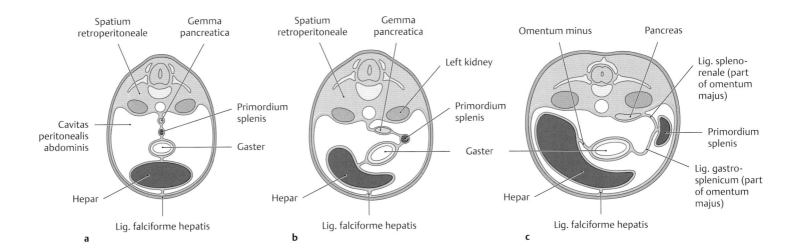

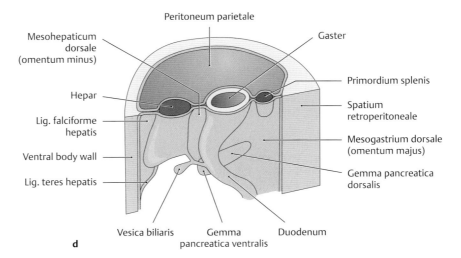

A Effects of gaster rotation on its mesenteria and on the position of organs in the caudal praeenteron region

a–c Horizontal section of the embryonic abdomen in successive stages of development; viewed from above; **d** Spatial representation of **a**, viewed from the left and above.

Duodenum: Gaster rotation moves the duodenum to the right and slightly up. By the time gaster rotation ends, the duodenum is bent into a C-shape with the open side facing left. As the duodenum rotates to the right its mesoduodenum ventrale rotates with it. This affects the position of the gemma pancreatica ventralis that is developing in the mesoduodenum. In addition to its migration as illustrated on page 43, this rotation moves the gemma pancreatica ventralis toward the gemma pancreatica dorsalis.

Pancreas: The gemmae pancreaticae ventralis and dorsalia fuse as the duodenum rotates clockwise. Initially they lie in the abdomen in an oblique position, but rotation further shifts the fused gemmae towards the posterior wall of the cavitas peritonealis. The peritoneum viscerale of the pancreas and duodenum then fuse with the peritoneum parietale on the posterior wall of the cavitas peritonealis. Thus, the pancreas and duodenum are secondarily retroperitoneal, and the anterior side of both organs is covered by peritoneum parietale.

Hepar: Since the developing hepar lies in the ventral mesogastrium, it is shifted to the right and upward along with the mesogastrium. Its peritoneal membrane is attached to the peritoneum covering the diaphragma. As the hepar grows it contacts the diaphragma and the peritoneum of both the hepar and diaphragma disintegrates at the area of contact. The portion of the hepar not covered by peritoneum is referred to as the area nuda. The portion on the diaphragma is called the hepatic surface of the diaphragma. The rest of the hepar remains intraperitoneal. However, due to its rapid growth, it moves dorsally and closer to the right ren, which keeps the right ren slightly more inferior than the left.

Bile ducts: The portion of the bile duct adjacent to the hepar will form the ductus hepatici. The portion of the bile duct that opens into the duodenum runs through the lateral edge of the omentum minus (the lig. hepatoduodenale). The extrahepatic ductus biliares are thus largely intraperitoneal, but portions become secondarily retroperitoneal after coursing through the pancreas to join with the ductus pancreatici close to the duodenum.

Splen: Gaster rotation moves the primordium splenis, which lies in the mesogastrium dorsale, to the left. It remains intraperitoneal within the mesogastrium.

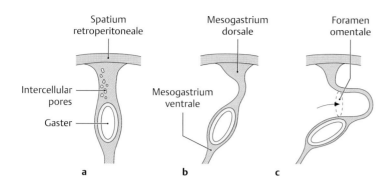
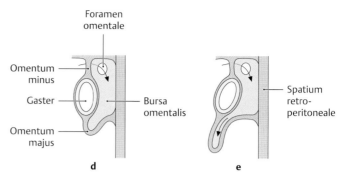

B Development of the bursa omentalis (after Sadler)

Gaster and mesogastria; **a–c** Horizontal sections of the abdomen, superior view; **d** and **e** Sagittal sections, viewed from the left. The upper arrows in **c–e** point to the foramen omentale, which is the only physiological opening into the bursa omentalis. The lower arrow in **e** shows the deepening pouch formed by the omentum majus.

As the gaster and mesogastria rotate, the originally right wall of the gaster is shifted posteriorly, and the left wall of the gaster anteriorly. The mesogastria dorsale and ventrale are still holding gaster in place, and as a result of the rotation, the original right side of the cavitas peritonealis becomes enclosed posterior to the stomach. This space is called the bursa omentalis, and its borders are demarcated

- posteriorly by the posterior wall of the cavitas peritonealis (anterior to the already retroperitonealized pancreas, see **Ac**),
- anteriorly by the posterior wall of the gaster and both of the mesogastria,
- to the right by the hepar,
- to the left by the splen,
- superiorly by the diaphragma (diaphragma not visible here),
- inferiorly by an outpouching of the mesogastrium dorsale (between layers of the omentum majus).

C Development of the caudal region of the praeenteron: Summary and peritonealization

The following processes are crucial for the formation of mature structures. They overlap in time, but are presented here in chronological order to aid clarification.

Organ primordia; gaster rotation and mesenteric rotation	Tilting of the gaster; shifting of the pancreas, hepar and splen	Differentiation of the mesenteria; peritoneal membranes of the organs
The gaster and upper duodenum have both dorsal and ventral mesenteria. Thus, at the level of these organs, the cavitas peritonealis is divided into left and right halves.	The gemmae pancreaticae ventralis and dorsalis move toward each other. This is partially due to the duodenum shifting right which causes the gemma pancreatica ventralis to move slightly dorsally. The two gemmae pancreaticae fuse.	The mesogastrium dorsale (along the curvatura major) becomes the omentum majus. The rapid growth of the hepar divides the mesogastrium ventrale into a mesohepaticum ventrale and dorsale.
Organ primordia develop in both mesenteries: • ventral: hepar, bile ducts and ventral pancreas; • dorsal: splen and dorsal pancreas.	Viewed from the front, the developing gaster tilts clockwise and grows asymmetrically: the curvaturae major (left) and minor (right) form with the mesogastria dorsale and ventrale still attached.	The mesohepaticum dorsale becomes the omentum minus (connects the hepar to the gaster and duodenum). The mesohepaticum ventrale becomes the ligg. falciforme and teres of the hepar (connects the hepar to the anterior abdominal wall)
Viewed from above, the gaster rotates 90 degrees clockwise. The duodenum follows the gaster in a clockwise rotation while acquiring its C-shaped loop.	The rotation and tilting of the gaster shifts the developing hepar to the right and upward where it becomes attached to the diaphragm. The primordium splenis shifts left and remains intraperitoneal.	The primordium splenis divides the upper portion of the mesogastrium dorsale into a mesosplenicum ventrale (becomes the lig. gastrosplenicum) and a mesosplenicum dorsale (becomes the lig. phrenicosplenicum).
The two mesenteries follow this rotation with the mesenterium ventrale being pulled right and the rapidly growing mesenterium dorsale pulled left.	The developing duodenum and the fused gemmae pancreaticae associated with it move dorsally along with their mesenterium dorsale and become secondarily retroperitoneal.	The bursa omentalis, a separated portion of the cavitas peritonealis, forms posterior to the gaster and omenta. The hepar, vesica biliaris, splen and gaster remain intraperitoneal. The pancreas and most of the duodenum become secondarily retroperitoneal.

6.5 Rotation of the Intestinal Loop and Development of Mesenteron and Metenteron Derivatives

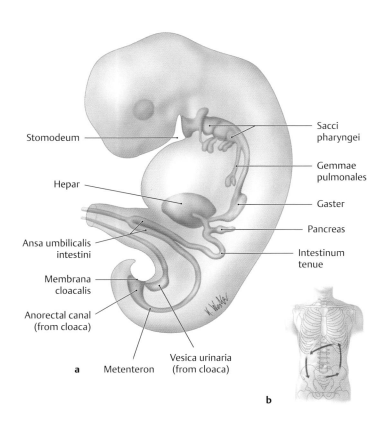

a   Metenteron

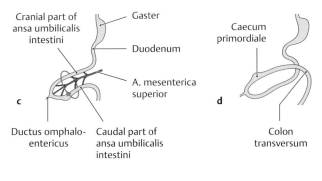

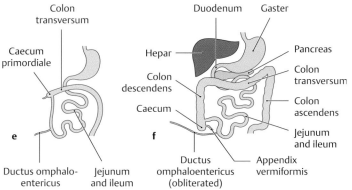

A Rotation and differentiation of the ansa umbilicalis intestini
(after Sadler)

a Overview of the ansa umbilicalis intestini: embryo viewed from left side, 5th week of embryonic development; **b** Direction of rotation of the ansa umbilicalis intestini: anterior view of abdomen; **c–e** Rotation of the ansa umbilicalis intestini, viewed from left side (in **c**, the gaster has not yet rotated); **f** Gastrointestinal tract after the rotations of the gaster and ansa umbilicalis intestini are complete, anterior view.

In the mesenteron and metenteron (at the level of intestinum tenue and crassum) a second rotation occurs between the 6th and 11th week of embryonic development, the "rotation of the ansa umbilicalis intestini." The entire ansa umbilicalis intestini rotates along an axis formed by the a. mesenterica superior and the ductus omphaloentericus (vitellointestinalis) (**c**). Viewed from the front, the rotation is counterclockwise (**d** and **e**). The ansa rotates 270 degrees as the canalis digestorius elongates. The crus proximale of the intestinal loop grows rapidly into the coiled jejunum and ileum (**e** and **f**). The caudal portion grows into the terminal portion of the ileum, the caecum, and appendix vermiformis (see **B**), and the intestinum crassum, which encloses the coils of the ansa umbilicalis intestini (**f**). Thus, rotation of the intestinal loop can be divided into three phases:

- the cranial and caudal parts of the ansa umbilicalis intestini rotation 90 degrees counterclockwise (**c**),
- the rotated loops shift to the right upper quadrant and rotate an additional 180 degrees (**d** and **e**);
- the region of the ileocecal junction and colon ascendens descends into right lower quadrant (**f**).

Note: The first phase in the rotation of the ansa umbilicalis intestini (the first 90 degrees) occurs outside the cavitas abdominis in the extraembryonic cavity in the funiculus umbilicalis at the start of the 6th week (**c**). This rotation outside of the body cavity is referred to as physiological umbilical herniation. In the 10th week, the intestinal coils return back to the cavitas abdominis.

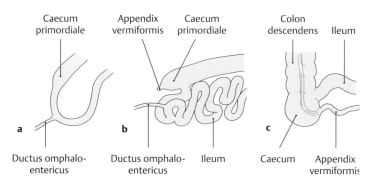

B Development of the caecum and appendix vermiformis
(after Sadler)

In the 6th week of development the caecum starts to form in the crus distale of the ansa umbilicalis intestini at the junction of the intestinum tenue and intestinum crassum (**a**). Between the 7th and 8th weeks, as the caecum is enlarging, the worm-like appendix vermiformis begins to form (**b**). The caecum develops into a blind sac at the beginning of the colon ascendens (**c**). The ileum opens perpendicularly into the junction of the caecum and colon ascendens. The development of the caecum occurs outside of the cavitas abdominis, and it is the last part of the intestinal tube to return to the cavitas abdominis.

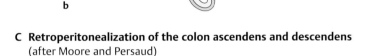

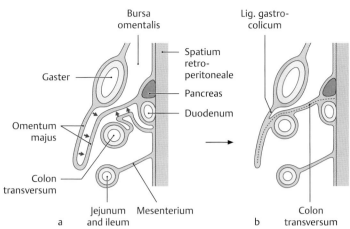

C Retroperitonealization of the colon ascendens and descendens
(after Moore and Persaud)

Horizontal sections of the abdomen, superior view.

Following rotation of the ansa umbilicalis intestini, the cola ascendens and descendens lie on the right and left sides of the cavitas abdominis (**a**). They are in direct contact with the posterior wall of the cavitas peritonealis, and they fuse to the posterior wall along with their mesenteria (**b**). Thus, the cola ascendens and descendens become secondarily retroperitoneal. However, the colon transversum, positioned anterior to portions of the intestinum tenue, remains intraperitoneal and retains its mesenterium (the mesocolon transversum). The jejunum and ileum also remain intraperitoneal and retain their mesenteric connection to the posterior wall of the cavitas peritonealis.

D Fusion of the omentum majus (after Moore and Persaud)

Sagittal sections of the abdomen, viewed from the left. The omentum majus (derived from the mesogastrium dorsale, see p. 43) extends down from the curvatura major of the gaster. As it grows downward, its two layers partially fuse with one another and with the colon transversum and the mesocolon transversum (**a**). This forms a pouch-like space between the bottom part of the gaster and the upper part of the colon transversum (**b**), which marks the inferior boundary of the bursa omentalis (see p. 45). The fused part of the omentum majus, which connects the gaster with the colon transversum, is called the lig. gastrocolicum.

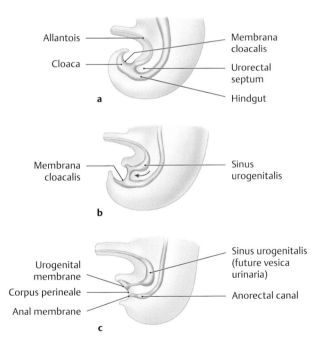

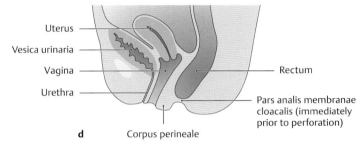

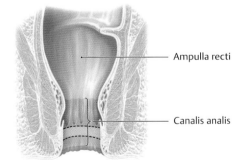

E Development of the cloaca (after Sadler and Moore/Persaud)

a–d Pelvic viscera of the fetus, viewed from the left side; **e** Anterior view of the mature anorectal canal.

Together with the urinary tract, the terminal portion of the metenteron enters into the cloaca. A transverse ridge of mesenchyma called the septum urorectale grows toward the membrana cloacalis (which is closing off the cloaca) (**a** and **b**). In about the 7th week of development the septum urorectale divides the cloaca into an anterior sinus urogenitalis, which gives rise to parts of the urogenital system, and posterior anorectal canal (**c**). Both are still closed by the membrana cloacalis, which is now divided into an anterior urogenital membrane and a posterior analis. The corpus perineale forms at the junction of membranae urogenitalis and anal membranes. Mesenchymal swellings form at the margins of the pars analis membranae cloacalis and, as a result, the pars analis membranae cloacalis lies in a depression called the fovea analis (**d**). By the end of the 9th week, the pars analis membranae cloacalis ruptures and the rectum is in open communication with the body's exterior (**e**). Thus, the rectum consists of two parts: the upper portion that develops from the metenteron, and the lower portion that develops from the cloaca.

6.6 Summary of the Development of the Mesenteron and Metenteron; Developmental Anomalies

A Development of the mesenteron and metenteron: Summary and peritonealization

The development of the midgut and metenteron can be divided into two processes: "rotation of the ansa umbilicalis intestini" and "peritoneal relationships and formation of the cloaca."

Rotation of the ansa umbilicalis intestini
The ansa umbilicalis intestini rotates around a virtual axis formed by the a. mesenterica superior and the ductus vitellointestinalis. As it rotates, it continues to grow and differentiate.
Viewed from the front, the ansa umbilicalis intestini undergoes a 270 degree counterclockwise rotation. The first 90 degrees take place outside of the body cavity during physiological umbilical herniation. The intestinal coils retract back into the abdomen by the 11th week.
The crus proximale of the ansa umbilicalis intestini elongates rapidly forming the numerous coils of the jejunum and ileum. They remain attached to the posterior wall of the cavitas peritonealis by their mesenterium.
As the ansa rotates, its crus distale forms a frame around the coils of the jejunum and ileum, thereby dividing the colon into individual sections, which assume their definitive position in the abdomen.
A lateral protrusion forms in the crus distale of the ansa umbilicalis intestini close to the axis of the a. mesenterica superior. This protrusion differentiates into the caecum, and the appendix vermiformis develops from it.
When rotation is complete, the intestina tenue and crassum have reached their definitive position, with the intestinum crassum forming a frame around the intestinum tenue. The subsequent retroperitonealization determines the final peritoneal relationships of the canalis digestorius.

Peritoneal relationships and formation of the cloaca
Rotation of the loop moves the caecum to the lower right quadrant, and the cola ascendens and descendens move dorsally and become secondarily retroperitoneal. The colon transversum and colon sigmoideum remain intraperitoneal with a mesocolon.
The colon transversum and mesocolon transversum fuse and become attached to the omentum majus, which originally was the mesogastrium dorsale (along the curvatura major of the gaster). Thus, the bursa omentalis, located behind the gaster, is almost completely closed off.
The septum urorectale divides the enlarged end of the metenteron, the cloaca, into an anterior sinus urogenitalis and a posterior anorectal canal. The septum grows caudally until it contacts the cloacal membrane.
The division of the cloaca leads to the division of the membrana cloacalis into an anterior urogenital membrane and a posterior pars analis membranae cloacalis. Mesenchymal tissue surrounding the pars analis membranae cloacalis proliferates and forms a depression called the fovea analis.
The fovea analis deepens toward the metenteron and gives rise to the canalis analis. As the pars analis membranae cloacalis ruptures in the 9th week, the rectum, which is derived from the cloaca, becomes open to the outside of the body.
The rectum lies deep within the pelvis. It moves posteriorly and becomes retroperitonealized along most of its length. The canalis analis derived from the proctodeum does not have any peritoneal relationships.

B Summary of the rotational motion of the canalis digestorius and peritoneal relationships

Organ rotation	Leads to the following organ positions	Which results in the following peritoneal relationships
Rotation of the gaster along with its mesogastria ventrale and dorsale	• Hepar and vesica biliaris in the right upper quadrant • Splen in the left upper quadrant • Most of the duodenum and the entire pancreas become attached to the posterior wall of the cavitas peritonealis	• Intraperitoneal with omentum minus, lig. falciforme and lig. teres hepaticum • Intraperitoneal • Secondarily retroperitoneal
Rotation of the ansa umbilicalis intestini along with its mesenteria	• Crus proximale of the ansa forms two segments of the intestinum tenue, the jejunum and ileum, along with their mesenteria • Crus distale forms the intestinum crassum and rectum along with their mesocolon and mesorectum: the inestinum crassum and rectum form a frame around the intestinum tenue • Colon ascendens, colon descendens, and rectum become attached to the posterior wall of the cavitas peritonealis	• Mesenterium remains and the jejunum and ileum are intraperitoneal • Colon transversum and colon sigmoideum retain their mesocola and remain intraperitoneal • Colon ascendens, colon descendens, and rectum lose their mesenteria and are secondarily retroperitoneal

C Developmental anomalies of the gastrointestinal tract

The anomalies listed here, some of which are quite rare except for Meckel's diverticulum, vary considerably in their pathological significance. A complete occlusion or extreme narrowing of the lumen in the gastrointestinal tract is usually fatal without treatment. Mild degrees of narrowing can remain asymptomatic. The twisting of intestinal segments can cause obstructions that often lead to life-threatening conditions.

Duodenal atresia	Solid duodenum without lumen
Duodenal stenosis	Narrowing of the duodenal lumen (e.g., by an annular pancreas)
Biliary atresia	Congenital or acquired obstruction of some or all extrahepatic bile ducts
Annular pancreas	Duodenal stenosis (see above) caused by a circle of pancreatic tissue
Omphalocele	Extracorporeal protrusion of the intestinum tenue at the umbilicus due to failure of the rotated intestinal loop to retract
Malrotation	Abnormal or failed rotation of the intestinal loop (see **E**)
Volvulus	Twisting of intestinal segments caused by failure of fixation of the mesenterium; risk of getting ileus
Intestinal stenosis	Narrowing of the intestinal lumen
Intestinal atresia	Complete occlusion of the intestinal lumen, if not treated this is incompatible with life
Meckel's diverticulum	Failure of regression of the ductus vitellointestinus with potential ileal diverticulitis (see **D**)

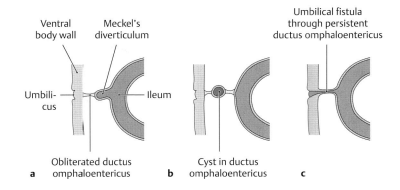

a Obliterated ductus omphaloentericus b Cyst in ductus omphaloentericus c

D Remnants of the ductus vitellointestinalis (after Sadler)

The ductus vitellointestinalis, initially patent in the embryo, usually is completely obliterated and lost as a connection between the ileum and trunk wall. Occasionally, however, the obliteration is incomplete or leaves a cord of connective tissue that attaches the ileum to the anterior trunk wall. This can have various manifestations:

a The wall of the ileum is partially outpouched and a fibrous cord remains. A **Meckel's diverticulum** forms (usually located 40–60 cm cranial to the valva ileocaecalis), which is subject to inflammatory changes and often contains ectopic gastric or pancreatic tissue.
b A cyst remains within the fibrous cord. This cyst may cause complaints and must be differentiated from a tumor.
c The ductus vitellointestinalis remains patent over its entire length, resulting in an **umbilical (or vitelline) fistula**. In extreme cases, portions of the intestinum tenue may herniate at the umbilicus and become inflamed. If a remnant of the ductus vitellointestinalis persists as a fibrous cord between ileum and umbilicus, mobile small intestinal loops may wrap around it and become strangulated (intestinal paralysis, or ileus, which is often fatal if untreated).

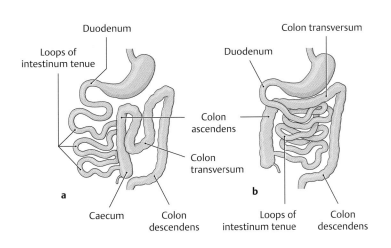

E Developmental anomalies of the gastrointestinal tract: Malrotation (after Sadler)

Ventral view. As long as the intestinal segments do not become twisted and do not lose gastrointestinal motility (see **C**, volvulus), the following types of malrotations may remain asymptomatic.

a Rotation of only 90 degrees instead of 270. The intestinum crassum remains to the left of the intestinum tenue and doesn't form a frame around the intestinum tenue.
b Clockwise rotation (viewed from the front). The intestinal loop rotates clockwise instead of counterclockwise. The initially caudal part of the loop comes to lie behind the cranial part and the colon transversum crosses posterior to the intestinum tenue.

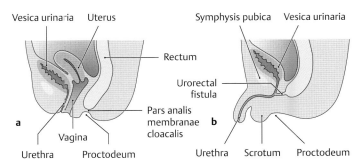

F Malformation of the canalis analis (after Sadler)

Pelvic viscera, viewed from the left side. In 1 out of 5000 births, the pars analis membranae cloacalis fails to rupture. As a result, the rectum is not connected to the outside environment. The two most frequent developmental anomalies are presented below:

a Imperforate anus: The pars analis membranae cloacalis fails to break down.
b Anorectal atresia (with fistula formation): Malformations of the septum urorectale, with the canalis analis missing, may create a nonphysiological fistula between the rectum and the perineum or the urogenital system, and in females between the rectum and the vagina.

Both of these conditions require surgical correction.

49

7.1 Overview of the Urinary System

Introduction

The urinary organs extend from the abdomen through the pelvis. Since they are closely related to the genital organs, both groups of organs are often referred to collectively as *urogenital organs*. For didactic reasons, both systems will be discussed separately in the following chapters.

The urinary organs help regulate the level of water and minerals in the body, and thus help regulate osmotic pressure. They excrete end products of body metabolism and harmful substances into a watery fluid, the *urine* (the excreted metabolites are dissolved in the water component of urine). By regulating the amount of water in the body, the renes also influence blood pressure. Through excreting or retaining sodium, potassium, calcium and chloride ions, they are involved in regulating the level of these important electrolytes in blood. In addition, the blood's acid-base balance is influenced by the excretion or retention of hydrogen ions. Many pharmaceutical substances are excreted through the renes. The renes also influence blood pressure by producing the enzyme renin, and the formation of red blood cells by producing the hormone erythropoietin. Lastly, they also play an important role in vitamin D metabolism.

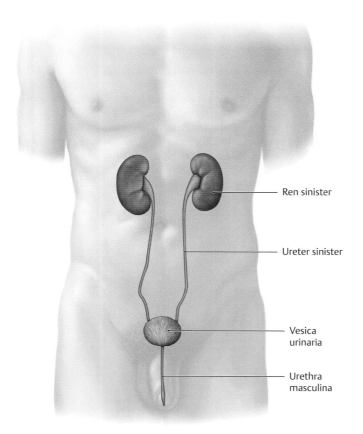

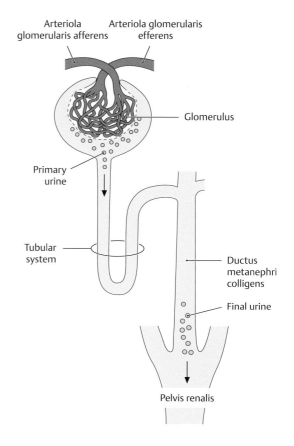

A Overview of the urinary organs

Male urinary organs, anterior view. The urinary system consists of the following organs:

* the paired renes, which continuously produce urine;
* the paired ureteres, which transport urine from the renes to the vesica urinaria;
* the unpaired vesica urinaria, which temporarily stores and discharges urine in a controlled manner; and
* the unpaired urethra. In women it is called the urethra feminina and it is solely a urinary organ, whereas in men it is called the urethra masculina and it is also a genital organ. In the urinary system, the urethra is involved in discharging urine from the vesica urinaria to the outside of the body. In men it is also serves as a passageway for sperm.

B Basics of urine production

The nephron, illustrated above, is the smallest functional unit of the renes (see p. 54).

In the glomeruli, richly branched capillary loops, which are supplied by branches of the aa. renales, drain an ultrafiltrate of blood called primary urine into a system of tubules. Adults produce approximately 170 liters of *primary urine* in 24 hours. However, in the tubular system, the primary urine is concentrated to 1% of its volume (by reabsorption of electrolytes and water back into the blood), and based on its composition, further modified with electrolytes and hydrogen ions. The volume of *final urine* formed in 24 hours is 1–2 liters. The final urine drains through ductus metanephrici colligentes into the pelvis renalis and then it is carried by the ureteres to the vesica urinaria.

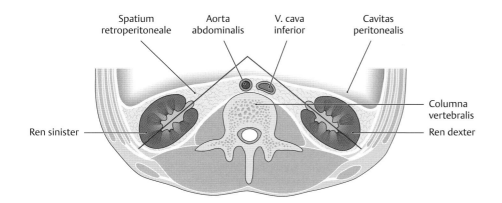

Spatium retroperitoneale | Aorta abdominalis | V. cava inferior | Cavitas peritonealis

Ren sinister

Columna vertebralis

Ren dexter

C Location of the renes and ureteres

Horizontal section of the body at the level of the first vertebra lumbalis, viewed from above. Both renes are embedded in a fatty, connective tissue capsule (capsula adiposa). They are located in the spatium retroperitoneale with one on either side of the columna vertebralis. The spatium retroperitoneale also contains the ureteres (not visible in this section), which extend downward to the pelvis minor to reach the vesica urinaria. The hilum of each ren faces medially and anteriorly (red axes).

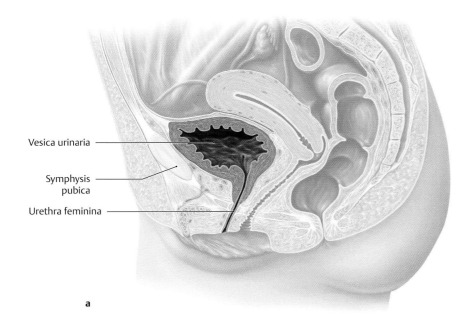

Vesica urinaria

Symphysis pubica

Urethra feminina

a

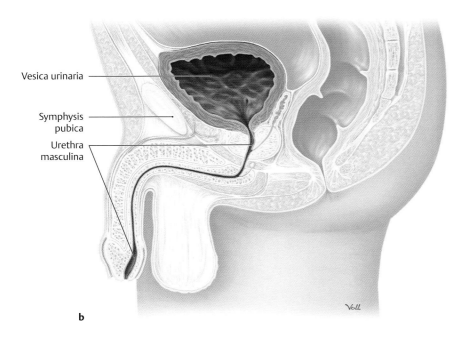

Vesica urinaria

Symphysis pubica

Urethra masculina

b

D Location of the vesica urinaria and urethra

Midsagittal section of a female (**a**) and male (**b**) pelvis, each viewed from the left side.

In both sexes, the vesica urinaria is located in the pelvis minor behind the symphysis pubica. In females it is situated in front of both the vagina and the uterus, and in males it is in front of the rectum. Depending on its degree of distension, the vesica urinaria is flattened or spherical. The vesica urinaria is straight and short, while the urethra masculina traverses the penis and bends multiple times along its course.

7.2 Development of the Renes, Pelvis Renalis, and Ureteres

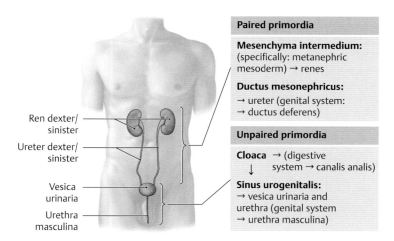

Paired primordia
Mesenchyma intermedium: (specifically: metanephric mesoderm) → renes
Ductus mesonephricus: → ureter (genital system: → ductus deferens)
Unpaired primordia
Cloaca → (digestive ↓ system → canalis analis)
Sinus urogenitalis: → vesica urinaria and urethra (genital system → urethra masculina)

Ren dexter/ sinister
Ureter dexter/ sinister
Vesica urinaria
Urethra masculina

A Overview of the embryonic development of the urinary organs

The embryonic development of the urinary organs is complex and overlaps with the development of the genital and digestive organs:

- overlap with the genital system: the development of some parts of the male reproductive system (see p. 62) is closely related to the development of the ductus mesonephrici, ureteres, and sinus urogenitalis.
- overlap with the digestive system: the canalis analis is derived from the cloaca.

The development of the urinary system can be divided into the development of the paired renes and ureteres, and development of the unpaired vesica urinaria and urethra. The renes and ureteres arise from the mesenchyma intermedium. The vesica urinaria and urethra develop from the sinus urogenitalis, which formed from the ventral portion of the cloaca in the region of the future pelvic floor (see p. 47). The sinus urogenitalis is derived from endoderma. Thus, the urinary organs are derived from two germ layers. Over the course of development the two sets of urinary organs will connect with each other.

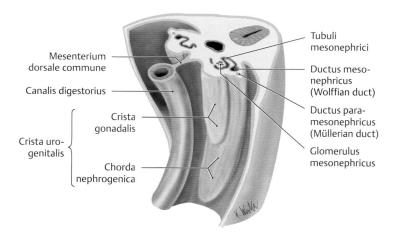

Mesenterium dorsale commune
Canalis digestorius
Crista gonadalis
Crista uro-genitalis
Chorda nephrogenica
Tubuli mesonephrici
Ductus meso-nephricus (Wolffian duct)
Ductus para-mesonephricus (Müllerian duct)
Glomerulus mesonephricus

B The urogenital ridge (crista mesonephrica)

Posterior body wall of the embryo, viewed from the front and above. The renal and internal genital primordia border each other. They bulge ventrally into the body cavity in the form of two ridges: the chorda nephrogenica and the crista gonadalis or crista mesonephrica. The developing gonadae lie anteromedially to the developing ren systems. The ductus paramesonephrici (Müllerian ducts), which in females develop into the tubae uterinae and uterus, lie anterolaterally to the renal primordia.

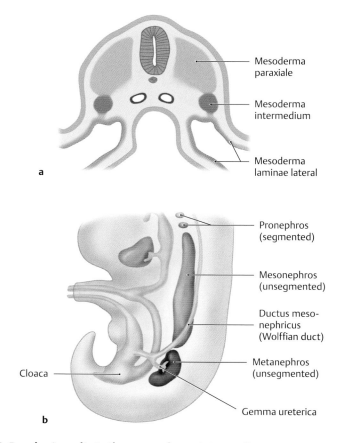

Mesoderma paraxiale
Mesoderma intermedium
Mesoderma laminae lateral
a

Pronephros (segmented)
Mesonephros (unsegmented)
Ductus meso-nephricus (Wolffian duct)
Metanephros (unsegmented)
Cloaca
Gemma ureterica
b

C Renal primordia in the mesenchyma intermedium

a Cross-section of an embryo, approx. 21 days, cranial view; **b** Embryo viewed from the left (unlike a, this figure does not depict a stage in the embryonic development but rather shows the location of the developing renal primordia and what it would look like if they all existed in the embryo at the same time).

The renes develop as pairs in a specialized region of the mesoderma, the mesenchyma intermedium, which becomes further differentiated in the posterior body cavity. In cervical and upper thoracic regions it becomes segmented and forms nephrotomi. It remains unsegmented in lower thoracic and abdominal regions and forms chordae nephrogenicae. Renal development within the mesenchyma proceeds in three successive steps. From cranial to caudal the three systems formed are as follows:

- Pronephros in the cervical and upper thoracic regions
- Mesonephros in the lower thoracic and abdominal regions
- Metanephros in the abdominal and pelvic regions

The pronephros is nonfunctional and completely degenerates while the mesonephros is developing. During development, the mesonephros produces urine for a short period. Most of the mesonephros system also degenerates. The portions that remain are the tubuli mesonephrici, which form the ductuli efferentes testis (see p. 54), and the ductus mesonephricus (Wolffian duct). Initially, the ductus mesonephricus develops adjacent to the pronephros, but soon becomes associated with the mesonephros. While the pronephros is still degenerating, the caudally located metanephros develops. Together with part of the ductus mesonephricus it forms the definitive ren.

Note: The definitive ren, which in adults sits just below the diaphragma, develops in the pelvic region and ascends only secondarily (ascent of the renes, see **D**).

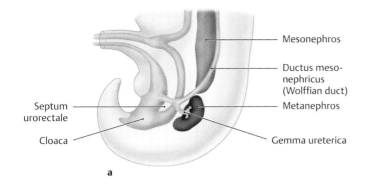

Mesonephros

Ductus meso-
nephricus
(Wolffian duct)

Metanephros

Septum
urorectale

Cloaca

Gemma ureterica

a

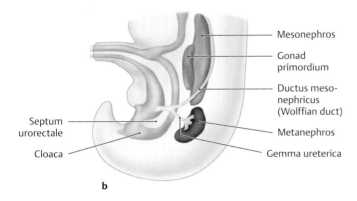

Mesonephros

Gonad
primordium

Ductus meso-
nephricus
(Wolffian duct)

Metanephros

Septum
urorectale

Cloaca

Gemma ureterica

b

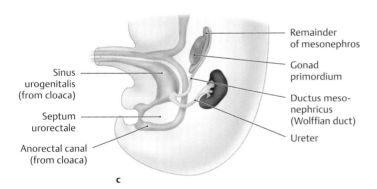

Remainder
of mesonephros

Gonad
primordium

Ductus meso-
nephricus
(Wolffian duct)

Ureter

Sinus
urogenitalis
(from cloaca)

Septum
urorectale

Anorectal canal
(from cloaca)

c

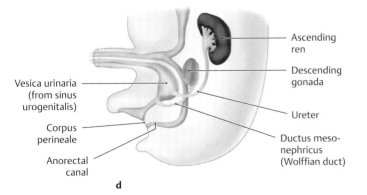

Ascending
ren

Descending
gonada

Ureter

Ductus meso-
nephricus
(Wolffian duct)

Vesica urinaria
(from sinus
urogenitalis)

Corpus
perineale

Anorectal
canal

d

D Development of the ureter and ren

Gemma ureterica and metanephros (**a**), as well as ascent of the renes (**b–d**), viewed from the left side; **e–h** Further development of the metanephros (for location of the crista mesonephrica see **B**).

a The metanephros develops during the 5th week in the most caudal portion of the mesenchyma intermedium. It is also called the *blastema metanephrogenicum*. The *gemma ureterica* sprouts from the ductus mesonephricus adjacent to the blastema and grows into the metanephros. The initially short stalk of the **gemma ureterica** elongates further and develops into the *ureter*. The tip of the gemma, which has entered into the metanephros, differentiates into components of the definitive ren (the *pelvis renalis* with its calices, and the ductus metanephrici colligentes system) (**e–h**).
Note: At this stage, the ureter is not in direct contact with the cloaca, which gives rise to the vesica urinaria. Rather, the ureter opens indirectly into the cloaca via the ductus mesonephricus. However, the other end of the ureter is already connected to the ren.

b–d The metanephros and gemma ureterica grow from the pelvic region in a cranial direction and later come to lie just below the diaphragma (ascent of the renes). This ascent is partially the result of a reduction of bending and increased growth of the sacro-lumbar region of the embryo. If a ren fails to ascend the result is referred to as a ren pelvicus. While the renes are ascending, the gonadae descend along with the remnants of the mesonephri (descent of the gonadae).

e–h The gemma ureterica enlarges after invading the metanephros and develops into the pelvis renalis with 2–3 calices renales majores (**f**). In the course of continuous branching into numerous tubuli, the gemma enters deeper into the metanephros (**g**). Within the ren, the "tubuli" form ductus metanephrici colligentes (**h**), which converge into groups close to the calices and empty into them through papillae renales. The last generation of ductus metanephrici colligentes does not divide further. Thus, the gemma ureterica gives rise to the following:

- Ureter
- Pelvis renalis
- Calices renales
- Papillae renales with ducts
- Ductus metanephrici colligentes with tubuli metanephrici conglutinati cum ampullis tubulorum colligentium (see p. 54)

Note: The blastema metanephrogenicum forms the urine producing part of the definitive ren, and the gemma ureterica forms the collecting system.

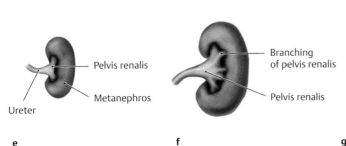

Pelvis renalis

Ureter

Metanephros

e

Branching
of pelvis renalis

Pelvis renalis

f

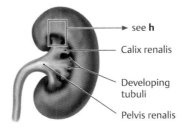

see **h**

Calix renalis

Developing
tubuli

Pelvis renalis

g

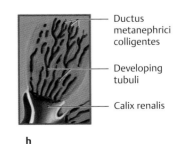

Ductus
metanephrici
colligentes

Developing
tubuli

Calix renalis

h

53

7.3 Development of Nephrons, and the Vesica Urinaria and Ureteres; Developmental Anomalies

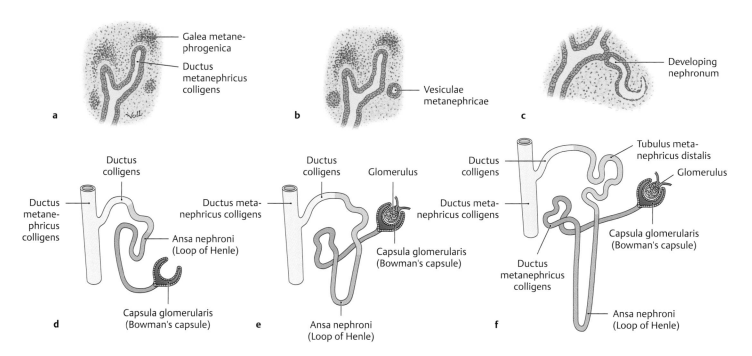

A Development of nephrona
The nephronum is the smallest functional unit of the ren. It consists of a capillary tuft, through which primary urine is discharged into the renal tubular system in a process called ultrafiltration. Within this tubular system, primary urine is concentrated into secondary or final urine through reabsorption of electrolytes and water (see p. 50). Nephron development is the final step necessary for the metanephros to become functional and proceeds in two stages:

- A vascular system is connected to the renal tubular system (for urine formation).
- The tubular system is connected to the collecting duct system (for urine discharge).

Nephron formation is induced by branching of the gemma ureterica, with each terminal ductus colligens being covered by a *galea*

metanephrogenica (**a**). Cells of the galea metanephrogenica move laterally and develop into vesiculae renales (**b**). Each vesicula gives rise to a small tubulus metanephricus sigmoideus (**c**). While segments of the tubulus continue to differentiate and elongate, its distal end, connects it to a ductus colligens (**d**). Its proximal end (capsula glomerularis, *Bowman's capsule*) becomes invaginated by a tuft of vasa capillaria (the *glomerulus*), which is supplied by a branch of the a. renalis (**e**). Continuous lengthening and differentiation of the tubuli result in the formation of the *tubular system* including the ansa nephroni (loop of Henle) (**f**). The ansa nephroni helps to concentrate primary urine (approximately 170 liters of primary urine is produced in 24 hours) to 1% of its volume to produce the final urine. At the start of the 13th week, almost 20% of nephrona are functional and can form urine.

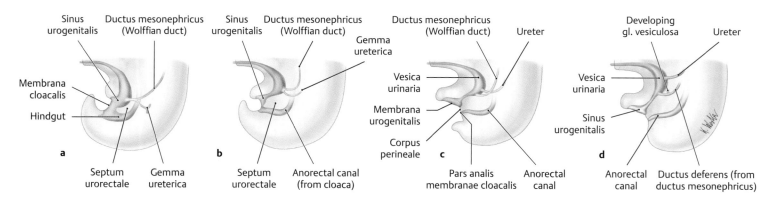

B Development of the vesica urinaria and urethra
Embryo viewed from the left side at 5 (**a**), 7 (**b**), and 8 weeks (**c**), **d** approx. 10 weeks.
The development of the vesica urinaria and urethra leads to a system concerned with the temporary storage and release of urine. Both structures are derived from the *cloaca*, the common excretory organ of the urinary and digestive systems. The *septum urorectale*, a wedge of caudally growing connective tissue, completely divides the cloaca into two parts; an anteriorly located *sinus urogenitalis* and a posteriorly located

anorectal canal (**a–c**). As the *septum urorectale* grows caudally it fuses with the membrana cloacalis, dividing it into an anteriorly located *urogenital membrane* and a posteriorly located *pars analis membranae cloacalis*. The point of fusion becomes the *corpus perineale*. As the membrana cloacalis disintegrates, the sinus urogenitalis and anorectal canal become connected to the outside of the body. The cranial part of the sinus urogenitalis gives rise to the vesica urinaria, and the pelvic part to the urethra (**d**).

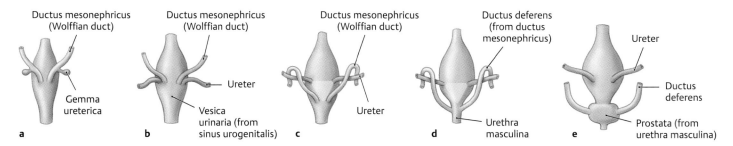

a Ductus mesonephricus (Wolffian duct) — Gemma ureterica

b Ductus mesonephricus (Wolffian duct) — Ureter — Vesica urinaria (from sinus urogenitalis)

c Ductus mesonephricus (Wolffian duct) — Ureter

d Ductus deferens (from ductus mesonephricus) — Urethra masculina

e Ureter — Ductus deferens — Prostata (from urethra masculina)

C Development of the connection between the ureteres and vesica urinaria

Dorsal view of the vesica urinaria and ductus mesonephrici. Initially, the ureteres are not in direct contact with the cloaca but open into it via the ductus mesonephrici (**a**). As the vesica urinaria further differentiates and grows, the caudal portions of the ductus mesonephrici get incorporated into the wall of the vesica urinaria as they continue to move caudally. For a short period of development, the ductus mesonephrici and ureteres share a common opening into the vesica urinaria (**b**). After further incorporation of the ductus mesonephrici into the wall of the vesica urinaria, the ductus mesonephrici and ureteres are no longer in contact, and the ureteres open into the posterior wall of the vesica uri-

naria through their own connection (**c**). The ductus mesonephrici continue to move caudally until they reach the region of the urethra (**d**). In males the *prostata* arises as an outgrowth of the urethra in the region of the ductus mesonephrici (**e**), and the ductus mesonephrici differentiate into the *ductus deferens* (see **E** and p. 62 and 64). In females, the ductus mesonephrici regress after the ureteres have become embedded in the wall of the vesica urinaria, and only two remnants, the epoophoron and paroophoron, remain (see p. 62 and 64).

Note: The incorporation of the mesodermal ductus mesonephrici and ureteres into the posterior wall of the vesica urinaria takes place over a broad, triangular area (**c, d**). As a result mesodermal tissue grows into the endodermally lined vesica urinaria.

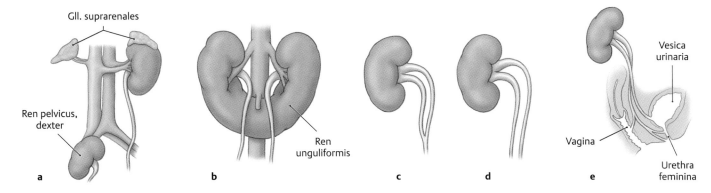

a Gll. suprarenales — Ren pelvicus, dexter

b Ren unguliformis

c

d

e Vesica urinaria — Vagina — Urethra feminina

D Developmental anomalies of the urinary system

a A ren fails to ascend resulting in a ren pelvicus.

Note: The gll. suprarenales develop in the upper gll. suprarenales, and the ascending renes stop just below the gll. suprarenales. Thus, in this figure, the right ren remains in the pelvis, and the right gl. suprarenalis is in its correct location.

b The two chordae nephrogenicae fuse resulting in a ren ungulifor-mis (horseshoe kidney); **c** Duplicated ureter (ureter bifidus; the gemma ureterica splits, resulting in two ureteres); **d** Split ureter (ureter duplex); **e** Ureter ectopicus (there are two gemmae uretericae; the ureter ectopicus atypically drains into the urethra or vagina).

These developmental anomalies may lead to hydronephrosis and subsequent bacterial pyelonephritis. The flow of urine can be obstructed which leads to bacteria migrating from the vesica urinaria to the pelvis renalis. Additionally, an atypical ureter, for instance one that drains into the vagina instead of the vesica urinaria, can lead to irritation of the vagina due to the continuous release of urine. The vaginal epithelium may become inflamed by hypertonic urine, leading to infection. In this case, bacteria migrating up the ureter may lead to bacterial pyelonephritis.

E Summary: Development of the urinary organs

Summary of the embryonic structures and the definitive body parts and organs they give rise to. Only functionally relevant structures are listed.

Embryonic structure	Definitive structure in the male	Definitive structure in the female
Blastema metanephrogenicum	Definitive nephronum	
Ductus mesonephricus	Pelvis renalis, calices, tubuli metanephrici colligentes, ureteres	
	Epididymis	
	Ductus deferens	
	Ductus ejaculatorii	
	Vesiculae seminales	
Tubuli mesonephrici	Ductuli efferentes testis	–
Sinus urogenitalis	Vesica urinaria	
	Urethra masculina	Urethra feminina
	Prostata	
	Gll. bulbourethrales	Gll. vestibulares majores
	Gll. urethrales	

8.1 Overview of the Genital System

Introduction

Function and terms: The genital organs, which in humans are sex-specific, are responsible for producing offspring. In mammals, including humans, the primary function of the reproduction system in males and females is to produce haploid cells (gametes) in specialized organs (the *gonadae*), which then fuse in the female organism to form a diploid zygote. During *sexual intercourse*, male gametes are propelled out of the male's reproductive tract and into the female reproductive tract where they fuse with the female gametes (*conception*). The initially single-celled organism, the *zygote*, is transported to the uterus where further embryonic development takes place. At the end of pregnancy (*gestation*), the baby is delivered through the birth canal. In mammals, the male is only involved in conception, whereas the female reproductive system helps create optimal conditions for the fetus to grow and to ensure a timely delivery. In both sexes, gender-specific hormones (sex hormones), which are produced in the gonadae, control these functions. These hormones determine the development and function of both the reproductive organs and the secondary sex characteristics of the individual organism.

Classification: The organization of the male and female reproductive systems can be classified in various ways:

- Topographically (see **A**): the internal genital organs (within the body cavity) and the external genital organs (outside of the body cavity).
- Functionally (**B** and **C**): as organs responsible for producing gametes and hormones (the gonadae), as organs involved in transport (of gametes), as organs involved with incubation and copulation, and as glands associated with the organs.
- Ontogenetically (see p. 4).

Functional differences between male and female genital systems: Both sexes produce gametes, which in males are referred to as *spermatozoa* and in females as *oocytes*. While spermatozoa are continuously produced from primordial germ cells (spermatogonia) from puberty until old age (several dozen millions per day), the number of oocytes is already determined at birth (they can only differentiate into fertilizable germ cells—one egg ripens each menstrual cycle). The production of spermatozoa, and thus offspring, in males is possible from puberty until old age. In females the ability to reproduce is limited to a period ranging from the differentiation of the first ovum in the woman's first menstrual cycle (menarche, onset around ages 13–14) to the differentiation of the last ovum (menopause, onset varies considerably, approx. between ages 40–60). It is important to keep in mind that mature eggs released in one of the first or last menstrual cycles may be less fertilizable.

A Male and female internal and external genitalia*

	Male	Female
Internal genitalia	Testis Epididymis Ductus deferens Prostata Gl. vesiculosa Gl. bulbourethralis	Ovarium Uterus Tuba uterina Vagina (upper portion)
External genitalia	Penis and urethra Scrotum and coverings of the testis	Vestibulum vaginae Labia majora and minora Mons pubis Gll. vestibulares majores and minores Clitoris

* The *female* external genitalia (pudendum femininum) are known clinically as the *vulva*.

B Functions of the male genital organs

Organ	Function
Testis	Germ-cell production Hormone production
Epididymis	Reservoir for sperm (sperm maturation)
Ductus deferens	Transport organ for sperm
Urethra	Transport organ for sperm and urinary organ
Accessory sex glands (prostata, vesiculae seminales, and gll. bulbourethrales)	Production of secretions (semen)
Penis	Copulatory and urinary organ

C Functions of the female genital organs

Organ	Function
Ovaria	Germ-cell production Hormone production
Tuba uterina	Site of conception and transport organ for zygote
Uterus	Organ of incubation and parturition
Vagina	Organ of copulation and parturition
Labia majora and minora	Copulatory organ
Gll. vestibulares majores and minores	Production of secretions

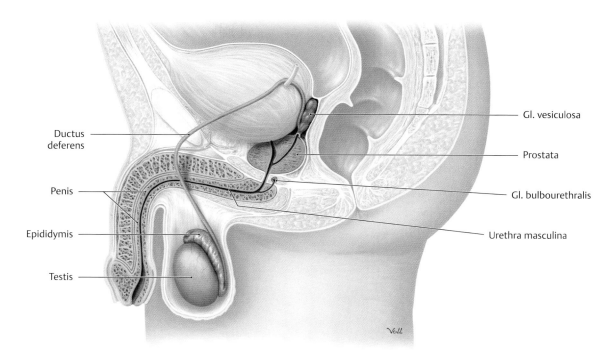

D Overview of the male genital organs
Schematic representation of the male genital organs, viewed from the left side.

Note: The urethra masculina is part of both the male urinary system and the male reproductive system. The male gonadae, the testes, lie outside the body cavity in a pouch of skin called the scrotum.

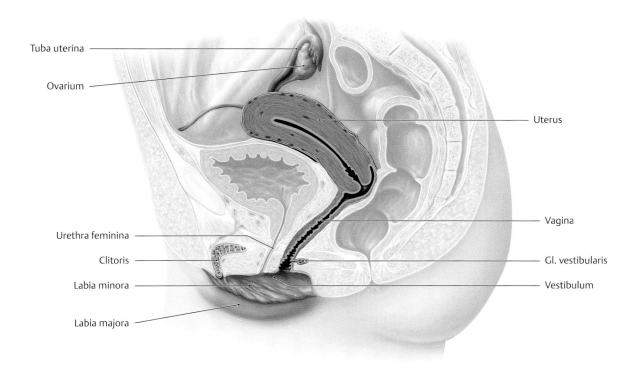

E Overview of the female genital organs
Schematic representation of the female genital organs, viewed from the left side.

Note: The urethra feminina opens into the vestibulum vaginae. However, unlike in males, the urethra feminina is not part of the female reproductive system. The female gonadae, the ovaria, are located in the cavity of the pelvis minor.

8.2 Development of the Gonadae

Ontogeny-based classification of the genital organs

Embryological structures involved in the formation of male and female genital organs:

- Derivatives of the gonadal primordia: They give rise to the gonads and develop from epithelium coelomicum and mesoderm in the crista gonadalis (see **A–C**).
- Derivatives of the ductus mesonephrici and paramesonephrici (see p. 60). They give rise to major parts of the genital tracts:
  - in males the ductus mesonephricus gives rise to the ductus deferens;
  - in females the ducti paramesonephrici gives rise to the tubae uterinae, uterus and part of the vagina
- Derivatives of the perineal region: The tubercula genitalia, plicae cloacales, and tubercula labioscrotalia give rise to the external genitalia (see p. 65).

- Derivatives of the sinus urogenitalis adjacent to the perineal region:
  - in both sexes the sinus urogenitalis gives rise to the urethra. In males the urethra and the associated prostata are also part of the genital system;
  - in females the sinus urogenitalis gives rise to part of the vagina.

Note: In males and females, the development of both the gonadae and the duct system initially pass through an indifferent stage (stadium neutrale) in which gender is not morphologically distinguishable. Over subsequent stages, only one gender-specific duct system fully develops in each sex, while the other regresses. In some people, nonfunctioning remnants of the regressed duct system can become clinically significant (e.g., Gärtner's duct cyst, see p. 64).

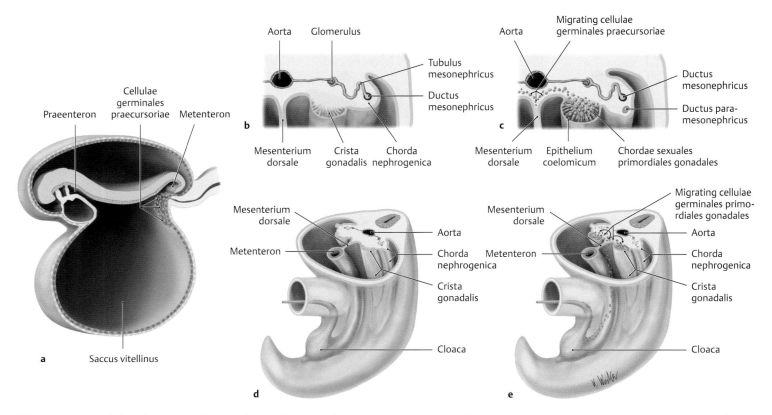

A Development of the cristae gonadales and gonada primordia; Germ cell migration

Schematic view of embryo: **a** With saccus vitellinus, viewed from the left side; **b–c** Horizontal sections, superior view; **d** and **e** Spatial representations of **b** and **c**.

a At the beginning of the 4th week, the spherical **cellulae germinales praecursoriae** are recognizable for the first time in the saccus vitellinus.

b and d Cristae gonadales and gonad primordia: The initial primordia of the gonadae, which will develop into testes in males and ovaria in females, are the paired, morphologically indifferent *cristae gonadales*. However, their future differentiation into testes or ovaria has already been genetically determined. The cristae gonadales lie along the posterior wall of the body cavity medial to the mesonephric region of the chordae nephrogenicae. Together, the chordae nephrogenicae and cristae gonadales protrude into the coelomic cavity as the *cristae urogenitales*.

Note: The initial gonada primordia do not yet contain germ cells. They migrate secondarily from the wall of the saccus vitellinus starting in the 6th week.

c and e Development of the gonadae and migration of germ cells: After the 3rd week, the cristae gonadae start to develop as a result of proliferation of the epithelium coelomicum and the underlying embryonic connective tissue called mesenchyma (**c**). The epithelial cells invade the mesenchyma and form chordae sexuales primordiales gonadales, which in both males and females are still in contact with the epithelium coelomicum. In the 6th week, the *cellulae germinales praecursoriae* in the wall of the saccus vitellinus (**a**), migrate to the gonada primordia by way of the mesenterium dorsale. Germ cell migration (**c** and **e**), leads to the formation of the indifferent gonadae in males and females. At the start of the 7th week, the morphological differentiation of the gonadae becomes apparent as they begin to develop into testes (male embryo) or ovaria (female embryo, see **C**).

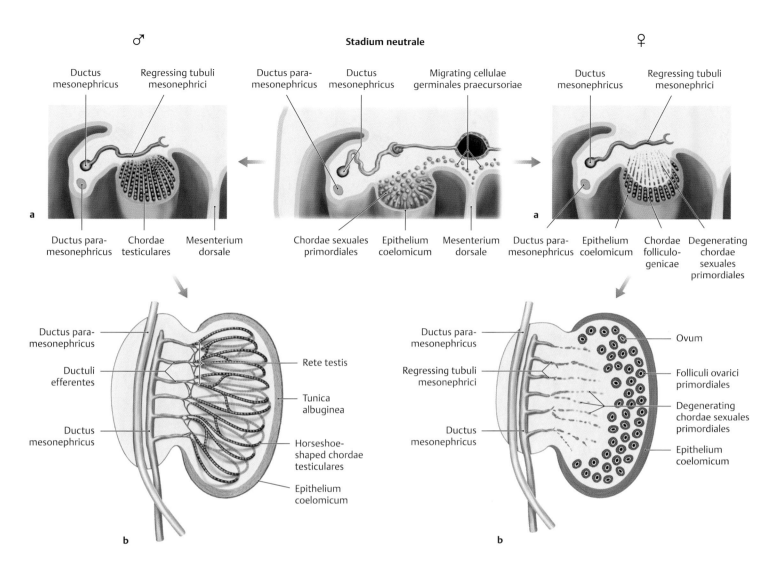

Stadium neutrale

B Development of the testes

Cross-section of the developing testis and ductus genitales in the male embryo, viewed from above (**a**) and from the front (**b**).

The chordae sexuales primordiales continue to grow and extend into the medulla of the gonadal primordia where they form the *chordae sexuales primordiales testis (chordae testiculares)*. The chordae adjacent to the hilum anastomose to form a network of tubules, the future rete testis. The chordae testiculares lose contact with the epithelium coelomicum and are separated from it by a connective tissue layer called the tunica albuginea. Around the 4th month, the ends of the chordae testiculares opposite from the hilum form horseshoe-shaped loops, which become continuous with the rete testis at the hilum. The solid chordae testiculares are now composed of spermatogonia (from the cellulae germinales praecursoriae) and sustentocyti (Sertoli cells) (from the surface epithelium of the gonadal primordium). Around the 7th—8th week, endocrinocyti interstitiales (Leydig cells) in the interstitial mesenchyme between the chordae start producing the gender-specific hormone testosterone. The testosterone induces the gender-specific development of the ductus genitales. The testis starts to descend from its position high up in the cavitas abdominis, through the canalis inguinalis and into the scrotum. Its location in the scrotum indicates mature development in the male newborn. At the onset of puberty (around age 12–13) the chordae testiculares become canalized and are now called tubuli seminiferi. The tubuli seminiferi are now connected to the rete testis, which in turn connect with the ductuli efferentes testis (remnants of the tubuli mesonephrici). The ductuli efferentes open into the ductus deferens, which was derived from the ductus mesonephricus (induced by testosterone).

C Development of the ovarium

Cross-section of developing ovarium and ductus genitales in a female embryo, viewed from above (**a**) and from the front (**b**).

Chordae sexuales primordiales also grow into the ovarium. Ingrowths of mesenchyma penetrate the chordae and divide them into cell clusters of various sizes. The cell clusters shift to the center of the ovarium and are replaced by a highly vascularized tissue, which will form the *medulla ovarii*. Around the 7th week, epithelial extensions from the epithelium coelomicum of the ovarian primordia again penetrate into the ovarian mesenchyme and form a second generation of cords called the *chordae folliculogenicae*. These cords, unlike the chordae sexuales primordiales, remain closer to the surface. In the 4th month, the chordae folliculogenicae are divided by ingrowths of mesenchyme into single, smaller cell clusters. These cell clusters then surround one or more germ cells. The germ cells become oogonia, and the surrounding layer consisting of chorda folliculogenica epithelial cells develops into the *folliculocyti primordiales* (**b**). Surrounding mesenchyma forms the theca folliculi around the follicles. Over the course of development, the ovarium descends into the pelvis minor to its definitive position. The tubuli and ductus mesonephrici located close to the hilum of the ovarium largely degenerate (the nonfunctioning remnants form the paroophoron and epoophoron, see p. 64).

59

8.3 Development of the Ductus Genitales

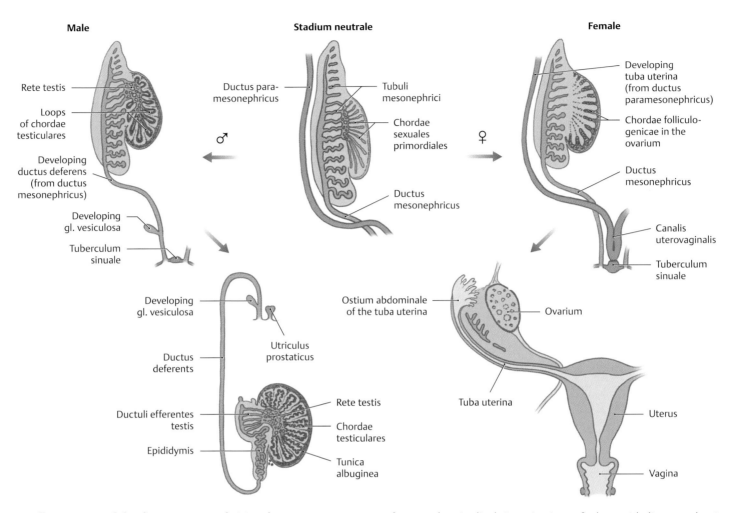

A Differentiation of the ductus mesonephrici and paramesonephrici

Cross-section of the developing gonadae and ductus genitales, viewed from the front

Similar to the gonadae, the ductus genitales pass through an indifferent stage (stadium neutrale). The embryo has two pairs of ducts: the ductus mesonephrici (Wollffian ducts) and the ductus paramesonephrici (Müllerian ducts), both of which develop in the crista urogenitalis. Both ducts eventually connect with the wall of the sinus urogenitalis. The *ductus mesonephricus* is a derivative of the mesenchyma intermedium, while the *ductus paramesonephricus* develops from a longitudinal invagination of the epithelium coelomicum. Two hormones from the developing testis, testosterone and anti-Müllerian hormone (AMH), largely determine the fate of both ducts. In male fetuses, testosterone stimulates the differentiation of the ductus mesonephrici, while AMH causes degeneration of the ductus paramesonephrici. Absence of these hormones leads to degeneration of the non-urinary portions of the ductus mesonephrici, and to persistence of the ductus paramesonephrici.

Note: In both male and female embryos the ductus mesonephrici give rise to the ureteres.

Male embryo

- Chordae sexuales primordiales testis (chordae testiculares) form the rete testis.

- *Some* tubuli mesonephrici connect with the rete testis.

- The remaining tubuli mesonephrici degenerate. Remnants form the nonfunctioning paradidymis.

- The ductus mesonephricus gives rise to the ureter, and to the epididymis and ductus deferens (which gives rise to the gl. vesiculosa and ductus ejaculatorius).

- The prostata develops from urethral epithelium (not shown). The ductus deferens and gl. vesiculosa connect with the ductus excretorius of the prostata. The colliculus seminalis is a remnant of the tuberculum sinuale, the utriculus prostaticus is a remnant of the ductus paramesonephricus.

- AMH causes degeneration of the ductus paramesonephrici.

Female embryo

- Chordae sexuales primordiales ovarii degenerate.

- Tubuli mesonephrici don't connect with other structures.

- All tubuli mesonephrici degenerate. Remnants form the nonfunctioning epoophoron and paroophoron.

- The ductus mesonephricus gives rise to the ureter, and the remaining parts of the duct degenerate. Nonfunctioning remnants may persist adjacent to the vagina in the form of a Gärtner's duct (ductus longitudinalis epoophori).

- Parts of the ductus paramesonephrici fuse: the upper portions form the paired tubae uterinae, the lower portions form the uterus (see **C**).

- The ductus mesonephrici degenerate in the absence of testosterone.

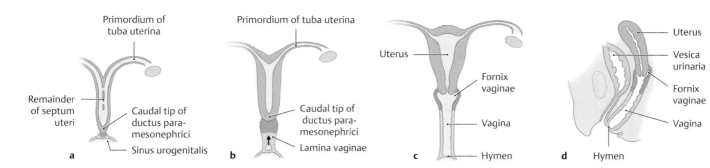

B Development of the ductus genitales in the female embryo:
Development of the uterus, tubae uterinae, and vagina
Anterior view (**a–c**) and view from the left side (**d**) of the developing tubae uterinae, uterus and vagina.

As development continues, the upper part of the ductus paramesonephrici become horizontal in position while the lower parts remain in vertical. The horizontal parts remain separated and develop into the tubae uterinae. The end of the upper part of the ductus paramesonephrici retains its open connection with the cavitas coelomica (which later becomes the cavitas peritonealis). This distal opening is called the ostium abdominale tubae uterinae and it projects toward the ovarium. The lower parts of the ducts fuse, forming the canalis uterovaginalis. The septum that initially separated the ducts resorbs resulting in a single cavitas uteri. The lower part of the fused ducts further grows caudally toward the sinus urogenitalis. Shortly before reaching

it, they merge with a cranial evagination of the sinus urogenitalis called the bulbi sinuvaginales. The bulbi sinovaginales form the solid lamina vaginae (**b**). The lamina vaginae continues to extend upward. Canalization of the lamina vaginae proceeds from the caudal end toward the cranial end and is completed by the 5th month (**b**). As a result of the upward growth, the distance between the developing uterus and sinus urogenitalis increases. The lamina vaginae forms the lower vagina, and the ductus paramesonephrici form the upper vagina. A thin membrane of connective tissue called the hymen separates the vagina from the sinus urogenitalis (**c, d**). Failure of the ductus paramesonephrici to fuse completely, or of the septum between them to degenerate completely, results in a uterus duplex or uterus septatus (for possible variations see **D**). Failed canalization of the lamina vaginae leads to partial or complete vaginal atresia.

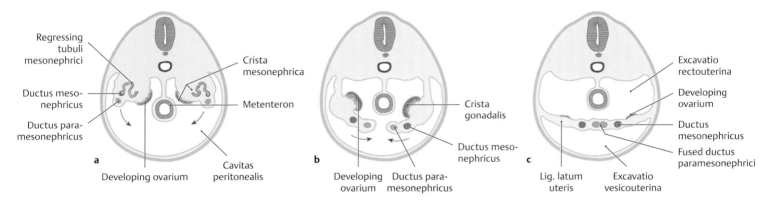

C Fusion of the cristae mesonephricae in the female embryo
Horizontal sections of the abdomen in a female embryo, viewed from above. **a** Protruding cristae mesonephricae; **b** Cristae mesonephricae approaching each other; **c** Fusion of the cristae mesonephricae.

As a result of continuous proliferation of mesodermal tissue, the cristae mesonephricae protrude into the cavitas coelomica. At the same time, both ductus paramesonephrici shift medially until they are in contact with each other. The ductus paramesonephrici fuse to form the canalis uterovaginalis, which together with the fusion of the cristae mesonephricae results in a layer of connective tissue located in the pelvis minor. This sheet of connective tissue extends laterally from the developing uterus and is called the plica lata uterina. The plica lata divides the cavitas peritonealis in the pelvis minor into anterior and posterior pouches:

- Anterior to the uterus (and posterior to vesica uterina, not shown here): the excavatio vesicouterina

- Posterior to the uterus (and anterior to rectum): the excavatio rectouterina.

Note: As the cristae mesonephricae shift position, the developing ovaria shift from an anterior position to a medial position and finally to a posterior position. Thus the definitive ovaria lie in the posterior aspect of the plica lata.

The ductus paramesonephrici originally develop lateral to the ductus mesonephrici. As a result of the shifting cristae mesonephricae and the fusion of their caudal portions, the fused ductus paramesonephrici lie medial to the ductus mesonephrici in the lower part of the cavitas coelomica. The ductus mesonephrici give rise to the ureteres, which thus traverse the plica lata on their way from the renes to the vesica urinaria.

D Developmental anomalies
Anterior view of the developing uterus and vagina. Several defects can arise from failed fusion of the ductus paramesonephrici. Incomplete fusion (**a–c**) with uterus duplex (and/or vagina duplex); rudimentary horn on one side of the uterus (**d**); atresia of the cervix (**e**); vaginal atresia (**f**). Developmental defects of the developing vagina, mainly atresia, may result from anomalies of the sinus urogenitalis.

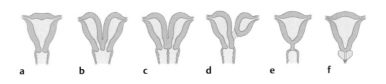

8.4 Comparison of Gender Differences and Relationship to the Urinary System

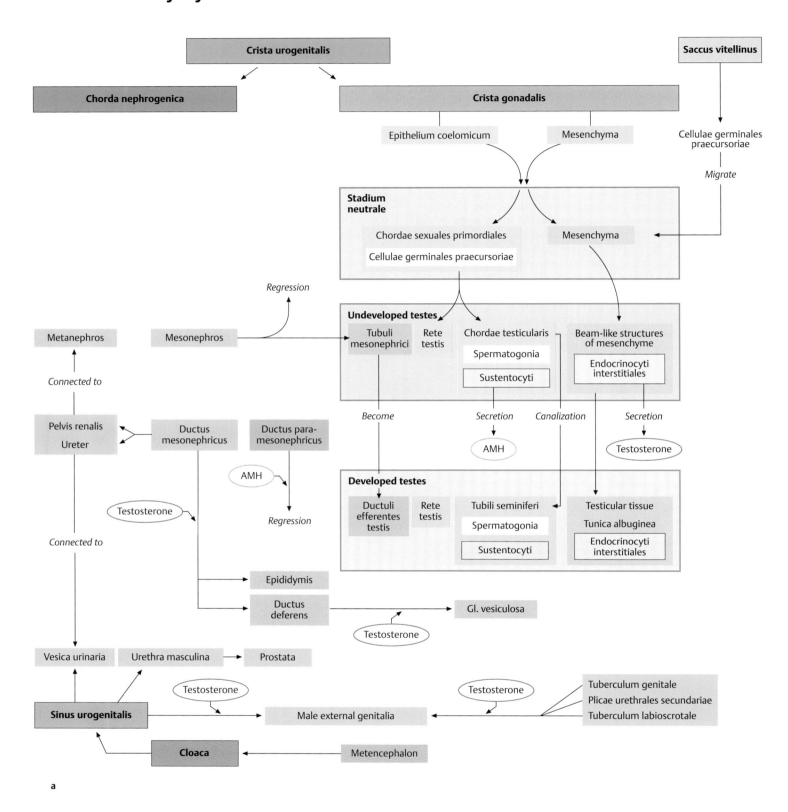

a

A Comparison of genital development in both sexes, and relationships to the urinary system

Schematic representation of the development of the male (**a**) and female (**b**) genital systems. Nonfunctioning embryonic remnants are not shown here (see **A**, p. 64). The relationship of the genital system to the urinary system, which is similar in both sexes, is shown here to illustrate the close relationship between the two systems.

Note: Chordae sexuales primordiales develop in both the male and female gonadal primordia. They degenerate in females and are replaced by secondary cords, the chordae folliculogenicae, which are involved

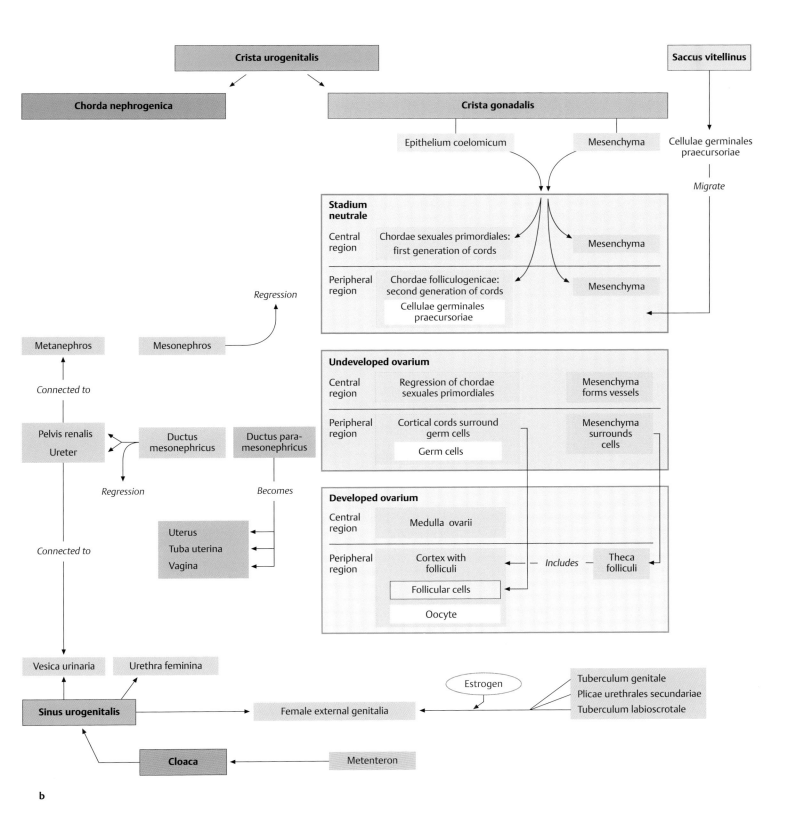

b

in the development of folliculi. In males, the chordae sexuales primordiae become chordae testiculares, which develop into the tubuli seminiferi. Chordae folliculogenicae don't develop in the testes. Development of a male phenotype requires testosterone (development of the male ductus genitales) and anti-Müllerian hormone (AMH, causes regression of the ductus paramesonephrici). If these two hormones are absent—or the ducts don't respond to them due to a lack of hormone receptors—a female phenotype develops even in the absence of estrogen.

8.5 Comparison of Embryonic and Mature Structures

A Comparison of embryonic and mature structures
Overview of development in both sexes. Some embryonic structures develop into functionally active mature structures, while others form nonfunctioning remnants. A male vs. female comparison of the structures listed in the following table is illustrated on the following page.

Embryonic primordium	Definitive structure in the male	Definitive structure in the female	Nonfunctioning remnants in the male	Nonfunctioning remnants in the female
Indifferent gonad with • Cortex • Medulla	Testis with • Tubuli seminiferi • Rete testis	Ovarium with • Follicles • Stroma ovarii		
Tubuli mesonephrici	Ductuli efferentes		Paradidymis	Epo- and paroophoron
Ductus mesonephricus (Wolffian duct)	• Epididymis • Ductus deferens • Ductus ejaculatorius • Gl. vesiculosa • Ureter • Pelvis renalis and calices renales, ductus metanephrici colligentes	• Ureter • Pelvis renalis and calices renales, ductus metanephrici colligentes	Appendix epididymidis	Ductus longitudinalis epoophori (Gärtner's duct)
Ductus paramesonephricus (Müllerian duct)		• Tuba uterina • Uterus • Superior portion of vagina	Appendix testis	Appendix vesiculosa (hydatid of Morgagni)
Sinus urogenitalis	• Prostata • Gl. bulbourethralis • Vesica urinaria • Urethra masculina	• Inferior portion of vagina • Gll. vestibulares majores and minores • Vesica urinaria • Urethra feminina	Utriculus prostaticus	
Tuberculum genitale (Phallus)	Corpus cavernosum penis	Clitoris, glans clitoridis		
Plicae urethrales secundariae	• Corpus spongiosum penis • Glans penis	• Labia minora • Bulbus vestibularis		
Tubercula labioscrotalia	Scrotum	Labia majora		
Gubernaculum		• Lig. ovarii proprium • Lig. teres uteri	Gubernaculum testis	
Tuberculum sinuale			Colliculus seminalis	Hymen

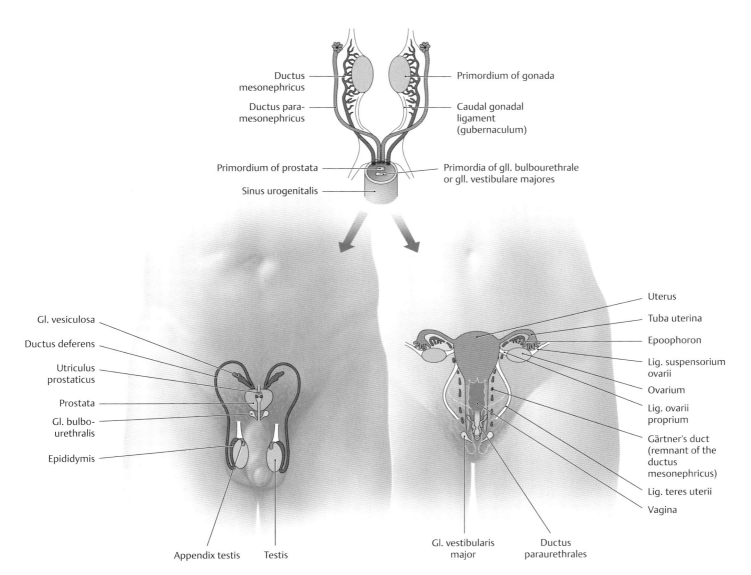

B Development of the internal genitalia
Embryonic primordia of the genital organs, and the mature organs, anterior view. For clarity, the representation of the primordia and the mature organs does not correspond with their actual sizes.
Note: The internal genital organs are located in the pelvis minor or outside the body in the scrotum. With the descent of the gonadae, the genital tracts, which develop from the ductus mesonephrici in males and the ductus paramesonephrici in females, move downward as the gonadae descend. Thus, the ducts shift from a craniocaudal orientation to a horizontal position (the tuba uterina in females) or to an almost upside-down position (the ductus deferens in males).

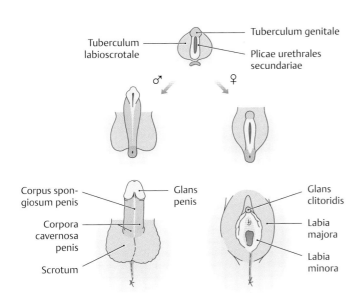

C Development of the external genitalia
Schematic representation of the developing external genitalia, inferior view.
In both sexes, the urethra develops from the sinus urogenitalis. In the male the urethra becomes part of both the urinary and reproductive systems. In the female the urethra is only a urinary organ, even though it is located directly anterior to the vaginal opening and between the labia of the external genitalia. The female internal and external genitalia are completely separated from the urinary organs; however, due to their close topographical relationship, developmental anomalies of one system may affect the other (such as a urethral-vaginal fistula where there is an abnormal connection between the urethra and vagina).

9.1 Overview of the Endocrine System

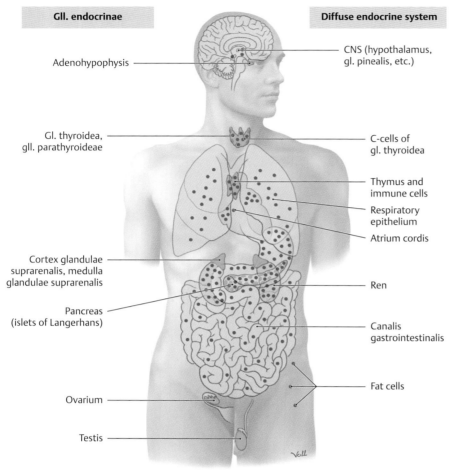

Gll. endocrinae		Diffuse endocrine system

Adenohypophysis

CNS (hypothalamus, gl. pinealis, etc.)

Gl. thyroidea, gll. parathyroideae

C-cells of gl. thyroidea

Thymus and immune cells

Respiratory epithelium

Atrium cordis

Cortex glandulae suprarenalis, medulla glandulae suprarenalis

Ren

Pancreas (islets of Langerhans)

Canalis gastrointestinalis

Fat cells

Ovarium

Testis

Voll

A The endocrine system

By secreting hormones, the endocrine system enables cells to communicate with other cells and coordinates bodily functions. Thus, the endocrine system is closely related to the nervous system, which has a similar coordinating function. The endocrine system includes the classic gll. endocrinae, which are visible *macroscopically* (left). Additionally, it includes individual cells or small groups of cells, which also secrete hormones, but are only visible histologically. These cells constitute the diffuse endocrine system (right), and they are located in a number of organs, including the gll. endocrinae.

The hormones produced by endocrine organs affect other cells in very low doses, and the organs themselves are usually small and difficult to dissect. In addition, they are difficult to classify histologically because they produce a number of different types of hormones (see **C**). Thus, this chapter will focus on the functional and biochemical aspects of the endocrine system.

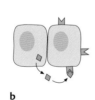

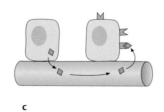

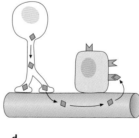

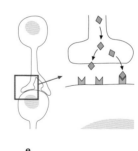

a　　b　　　　c　　　　　d　　　　e

B Types of hormonal communication

In hormonal communication a cell secretes a hormone, and a receptor recognizes the hormone and triggers a signal transduction cascade leading to changes in the cell that bears the receptor. There are several types of hormonal communication.

a Autocrine secretion: The hormones are synthesized and secreted by the same cells that possess the receptors. Thus, the cell stimulates itself. Autocrine secretion plays a particularly important role in tumor development.

b Paracrine secretion: The hormones are released into the interstitial fluid and diffuse to neighboring cells that have the hormones' receptors. This is the most primitive form of hormonal effect; it developed early in evolution and it still plays a major role in the human endocrine system. Diffuse endocrine cells (see above) act this way, and the immune system uses paracrine signaling with interleukins to enable communication between cells.

c Endocrine secretion: The secreting cell releases the hormone into the blood, where it is transported to the receptor-bearing cells. All major gll. endocrinae utilize this mechanism.

d Neurosecretion: The secreting cell, a neuron, releases its neurotransmitter, which acts as a hormone, directly into the blood stream. Neurosecretion is a transitional type of communication between endocrine signaling and synaptic transmission. It illustrates the close relationship between nervous system and endocrine system.

e Synaptic transmission (neurocrine secretion): Synaptic transmission is a special form of paracrine signaling. The neurotransmitter (hormone) is released by a neuron from its presynaptic membrane. The transmitter diffuses across the synaptic cleft to receptors on the postsynaptic membrane.

C Classification of hormones as lipophilic or hydrophilic molecules (after Karlson)

Hormones can be either lipophilic or hydrophilic, which helps explain the substantial differences in their synthesis and function. Lipophilic hormones such as the steroid hormones are synthesized in smooth endoplasmic reticulum, while hydrophilic hormones such as the protein hormones are synthesized in rough endoplasmic reticulum. These differences in synthesis are reflected in the varying amounts of the organelles in hormone-producing cells.

	Lipophilic hormones	Hydrophilic hormones
Signaling molecule	• Steroid hormones • Thyroid hormones • Retinoic acid	• Amino acids and their derivatives • Peptide hormones • Protein hormones
Plasma transport	Bound	Mostly unbound
Half-life	Long (hours to days)	Short (minutes)
Receptors	Intracellular	Membranous
Effect	Transcription control	Intracellular signaling cascades via membrane proteins

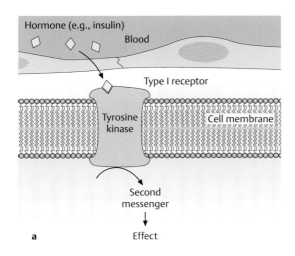

a

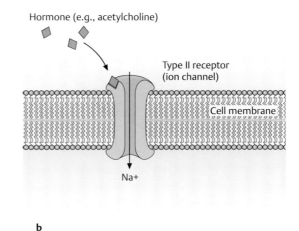

b

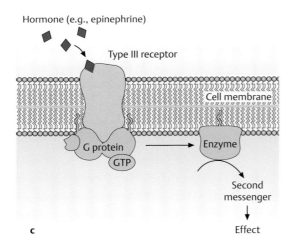

c

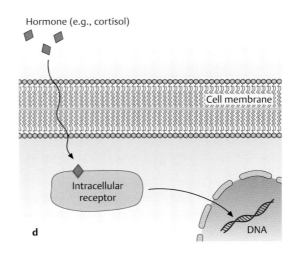

d

D Types of hormone receptors

There are 4 general types of hormone receptors.

a Type I receptors: The receptor protein, which is an enzyme, is embedded in the lipid bilayer of the cell membrane. The hormone binds to cell-surface receptors. However, the enzymatic reaction occurs on the cytoplasmic side of the membrane, where the substrate-binding site for the enzymatic reaction is located. Generally, the enzyme is a tyrosine kinase that phosphorylates substrates when activated. *Example: insulin receptors.*

b Type II receptors: The receptors are ion channels, which change their conductance depending on ligand-binding. Example: *Acetylcholine receptors* in neurons (another example of the close relationship between the endocrine and nervous systems).

c Type III receptors: The hormone receptors activate G proteins (guanine nucleotide-binding proteins), which in turn activate intracellular proteins (indirect activation). This is the largest group of hormone receptors. *Example: epinephrine receptors.*

d Intracellular receptors: Lipophilic hormones pass directly through the cell membrane and activate intracellular receptors. The primary function of these receptors is regulation of gene expression. *Example: cortisol receptors.*

Note: The hormonal effects regulated by gene expression are characterized by a slower response compared to the fast effects regulated by type II receptors.

67

9.2 Metabolism and Feedback Loop Regulation in the Endocrine System

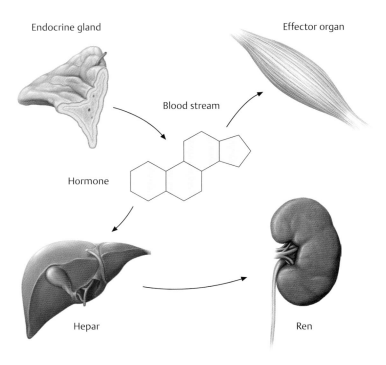

A Metabolism of hormones

The hormone is produced by the cells of a gl. endocrina (in this example a steroid hormone from the cortex glandulae suprarenalis) and released into the blood as needed. The hormone is transported in the bloodstream to the effector organ (here: skeletal muscle), where it binds to receptors that mediate the cellular effects of the hormone. The hormone is broken down in the hepar and the metabolites are excreted via the renes.

B Feedback loops in the endocrine system

Inhibitory (red) and stimulatory (green) pathways from higher centers of the brain modulate the hypothalamus, which is part of the diencephalon and serves as a master control center for a large part of hormone regulation. A preponderance of inhibitory input leads to the release of inhibiting hormones and a preponderance of stimulatory input leads to the release of releasing hormones. If releasing hormones outweigh inhibiting hormones, the adenohypophysis (anterior pituitary) will release a glandotropic hormone (a hormone that affects a peripheral endocrine gland, e.g., gl. suprarenalis or thyroidea). This hormone stimulates the gland to release its hormones, which stimulate the effector organ. At the same time the hormone inhibits the adenohypophysis and hypothalamus, which leads to a reduction in further hormone production and release (a negative feedback loop). Thus, in the regulation of hormone production and release, multiple hormones can be thought of being serially connected in a chain with a feedback mechanism incorporated into the links.

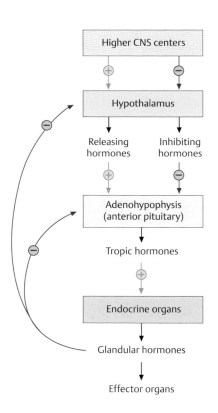

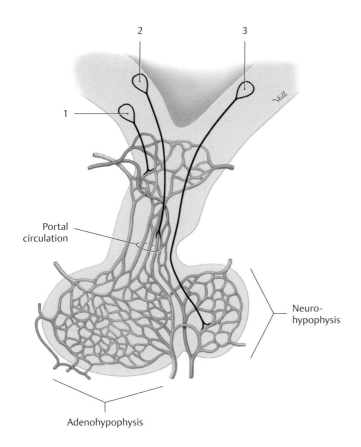

Portal circulation

Neuro-hypophysis

Adenohypophysis

C The hypothalamic-pituitary axis and hormone regulation

The hypothalamus and hypophysis function as higher control centers for hormone release by other gll. endocrinae. They are connected to each other through the infundibulum hypophysis by a venous portal system and a long axon system:

- Regulation via the portal system: Neuronal cell bodies in the hypothalamus (neurons 1 and 2) synthesize releasing and inhibiting hormones, and, via short axons, release them into the portal blood vessels. They are then transported in the vessels to cells in the *anterior* pituitary (*adenohypophysis*). These cells then produce hormones, which are released into the systemic circulation. The first neurons (neurons 1 and 2) are called neuroendocrine transducers because they transform neural information into hormonal information by releasing their transmitters into the portal circulation. They do not terminate at other nerve cells.
- Regulation via *long* axons: Neurons located in the hypothalamus (neuron 3) project to the *posterior* pituitary (*neurohypophysis*), where they release their hormones directly into the blood vessels of the neurohypophysis (neurosecretion). This system bypasses the portal circulation, and the neurons themselves (neuron 3) are the neuroendocrine transducers. The hormones oxytocin and vasopressin (ADH) are released in this way.

Note: The secretions of the disseminated endocrine cells in the digestive and respiratory tracts is not regulated by the hypothalamic-pituitary axis.

D Principal sites where hormones and hormone-like substances are formed

Hormones are vitally important chemical messengers that enable cells to communicate with one another. Usually, very small amounts of these messengers act on metabolic processes in their target cells. Different hormones can be classified on the basis of their

- site of formation,
- site of action,
- mechanism of action, or
- chemical structure.

Examples are steroid hormones (e.g., testosterone, aldosterone), amino acid derivatives (e.g., epinephrine, norepinephrine, dopamine, serotonin), peptide hormones (e.g., insulin, glucagon), and fatty acid derivatives (e.g., prostaglandins).

Principal sites of formation	Hormones and hormone-like substances
Classic endocrine hormonal glands	
Hypophysis (anterior and posterior lobes)	ACTH (adrenocorticotropic hormone, corticotropin) TSH (thyroid-stimulating hormone, thyrotropin) FSH (follicle-stimulating hormone, follitropin) LH (luteinizing hormone, lutropin) STH (somatotropic hormone, somatotropin) MSH (melanocyte-stimulating hormone, melanotropin) PRL (prolactin) ADH (antidiuretic hormone or vasopressin) Oxytocin (formed in the hypothalamus and secreted by the posterior pituitary)
Gl. pinealis	Melatonin
Gl. thyroidea	Thyroxine (T4) and triiodothyronine (T3)
C cells of the gl. thyroidea	Calcitonin
Gll. parathyroideae	Parathyroid hormone
Gll. suprarenales	Mineralocorticoids and glucocorticoids Androgens Epinephrine and norepinephrine
Insulae pancreaticae (islets of Langerhans)	Insulin, glucagon, somatostatin, and pancreatic polypeptide
Ovarium	Estrogens and progestins
Testis	Androgens (mainly testosterone)
Placenta	Chorionic gonadotropin, progesterone
Hormone-producing tissues and single cells	
Central and autonomic nervous system	Neuronal transmitters
Parts of the diencephalon (e.g., the hypothalamus)	Releasing and inhibitory hormones
System of gastrointestinal cells in the GI tract	Gastrin, cholecystokinin, secretin
Atria cordis	Atrial natriuretic peptide
Ren	Erythropoietin, renin
Hepar	Angiotensinogen, somatomedins
Immune organs	Thymus hormones, cytokines, lymphokines
Tissue hormones	Eicosanoids, prostaglandins, histamine, bradykinin

10.1 The Sympathetic and Parasympathetic Nervous Systems

The autonomic, or visceral nervous system innervates the internal organs. It is divided into three parts: the pars sympathica, pars parasympathica, and plexus entericus. For didactic reasons these systems are discussed separately; however, they represent one functional unit.

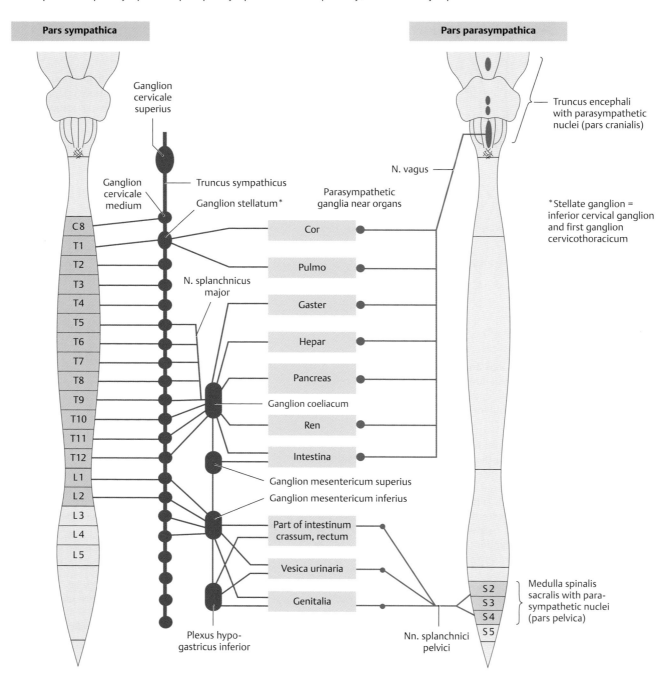

Pars sympathica

Pars parasympathica

Ganglion cervicale superius

Truncus sympathicus

Ganglion cervicale medium

Ganglion stellatum*

N. splanchnicus major

Ganglion coeliacum

Ganglion mesentericum superius

Ganglion mesentericum inferius

Plexus hypo-gastricus inferior

Truncus encephali with parasympathetic nuclei (pars cranialis)

N. vagus

Parasympathetic ganglia near organs

*Stellate ganglion = inferior cervical ganglion and first ganglion cervicothoracicum

Cor — Pulmo — Gaster — Hepar — Pancreas — Ren — Intestina — Part of intestinum crassum, rectum — Vesica urinaria — Genitalia

Medulla spinalis sacralis with para-sympathetic nuclei (pars pelvica)

Nn. splanchnici pelvici

C8, T1, T2, T3, T4, T5, T6, T7, T8, T9, T10, T11, T12, L1, L2, L3, L4, L5

S2, S3, S4, S5

A Structure of the pars sympathica (red) and pars parasympathica (blue)

Both the partes sympathica and parasympathica utilize a two-neuron pathway between the CNS and their targets. The first neuron is called the preganglionic neuron, and the second neuron is the postganglionic neuron. The preganglionic sympathetic neurons are located in the cornu laterale of lower pars cervicalis, pars thoracica, and upper pars lumbalis of the medulla spinalis. The preganglionic parasympathetic neurons are located in nuclei nervorum cranialium and the pars sacralis of the medulla spinalis. The n. vagus, a n. cranialis, contains the preganglionic parasympathetic neurons that will innervate cervical, thoracic, and abdominal viscera. In both the partes sympathica and parasympathica, the preganglionic neurons of the CNS synapse with the postganglionic neurons in ganglia of the peripheral nervous system (see **C** and **D**).

- In the pars sympathica of the nervous system, the preganglionic neuron synapses with the postganglionic neuron in ganglia of the truncus sympathicus (for trunk and limbs), in prevertebral ganglia (for viscera) or directly in the organs (only gll. suprarenales).
- In the pars parasympathica of the nervous system, the n. vagus terminates at ganglia close to or in the walls (intramural ganglia) of the organs.

According to Langley (1905), the terms pars sympathica and parasympathica originally referred only to efferent neurons and their axons (visceral efferent fibers, as shown above). It has now been shown that the partes sympathica and parasympathica contain afferent fibers (visceral afferent fibers, pain and stretch receptors not shown here, see p. 72).

B Synopsis of the partes sympathica and parasympathica of the nervous system

1. The pars sympathica can be considered the excitatory part of the autonomic nervous system that prepares the body for a *"fight or flight"* response.
2. The pars parasympathica is the part of the autonomic nervous system that coordinates the *"rest and digest"* responses of the body.
3. Although there are separate control centers for the two divisions in the truncus encephali and medulla spinalis, they have close anatomic and functional ties in the periphery.
4. The principal transmitter at the target organ is *acetylcholine* in the pars parasympathica and *norepinephrine* in the pars sympathica.
5. Stimulation of the partes sympathica and parasympathica produces the following different effects on specific organs:

Organ	Pars sympathica	Pars parasympathica
Cor	Increased heart rate	Decreased heart rate
Pulmones	Bronchodilation and decreased bronchial secretions	Bronchoconstriction and increased bronchial secretions
Gastrointestinal tract	Decreased secretions and motor activity	Increased secretions and motor activity
Pancreas	Decreased endocrine and exocrine secretions	Increased exocrine secretions
Male genitalia	Ejaculation	Erection

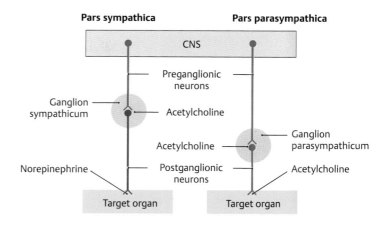

C Circuit diagram of the divisio autonomica of the nervous system

The synapse of the central, preganglionic neuron uses *acetylcholine* as a transmitter in both the partes sympathica *and* parasympathica (cholinergic neuron, shown in blue). In the pars sympathica, the transmitter changes to *norepinephrine* at the synapse of the postganglionic neuron with the target organ (adrenergic neuron, shown in red), while the pars parasympathica continues to use acetylcholine at that level.
Note: Various types of receptors for acetylcholine (neurotransmitter sensors) are located in the membrane of the target cells. As a result, acetylcholine can produce a range of effects depending on the receptor type.

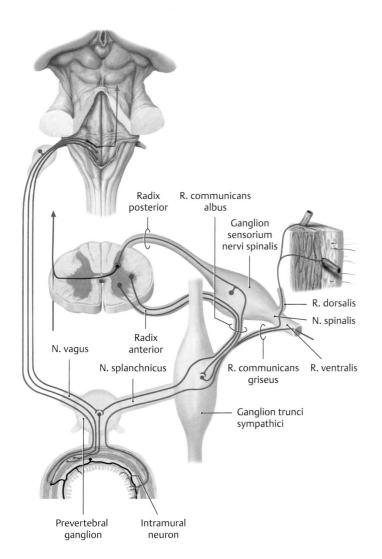

D Circuitry of the autonomic nervous system

Although the partes sympathica and parasympathica emerge from two different regions of the CNS (see **A**), they form a close structural and functional unit close to the organs. The perikarya of the preganglionic **sympathetic** neurons are located in the cornu laterale of the medulla spinalis. Their axons exit the medulla spinalis through the radix anterior and travel in the rr. communicantes albi (white because they are myelinated) to the ganglia sympathica. The axons synapse with the postganglionic neurons at three different levels:

- For the sympathetic fibers going to the limbs and trunk wall, the preganglionic sympathetic neurons synapse with the postganglionic neurons in the ganglia sympathica. The postganglionic fibers travel in the rr. communicantes grisei (gray because they are unmyelinated) back to the nn. spinales.
- For the sympathetic fibers going to the viscera, the preganglionic sympathetic fibers usually pass through the ganglia sympathica as nn. splanchnici. They synapse with the postganglionic sympathetic neurons in ganglia close to the organs (prevertebral ganglia). From there, the postganglionic fibers travel to the organs. The pars sympathica also influences the plexus entericus, which is referred to as the third part of the autonomic nervous system (see p. 73). In the colon, for example, sympathetic fibers will contact intramural neurons of the enteric system.
- For the sympathetic fibers going to the medulla glandulae suprarenalis, the preganglionic sympathetic fibers terminate on the cells of the medulla (not shown here).

The preganglionic **parasympathetic** neurons of the viscera located in the body cavities originate from truncus encephali nuclei of the n. vagus or from segmenta sacralia of the medulla spinalis (not shown). They synapse in ganglia that are either very close to or embedded in the organ (intramural ganglia). Afferent pain fibers (marked in green) accompany both sympathetic and parasympathetic nerve fibers. The axons of these fibers originate in pseudounipolar neurons, which are located either in ganglia sensoria nervorum spinalium or in ganglia of the n. vagus (see p. 72).

10.2 Afferent Pathways of the Autonomic Nervous System and the Enteric Nervous System

A Pain afferents from the viscera conducted by the sympathetic and parasympathetic pathways (after Jaenig)
a Sympathetic pain fibers, **b** Parasympathetic pain fibers.

Both nervous systems also carry axons of afferent pain fibers, which run parallel to the efferent pathways. They only make up about 5% of all afferent pain fibers and thus, quantatively, they play a minor role and become active mainly in response to organ lesions.

a The pain conducting (nociceptive) axons from the viscera run along with the nn. splanchnici to the ganglia sympathica and reach the nn. spinales by way of the rr. communicantes albi. They then run in the radices posteriores of the nn. spinales to the ganglia sensoria nervorum spinalium, where their perikarya are located. From the ganglia, their axons pass through the radices posteriores to the cornu posterius of the medulla spinalis, where they synapse and establish connections with ascending pain pathways.
Note: Unlike the efferent system, the afferent nociceptive fibers do not synapse in peripheral ganglia.

b The perikarya of the pain-conducting pseudounipolar neurons in the *cranial part* of the pars parasympathica of the autonomic nervous system are located in the ganglia inferiora or superiora of the nn. vagi. Those of the sacral part of the pars parasympathica are located in ganglia sensoria of sacral medulla spinalis levels S2–S4. Their fibers run parallel to the efferent vagal, or spinal, fibers and establish a central connection with the pain-processing systems.

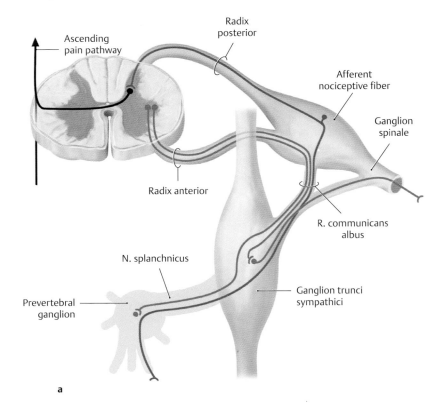

a

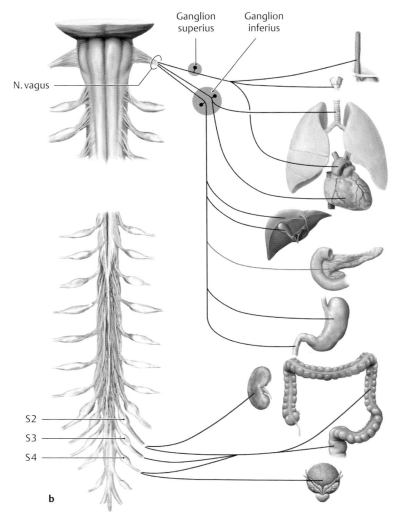

b

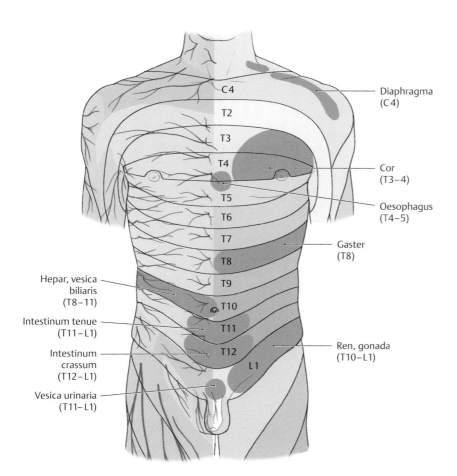

B Referred pain

Pain afferents from the viscera (visceral pain) and dermatomes (somatic pain) terminate at the same pain processing neurons in the cornu posterius of the medulla spinalis. The convergence of visceral and somatic afferent fibers confuses the relationship between the pain's origin and its perception. Thus, the cortex cerebri may register pain impulses from the gaster as coming from the abdominal wall. This phenomenon is known as referred pain. The pain impulses from a particular internal organ are consistently projected to the same well-defined skin area (see dermatome levels on figure). Thus, the area of skin that the pain is projected to provides crucial information regarding what organ is affected. The skin areas to which a particular internal organ projects its pain are referred to as Head-zones, named after their discoverer, the English neurologist Sir Henry Head. This model considers only the peripheral processing of impulses, which the cortex cerebri perceives as pain. It is not clear why somatic pain is not perceived as visceral pain.

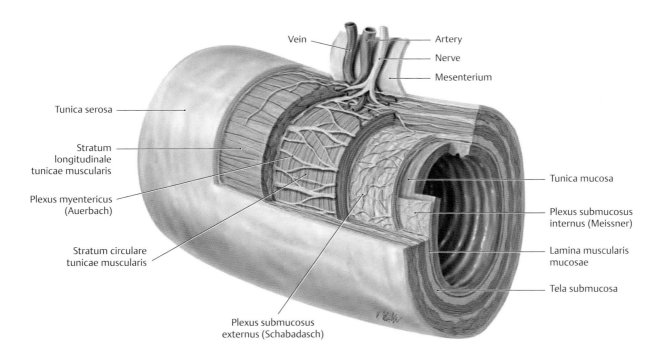

C The enteric nervous system (plexus entericus) in the intestinum tenue

The plexus entericus is considered a third and independent part of the autonomic nervous system ("The gut has a small brain"), and thus it is discussed separately after the partes sympathica and parasympathica of the autonomous nervous system. The plexus entericus consists of small groups of neurons that form interconnected, microscopically visible ganglia in the wall of the gut tube. The enteric system is organized into two plexuses: the *plexus myentericus* (Auerbach), located between the strata longitudina and circulare of the tunica muscularis, and the *plexus submucosus* (in the tela submucosa), which is subdivided into an external plexus (Schabadasch) and an internal plexus (Meissner). (For more details on the structure of the plexus entericus see histology textbooks.) These networks of neurons form the basis for autonomic reflex pathways. In principle, they can function without external innervation but their activity is greatly influenced by the partes sympathica and parasympathica of the nervous system. Activities regulated by the plexus entericus include gastrointestinal motility, secretions into the gut tube and local blood flow.

10.3 Paraganglia

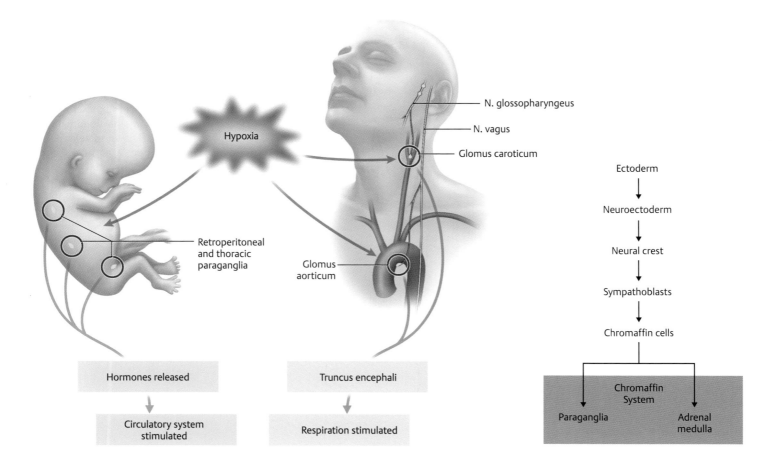

A Definition, function, and classification of paraganglia

Ganglia are aggregations of nerve cell bodies in the peripheral nervous system. Paraganglia are aggregations of specialized neurons in the peripheral nervous system which in part have an endocrine function. As such they are between the nervous system and the hormone system. Measuring only a few millimeters in size, the paraganglia act as an "early warning and control system" for lack of oxygen in arterial blood (hypoxia). They continuously measure the intra-arterial partial pressure of O_2 and CO_2 as well as the pH value. Thus they act as chemosensors. In the fetus, paraganglia respond to hypoxia by releasing hormones that increase circulatory activity. In the fully developed body after birth, certain paraganglia respond to hypoxia by transmitting a signal to the brainstem via nerves. The truncus encephali reflexively increases respiration, improving the supply of oxygen. This means that paraganglia are of paramount importance for regulating the supply of oxygen in the body. Two types are differentiated according to their location in the body:

- *Retroperitoneal ganglia:* In the embryo and small child they are found in large numbers in the thorax and in the *spatium retroperitoneale* of the abdomen next to

(= *para*) the ganglia of the truncus sympathicus. Such ganglia are also found in the genital region. Their number decreases markedly in the adult. In the fetal period and at birth, they respond to hypoxia by secreting the hormone norepinephrine, which increases the unborn child's blood pressure and pulse rate. Their functional significance in adults is the subject of discussion. A comparatively large group of paraganglia ususally located at the level of the origin of the a. mesenterica inferior where it arises from the abdominal aorta are known as the *ganglia praeaortica.*

- *Glomus bodies (especially the glomus caroticum and the glomus aorticum; glomus = ball):* These extravascular structures lie at the bifurcation of the common carotid artery (*glomus caroticum;* at the level of the C4 vertebra, one on each side) and at the aortic arch (usually multiple *aortic bodies* are present). Functionally, they are directly associated with the ninth cranial nerve (*n. glossopharyngeus; carotid body*) and the tenth cranial nerve (*n. vagus; aortic bodies*) through which their signal reaches the truncus encephali. The hypoxia signal of the glomus bodies leads to increased respiratory activity. In unborn fetuses, which do not

yet have independent respiration, they have no functional significance.

- A *jugular body* lying near the base of the skull along the internal v. jugularis interna is occasionally observed. Little is known about its function. It is not shown here.

B Origin of the paraganglia

Paraganglia arise from the neural crest and thus from the neuroectoderm. They share a key histologic characteristic with the adrenal medulla, which also arises from the neural crest: so-called "chromaffin cells" (see C). Chromaffin cells contains granules (chromaffin granules) in which catecholamines (adrenaline, norepinephrine, dopamine) are stored as hormones or neurotransmitters. If one histologically fixes such cells with chromic salts, the granules (and thus indirectly the cells) stain grayish brown. The histophysiologic term *chromaffin cell* is a synonym for *catecholamine-synthesizing cell*. As both the adrenal medulla and the paraganglia synthesize catecholamines and their cells contain chromaffin granules, both of them are histologically classified as belonging to the *chromaffin system*. Chromaffin cells arise in the embryo from a special neuroectodermal cell, the sympathoblast. Because of their embryonal relationship and their common histochemical characteristics, the adrenal medulla is generally understood to be a special form of paraganglia, although the literature is not consistent in this regard.

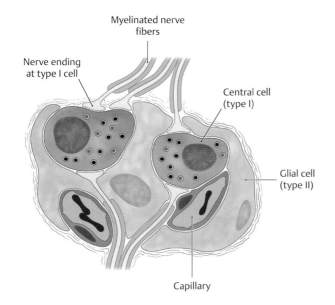

Myelinated nerve fibers

Nerve ending at type I cell

Central cell (type I)

Glial cell (type II)

Capillary

C Structure of the paraganglia

Schematic diagram of a glomus body. Paraganglia contain at least two types of cells:

- *Central cells* = type I cells (brown): They store catecholamines (especially dopamine), serotonin, and enkephalins in small granules and secrete the *neurotransmitter* dopamine. Functionally, they are the true chemosensors and morphologically they are the *chromaffin cells.* As *secondary* sensory cells, they have no axons but directly contact the afferent fibers of the glossopharyngeal or vagus nerves.
- *Glial cells* = type II cell (blue): They envelop the type I cells and are regarded as part of the peripheral glia. They are not chemosensitive but are thought to aid in signal transmission from the central cell to the nerve cell.
- Glomus bodies contain numerous sensory nerve endings (yellow) of the glossopharyngeal and vagus nerves and are connected via the *ganglion inferius nervi glossopharyngei (glomus caroticum)* or the *vagus nerve (glomus aorticum)* to the *nucleus tractus solitarii* which in turn projects onto neurons of the respiratory center of the medulla oblongata (see D). Glomus bodies are highly vascularized with a *fenestrated* epithelium. Their relative perfusion is 25 times as high as that of the brain. This extreme perfusion ensures that representative quantities of blood can continuously be evaluated for their O_2 and CO_2 content.

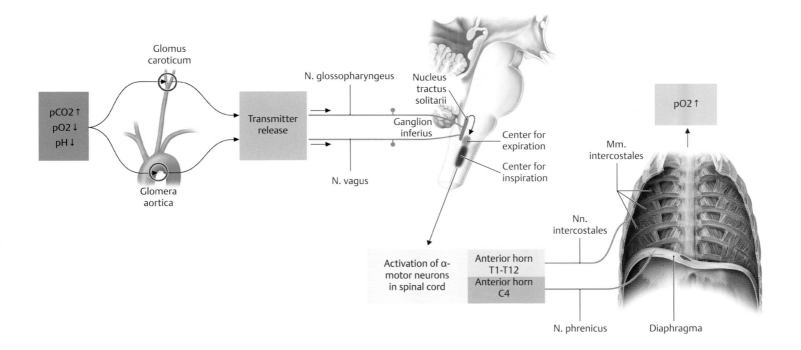

Glomus caroticum

N. glossopharyngeus

Nucleus tractus solitarii

pO2 ↑

pCO2 ↑
pO2 ↓
pH ↓

Transmitter release

Ganglion inferius

Center for expiration

Mm. intercostales

Center for inspiration

N. vagus

Glomera aortica

Nn. intercostales

Activation of α-motor neurons in spinal cord

Anterior horn T1-T12

Anterior horn C4

N. phrenicus

Diaphragma

D Functional synopsis of the glomus bodies

Type I cells detect a drop in intra-arterial O_2 partial pressure (actual value is below target value), a drop in the pH value, or an increase in intra-arterial CO_2 partial pressure. They then release the neurotransmitter dopamine from their granules. Afferent fibers of the n. glossopharyngeus (glomus caroticum) or the n. vagus (glomera aortica) project via the ganglion inferius of the respective cranial nerves to the nucleus tractus solitarii which in turn activates respiratory centers in the medulla oblongata. These act on α-motor neurons in the spinal cord. The respiratory musculature is activated via the nn. phrenici. The increased respiratory activity then leads to an increase in O_2 partial pressure and a decrease in CO_2 partial pressure.

Retroperitoneal paraganglia in the embryo stimulate the circulatory system because it is not possible to increase respiration in an embryo (see **A**). Little is known about the function of the retroperitoneal paraganglia in the fully developed body.

Clinical note: Similar to the adrenal medulla, tumors can also arise from the paraganglia (*pheochromocytomas or paragangliomas*). Their spontaneous release of catecholamines can lead to episodic blood pressure crises. The clinical course of such tumors in children is usually unfavorable. It is also thought that spontaneously occurring "incorrect readings" of the oxygen content of the blood reported by the glomus bodies can lead to a sensation of asphyxiation and panic attacks.

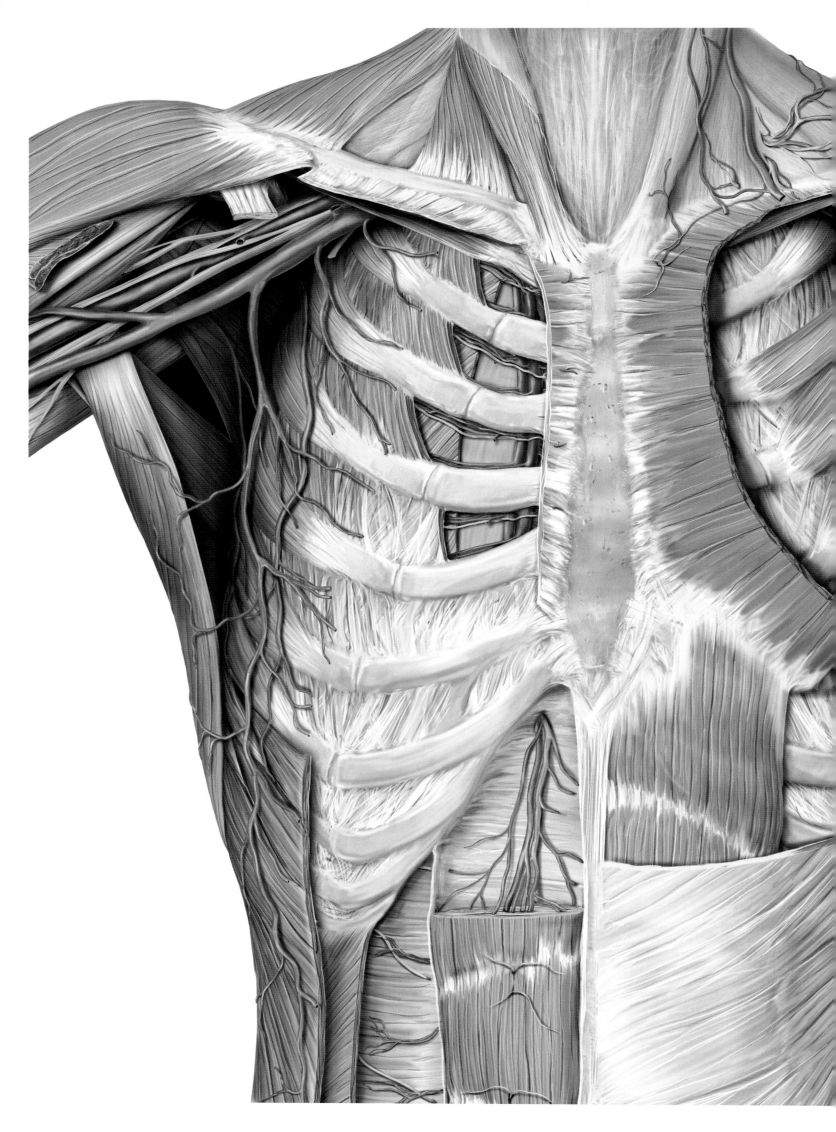

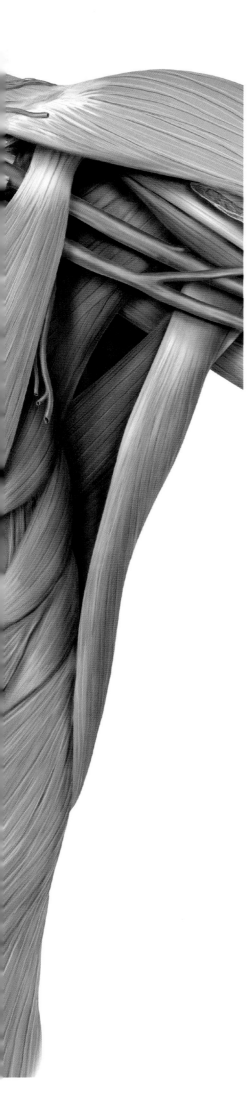

B Thorax

1.1 Divisions of the Cavitas Thoracica and Mediastinum

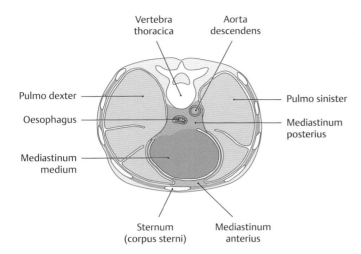

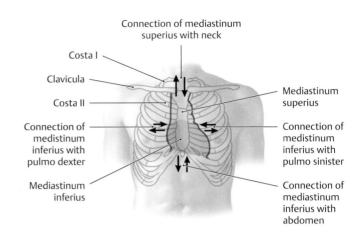

A Divisions of the cavitas thoracica and mediastinum
Transverse section, superior view.
The cavitas thoracica is divided into three large spaces:

- The **mediastinum**, in the midline, is divided into an upper, smaller *mediastinum superius* and a lower, larger *mediastinum inferius* (see **B**). The mediastinum inferius is further subdivided, from front to back, into the *mediastinum anterius, medium,* and *posterius*. The mediastinum anterius is an extremely narrow space between the sternum and pericardium, containing only small vascular components (see table, **C**).
- The **paired cavitates pleurales** on the left and right sides of the mediastinum are lined by tunica serosa (pleura parietalis) and contain the pulmones sinister and dexter. They are completely separated from each other by the mediastinum. The mediastinum extends further to the left than to the right owing to the asymmetrical position of the cor and pericardium. Because of this, the cavitas pleuralis (and pulmo) is smaller on the left side than on the right. The cavitates pleurales terminate blindly at their upper end, but the mediastinum is continuous with the connective tissue of the neck.

B Principal neurovascular structures that enter and leave the mediastinum

Mediastinum superius (borders the neck, yellow):
- The nn. vagus and phrenicus, veins (tributaries of the v. cava superior), oesophagus, and trachea enter the mediastinum superius from the neck.
- Arterial branches from the arcus aortae and the cervical part of the truncus sympathicus leave the mediastinum superius to enter the neck.

Mediastinum inferius (borders the abdomen and cavitates pleurales, red):
- The ductus thoracicus and ascending abdominal lumbar veins (the v. azygos on the right side, the v. hemiazygos on the left side) pass through the diaphragma to enter the mediastinum inferius.
- The nn. vagus and phrenicus, portions of the pars sympathica of the nervous system, the aorta, and the oesophagus descend from the mediastinum inferius and pass through the diaphragma to enter the abdomen.

Aa. and vv. pulmonales, vasa lymphatica, autonomic nerves (plexus pulmonalis), and the bronchi principales connect the mediastinum to the pulmones (and vice versa).

C Contents of the mediastinum (for divisions see **A**)

	Mediastinum superius	**Mediastinum inferius**		
		Mediastinum anterius	*Mediastinum medium*	*Mediastinum posterius*
Organs	• Thymus • Trachea • Oesophagus	• Thymus (in children)	• Cor • Pericardium	• Oesophagus
Arteries	• Arcus aortae • Truncus brachiocephalicus • Left a. carotis communis • Left a. subclavia	• Smaller arteries	• Pars ascendens aortae • Truncus pulmonalis and its branches • Aa. pericardiacophrenicae	• Pars thoracica aortae and its branches
Veins and vasa lymphatica	• V. cava superior • Vv. brachiocephalicae • V. hemizygos accessoria • Ductus thoracicus	• Smaller veins and vasa lymphatica • Smaller nodi lymphoidei	• v. cava inferior • V. azygos • Vv. pulmonales • Vv. pericardiacophrenicae	• V. azygos • V. hemiazygos • Ductus thoracicus
Nerves	• Nn. vagi • Left n. laryngeus recurrens • Nn. cardiaci • Nn. phrenici	–	• Nn. phrenici	• Nn. vagi • Truncus sympathicus

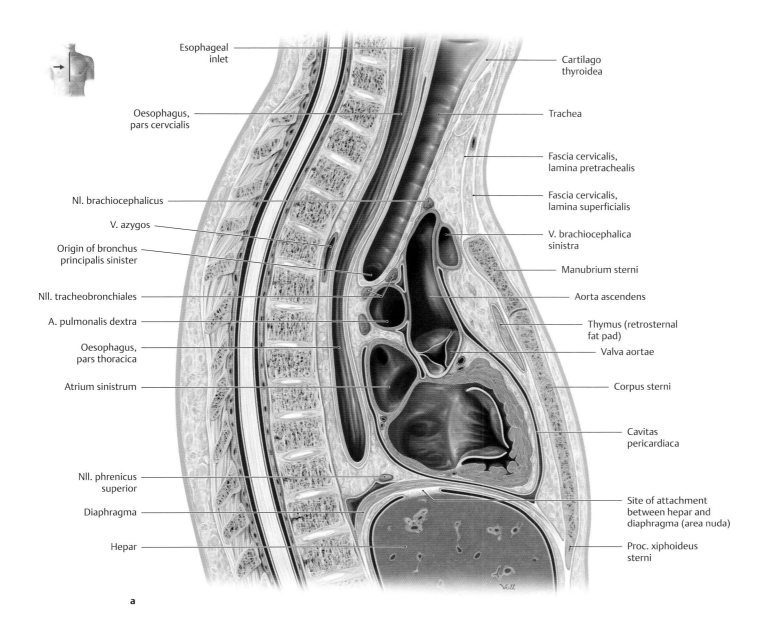

Esophageal inlet

Oesophagus, pars cervcialis

Nl. brachiocephalicus

V. azygos

Origin of bronchus principalis sinister

Nll. tracheobronchiales

A. pulmonalis dextra

Oesophagus, pars thoracica

Atrium sinistrum

Nll. phrenicus superior

Diaphragma

Hepar

Cartilago thyroidea

Trachea

Fascia cervicalis, lamina pretrachealis

Fascia cervicalis, lamina superficialis

V. brachiocephalica sinistra

Manubrium sterni

Aorta ascendens

Thymus (retrosternal fat pad)

Valva aortae

Corpus sterni

Cavitas pericardiaca

Site of attachment between hepar and diaphragma (area nuda)

Proc. xiphoideus sterni

a

D Subdivisions of the mediastinum
Midsagittal sections viewed from the right side.

a Detailed view: simplified drawing of the pericardium, cor, trachea, and oesophagus in midsagittal section. This lateral view demonstrates how the atrium sinistrum of the cor narrows the mediastinum posterius and abuts the anterior wall of the oesophagus. Because of this proximity, abnormal enlargement of the atrium sinistrum may cause narrowing of the esophageal lumen that is detectable by radiographic examination with oral contrast medium. Radiologists call the area between the images of the cor and columna vertebralis the *retrocardiac space*.

b Schematic view: subdivisions of the mediastinum (described in **A,** with contents listed in **C**).

Note: Single diagrams cannot adequately show the components and configuration of the mediastinum, because of its asymmetry and extensions in all three axes. The anatomical relations in this space are best appreciated when viewed from multiple directions, at different planes (see also pp. 190ff).

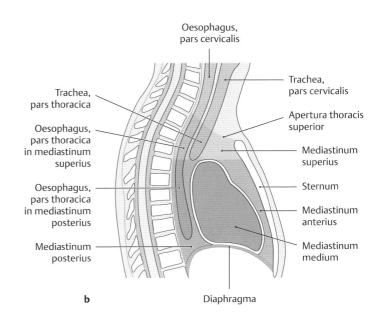

Oesophagus, pars cervicalis

Trachea, pars thoracica

Oesophagus, pars thoracica in mediastinum superius

Oesophagus, pars thoracica in mediastinum posterius

Mediastinum posterius

Trachea, pars cervicalis

Apertura thoracis superior

Mediastinum superius

Sternum

Mediastinum anterius

Mediastinum medium

Diaphragma

b

1.2 Diaphragma: Location and Projection onto the Trunk

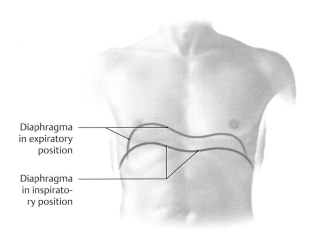

Diaphragma in expiratory position

Diaphragma in inspiratory position

A Projection of the diaphragma onto the trunk

Anterior view. The positions of the diaphragma in expiration (blue) and inspiration (red) are shown. The right hemidiaphragm rises as high as the fourth rib during expiration, and the diaphragma may fall almost to the level of the seventh rib at full inspiration.

Note:

- The exact position of the diaphragma depends on body type, sex, and age.
- The left diaphragma leaflet is lower than the right due to the asymmetrical position of the cor.
- Inspiration is marked by an overall depression of the diaphragma and also by a flattening of the diaphragm leaflets.
- The diaphragma is higher in the supine position (pressure from the intra-abdominal organs) than in the standing position.
- The degree of diaphragmatic movement during inspiration can be assessed by noting the movement of the hepatic border, which is easily palpated.
- The diaphragma in a cadaver occupies a higher level than the expiratory position in vivo due to the loss of muscular tone.

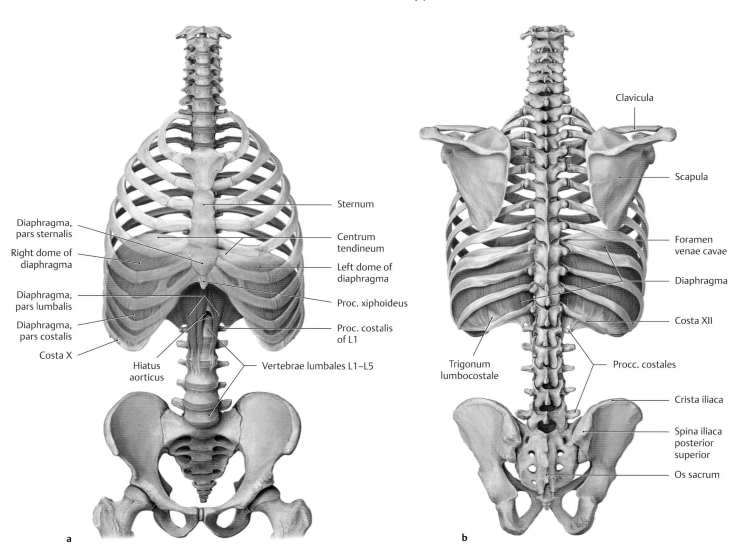

a

b

B Anterior (a) and posterior (b) views of the diaphragm

In **a**, the *anterior* rib segments in front of the diaphragma are shown transparent to demonstrate the location of the diaphragma; in **b** the *posterior* rib segments are not shown transparent.

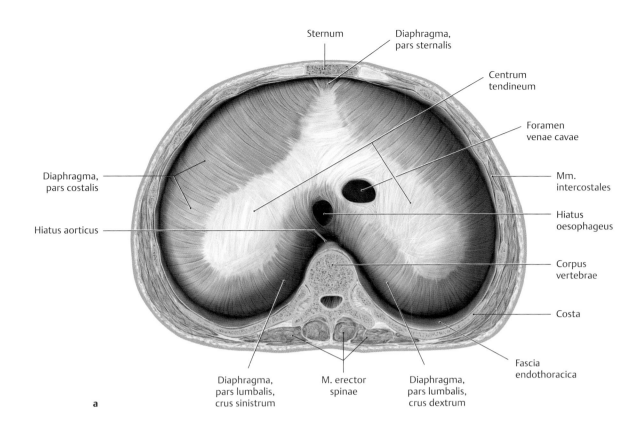

Sternum
Diaphragma, pars sternalis
Centrum tendineum
Foramen venae cavae
Mm. intercostales
Hiatus oesophageus
Corpus vertebrae
Costa
Fascia endothoracica
Diaphragma, pars costalis
Hiatus aorticus
Diaphragma, pars lumbalis, crus sinistrum
M. erector spinae
Diaphragma, pars lumbalis, crus dextrum

a

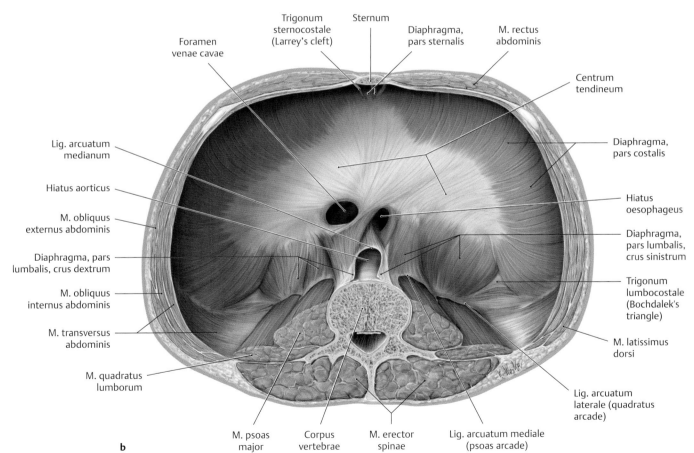

Trigonum sternocostale (Larrey's cleft)
Sternum
Diaphragma, pars sternalis
M. rectus abdominis
Foramen venae cavae
Centrum tendineum
Diaphragma, pars costalis
Lig. arcuatum medianum
Hiatus aorticus
Hiatus oesophageus
M. obliquus externus abdominis
Diaphragma, pars lumbalis, crus sinistrum
Diaphragma, pars lumbalis, crus dextrum
Trigonum lumbocostale (Bochdalek's triangle)
M. obliquus internus abdominis
M. transversus abdominis
M. latissimus dorsi
M. quadratus lumborum
Lig. arcuatum laterale (quadratus arcade)
M. psoas major
Corpus vertebrae
M. erector spinae
Lig. arcuatum mediale (psoas arcade)

b

C Superior (a) and inferior (b) views of the diaphragma
Fascias and serous membranes lining the superior and inferior surfaces of the diaphragma have been removed.

The muscular diaphragma closes the apertura thoracis inferior. It completely separates the cavitates thoracis and abdominis and has three openings for the oesophagus, aorta, and v. cava inferior.

1.3 Diaphragma: Structure and Main Openings

A Shape and structure of the diaphragma
a Inferior view; **b** Frontal section of the diaphragma, anterior view; **c** Midsagittal section with diaphragma in intermediate position.
The diaphragma is divided into three parts (**a**): pars costalis diaphragmatis (slate blue), pars lumbalis diaphragmatis (yellow green) and pars sternalis diaphragmatis (brown). For details about the origin of these three parts see **C**. For details about the location of the openings in the diaphragma see next page. Sections (**b** and **c**) show the location of the diaphragma between the cavitates thoracica and abdominis and illustrate the diaphragma's distinct dome-shaped structure: Recesses along the sides (**b**) and anterior and posterior margins (**c**) of the diaphragma vary in depth (Recesses, see p. 144 and 183). Flattening of the diaphragmatic domes and recesses play a central role in respiratory mechanics.

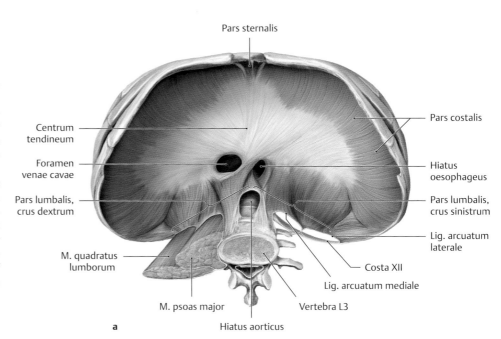

Pars sternalis

Centrum tendineum

Foramen venae cavae

Pars lumbalis, crus dextrum

M. quadratus lumborum

M. psoas major

Hiatus aorticus

Pars costalis

Hiatus oesophageus

Pars lumbalis, crus sinistrum

Lig. arcuatum laterale

Costa XII

Lig. arcuatum mediale

Vertebra L3

a

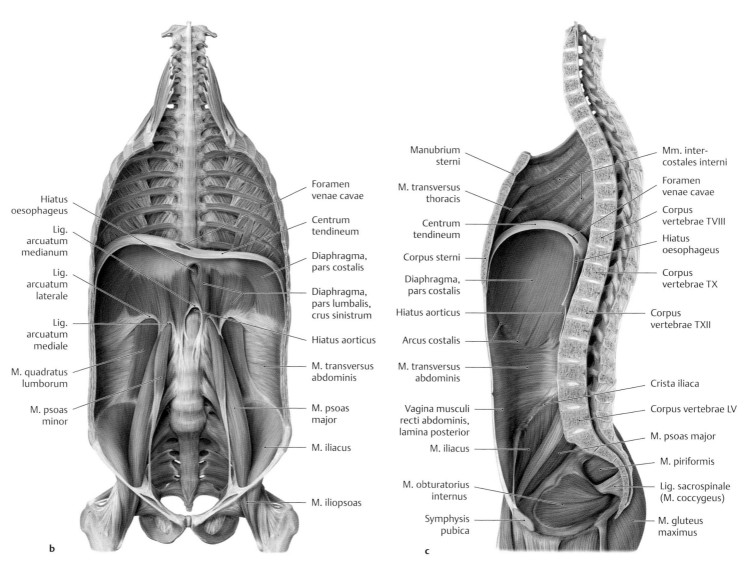

b

Hiatus oesophageus

Lig. arcuatum medianum

Lig. arcuatum laterale

Lig. arcuatum mediale

M. quadratus lumborum

M. psoas minor

Foramen venae cavae

Centrum tendineum

Diaphragma, pars costalis

Diaphragma, pars lumbalis, crus sinistrum

Hiatus aorticus

M. transversus abdominis

M. psoas major

M. iliacus

M. iliopsoas

c

Manubrium sterni

M. transversus thoracis

Centrum tendineum

Corpus sterni

Diaphragma, pars costalis

Hiatus aorticus

Arcus costalis

M. transversus abdominis

Vagina musculi recti abdominis, lamina posterior

M. iliacus

M. obturatorius internus

Symphysis pubica

Mm. intercostales interni

Foramen venae cavae

Corpus vertebrae TVIII

Hiatus oesophageus

Corpus vertebrae TX

Corpus vertebrae TXII

Crista iliaca

Corpus vertebrae LV

M. psoas major

M. piriformis

Lig. sacrospinale (M. coccygeus)

M. gluteus maximus

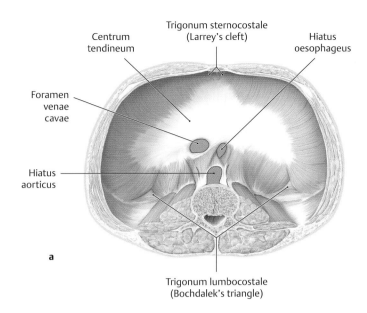

Trigonum sternocostale
(Larrey's cleft)

Centrum
tendineum

Hiatus
oesophageus

Foramen
venae
cavae

Hiatus
aorticus

a

Trigonum lumbocostale
(Bochdalek's triangle)

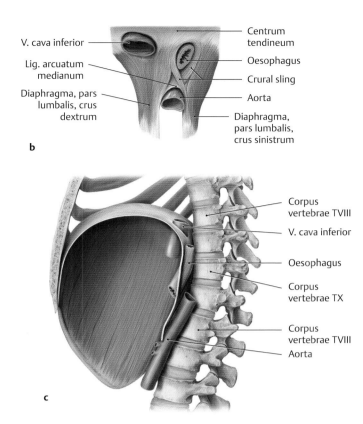

V. cava inferior

Centrum
tendineum

Lig. arcuatum
medianum

Oesophagus

Crural sling

Diaphragma, pars
lumbalis, crus
dextrum

Aorta

Diaphragma,
pars lumbalis,
crus sinistrum

b

Corpus
vertebrae TVIII

V. cava inferior

Oesophagus

Corpus
vertebrae TX

Corpus
vertebrae TVIII

Aorta

c

B Openings and gaps in the diaphragma and their clinical significance

a Inferior view; **b** Anterior view of the pars lumbalis diaphragmatis and portion of the centrum tendineum; location of the openings in the different parts of the diaphragma and their position relative to the median plane: foramen venae cavae in the centrum tendineum, to the right of the median plane; hiatus aorticus and hiatus oesophageus in the pars lumbalis, in or immediately to the left of the median plane; **c** Opened thorax viewed from the left side; projections of the openings onto the lower thoracic spine: foramen venae cavae: TVIII; hiatus oesophageus: TX; hiatus aorticus: TXII; **c** Diaphragma in resting expiratory position. Openings and gaps in the diaphragma develop

- because the oesophagus and large neurovascular structures pass through the muscle tissue and centrum tendineum of the diaphragma and extend from the thorax to abdomen or vice versa (*functional openings*, see above) and

- because gaps between the different parts of the diaphragma are closed only by connective tissue (e.g., apertures in the crus mediale that allow passage of neurovascular structures [nn. splanchnici; vv. lumbales ascendentes]).

The larger openings are clinically important because they create weak spots through which abdominal organs may herniate into the thorax (visceral or diaphragmatic hernias). The most common site for herniation is the hiatus oesophageus (hiatal hernias) which accounts for 90% of cases. Most hiatal hernias occur when the distal end of the oesophagus and the pars cardiaca of the gaster slide up into the thorax through the hiatus oesophageus (axial hiatal hernia; approximately 85% of all hiatal hernias). Typical complaints range from heartburn, belching, and pressure behind the sternum to nausea, vomiting, shortness of breath, and functional heart problems.

C Overview of the diaphragma

Origin:	• Pars costalis: inferior border of the ribs (inner surface of ribs 7 through 12)
	• Pars lumbalis (including crura dextrum and sinistrum):
	  – medial part: corpora vertebrarum LI–LIII and disci intervertebrales, lig. longitudinale anterius
	  – lateral parts: lig. arcuatum mediale (from corpus vertebrae LII to the respective processus transversus); lig. arcuatum laterale (from the processus transversus of LII to the tip of the 12th rib)
	• Pars sternalis: posterior surface of the processus xiphoideus

Insertion:	Centrum tendineum
Function:	Principal muscle of inspiration (diaphragmatic or abdominal breathing); involved in regulating abdominal pressure
Innervation:	N. phrenicus from the plexus cervicalis (C3–5)

D Openings in the diaphragma and transmitted structures

Openings	Transmitted structures
Foramen venae cavae (at the level of the TVIII vertebra)	V. cava inferior R. phrenicoabdominalis of right n. phrenicus (the left r. phrenicoabdominalis pierces the muscle)
Hiatus oesophageus (at the level of the TX vertebra)	Oesophagus Trunci vagales anterior and posterior (on the oesophagus)
Hiatus aorticus (at the level of the TXII/LI vertebrae)	Pars descendens aortae Ductus thoracicus
Apertures in the crus mediale	V. azygos, v. hemiazygos, nn. splanchnici major et minor
Apertures between the medial and lateral crura	Truncus sympathicus, n. splanchnicus minor (common variant)
Trigonum sternocostale	A. and v. thoracica interna/ epigastrica superior

83

1.4 Diaphragma: Innervation, Blood and Lymphatic Vessels

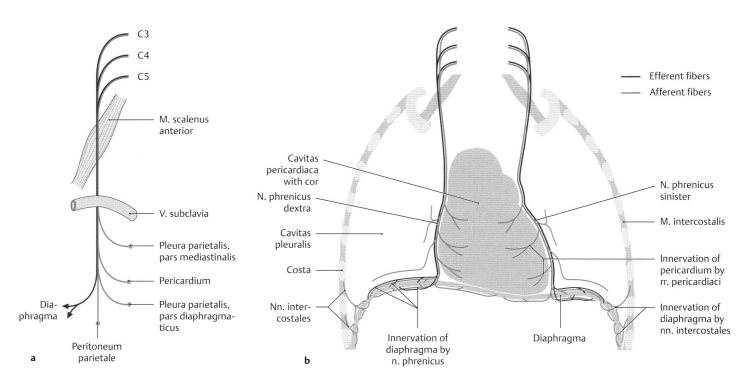

A Innervation

The diaphragma is largely innervated by the n. phrenicus, a somato-motor and somatosensory nerve that arises from the plexus cervicalis, specifically segmenta cervicalia C3–C5 medullae spinalis (mainly C4, see **a**). The n. phrenicus descends while giving off branches to the pars mediastinalis pleurae parietalis and the pericardium (rr. pericardiaci, see **b**). It contains more efferent (motor) than afferent (sensory) fibers; the latter being responsible for pain conduction from the tunicae serosae (pars diaphragmatica pleurae parietalis and peritoneum parietale) that cover the diaphragma. A r. phrenicoabdominalis passes through the diaphragma to the peritoneum on its inferior surface. The tunicae serosae covering the diaphragma near the ribs also receive somatosensory innervation from the tenth and eleventh nn. intercostales (see **b**) and from the n. subcostalis (T12, not shown). Occasionally, a n. phrenicus accessorius (not shown here) is observed as fibers from C5 (C6) join with the n. phrenicus via the n. subclavius. Similar to other blood vessels, those of the diaphragma receive an autonomic innervation.

Note: Bilateral disruption of the n. phrenicus (e.g., due to a high transection of the cervical medulla spinalis) leads to bilateral paralysis of the diaphragma. Because the diaphragma is the dominant muscle of respiration, bilateral diaphragmatic paralysis is usually fatal.

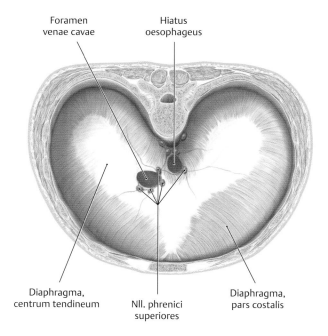

B Nodi lymphoidei and lymphatic drainage of the diaphragma

Superior view. The nodi lymphoidei of the diaphragma are divided into two groups based on their location:

• Nodi phrenici superiores on the superior surface of the diaphragma
• Nodi phrenici inferiores on the inferior surface of the diaphragma.

The **nodi phrenici superiores** are nodi lymphoidei *thoracis* that collect lymph from the diaphragma, lower oesophagus (see p. 172), pulmo, and also from the hepar (by a transdiaphragmatic route, see p. 91). The nodi phrenici superiores on the right side are involved in hepatic drainage. The nodi phrenici superiores drain to the truncus bronchomediastinalis. The **nodi phrenici inferiores** are nodi lymphoidei *abdominis*; they collect lymph from the diaphragma and usually convey it to a truncus lumbalis (see p. 223). They may also collect lymph from the lobi inferiores of the pulmones.

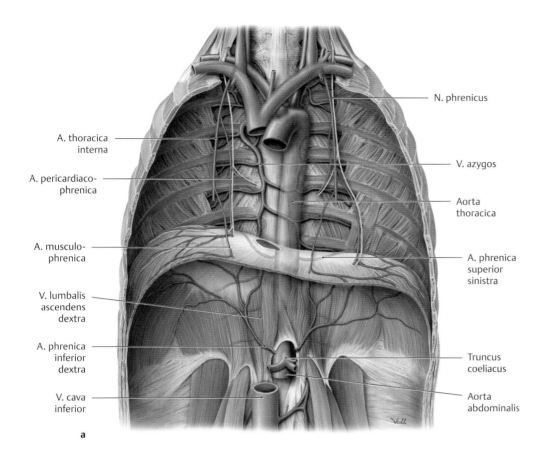

A. thoracica interna

A. pericardiaco-phrenica

A. musculo-phrenica

V. lumbalis ascendens dextra

A. phrenica inferior dextra

V. cava inferior

N. phrenicus

V. azygos

Aorta thoracica

A. phrenica superior sinistra

Truncus coeliacus

Aorta abdominalis

a

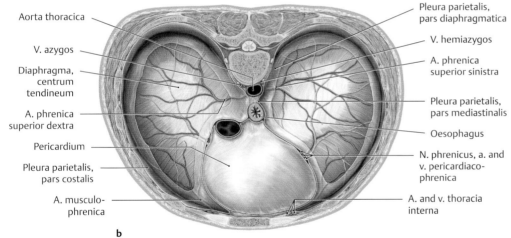

Aorta thoracica

V. azygos

Diaphragma, centrum tendineum

A. phrenica superior dextra

Pericardium

Pleura parietalis, pars costalis

A. musculo-phrenica

Pleura parietalis, pars diaphragmatica

V. hemiazygos

A. phrenica superior sinistra

Pleura parietalis, pars mediastinalis

Oesophagus

N. phrenicus, a. and v. pericardiaco-phrenica

A. and v. thoracica interna

b

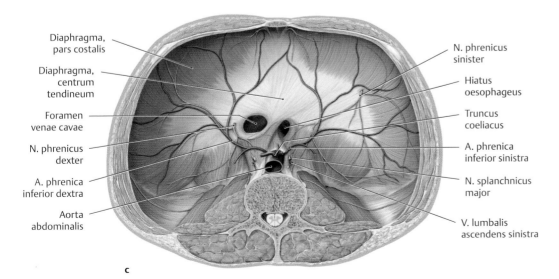

Diaphragma, pars costalis

Diaphragma, centrum tendineum

Foramen venae cavae

N. phrenicus dexter

A. phrenica inferior dextra

Aorta abdominalis

N. phrenicus sinister

Hiatus oesophageus

Truncus coeliacus

A. phrenica inferior sinistra

N. splanchnicus major

V. lumbalis ascendens sinistra

c

C Arteries of the diaphragma

a Anterior view of the opened thorax; organs, internal fascias and tunicae serosae have been removed. The n. phrenicus (for more details see p. 99) along with the a. pericardiacophrenica run lateral to the pericardium, which has been removed here. The long course of the a. pericardiacophrenica through the entire mediastinum is clearly visible.

b Superior surface of the diaphragma viewed from above. The pleura parietalis (pars diaphragmatica) has been removed over a broad area, leaving the pericardium in place. Three (pairs of) arteries supply the superior surface of the diaphragma:

- A. phrenica superior: arises from the aorta thoracica just above the diaphragma and supplies the largest area of the diaphragma.
- A. pericardiacophrenica: arises from the a. thoracica interna, runs close to the pericardium, and gives off branches to the diaphragma.
- A. thoracica interna: supplies the diaphragma by direct branches or via the a. musculophrenica.

c Inferior surface of the diaphragma viewed from below. The peritoneum parietale has been completely removed. The inferior surface of the diaphragma is supplied by the paired aa. phrenicae inferiores, the highest branches of the aorta abdominalis.

The **diaphragmatic veins** (not shown here) mainly accompany the arteries:

- Vv. phrenicae inferiores: open into the v. cava inferior.
- Vv. phrenicae superiores: usually open into the v. azygos on the right side and into the v. hemiazygos on the left side.

85

2.1 Arteries: Aorta Thoracica

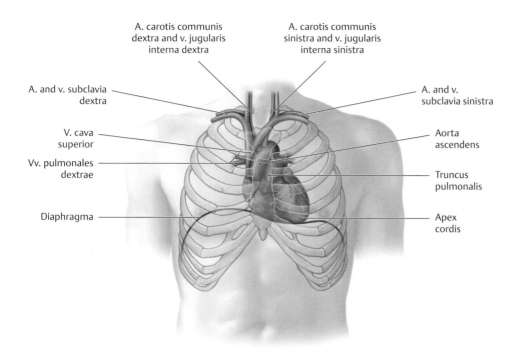

A. carotis communis dextra and v. jugularis interna dextra

A. carotis communis sinistra and v. jugularis interna sinistra

A. and v. subclavia dextra

A. and v. subclavia sinistra

V. cava superior

Aorta ascendens

Vv. pulmonales dextrae

Truncus pulmonalis

Diaphragma

Apex cordis

A Projection of the cor and vessels onto the chest wall

Anterior view. The two great arterial vessels in the thorax are the *aorta* and the *truncus pulmonalis*. Because the aa. pulmonales run a very short distance before entering the pulmones, they are discussed under the heading of the pulmonary vessels (see p. 150f).

The aorta *ascendens* is "in the shadow" of the sternum on the PA chest radiograph, while the arcus aortae ("aortic knob") forms the superior left portion of the left heart border. The aorta descendens is hidden by the cor itself.

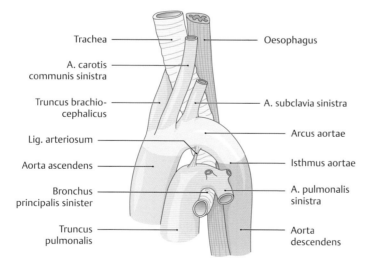

Trachea

Oesophagus

A. carotis communis sinistra

Truncus brachio-cephalicus

A. subclavia sinistra

Lig. arteriosum

Arcus aortae

Aorta ascendens

Isthmus aortae

Bronchus principalis sinister

A. pulmonalis sinistra

Truncus pulmonalis

Aorta descendens

B Parts of the aorta and their relationship to the trachea and oesophagus

Left lateral view. The aorta consists of three main parts:

- Aorta ascendens: arises from the ventriculus sinister, is dilated near the cor to form the bulbus aortae (not visible here).
- Arcus aortae: the arched portion of the aorta between the partes ascendens and

descendens, runs posteriorly and to the left. A constriction may persist as an embryonic remnant in this part of the aorta (the isthmus aortae, see p. 198).

- Aorta descendens: consists of the partes thoracica and abdominalis of the aorta (see **D**).

C Functional groups of arteries that supply the thoracic organs

These are mainly vessels that supply the *organs and internal structures* of the thorax. The intrathoracic branches of the aorta can be divided into four main functional groups:

Arteries to the head and neck or to the upper limb:

- Truncus brachiocephalicus with
  - Right a. carotis communis
  - Right a. subclavia
- A. thyroidea ima (present in only 10% of the population)
- Left a. carotis communis
- Left a. subclavia

Direct aortic branches that supply intrathoracic structures:

- Visceral branches to thoracic organs (cor, trachea, bronchi, and oesophagus):
  - Aa. coronariae dextra and sinistra
  - Rr. tracheales
  - Rr. pericardiaci
  - Rr. bronchiales
  - Rr. oesophageales
- Parietal branches to the internal (mainly posterolateral) chest wall and diaphragma:
  - Aa. intercostales posteriores
  - Right and left aa. phrenicae superiores

Indirect paired branches (not arising directly from the aorta) that are distributed primarily to the head and neck but give off branches, usually small, that enter the chest and supply intrathoracic organs:

- A. thyroidea inferior (from the truncus thyrocervicalis = branch of a. subclavia) with
  - Rr. oesophageales
  - Rr. tracheales

Indirect paired branches which supply the chest wall (mostly anterior, some inferior), usually in the form of parietal branches, and may give off other branches to intrathoracic organs (visceral sub-branches):

- A. thoracica interna (from the a. subclavia) with
  - Rr. thymici
  - Rr. mediastinales
  - Rr. intercostales anteriores
  - A. pericardiacophrenica (with branches to the pericardium and diaphragma)
  - A. musculophrenica (with a branch to the diaphragma)

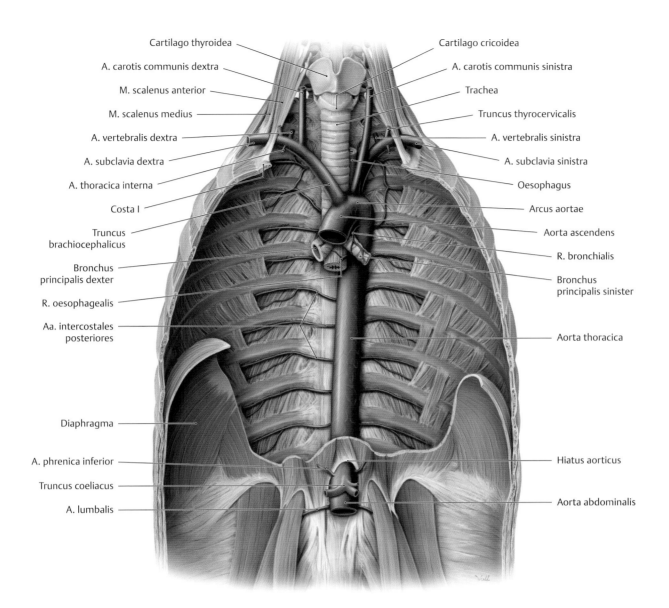

D Position of the aorta in the thorax

Anterior view. The pleura, internal fasciae, and most thoracic organs have been removed, and the diaphragma has been windowed to display more of the cavitas thoracis. The branches of the aorta (see **C** and p. 211) supply blood to all the organs, delivering almost 5 liters of blood per minute throughout the body. The aorta thoracica is thick-walled, particularly in its pars ascendens and arcus aortae, but these walls are also elastic. During the systolic wave of pressure as the ventriculus sinister contracts, these segments of the aorta dilate rapidly and then recoil. This serves to absorb and dissipate the pressure wave to produce a steadier, more even flow of blood in the arteries farther away from the cor. Because the arcus aortae runs posteriorly and to the left, the relationship of the aorta to the trachea and oesophagus changes as the vessel passes inferiorly through the chest (see also **B** and p. 170). The most anterior part of the aorta is the *aorta ascendens*. The *arcus aortae* then passes to the left side of the trachea, arching over the bronchus principalis sinister. It passes initially to the left of the oesophagus but then descends *posterior* to the oesophagus and anterior to the columna vertebralis. Because of this relationship, an abnormal outpouching of the aortic wall (aneurysm) may narrow the oesophagus and cause swallowing difficulties (dysphagia). The pars thoracica aortae pierces the diaphragma at the hiatus aorticus (junction of the T11/T12 vertebrae), becoming the aorta abdominalis.

Note: In rare cases the arcus aortae is constricted behind the lig. arteriosum (see **B**). This constriction is normal in the embryonic circulation, but its persistence after birth may produce the clinical manifestations of a *coarctation of the aorta*. This includes hypertension in the head, neck, and upper limbs, insufficient blood flow in the lower extremities, and left ventricular hypertrophy (due to chronic excessive workload and pressure) (see p.198f).

E Aortic Windkessel function

a During systole, part of the ventricular stroke volume is stored in the elastic wall of the aorta (blue arrows pointing outward) and discharged again during diastole (**b**) (blue arrows pointing inward).

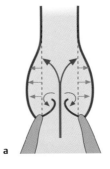
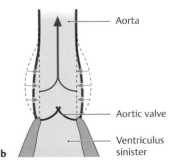

2.2   Veins: Vena Cava and Azygos System

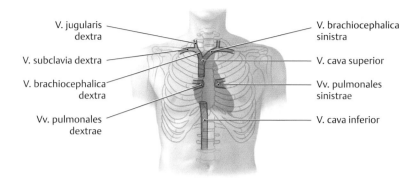

V. jugularis dextra
V. subclavia dextra
V. brachiocephalica dextra
Vv. pulmonales dextrae

V. brachiocephalica sinistra
V. cava superior
Vv. pulmonales sinistrae
V. cava inferior

C Functional groups of veins that drain the thoracic organs

These are mainly vessels that drain the *organs and internal structures* of the thorax. All of them drain ultimately to the v. cava superior, whose tributaries in the chest can be divided into four main functional groups:

Veins that drain the head and neck or the upper limb:

- Left and right vv. brachiocephalicae with
  – Right and left vv. subclaviae
  – Right and left vv. jugulares internae
  – Right and left vv. jugulares externae
  – Vv. intercostales supremae
  – Vv. pericardiacae
  – V. intercostalis superior sinistra

Veins that drain intrathoracic structures (open into the v. hemiazygos accessoria or v. hemiazygos on the left side, into the v. azygos on the right side). Blood from both territories is collected in the v. azygos, which empties into the v. cava superior. The tributaries can be grouped as follows:

- Visceral branches that drain the trachea, bronchi, and oesophagus:
  – Vv. tracheales
  – Vv. bronchiales
  – Vv. oesophageales
- Parietal branches that drain the inner chest wall and diaphragm:
  – Vv. intercostales posteriores
  – Right and left vv. phrenicae superiores
  – V. intercostalis superior dextra

Indirect paired tributaries of the v. cava superior that descend from the head and neck but receive smaller veins that drain thoracic organs:

- V. thyroidea inferior (tributaries of the v. brachiocephalica) with
  – Vv. oesophageales
  – Vv. tracheales

Indirect paired tributaries of the v. cava superior that mainly drain the anterior chest wall as parietal branches but may also receive tributaries (visceral subbranches) from organs:

- Vv. thoracicae internae (opens into the v. brachiocephalica) with
  – Vv. thymicae
  – Vv. mediastinales
  – Vv. intercostales anteriores
  – Vv. pericardiacophrenicae (with tributaries from the pericardium and diaphragma)
  – Vv. musculophrenicae (with a tributary from the diaphragma)

Note: Structures of the mediastinum superius may also drain directly to the vv. brachiocephalicae (e.g., via the vv. tracheales, vv. oesophageales, and vv. mediastinales).

A Projection of the venae cavae onto the skeleton

Anterior view. The v. cava *superior* lies to the right of the midline and appears at the right sternal border on radiographs. Formed by the confluence of the two vv. brachiocephalicae, the v. cava superior enters the atrium dextrum of the cor from above, forming its border in the PA chest radiograph (see p. 110). The v. cava *inferior* runs a very short distance within the thorax (approximately 1 cm, not shown here). Immediately after piercing the diaphragma (at the foramen venae cavae), it passes through the pericardium and ends by opening into the atrium dextrum of the cor from below. It has no tributaries within the chest (the vv. pulmonales are described on p. 150f).

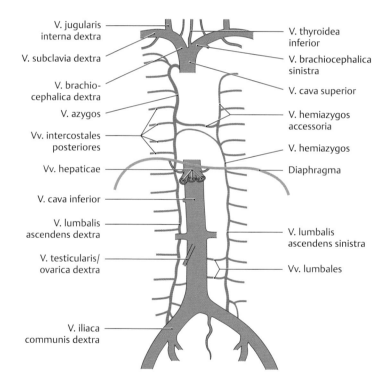

V. jugularis interna dextra
V. subclavia dextra
V. brachiocephalica dextra
V. azygos
Vv. intercostales posteriores
Vv. hepaticae
V. cava inferior
V. lumbalis ascendens dextra
V. testicularis/ ovarica dextra
V. iliaca communis dextra

V. thyroidea inferior
V. brachiocephalica sinistra
V. cava superior
V. hemiazygos accessoria
V. hemiazygos
Diaphragma
V. lumbalis ascendens sinistra
Vv. lumbales

B The azygos system

Anterior view. The venous drainage of the thorax is handled mainly by the long azygos system, which runs vertically through the chest. The *v. azygos* runs to the right of the columna vertebralis, the *v. hemiazygos* to the left. The v. hemiazygos empties into the v. azygos, which in turn empties into the v. cava superior. A *v. hemiazygos accessoria* is frequently present in the upper left thorax; it may open independently into the v. azygos or by way of the v. hemiazygos. The azygos system receives tributaries from the mediastinum and from portions of the chest wall, predominantly in the central and lower thorax.

Note: The v. azygos empties into the v. cava superior, while the vv. lumbales ascendentes on both sides open into the v. cava inferior via the vv. lumbales and the vv. iliacae communes. In this way the azygos system creates a shunt between the vv. cavae superior and inferior, called the "cavocaval anastomosis." If drainage from the v. cava inferior is obstructed, venous blood can still reach the v. cava superior and enter the right cor by passing through the azygos system (see **D** and p. 218).

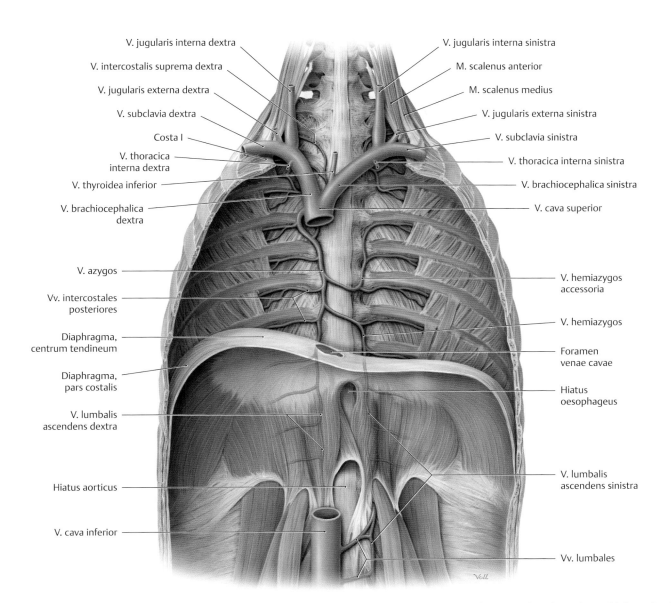

V. jugularis interna dextra

V. intercostalis suprema dextra

V. jugularis externa dextra

V. subclavia dextra

Costa I

V. thoracica interna dextra

V. thyroidea inferior

V. brachiocephalica dextra

V. azygos

Vv. intercostales posteriores

Diaphragma, centrum tendineum

Diaphragma, pars costalis

V. lumbalis ascendens dextra

Hiatus aorticus

V. cava inferior

V. jugularis interna sinistra

M. scalenus anterior

M. scalenus medius

V. jugularis externa sinistra

V. subclavia sinistra

V. thoracica interna sinistra

V. brachiocephalica sinistra

V. cava superior

V. hemiazygos accessoria

V. hemiazygos

Foramen venae cavae

Hiatus oesophageus

V. lumbalis ascendens sinistra

Vv. lumbales

D Vena cava superior and azygos system in the thorax
Anterior view. The thorax has been cut open and the organs, internal fasciae, and serous membranes have been removed. The v. cava inferior has been removed at the level of the L1/L2 vertebrae to display the right v. lumbalis ascendens. The **v. cava superior** is formed by the confluence of the two vv. brachiocephalicae at the approximate level of the T2/T3 junction, to the right of the median plane. Each v. brachiocephalica is formed in turn by the union of the v. jugularis interna and v. subclavia. The v. azygos ascends on the right side of the columna vertebralis and opens into the posterior right aspect of the v. cava superior just below the

union of the vv. brachiocephalicae. After the right and left vv. lumbales ascendentes pass through the diaphragma they form the **v. azygos** on the right side and the **v. hemiazygos** on the left side.
At the level of the T7 vertebra, the v. hemiazygos crosses over the columna vertebralis from the left side and opens into the v. azygos. In this dissection the v. hemiazygos accessoria drains separately into the v. azygos after crossing over the columna vertebralis from left to right. Not infrequently, however, the v. hemiazygos and v. hemiazygos accessoria are interconnected by anastomoses.

V. jugularis interna dextra

V. thyroidea inferior

V. jugularis interna sinistra

V. subclavia dextra

V. brachiocephalica dextra

Bronchus principalis

V. azygos

V. subclavia sinistra

V. brachiocephalica sinistra

Trachea

Bronchus principalis sinsister

V. hemiazygos accessoria

V. hemiazygos

E Relations of the trachea, vena cava superior, and azygos system
The v. cava superior lies to the right of the trachea. The left v. brachiocephalica passes anterior to the trachea from the left side to unite with the right v. brachiocephalica. The v. azygos ascends posterior to the bronchus principalis dexter and turns anteriorly to enter the v. cava superior from behind (the v. azygos "rides" upon the bronchus principalis dexter). The v. hemiazygos accessoria ascends behind the bronchus principalis sinister and may open independently into the v. azygos or may join the v. hemiazygos to form a common trunk that opens into the v. azygos.

2.3 Vasa Lymphatica

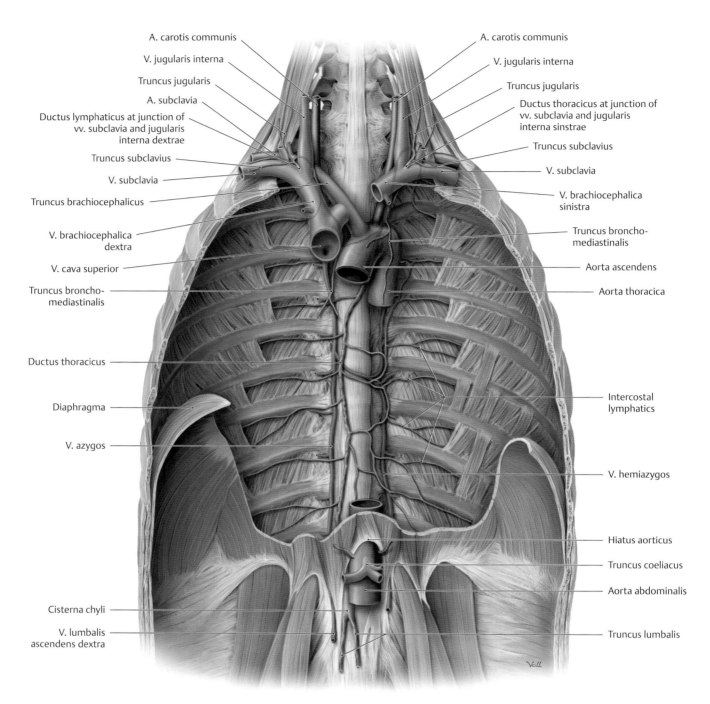

A. carotis communis

V. jugularis interna

Truncus jugularis

A. subclavia

Ductus lymphaticus at junction of vv. subclavia and jugularis interna dextrae

Truncus subclavius

V. subclavia

Truncus brachiocephalicus

V. brachiocephalica dextra

V. cava superior

Truncus broncho-mediastinalis

Ductus thoracicus

Diaphragma

V. azygos

Cisterna chyli

V. lumbalis ascendens dextra

A. carotis communis

V. jugularis interna

Truncus jugularis

Ductus thoracicus at junction of vv. subclavia and jugularis interna sinstrae

Truncus subclavius

V. subclavia

V. brachiocephalica sinistra

Truncus broncho-mediastinalis

Aorta ascendens

Aorta thoracica

Intercostal lymphatics

V. hemiazygos

Hiatus aorticus

Truncus coeliacus

Aorta abdominalis

Truncus lumbalis

A Trunci lymphatici in the thorax

Anterior view of the opened thorax with the pleura, internal fasciae, and organs removed. The diaphragma has been windowed, and the upper part of the abdomen can be seen. The principal trunks that convey lymph from all body regions to the venous system are the ductus thoracicus and ductus lymphaticus dexter. The **ductus thoracicus** begins in the abdomen at the upper end of a large sac, the cisterna chyli. It traverses the diaphragma through the hiatus aorticus, passing behind the aorta and in front of the columna vertebralis, and usually ascends just to the right of the midline. Just below the arcus aorticus it shifts to the left and terminates by opening into the junction of the left vv. subclavia and jugularis interna. It is joined in the neck by the *left truncus bronchomediastinalis, left truncus jugularis,* and *left truncus subclavius.* A number of small, unnamed lymphatic trunks that collect lymph from smaller groups of nodi lymphoidei convey lymph from the mediastinum and spatia intercostalia to the ductus thoracicus (lymph from the posterior portions of the lower right spatia intercostalia usually drains into the

ductus thoracicus rather than the short right truncus bronchomediastinalis). The **ductus lymphaticus dexter** is a short duct that receives the *right truncus bronchomediastinalis, right truncus jugularis,* and *right truncus subclavius* just before it opens into the junction of the right vv. subclavia and jugularis interna.

Note: All major trunci lymphatici pass through the cavitas thoracica. The intrathoracic pressure undergoes rhythmic variations with breathing, and these pressure changes are transmitted to the trunci lymphatici. These changes act mainly on the relatively large-caliber ductus thoracicus and have a significant impact on lymphatic return: the fall of intrathoracic pressure during inspiration causes a passive, transient swelling of the ductus thoracicus, which increases the flow of lymph through that vessel. This principle can be applied therapeutically in lymphedema patients by having the patient perform a slow, deep inhalation to create a sustained negative intrathoracic pressure that will promote lymphatic drainage.

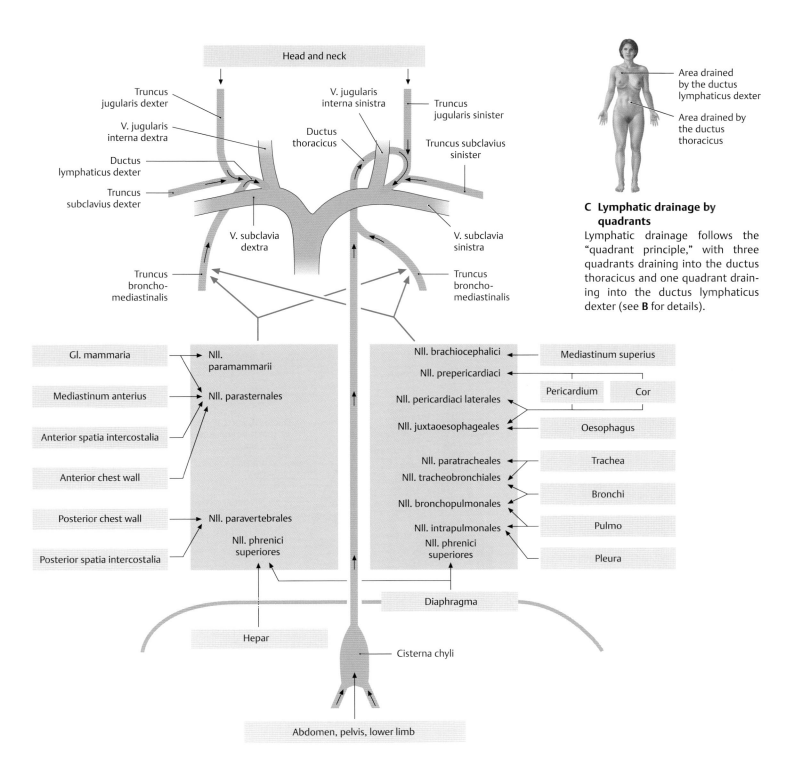

C Lymphatic drainage by quadrants

Lymphatic drainage follows the "quadrant principle," with three quadrants draining into the ductus thoracicus and one quadrant draining into the ductus lymphaticus dexter (see **B** for details).

B Overview of lymphatic pathways in the thorax

The lymph from all body regions is returned to the venous circulation at the junctions of the right and left vv. subclaviae and jugulares internae (sometimes called the right and left "venous angles"). The **ductus thoracicus** conveys lymph from the abdomen, pelvis, lower limb, left half of the thorax, left upper limb, and left half of the head and neck to the junction of the *left* vv. subclavia and jugularis interna (corresponding to three of the four quadrants shown in **C**). The **ductus lymphaticus dexter** is a short duct (only about 1 cm long) that conveys lymph from the right half of the thorax, portions of the hepar, the right upper limb, and the right half of the head and neck to the junction of the *right vv. subclavia* and jugularis interna (corresponding to one of the four quadrants).

Lymph from the posterior portions of the lower spatia intercostalia *on both sides* usually drains into the ductus thoracicus (see **A**). Both of the main trunks receive thoracic lymph from the **trunci bronchomediastinales sinister** and **dexter** and from smaller, unnamed trunks. The nodi lymphoidei (see p. 92) may be located close to the chest wall (e.g., the nll. parasternales, paramammarii, and prevertebrales), in the mediastinum (known clinically as the "mediastinal" nodi lymphoidei), or may be closely associated with the arbor bronchialis and named for their location. Overlapping patterns of lymphatic drainage are common in the chest due to the close topographical relationships of intrathoracic structures. Thus, for example, the nll. juxtaoesophageales collect lymph from the oesophagus *and* from the cor.

2.4 Nodi Lymphoidei Thoracis

A Overview of the nodi lymphoidei thoracis

Transverse section at the level of the bifurcatio tracheae (at approximately T4), viewed from above. Topographically, the nodi lymphoidei thoracis can be divided into three broad groups:

- Nodi lymphoidei in the chest wall (shown here in purple), which drain the chest wall.
- Nodi lymphoidei in the pulmo and at the divisions of the arbor bronchialis (nll. intrapulmonales and bronchopulmonales, shown here in blue). This group drains the pulmo and arbor bronchialis and conveys its lymph to the next group (see C and p. 91).
- Nodi lymphoidei associated with the central structures of the mediastinum (trachea, oesophagus, and pericardium, shown here in green).

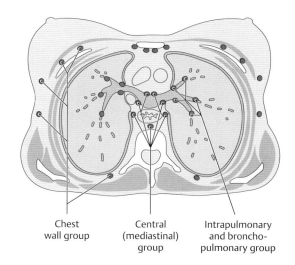

Chest wall group   Central (mediastinal) group   Intrapulmonary and broncho-pulmonary group

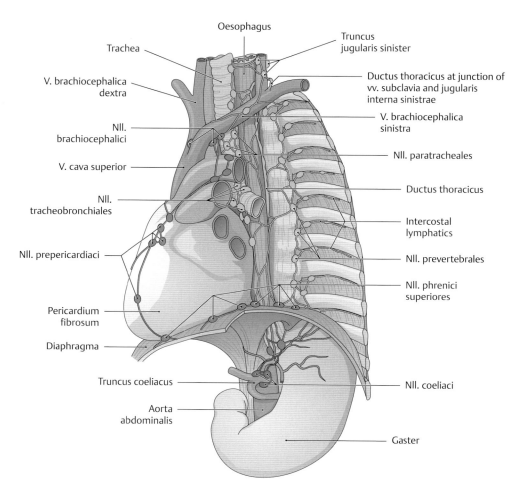

Oesophagus
Trachea
Truncus jugularis sinister
V. brachiocephalica dextra
Ductus thoracicus at junction of vv. subclavia and jugularis interna sinistrae
Nll. brachiocephalici
V. brachiocephalica sinistra
V. cava superior
Nll. paratracheales
Nll. tracheobronchiales
Ductus thoracicus
Intercostal lymphatics
Nll. prepericardiaci
Nll. prevertebrales
Nll. phrenici superiores
Pericardium fibrosum
Diaphragma
Truncus coeliacus
Nll. coeliaci
Aorta abdominalis
Gaster

B Nodi lymphoidei thoracis

Schematic, left anterior view (the gaster and v. brachiocephalica are not shown to scale). Part of the diaphragma has been cut away, and the v. brachiocephalica has been retracted posterosuperiorly to display the nodi lymphoidei and the junction of the left vv. subclavia and jugularis interna. There is no significant functional distinction between parietal and visceral nodi lymphoidei in the thorax (in sharp contrast with the segregated visceral lymphatic flow in the abdomen and pelvis (see p. 222).

The nodi lymphoidei thoracis are grouped in the mediastinum ("mediastinal" lymph nodes) around the pericardium, trachea, oesophagus, and bronchi and collect the lymph from these organs.

Note: There may be a transdiaphragmatic connection, varying in different individuals, by which the nodi lymphoidei thoracis communicate directly with nodi lymphoidei abdominis. This connection may allow a direct lymphatic metastasis of malignant tumors (e.g., gastric carcinoma) to the nodi lymphoidei thoracis.

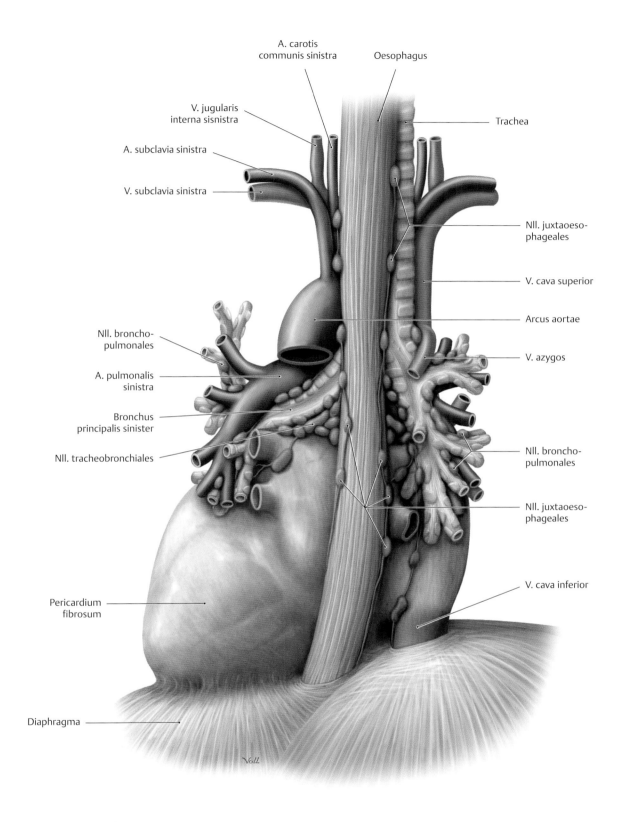

A. carotis
communis sinistra

Oesophagus

V. jugularis
interna sisnistra

Trachea

A. subclavia sinistra

V. subclavia sinistra

Nll. juxtaoeso-
phageales

V. cava superior

Arcus aortae

Nll. broncho-
pulmonales

V. azygos

A. pulmonalis
sinistra

Bronchus
principalis sinister

Nll. broncho-
pulmonales

Nll. tracheobronchiales

Nll. juxtaoeso-
phageales

V. cava inferior

Pericardium
fibrosum

Diaphragma

C Nodi lymphoidei thoracis, posterior view
The numerous nodi lymphoidei located at the divisions of the bronchi
principales into bronchi lobares are often called the "hilar" nodi lymphoidei because they are located in the region of the hilum pulmonis
(not shown here). Frequently they are the first group of nodi lymphoidei
to be affected by pulmonary disease (tuberculosis, malignant tumors).

2.5 Thoracic Innervation

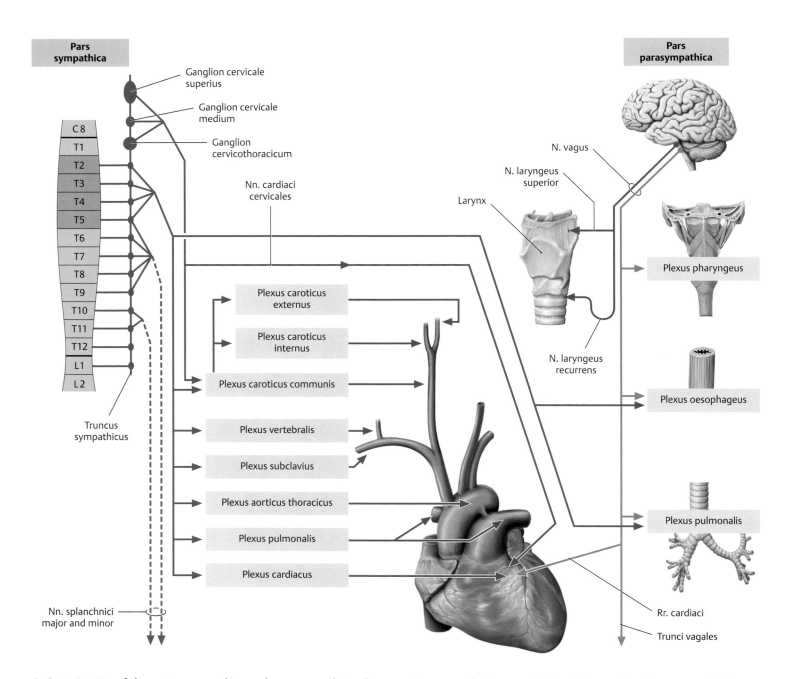

A Organization of the partes sympathica and parasympathica of the nervous systems in the thorax

With the prominent exceptions of the n. phrenicus and nn. intercostales (**B**), thoracic innervation is largely autonomic, arising from either the paravertebral trunci sympathici or the parasympathetic nn. vagi.

Sympathetic organization: The peripheral sympathetic system consists of a two-neuron relay, with presynaptic (preganglionic) fibers arising from neurons in the medulla spinalis. These axons synapse onto neurons in the paired paravertebral ganglia trunci sympathici, which send axons to innervate the thoracic viscera and blood vessels.

The cell bodies of the presynaptic motor neurons are located in the cornua lateralia of the thoracolumbar medulla spinalis (T1 to L2); the neurons involved in sympathetic innervation of the thorax are concentrated in upper thoracic levels. Axons from the paravertebral ganglion cells (postsynaptic [postganglionic] fibers) follow several courses: some fibers follow nn. intercostales to innervate blood vessels and glands in the chest wall; others accompany arteries to visceral targets; other groups of postganglionic axons gather in the nn. splanchnici major and minor and enter the abdomen (see p. 226).

Parasympathetic organization: The peripheral parasympathetic nervous system has a similar two-neuron relay, but its presynaptic neurons are in the truncus encephali and the ganglion cells are scattered in microscopic groups in their target organs. The n. vagus (CN X) carries presynaptic parasympathetic motor axons from truncus encephali neurons into the thorax and gives off the following branches:

- Rr. cardiaci to the plexus cardiacus (cor)
- Rr. oesophagei to the plexus oesophageus (oesophagus)
- Rr. tracheales (trachea) and rr. bronchiales to the plexus pulmonalis (bronchi, pulmonary vessels)

The nn. vagi continue beyond these branches, following the oesophagus into the abdomen (see p. 227).

Note: The n. vagus also carries visceral sensory axons (mostly pressure sensation) for thoracic organs. The sensory neuron cell bodies are in the ganglion inferius nervi vagi (nodose); the first synapse in this sensory pathway is in the truncus encephali.

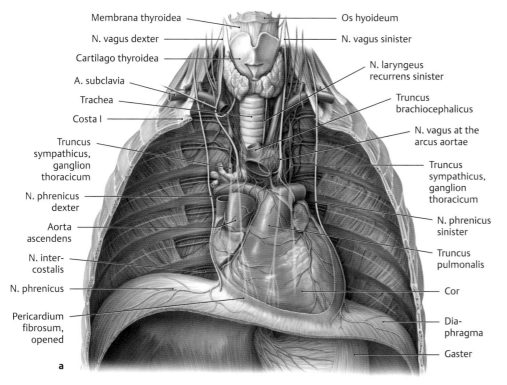

Membrana thyroidea — Os hyoideum
N. vagus dexter — N. vagus sinister
Cartilago thyroidea — N. laryngeus recurrens sinister
A. subclavia — Truncus brachiocephalicus
Trachea —
Costa I —
Truncus sympathicus, ganglion thoracicum — N. vagus at the arcus aortae
N. phrenicus dexter — Truncus sympathicus, ganglion thoracicum
Aorta ascendens — N. phrenicus sinister
N. inter-costalis — Truncus pulmonalis
N. phrenicus — Cor
Pericardium fibrosum, opened — Dia-phragma
— Gaster

a

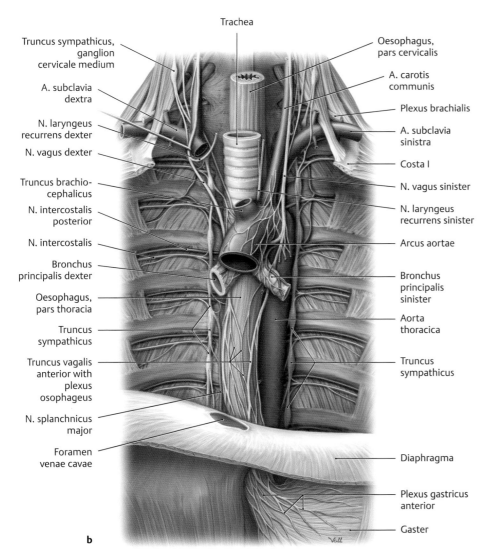

Trachea

Truncus sympathicus, ganglion cervicale medium — Oesophagus, pars cervicalis
A. subclavia dextra — A. carotis communis
N. laryngeus recurrens dexter — Plexus brachialis
N. vagus dexter — A. subclavia sinistra
Truncus brachio-cephalicus — Costa I
N. intercostalis posterior — N. vagus sinister
N. intercostalis — N. laryngeus recurrens sinister
Bronchus principalis dexter — Arcus aortae
Oesophagus, pars thoracica — Bronchus principalis sinister
Truncus sympathicus — Aorta thoracica
Truncus vagalis anterior with plexus osophageus — Truncus sympathicus
N. splanchnicus major —
Foramen venae cavae — Diaphragma
— Plexus gastricus anterior
— Gaster

b

B Overview of nerves in the thorax

Anterior view. **a** The cor and part of the pericardium have been left in place in the mediastinum medium to display the location and course of the nn. phrenici; **b** All organs, except for the oesophagus and part of the trachea, and the nn. phrenici have been removed in order to display the trunci sympathici, nn. intercostales and plexus oesophageus.

The **truncus sympathicus** runs alongside the columna vertebralis in the thorax. Postsynaptic branches of the truncus sympathicus usually accompany the intrathoracic arteries to their target organ in the chest, where they enter the plexus associated with that organ (see p. 94). The **nn. intercostales** are all posterior. They arise from segmenta T1–T12 medullae spinalis (the paired nerves arising from segmentum T12 are called the *nn. subcostales* because they run below the twelfth rib; not shown here) and they emerge below the T1 through T12 vertebra. They initially course with the intercostal vessels along the inferior border of the associated rib. They supply motor innervation to the mm. intercostales and give sensory innervation to the T1–T12 dermatomes. Each n. intercostalis receives postsynaptic sympathetic fibers for the autonomic innervation of glands and vessels in the skin of the dermatomes (see Vol. I, *General Anatomy and Musculoskeletal System*). The thoracic portions of the **nn. vagi** initially run in the plane of the trachea, pass posterior to the two bronchi principales while giving off branches, and then descend on the oesophagus, passing with it through the hiatus oesophageus into the abdomen.

Note: The left and right nn. vagi are organized around the oesophagus to form the trunci vagales anterior and posterior. Topographically, these trunks are a continuation of the plexus oesophageus. Both trunks contain fibers from both nn. vagi: the truncus vagalis *anterior* contains more fibers from the *left* n. vagus, while the truncus vagalis *posterior* contains more fibers from the *right* n. vagus. The left n. vagus gives off the *left n. laryngeus recurrens* at the arcus aorticus, while the right n. vagus gives off the *right n. laryngeus recurrens* at the right a. subclavia. Each of these nerves is a recurrent branch of the n. vagus that ascends into the neck. It is not uncommon for the nn. laryngei recurrentes to run more posteriorly in the neck than shown here, occupying the groove between the trachea and oesophagus where they are vulnerable during operations on the nearby gl. thyroidea. For clarity, the nn. laryngei recurrentes have been retracted slightly forward in this dissection.

Note: The pericardium and diaphragma do not have an autonomic nerve supply (except their blood vessels).

3.1   Location of the Heart (Cor) in the Thorax

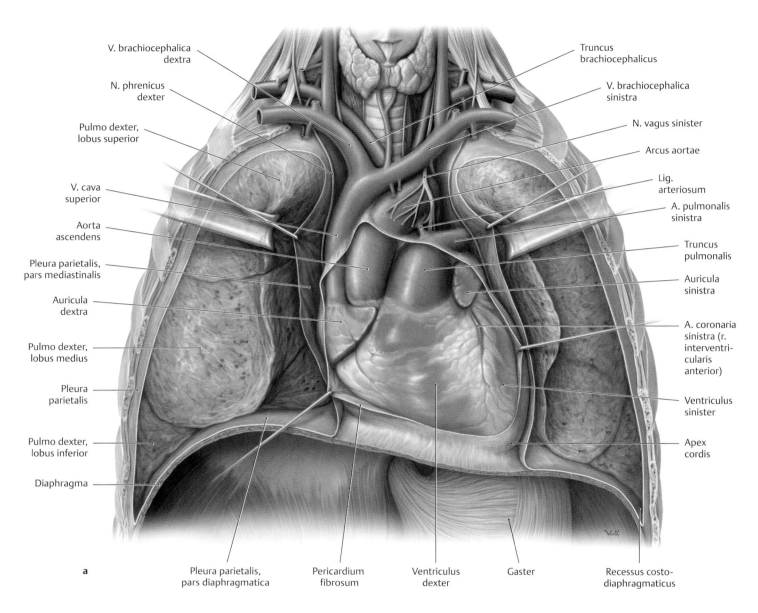

V. brachiocephalica dextra

N. phrenicus dexter

Pulmo dexter, lobus superior

V. cava superior

Aorta ascendens

Pleura parietalis, pars mediastinalis

Auricula dextra

Pulmo dexter, lobus medius

Pleura parietalis

Pulmo dexter, lobus inferior

Diaphragma

Truncus brachiocephalicus

V. brachiocephalica sinistra

N. vagus sinister

Arcus aortae

Lig. arteriosum

A. pulmonalis sinistra

Truncus pulmonalis

Auricula sinistra

A. coronaria sinistra (r. interventricularis anterior)

Ventriculus sinister

Apex cordis

a   Pleura parietalis, pars diaphragmatica   Pericardium fibrosum   Ventriculus dexter   Gaster   Recessus costo-diaphragmaticus

A   The cor in situ, anterior view
a Simplified illustration. The chest has been widely opened, and the cavitates pleurales and pericardium fibrosum have been cut open. The connective tissue has been removed from the mediastinum anterius to display the cor. Although the cavitates pleurales have been opened, the pulmones are not shown in a collapsed state. **b** Projection of the cor on the bony thorax. The cor lies within the pericardium, which is firmly attached to the diaphragma (see p. 98) but is mobile in relation to the pleura parietalis. A longitudinal axis drawn from the basis cordis to the apex cordis demonstrates that this "long axis" is directed forward and downward from right to left. Thus the cor, when viewed from the front, has an oblique orientation and is tilted counterclockwise within the chest. Along this axis it appears slightly "rolled" in a posterior direction. Thus the ventriculus dexter faces forward, as pictured here, while the ventriculus sinister is only partly visible. As a result, all of the great vessels cannot be seen even when the basis cordis is viewed from the front. The short vv. pulmonales are covered by the cardiac silhouette because they terminate at the atrium sinistrum, which is directed posteriorly. The auriculae dextra and dextra (atrial appendages) are clearly visible. The apex cordis points downward and to the left. Most of it is still covered by pericardium in this dissection. Its movement, called the

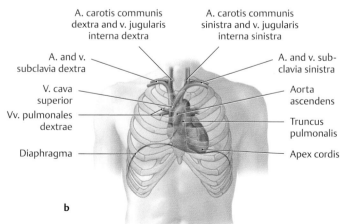

A. carotis communis dextra and v. jugularis interna dextra

A. carotis communis sinistra and v. jugularis interna sinistra

A. and v. subclavia dextra

V. cava superior

Vv. pulmonales dextrae

Diaphragma

A. and v. subclavia sinistra

Aorta ascendens

Truncus pulmonalis

Apex cordis

b

apical beat, is palpable as a fine motion in the fifth spatium intercostale on the left midclavicular line (see p. 109). The thin tunica serosa of the lamina visceralis pericardii serosi (see p. 98) gives the surface of the heart a shiny appearance. Under this membrane are clusters of fatty tissue in which the coronary vessels are embedded.

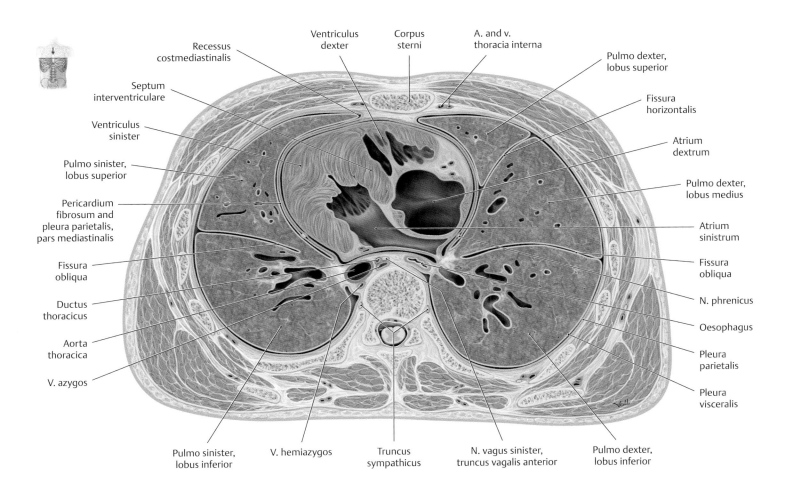

Ventriculus dexter

Corpus sterni

A. and v. thoracia interna

Recessus costmediastinalis

Pulmo dexter, lobus superior

Septum interventriculare

Fissura horizontalis

Ventriculus sinister

Atrium dextrum

Pulmo sinister, lobus superior

Pulmo dexter, lobus medius

Pericardium fibrosum and pleura parietalis, pars mediastinalis

Atrium sinistrum

Fissura obliqua

Fissura obliqua

N. phrenicus

Ductus thoracicus

Oesophagus

Aorta thoracica

Pleura parietalis

V. azygos

Pleura visceralis

Pulmo sinister, lobus inferior

V. hemiazygos

Truncus sympathicus

N. vagus sinister, truncus vagalis anterior

Pulmo dexter, lobus inferior

B The cor in situ, superior view

Transverse section through the thorax at the level of T8 vertebra. Viewing the transverse section demonstrates the asymmetrical position of the cor in the mediastinum medium and its slight degree of physiologic counterclockwise rotation: the *ventriculus sinister* faces downward and to the left, while the ventriculus dexter faces forward and to the right. The *ventriculus dexter* thus lies almost directly behind the posterior wall of the sternum (with only the narrow mediastinum anterius intervening, see p. 79). The *atrium sinistrum* is in very close relationship to the oesophagus. The recessus costomediastinalis is interposed between the cor and *sternum* on the right and left sides. A relatively small space remains between the cor and *columna vertebralis* for the passage of neurovascular structures and organs: pars thoracica aortae, oesophagus, ductus thoracicus, vv. azygos and hemiazygos, and portions of the autonomic nervous system. Each pulmo bears an indentation from the cor called the impressio cardiaca. This impression is larger in the pulmo sinister than in the pulmo dexter because of the cor's asymmetric position. The potential spaces between the pleural layers and the pericardium serosum are considerably smaller than pictured here.

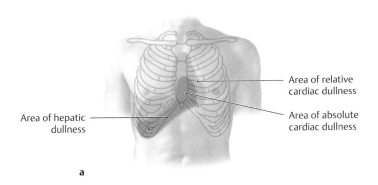

Area of relative cardiac dullness

Area of hepatic dullness

Area of absolute cardiac dullness

a

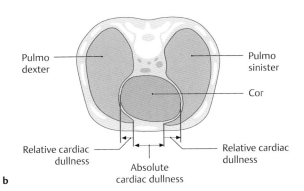

Pulmo dexter

Pulmo sinister

Cor

Relative cardiac dullness

Relative cardiac dullness

Absolute cardiac dullness

b

C Cardiac dullness on percussion of the chest

Anterior view (**a**) and transverse section viewed from above (**b**). In contrast to the sonorous sound that is produced by the percussion of *airfilled* pulmo (see p. 136), the *fluid-filled* cor produces a flat sound on percussion known as *cardiac dullness*. The dullness may be *absolute* (at sites where there is no pulmo tissue to moderate cardiac dullness) or *relative* (at sites where pulmo tissue overlies the cor and adds resonance to the percussion sound). Accordingly, the area of absolute cardiac dullness is located between the chest wall and cor while the area of relative cardiac dullness is located over the recessus costomediastinales dexter and sinister, which contain small expansions of pulmo tissue (see **B**).
Note: Cardiac dullness gives way to hepatic dullness in the epigastrium and right hypochondriac region due to the anatomical extent of the hepar (see **a**). The boundaries of the cor can be roughly estimated from the area of cardiac dullness because the sound characteristics at the cardiac borders contrast with the more resonant pulmo sounds.

97

3.2 Pericardium: Location, Structure, and Innervation

A Location of the pericardium in the thorax, anterior view

The chest has been opened to display the pericardium, which is the dominant structure in the mediastinum inferius. It is attached inferiorly to the fascia diaphragmatica by connective tissue. Anteriorly, it is separated from the posterior surface of the sternum only by connective tissue of the mediastinum anterius (removed here, see p. 79). The pericardium is bounded laterally by the cavitates pleurales, from which it is separated by pars mediastinalis pleurae.

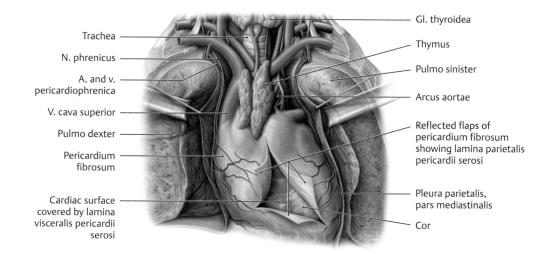

- Trachea
- N. phrenicus
- A. and v. pericardiophrenica
- V. cava superior
- Pulmo dexter
- Pericardium fibrosum
- Cardiac surface covered by lamina visceralis pericardii serosi
- Gl. thyroidea
- Thymus
- Pulmo sinister
- Arcus aortae
- Reflected flaps of pericardium fibrosum showing lamina parietalis pericardii serosi
- Pleura parietalis, pars mediastinalis
- Cor

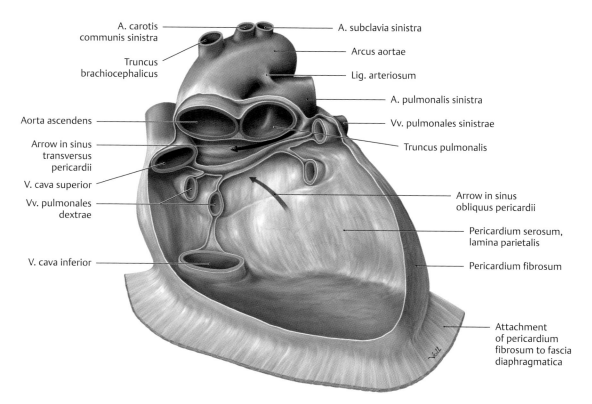

- A. carotis communis sinistra
- Truncus brachiocephalicus
- Aorta ascendens
- Arrow in sinus transversus pericardii
- V. cava superior
- Vv. pulmonales dextrae
- V. cava inferior
- A. subclavia sinistra
- Arcus aortae
- Lig. arteriosum
- A. pulmonalis sinistra
- Vv. pulmonales sinistrae
- Truncus pulmonalis
- Arrow in sinus obliquus pericardii
- Pericardium serosum, lamina parietalis
- Pericardium fibrosum
- Attachment of pericardium fibrosum to fascia diaphragmatica

B Cavitas pericardiaca and structure of the pericardium

Anterior view of the empty pericardial sac. The pericardium consists of two **layers**, one within the other, that enclose and protect the heart:

- Lamina parietalis. The lamina parietalis pericardii forms a sac with an outer surface, the *pericardium fibrosum*, composed of tough and indistensible connective tissue which is partially attached to the diaphragma. Its inner surface, facing the heart, is lined with a serous membrane.
- Lamina visceralis (*epicardium*). This is a thin serous membrane which covers, and is firmly adherent to, the cor itself and the proximal parts of the great vessels.

The two tunicae serosae of the laminae parietalis and visceralis are closely apposed, but move freely over one another, allowing a gliding motion during the heartbeat. These two tunicae serosae are referred to together as the *pericardium serosum*.

In the locations where the lamina parietalis is folded back onto the lamina visceralis covering the vessels, two **sinuses** are formed (see arrows):

- The sinus transversus pericardii located between the arteries and veins
- The sinus obliquus pericardii located between the vv. pulmonales sinistrae and dextrae

Note: Because the pericardium cannot expand significantly, bleeding into the cavitas pericardii (e.g., from a ruptured myocardial aneurysm) will place increasing pressure on the cor as the blood accumulates within the sac. This condition, called cardiac tamponade, seriously compromises the ability of the ventriculi to fill and pump blood, creating a threat of cardiac arrest. Similar problems may arise from inflammation of the pericardium (pericarditis).

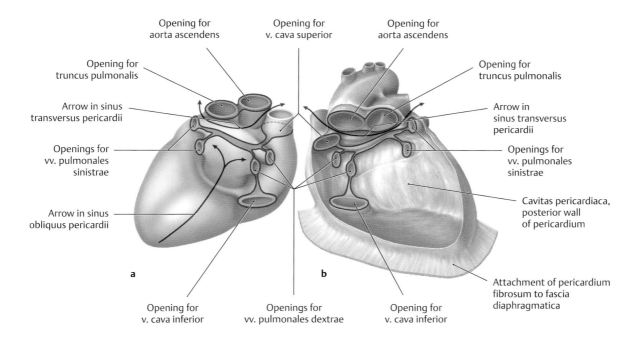

C Openings in the pericardium
a Posterior view of the cor with the epicardium. **b** Anterior view of the "empty" cavitas pericardiaca. An empty pericardium typically has eight openings by which vessels enter and leave the cor:

- One opening for the aorta ascendens
- One opening for the truncus pulmonalis
- Two openings for the two venae cavae
- Up to four openings for the four vv. pulmonales

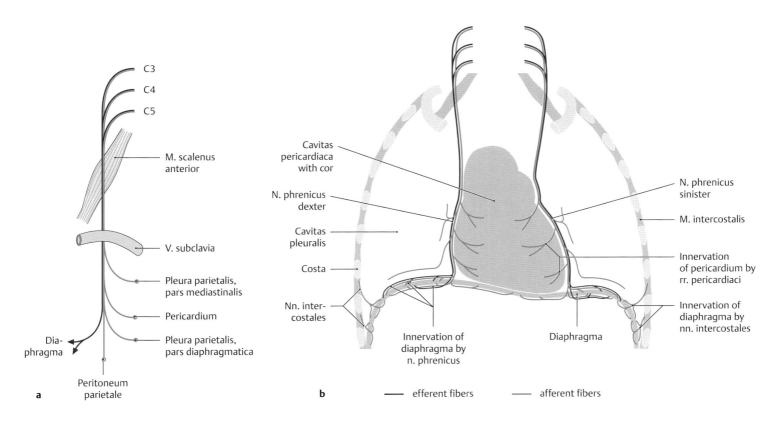

D Innervation of the pericardium
a Somatosensory and somatomotor components of the n. phrenicus
b Sensory and motor distribution of the n. phrenicus

Like the serous membranes of the diaphragma (pars diaphragmatica pleurae and peritoneum parietale), the pericardium (pericardium fibrosum and lamina parietalis of pericardium serosum) is innervated by the nn. phrenici, which arise from segmenta cervicales C3–5 medullae spinalis.

3.3 Cor: Shape and Structure

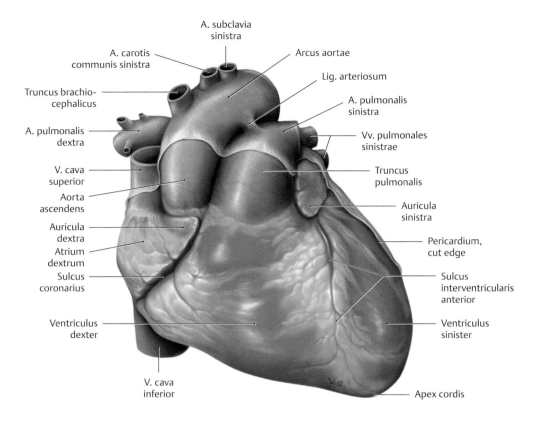

A. subclavia sinistra

A. carotis communis sinistra

Arcus aortae

Lig. arteriosum

Truncus brachio-cephalicus

A. pulmonalis sinistra

A. pulmonalis dextra

Vv. pulmonales sinistrae

V. cava superior

Truncus pulmonalis

Aorta ascendens

Auricula sinistra

Auricula dextra

Pericardium, cut edge

Atrium dextrum

Sulcus coronarius

Sulcus interventricularis anterior

Ventriculus dexter

Ventriculus sinister

V. cava inferior

Apex cordis

A Cor, facies sternocostalis

Anterior view. The cor is a muscular hollow organ shaped approximately like a flattened cone. It consists topographically of a base, apex, and three surfaces:

- The basis cordis, which is occupied by entering and emerging vessels, is directed superiorly, posteriorly, and to the right.
- The apex cordis is directed inferiorly, anteriorly, and to the left.
- The surfaces are described as facies anterior (sternocostalis), facies posterior, and facies inferior (diaphragmatica) (see **B**).

The facies sternocostalis of the cor is formed chiefly by the ventriculus dexter, whose boundary with the ventriculus sinister is marked by the sulcus interventricularis anterior. The ventriculus sinister (occupying the inferior and posterior cordis) forms the left border and apex cordis.

The *sulcus interventricularis anterior* contains the r. interventricularis anterior of the a. coronaria sinistra (see p. 120) and the v. interventricularis anterior (v. cardiaca magna). Both vessels are embedded in fat and almost completely occupy the groove, so that the facies anterior of the cor appears nearly smooth. The atria sinistrum and dextrum are separated from the ventriculi by the *sulcus coronarius*, which also transmits coronary vessels (the intrinsic vessels of the cor, see pp. 120–123) The right auricula atrii lies at the root of the aorta ascendens, the auricula sinistra at the root of the truncus pulmonalis. The origin of the a. pulmonalis dextra from the truncus pulmonalis is hidden by the pars ascendens aortae. For clarity, all three illustrations in this series (**A, C, D**) show sites where the lamina visceralis of the pericardium is reflected to form the lamina parietalis. The pericardium extends onto the roots of the great arteries.

B Facies of the cor

Surface	Orientation	Cardiac chambers that form the surface (with vessels)
Facies anterior (sternocostalis)	Directed anteriorly toward the posterior surface of the sternum and the ribs	• Atrium dextrum with auricula dextra • Ventriculus dexter • Small part of ventriculus sinister with apex cordis • Auricula sinistra • Pars ascendens aortae, v. cava superior, truncus pulmonalis
Facies posterior	Directed posteriorly toward the mediastinum posterius	• Atrium sinistrum with termination of four vv. pulmonales • Ventriculus sinister • Part of atrium dextrum with termination of vv. cavae superior and inferior
Facies inferior (diaphragmatica) (clinically: the posterior wall)	Directed inferiorly toward the diaphragma	• Ventriculus sinister with apex cordis • Ventriculus dexter • Part of atrium dextrum with termination of v. cava inferior

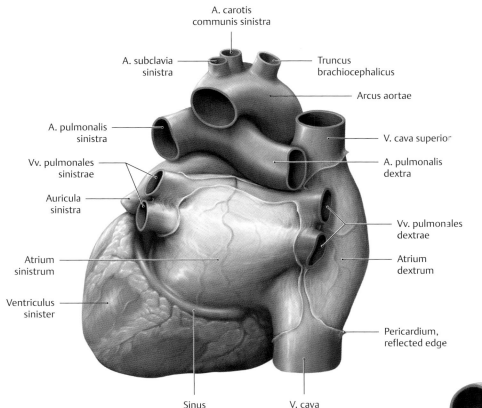

A. carotis
communis sinistra

A. subclavia
sinistra

Truncus
brachiocephalicus

Arcus aortae

A. pulmonalis
sinistra

V. cava superior

Vv. pulmonales
sinistrae

A. pulmonalis
dextra

Auricula
sinistra

Vv. pulmonales
dextrae

Atrium
sinistrum

Atrium
dextrum

Ventriculus
sinister

Pericardium,
reflected edge

Sinus
coronarius

V. cava
inferior

C Cor, facies posterior
Posterior view. This dissection shows how the arcus aortae crosses over the truncus pulmonalis at the point where the trunk divides into the aa. pulmonales sinistra and dextra. At that site the aorta gives off the three major arteries to the upper limbs, neck, and head: the truncus brachiocephalicus, left a. carotis communis, and left a. subclavia. This view also clearly shows the terminations of the vv. pulmonales (usually four in number) in the atrium *sinistrum* and the terminations of the two vv. cavae in the atrium *dextrum*. Note also the sinus coronarius in the posterior part of the sulcus coronarius, which runs between the ventriculus sinister and atrium sinistrum. This sinus is the collecting vessel for venous blood returned from the heart by the vv. cardiacae.

Arcus aortae

V. cava superior

A. pulmonalis
sinistra

A. pulmonalis
dextra

Vv. pulmonales
sinistrae

Vv. pulmonales
dextrae

Atrium
sinistrum

Atrium
dextrum

Sinus
coronarius

V. cava
inferior

D Cor, facies diaphragmatica
Posteroinferior view. The cor is tilted forward to give a better view of its facies diaphragmatica, which is formed by both ventriculi and the atrium dextrum with the termination of the v. cava inferior. If the cor were viewed from below, from the perspective of the diaphragma (not shown here), it would be obvious that both vv. cavae are in alignment: Looking into the v. cava inferior, one can see through the terminal part of the v. cava superior.

Ventriculus
sinister

Ventriculus
dexter

Sulcus
interventricularis
posterior

Apex cordis

E Structure of the cardiac wall

Layer	Location	Composition
Endocardium	Innermost layer, lines the cavities of the cor and lines the cuspides and pockets of the cardiac valves	Single layer of epithelial cells with a subendothelial layer composed of collagen and elastic fibers; both layers are continuous with the intima of the vessels
Myocardium	Middle layer and thickest part of the cardiac wall; motor for the pumping action of the cor (see pp. 102 and 103)	Complex arrangement of muscle fibers
Epicardium	Outermost layer of the cardiac wall; part of the pericardium (see p. 98), forming its lamina visceralis	Serous membrane (single layer of epithelial cells with underlying layer of connective tissue)

3.4   Structure of the Cardiac Musculature (Myocardium)

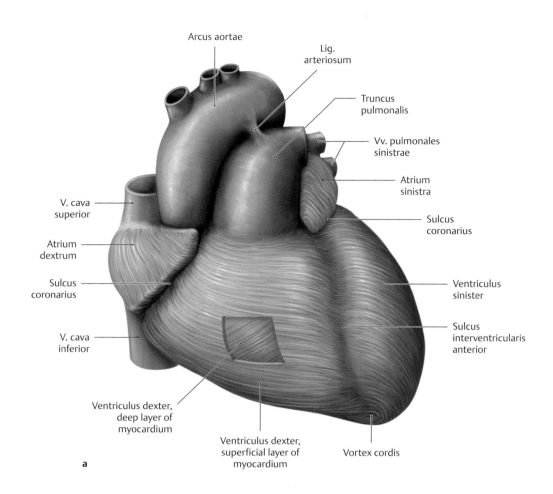

Arcus aortae

Lig. arteriosum

Truncus pulmonalis

Vv. pulmonales sinistrae

Atrium sinistra

V. cava superior

Atrium dextrum

Sulcus coronarius

Sulcus coronarius

Ventriculus sinister

V. cava inferior

Sulcus interventricularis anterior

Ventriculus dexter, deep layer of myocardium

Ventriculus dexter, superficial layer of myocardium

Vortex cordis

a

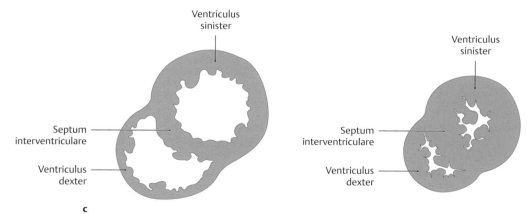

Ventriculus sinister

Ventriculus sinister

Septum interventriculare

Septum interventriculare

Ventriculus dexter

Ventriculus dexter

c

A Myocardial architecture

a, b External musculature of the cor, simplified anteroinferior view. The muscular walls of the ventriculi dexter and sinister have been windowed to display the deeper fibers.

Note: The epicardium has been removed in **a** and **b** along with the subepicardial fat. The coronary vessels are not shown in order to display more clearly the cardiac surface grooves (sulci interventriculares anterior and posterior).

The **musculature of the atria** is arranged in two layers, superficial and deep. The superficial layer (shown here) extends over the atria and is common to both, whereas each atrium has its own deep layer.

Looped and annular muscle fibers extend down to the atrioventricular boundary and also encircle the ostia venarum. The **ventricular musculature** has a complex arrangement, consisting basically of a superficial (subepicardial), middle, and deep (subendocardial) layer. The superficial layer joins apically with the deeper layers to form a whorled arrangement of muscle fibers around the apex cordis (vortex cordis). The ventriculus dexter, which is a low-pressure system (see **c**), is less muscular than the ventriculus sinister and almost completely lacks a middle layer. The subendocardial layer forms the trabeculae carneae and mm. papillares (see **d** and p. 109).

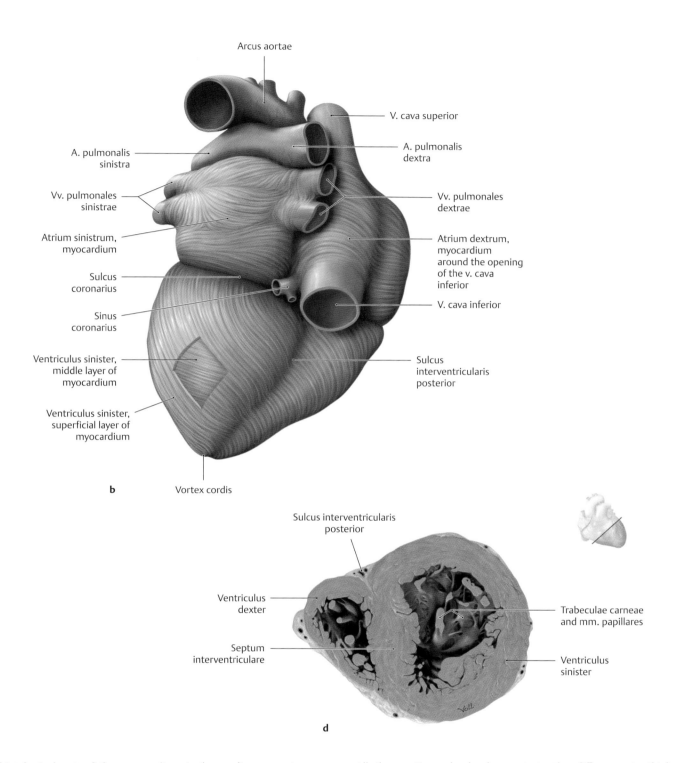

Arcus aortae

V. cava superior

A. pulmonalis
sinistra

A. pulmonalis
dextra

Vv. pulmonales
sinistrae

Vv. pulmonales
dextrae

Atrium sinistrum,
myocardium

Atrium dextrum,
myocardium
around the opening
of the v. cava
inferior

Sulcus
coronarius

Sinus
coronarius

V. cava inferior

Ventriculus sinister,
middle layer of
myocardium

Sulcus
interventricularis
posterior

Ventriculus sinister,
superficial layer of
myocardium

b   Vortex cordis

Sulcus interventricularis
posterior

Ventriculus
dexter

Trabeculae carneae
and mm. papillares

Septum
interventriculare

Ventriculus
sinister

d

The histological unit of the myocardium is the cardiac myocyte, a specialized form of cardiac muscle cell. Unlike their electronically isolated counterparts in skeletal muscle, cardiac myocytes form a syncytium in which membrane depolarization and contraction spread in a wave.

c, d Myocardial cross-sections perpendicular to the long axis of the cor, viewed from above. **c** Schematic representation: The ventriculi in an expanded state (diastole, left figure), and in a contracted state (systole, right figure). **d** Transverse section through a specimen during diastole.

All the sections clearly demonstrate the difference in thickness between the left and right ventricular myocardia: The ventriculus sinister is part of the high-pressure system, and therefore its myocardium must generate a significantly higher pressure (120–140 mmHg during ventricular contraction) than the ventriculus dexter (approximately 25–30 mmHg). The difference in thickness is most pronounced during ventricular contraction (see **c**). Section **d** shows how the coronary vessels and subepicardial fat fill the sulci in the cor.

3.5 Cardiac Chambers

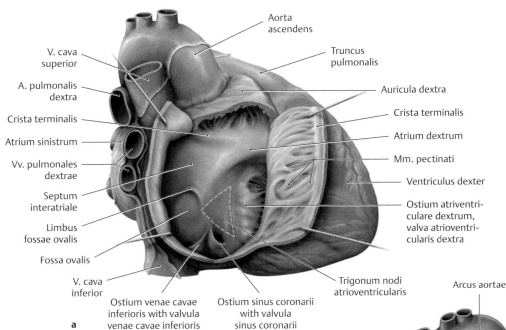

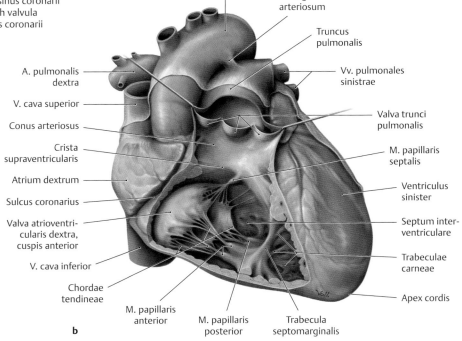

A Chambers of the right heart

a Right view of the atrium. **b** Anterior view of the ventriculus. The ventricular and atrial walls have been opened widely, and the heart wall has been cut open to display the internal chambers.

The **atrium dextrum** (see **a**) consists of:

- the anterior segment, which comprises the actual atrium with the auricle, and
- the posterior segment with the sinus venarum cavarum (not visible here). It bears the ostia venarum cavarum superioris et inferioris.

The ostia venae cavae inferioris et sinus coronarii and the margin of the cuspis septalis valvae tricuspidalis leaflet define what is known as the trigonum nodi atrioventricularis, an area on the wall of the atrium dextrum. This is the location of the nodus atrioventricularis. A small valve at the ostium venae cavae inferioris (valvula vena cavae inferioris) directs blood in the prenatal circulation through the foramen ovale septum interatriale. The foramen ovale is sealed shut postnatally, becoming the fossa ovalis (surrounded by a rounded margin, the limbus). The ostium sinus coronarii also bears a small crescent-shaped valve (valvula sinus coronarii). The anterior segment, which comprises the actual atrium with the auricula, is separated from the posterior segment by a ridge, the crista terminalis. Small muscular trabeculae, the mm. pectinati, arise from this ridge, giving this segment an irregular wall texture. In contrast, the wall of the posterior segment is smooth.

The **right ventricle** is characterized by two muscular ridges, the supraventricular crest and the septomarginal trabecula. It is also divided into two sections:

- the inflow tract posteroinferiorly (with the heart positioned in situ) and
- the outflow tract anterosuperiorly (see also p. 119).

The muscular ridges of the trabeculae carneae are visible on the wall of the ventricular inflow tract. Specialized extensions of the trabeculae, the papillary muscles, are attached to the cusps of the right atrioventricular valve by collagenous cords, the chordae tendineae (see p. 109). The *outflow tract* is cone-shaped and consists mainly of the conus arteriosus, which has a smooth wall. The right ventricular outflow tract expels blood into the pulmonary trunk, whose orifice is guarded by the pulmonary valve. The wall of the right ventricle is relatively thin (low-pressure system). All of the cardiac chambers are lined with endocardium.

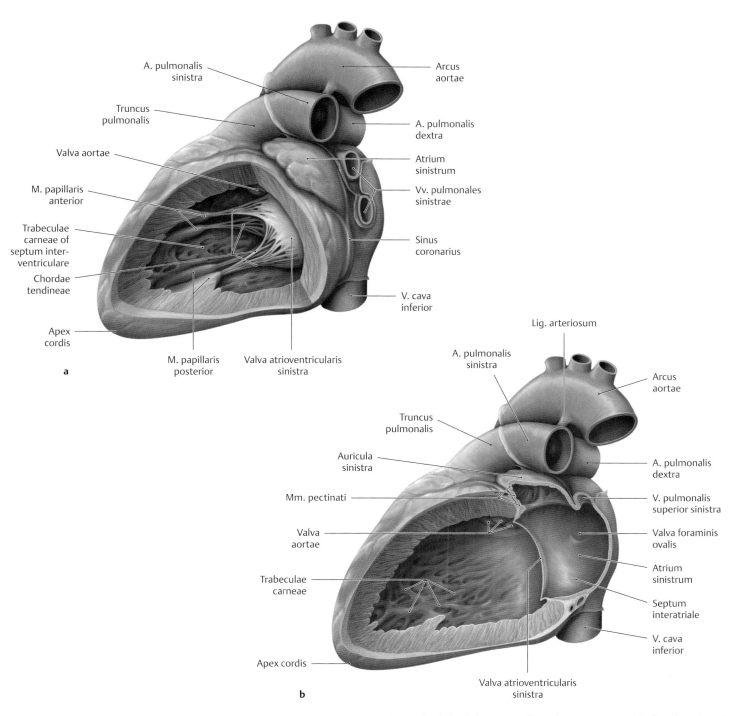

A. pulmonalis sinistra

Truncus pulmonalis

Valva aortae

M. papillaris anterior

Trabeculae carneae of septum inter-ventriculare

Chordae tendineae

Apex cordis

Arcus aortae

A. pulmonalis dextra

Atrium sinistrum

Vv. pulmonales sinistrae

Sinus coronarius

V. cava inferior

a

M. papillaris posterior · Valva atrioventricularis sinistra

Lig. arteriosum

A. pulmonalis sinistra

Truncus pulmonalis

Auricula sinistra

Mm. pectinati

Valva aortae

Trabeculae carneae

Apex cordis

Arcus aortae

A. pulmonalis dextra

V. pulmonalis superior sinistra

Valva foraminis ovalis

Atrium sinistrum

Septum interatriale

V. cava inferior

b

Valva atrioventricularis sinistra

B Chambers of the left cor

Left lateral view. **a** Ventriculus, **b** ventriculus and atrium. The ventricular and atrial walls have been opened.

The **atrium sinistrum** is smaller than the atrium dextrum (see **Aa**). Its muscular wall is thin (low-pressure system) and is smooth in areas derived embryologically from the ostia venarum pulmonalium. The rest of the atrium is lined by mm. pectinati. The vv. pulmonales, usually four in number, terminate in the atrium sinistrum. Occasionally a narrow tissue fold (valvula foraminis ovalis) is found on the septum interatriale, formed by a protrusion of the fossa ovalis into the atrium sinistrum. It marks the site of fusion between the embryonic septum primum and septum secundum.

The **ventriculus sinister** has an *inflow tract* and outflow tract. The inflow tract begins at the left ostium atrioventriculare, which is guarded by the valva atrioventricularis sinistra (see p. 107). As in the ventriculus dexter,

the wall of the left ventricular *inflow tract* is studded with trabeculae carneae, and mm. papillares are attached by chordae tendineae to the valva atrioventricularis sinistra. The *outflow tract* of the ventriculus sinister has smooth inner walls and lies close to the septum interventriculare. It leads to the aorta and is capped by the valva aortae at the root of the aorta ascendens (see p. 107). The septum interventriculare consists largely of muscle tissue (pars muscularis), and only a small portion near the aorta consists entirely of connective tissue (pars membranacea). The placement of the septum interventriculare between the cardiac chambers is marked externally by the sulci interventriculares anterior and posterior on the cardiac surface. The muscular wall of the ventriculus sinister is thick (high-pressure system), having approximately three times the thickness of the right ventricular wall (see **Ab**). The chambers of the left (and right) cor are lined by endocardium.

3.6 Overview of the Cardiac Valvae (Valve Plane and Cardiac Skeleton)

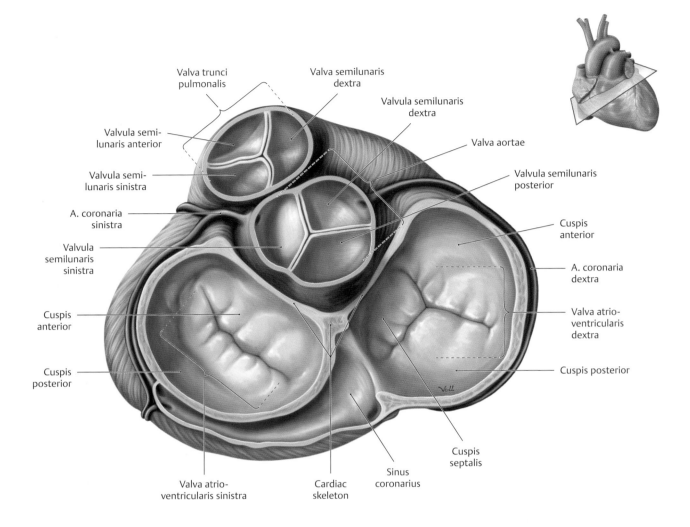

Valva trunci pulmonalis

Valvula semilunaris anterior

Valvula semilunaris sinistra

A. coronaria sinistra

Valvula semilunaris sinistra

Cuspis anterior

Cuspis posterior

Valva atrioventricularis sinistra

Cardiac skeleton

Valva semilunaris dextra

Valvula semilunaris dextra

Valva aortae

Valvula semilunaris posterior

Cuspis anterior

A. coronaria dextra

Valva atrioventricularis dextra

Cuspis posterior

Cuspis septalis

Sinus coronarius

A Overview of the cardiac valvae
Plane of the cardiac valvae viewed from above. The atria have been removed, and the great arteries have been transected at their roots. The cardiac valvae are classified into two types—atrioventricular and semilunar. All heart valves lie in a plane, the valve plane. The cardiac valvae function as one-way valves. They ensure the unidirectional flow of blood between the atria and ventriculi (valvae atrioventriculares sinistra and dextra), and out of the heart (valva aortae and valva trunci pulmonalis).
Valvae atrioventriculares. Located between the atria and ventriculi, the valvae atrioventriculares sinistra and dextra are composed of thin, avascular connective tissue covered by endocardium. They are classified mechanically as *sail valves* (see **C**) because the chordae tendineae (see **C**) constrain the movement of each cuspis like the tethering ropes on a sail. The function of these valvae is to prevent the reflux of blood from the ventriculi into the atria.

- The *valva atrioventricularis sinistra* (valva mitralis) has two cuspides (*bicuspid valve*): a cuspis anterior (anteromedial) and a cuspis posterior (posterolateral). The cuspis anterior is continuous with the wall of the aorta. The alternate term *valva mitralis* is derived from the two major cuspides, which are similar in shape to a bishop's miter. Subdivisions in the lateral margins of the otherwise smooth valve

have led some anatomists to describe small accessory cusps called the cuspides commissurales (usually two). These are not true cuspides, however, and are not connected to the anulus fibrosus sinister of the cardiac skeleton (see **B**). The cuspides are tethered by mm. papillares (see **C**).
- The *valva atrioventricularis dextra* has three cuspides (*valva tricuspidalis*): cuspides anterior, posterior, and septalis. One or two small accessory cusps may also be found; they do not extend to the anulus fibrosus dexter.

Semilunar valves. These valves have three crescent-shaped valvulae of approximately equal size placed at the ostia of the truncus pulmonalis (valva trunci pulmonalis) and aorta (valva aortae). Like the valvae atrioventriculares, they are composed of thin connective tissue covered by endocardium. The semilunar valves are classified mechanically as *pocket valves* because their valvulae pouch into the ventriculus like bulging pockets. The wall of the aorta and truncus pulmonalis show slight dilations just above the valve (the sinus trunci pulmonalis and sinus aortae). The sinus aortae expand the cross-section of the aorta, forming the bulbus aortae. The aa. coronariae dextra and sinistra branch off the base of the aorta just past the valva aortae (see pp. 120–123 for details).

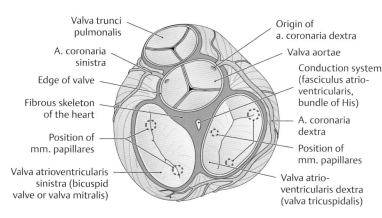

B Skeleton of the cor

The skeleton of the cor is a layer of connective tissue (often with considerable fat) that completely separates the myocardium of the ventriculi from that of the atria. The components of the cardiac skeleton in a *narrow sense* are as follows:

- The anuli fibrosi dexter and sinister and intervening trigona fibrosa
- The anulus fibrosus of the valva aortae, which is connected to both anuli fibrosi
- The pars membranacea of the septum interventriculare (not shown here).

In a *broad sense*, the anulus fibrosus of the valva trunci pulmonalis also contributes to the cardiac skeleton. It is connected by a collagenous band (tendo infundibuli) to the anulus fibrosus of the valva aortae. The valvae atrioventriculares are anchored to the anuli fibrosi, while the semilunar valves are each attached by connective tissue to their valvular anuli fibrosi. Thus, the cardiac skeleton in the broad sense provides a mechanical framework for all the cardiac valvae. Besides *mechanically stabilizing* the heart, the fibrous skeleton also functions as an *electrical insulator* between the atria and ventriculi. The electrical impulses that stimulate cardiac contractions (see p. 116 f) can pass from the atrium to the ventriculus only through the fasciculus atrioventricularis (bundle of His), and there is only one opening in the fibrous skeleton (in the trigonum fibrosum dextrum) which transmits that bundle).

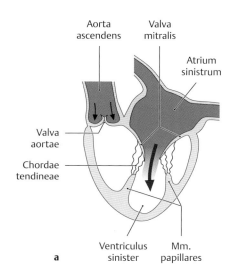

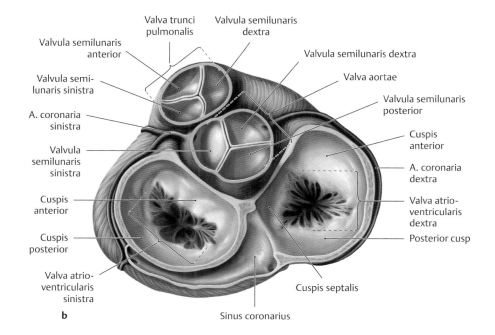

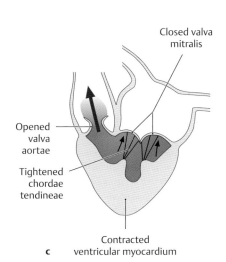

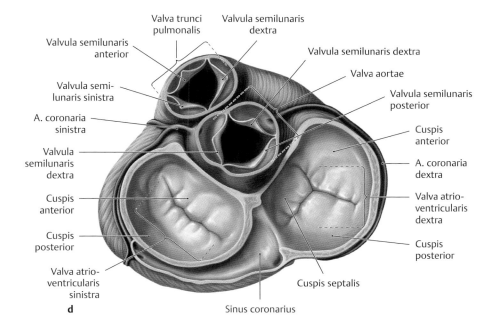

C Function of the valvae cordis during the cardiac cycle

a and **b** Ventricular diastole; **c** and **d** Ventricular systole. **a** and **c** Direction of blood flow in the left cor; **b** and **d** Valve plane viewed from above.

3.7 Cardiac Valves and Auscultation Sites

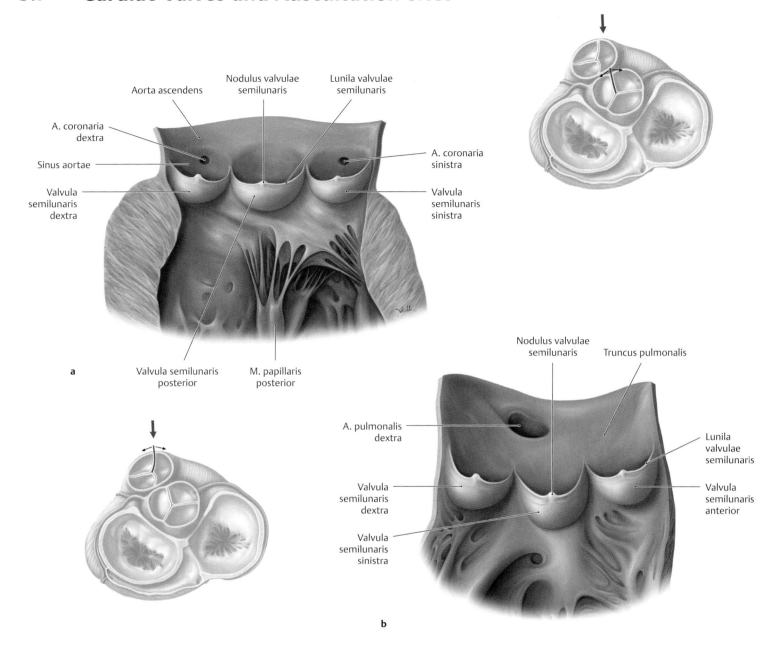

a

Aorta ascendens

Nodulus valvulae semilunaris

Lunila valvulae semilunaris

A. coronaria dextra

A. coronaria sinistra

Sinus aortae

Valvula semilunaris dextra

Valvula semilunaris sinistra

Valvula semilunaris posterior

M. papillaris posterior

Nodulus valvulae semilunaris

Truncus pulmonalis

A. pulmonalis dextra

Lunila valvulae semilunaris

Valvula semilunaris dextra

Valvula semilunaris anterior

Valvula semilunaris sinistra

b

A Semilunar valves of the outflow tracts (valva aortae and valva trunci pulmonalis)

The valva aortae (**a**) and valva pulmonalis (**b**) have been displayed by cutting open the pars ascendens aortae and truncus pulmonalis and opening them up like a book. The valva aortae and valva trunci pulmonalis close the ventricular outflow tracts during diastole:

- The valva aortae closes the left ventricular outflow tract.
- The valva trunci pulmonalis closes the right ventricular outflow tract.

These valves almost completely prevent the regurgitation of blood expelled by the ventriculi. The origins of the arteriae coronariae sinistra and dextra can be clearly identified in the sinus aortae past the valvulae semilunares (**a**), and the origin of the a. pulmonalis dextra can be identified in the truncus pulmonalis (**b**). The free margin of each valvula semilunaris is thickened centrally to form a nodulus valvulae semilunaris, and on each side of the nodulus is a fine rim called the lunula valvae semilunaris. The nodulus and lunula ensure that the margins of the valvulae appose tightly and completely during valva closure. Both

the valvae atrioventriculares (see p. 106) and the semilunar valvae may undergo pathological changes, usually due to inflammation (endocarditis). Inflammation may result in secondary vascularization of the initially avascular valvae, causing them to undergo fibrotic changes that stiffen the valvae and compromise their function. There are two main abnormalities of valvular mechanics, which may coexist in the same valva:

- Valvular stenosis: *Opening* of the valve is impaired, causing a reduction of blood flow across the valve. Usually this creates a pressure overload on the chamber proximal to the obstruction.
- Valvular insufficiency: *Closure* of the valve is impaired, allowing blood to regurgitate into the chamber proximal to the valve. Such a pathological reflux creates a volume overload on the affected cardiac segments. When the load exceeds a certain magnitude, surgical replacement of the valve may be necessary to prevent further damage to the cor.
- Stenosis and insufficiency may coexist: A valva may become stuck in an intermediate position, unable to open or close completely.

Cuspis commissuralis

Atrium sinistrum

Valva atrio-ventricularis sinistra, cuspis posterior

Valva atrio-ventricularis dextra, cuspis anterior

Valva atrio-ventricularis dextra, cuspis septalis

Valva atrioventri-cularis sinistra, cuspis anterior

Septum interatriale

Septum inter-ventriculare, pars membranacea

M. papillaris anterior

Septum interventriculare, pars muscularis

Valva atrio-ventricularis dextra, cuspis posterior

Chordae tendineae

M. papillaris posterior

M. papillaris septalis

Septum inter-ventriculare

M. papillaris anterior

Trabecula septomarginalis

a

Apex cordis

b

B Valvae atrioventriculares and musculi papillares

Anterior view of the valvae atrioventriculares sinistra (**a**) and dextra (**b**). The drawings represent a very early phase of ventricular contraction in which the valvae atrioventriculares have just closed. The mm. papillares are clearly displayed. There are *three* mm. papillares for the *three* cuspides of the valva atrioventricularis dextra (mm. papillares anterior, posterior, and septalis) and *two* mm. papillares for the *two* cuspides of the valva atrioventricularis sinistra (mm. papillares anterior and posterior). The mm. papillares (specialized extensions of the trabeculae carneae) are attached to the free margins of the valve cuspides by chordae tendineae. When the mm. papillares contract (valva closure), the chordae tendineae

are shortened to restrict the motion of the valve cuspides. This keeps the cuspides from opening into the atria during ventricular contraction (systole), thereby preventing the regurgitation of blood back into the atria. *Note:* Like other myocardial regions, the myocardium of the mm. papillares may suffer necrosis due to a myocardial infarction, leaving the corresponding cuspis prone to prolapse into the atrium. Conversely, pathological shortening of the chordae may also prevent the valve from closing completely. This also would allow blood to regurgitate into the atrium during ventricular systole, producing an audible heart murmur (see p. 118).

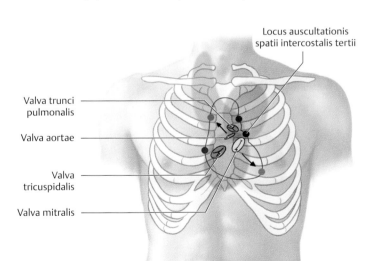

Locus auscultationis spatii intercostalis tertii

Valva trunci pulmonalis

Valva aortae

Valva tricuspidalis

Valva mitralis

C Auscultation of the valvae cordis

The diagram shows the anatomical projection of the valvae onto the thorax and the auscultation sites (the areas to which abnormal heart murmurs of the respective valves are transmitted). In the healthy heart, blood does not generate a perceptible sound as it flows across thevalvae cordis (see p. 118 for the physiologic heart sounds). But if the valvae are functionally impaired as a result of disease, the blood flow at the valvae cordis becomes turbulent. This type of flow produces audible sounds that are transmitted via the bloodstream. As the thick cardiac wall muffles these sounds, they are not heard best over the anatomical projections of the valvae on the chest wall, but are heard more clearly at sites located downstream from the valvae (see **D**).

D Anatomical projections and auscultation sites of the cardiac valves

Valve	Anatomical projection	Auscultation site
Valva aortae	Left sternal border at the level of the third spatium intercostale	Right second spatium intercostale close to the sternum
Valva trunci pulmonalis	Left sternal border at the level of the costa III	Left second spatium intercostale close to the sternum
Valva atrioventricularis dextra (valva tricuspidalis)	Sternum at the level of the costa V	Right fourth spatium intercostale close to the sternum*
Valva atrioventricularis sinistra (valva mitralis)	Left fourth or costa V	Left fifth spatium intercostale in the linea medioclavicularis

*The left lower sternal border is also a common site for auscultation of the right valva atrioventricularis.

109

3.8 Radiographic Appearance of the Cor

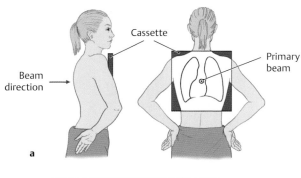

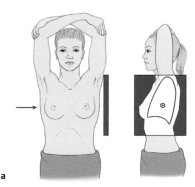

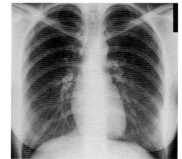

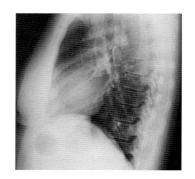

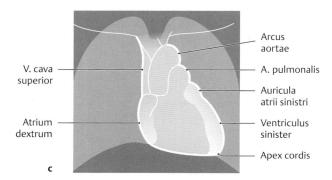

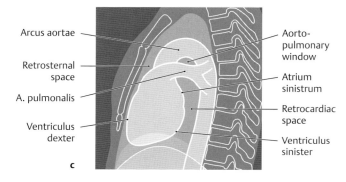

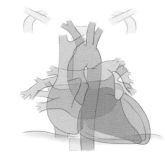

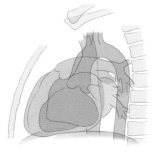

A Postero-anterior (PA) chest radiograph

a The patient stands with the anterior chest wall on the cassette (the beam "passes" through the patient in a posterior-to-anterior direction with the central beam targeted at the level of the T6 vertebra). The radiographs are taken with the patient keeping the mouth open, breathing in and holding the breath. The back of the hands are placed on the hips with the elbows turned forward;

b Posterior-anterior radiograph (viewed from an anterior to posterior direction);

c Heart shadow (cardiac silhouette) with structures that form the cardiac borders;

d Topography of the cardiac shadow: right cor with inflow and outflow tract (gray); ventriculus sinister with outflow tract (red), atrium sinistrum with inflow tract (blue).

B Lateral chest radiograph

a The patient is standing with his or her left side against the cassette (thus preventing the appearance of an enlarged cor), with the arms raised and crossed above the head. The central beam is targeted a hand's width below the left armpit;

b Left lateral radiograph;

c Heart shadow with structures that form the cardiac borders;

d Topography of the cardiac shadow: right cor with inflow and outflow tract (gray); ventriculus sinister with outflow tract (red), atrium sinistrum with inflow tract (blue).

(Radiographs shown on this page are from Lange, S.: Radiologische Diagnostik der Thoraxerkrankungen, 3. Aufl./Diagnostic Thoracic Radiology, 3rd edition Thieme, Stuttgart 2005)

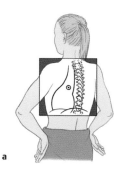
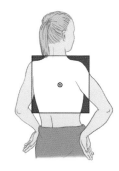

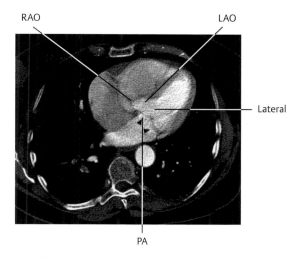

C Oblique chest radiograph

An oblique radiograph is taken with the patient turned 45 degrees toward the cassette. For optimal results, the distance between the cassette and the side of the columna vertebralis furthest away from it ("2" fig. **Eb** and **Fb**) should be two times the distance of the side closest to the cassette ("1" fig. **Eb** and **Fb**).

a Right anterior oblique view (RAO): the right chest touches the cassette (the fencing position);
b Left anterior oblique view (LAO): the left chest touches the cassette (the boxing position).

Note: The direction of the X-ray beam is from posterior to anterior. However, the radiograph is viewed from the front.

D Illustration of the various X-ray projections (LAO, RAO, PA, lateral) in a transverse (axial) CT scan

Note: axial images are always displayed from an inferior view (see p. 114).

(CT scans and radiographs on this page are from: Reiser, M. et al.: Radiologie [Duale Reihe], 2. Aufl./Radiology, 2nd edition Thieme, Stuttgart 2006)

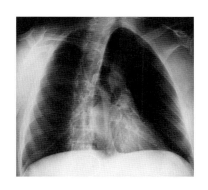
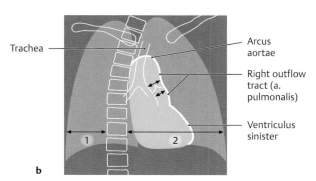
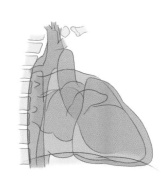

E Right anterior oblique (RAO) chest radiograph

a Radiograph (cor located on the right side of the columna vertebralis when viewed by examiner);
b Heart shadow with structures forming the cardiac borders: the right anterior oblique view is along the longitudinal axis of the cor and is thus a *lateral view*. The ROA view mainly demonstrates the

ventriculus dexter, its outflow tract, and the margin of the truncus pulmonalis.
c Topography of the cardiac shadow: right cor with inflow and outflow tract (gray); ventriculus sinister with outflow tract (red), atrium sinistrum with inflow tract (blue).

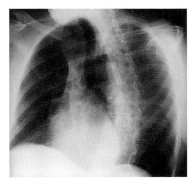
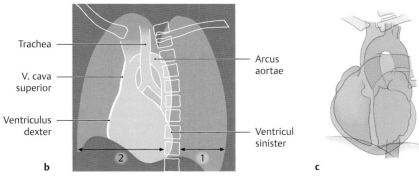

F Left anterior oblique (LAO) chest radiograph

a Radiograph (cor located on the *left side* of the columna vertebralis when viewed by examiner);
b Heart shadow with structures forming the cardiac borders: the left anterior oblique radiograph is a true *frontal view* (perpendicular to the RAO projection). The LAO projection is also referred to as the

"opened up aortic arch" view, since it shows the entire length of the arcus aortae. Structures that form the cardiac borders mainly include the ventriculi dexter and sinister.
c Topography of the cardiac shadow: right cor with inflow and outflow tract (gray); ventriculus sinister with outflow tract (red), atrium sinistrum with inflow tract (blue).

111

3.9 Sonographic Appearance of the Cor: Echocardiography

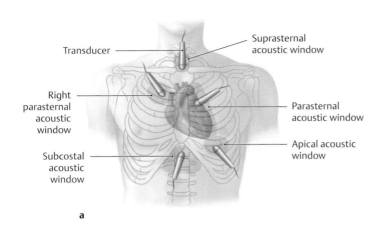

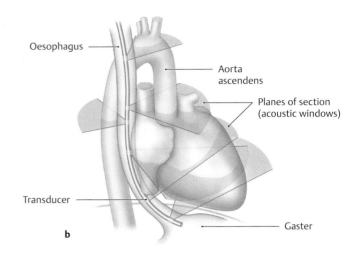

a

b

A Transthoracic echocardiography (TTE) and transesophageal echocardiography (TEE)

Echocardiography (cardiac ultrasound) is one of the most common procedures in the diagnosis of heart disease and is considered the most important, noninvasive imaging technique in cardiology. An essential component of every echocardiography device is the transducer. Through its piezoelectric crystals, the transducer generates ultrasonic waves, passes them into the body and receives the reflected ultrasound signal. Modern transducers contain many single crystals, which work in parallel and generate wave fronts resulting in a two-dimensional image (B-mode ultrasound). An echocardiogram is usually done with the patient lying down. The site where the transducer is placed is called the "acoustic window," a place on the body where the passage of sonic waves cannot be impeded by tissue of the pulmones or ribs (for example in the spatia intercostalia). It is worth noting that the acoustic window is not an exactly determined anatomical landmark but rather refers to an area, within which the optimum transducer location has to be determined individually for every patient. Depending on the acoustic window, one distinguishes between transthoracic (TTE) and transesophageal (TEE) echocardiography:

- In **transthoracic echocardiography** (**a**), the acoustic window is located with the patient in the left lateral position (for parasternal and apical acoustic windows), with the patient lying flat on their back (for suprasternal and subcostal acoustic windows), or with the patient in the right lateral position (for the right parasternal acoustic window). In the lateral position, the respective arm is placed under the head to spread the spatia intercostalia as much as possible. A disadvantage of this echocardiographic examination is that thoracic and pulmo structures such as ribs, muscle, fat and even pulmonary diseases (such as emphysema) may impede the diagnosis.

- In contrast to the conventional acoustic windows used in TTE, **transesophageal echocardiography** (**b**) uses part of the oesophagus as the acoustic window. Similar to gastroscopy, a miniaturized transducer is inserted through the cavitas oris and pharynx and into the oesophagus or fundus of the gaster. This places the probe close to the cor. Due to the short distance to the cor and the absence of interference from pulmo or thoracic structures, TEE provides better image quality than TTE. TEE clearly depicts the dorsal surface of the cor, the cardiac valvae, and the pars descendens aortae thoracicae. Using a multiplane transducer (which can be rotated throughout 180 degrees), pulling the transducer forward, backward, left and right, allows for a wide variety of sectional planes within the transesophageal acoustic window.

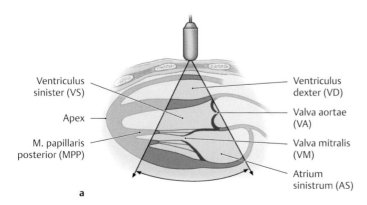

a

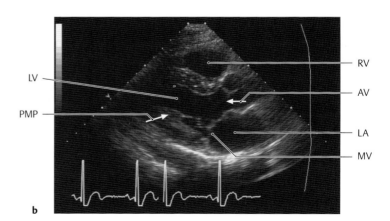

b

B Transthoracic echocardiography: Parasternal acoustic window (long-axis view)

a Schematic representation (Note, the apex of the ventriculus sinister is not shown); **b** Parasternal longitudinal view during isovolumic relaxation (from: Flachskampf, F.: Kursbuch Echokardiografie, 4. Aufl./Textbook Echocardiography, 4th edition, Thieme, Stuttgart 2008).

The echocardiographic examination usually begins with the parasternal longitudinal view. It is defined by the appearance of the valva aortae and valva mitralis, the septum interventriculare, which runs horizontally, the posterior wall of the ventriculus sinister and part of the ventriculus dexter. Short axis parasternal views of the cor can be obtained by rotating the transducer 90 degrees (see **C**).

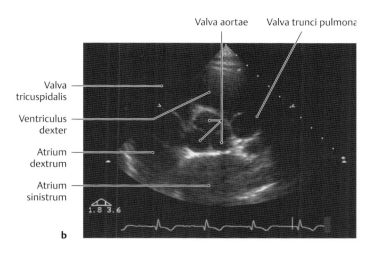

a Aortic valve **b**

1.8 3.6

C Transthoracic echocardiography: Parasternal acoustic window (short axis view)

a Schematic representation of the major short-axis views (imaging planes A, B, C, and D relative to a long-axis view); **b** Basal short-axis view at the level of the valva aortae (from: Flachskampf, F.: Kursbuch Echokardiografie, 4. Aufl./Textbook Echocardiography, 4th edition, Thieme, Stuttgart 2008).

This imaging plane shows at its center the valva aortae along with its three valvulae (valvulae semilunares sinistra, dextra and posterior [valvula non coronaria], see **B**, p. 128). In this scan, the valva aortae is surrounded by the following structures from clockwise: outflow tract of the ventriculus dexter (12 o'clock), valva trunci pulmonalis (2 o'clock), atrium sinistrum (5–7 o'clock), atrium dextrum (7–10 o'clock) and valva tricuspidalis (10 o'clock).

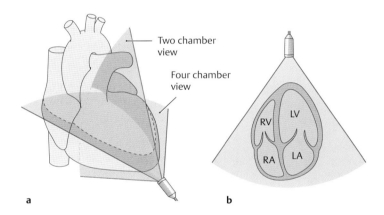

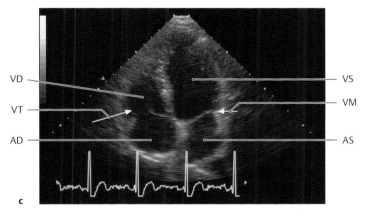

a **b** **c**

D Transthoracic echocardiography: Apical acoustic window (two- and four chamber views)

a and **b** Schematic representation (four- and two chamber views are perpendicular to each other; **c** Apical four chamber view at the beginning of systole (from: Flachskampf, F.: Kursbuch Echokardiografie, 4. Aufl./Textbook Echocardiography, 4th edition, Thieme, Stuttgart 2008).

The apical acoustic window is located approximately at the level of the apical impulse. The apical four-chamber view displays both ventriculi (VS, VD), both atria (AS, AD) and the valvae mitralis and tricuspidalis (VM, VT). Additionally, this window allows for the visualization of individual structures such as the septum and lateral portions of the myocardium during contraction.

E Transesophageal echocardiogram for atrial septal defect

Color-coded Doppler echocardiography displays a left-to-right shunt, esophageal acoustic window (four-chamber view). The atrial septal defect measures 1 cm in diameter. The Doppler echocardiography allows simultaneous imaging of the two-dimensional ultrasound scan and the color-coded Doppler technique. The blood flow is color-coded according to its direction and velocity. In this way, valva insufficiency and shunting of blood can be detected. (from: Reiser, M. et al.: Radiologie [Duale Reihe], 2. Aufl./Radiology, 2nd edition, Thieme, Stuttgart 2006).

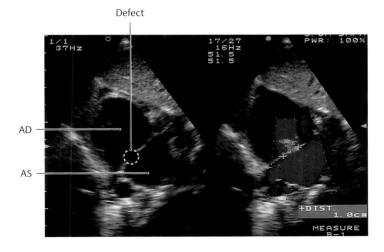

3.10 Magnetic Resonance Imaging (MRI) of the Cor

A Examination of cross-sectional images
Examination of **axial** or **transverse** cross-sectional images is done from an inferior view as if the patient is lying flat on his or her back. Thus, the planes of section are displayed with the columna vertebralis, located posteriorly, pointing downward and the skeleton thoracis, located anteriorly, pointing upward. Additionally, anatomical structures located on the right side appear on the left side of the image and vice versa.
The examination of **frontal** or **coronal** cross-sectional images is done as if the patient is standing in front of, and facing, the examiner.

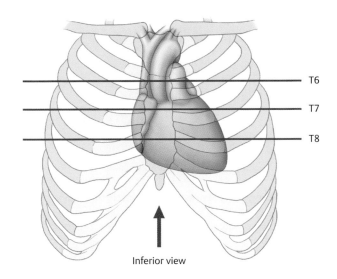

Inferior view

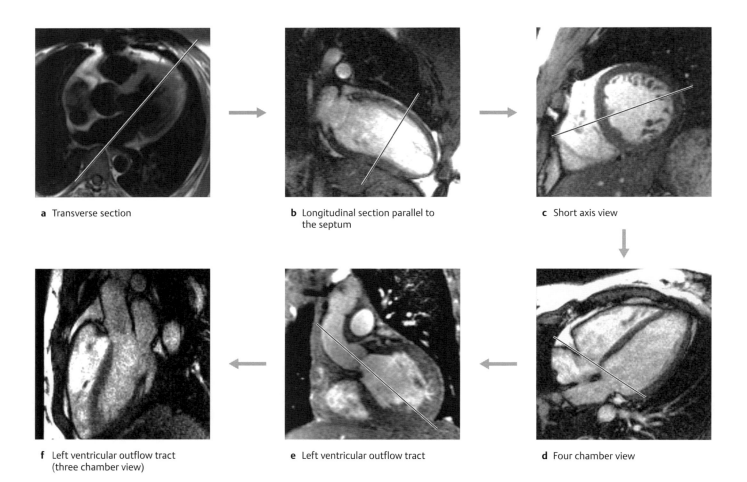

a Transverse section

b Longitudinal section parallel to the septum

c Short axis view

f Left ventricular outflow tract (three chamber view)

e Left ventricular outflow tract

d Four chamber view

B Overview of the standard views of a cardiac MRI
Cross-sectional imaging techniques for diagnosis of the heart use certain standard views obtained in multiple planes (**a–d**). In the single cross-sectional images, the plane of section for the following image has been marked (e.g., **a** shows a transverse section of the cor and the line corresponds to a longitudinal section of the ventriculus sinister parallel to the septum (**b**), etc.).

(All MRIs in this chapter are from Claussen, C. D. et al.: Pareto Reihe Radoiologie. Herz/Pareto series Radiology, Heart, Thieme, Stuttgart 2007.)

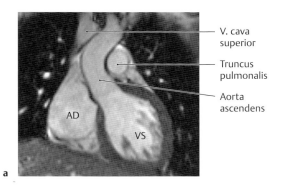

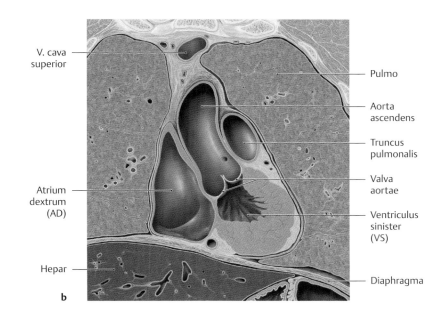

V. cava superior

Truncus pulmonalis

Aorta ascendens

AD

VS

a

V. cava superior

Atrium dextrum (AD)

Hepar

b

Pulmo

Aorta ascendens

Truncus pulmonalis

Valva aortae

Ventriculus sinister (VS)

Diaphragma

C Coronal MRI of the cor (SSFP sequence)

a Image displays left ventricular outflow tract (LVOT) during diastole.

b Corresponding coronal (frontal) anatomical cross-section of the cor, anterior view.

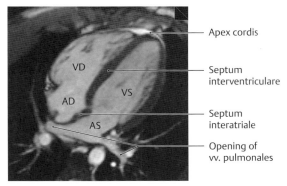

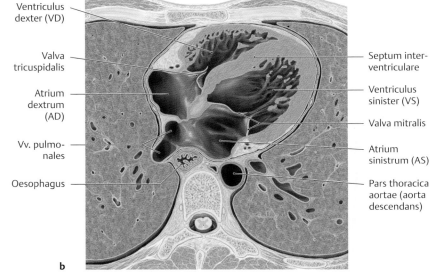

Apex cordis

Septum interventriculare

Septum interatriale

Opening of vv. pulmonales

VD

AD

VS

AS

a

Ventriculus dexter (VD)

Valva tricuspidalis

Atrium dextrum (AD)

Vv. pulmonales

Oesophagus

b

Septum interventriculare

Ventriculus sinister (VS)

Valva mitralis

Atrium sinistrum (AS)

Pars thoracica aortae (aorta descendans)

D Axial MRI of the cor (SSFP sequence)

a Image displays the atrioventricular connections of both the right and left sides of the cor during diastole (four-chamber view).

b Corresponding transverse anatomical cross section of the cor, inferior view.

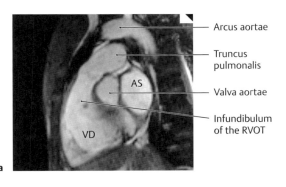

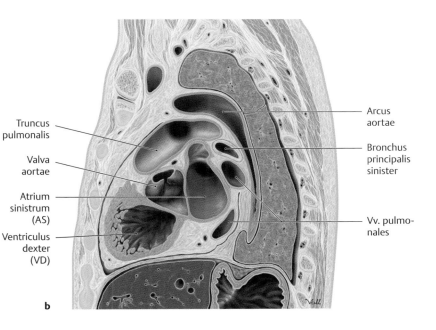

Arcus aortae

Truncus pulmonalis

Valva aortae

Infundibulum of the RVOT

AS

VD

a

Truncus pulmonalis

Valva aortae

Atrium sinistrum (AS)

Ventriculus dexter (VD)

b

Arcus aortae

Bronchus principalis sinister

Vv. pulmonales

E Sagittal MRI of the cor (SSFP sequence)

a Image displays the right ventricular outflow tract (RVOT) during diastole.

b Corresponding sagittal anatomical cross-section of the cor, viewed from the left side.

3.11 Impulse Formation and Conduction System of the Cor; Electrocardiogram

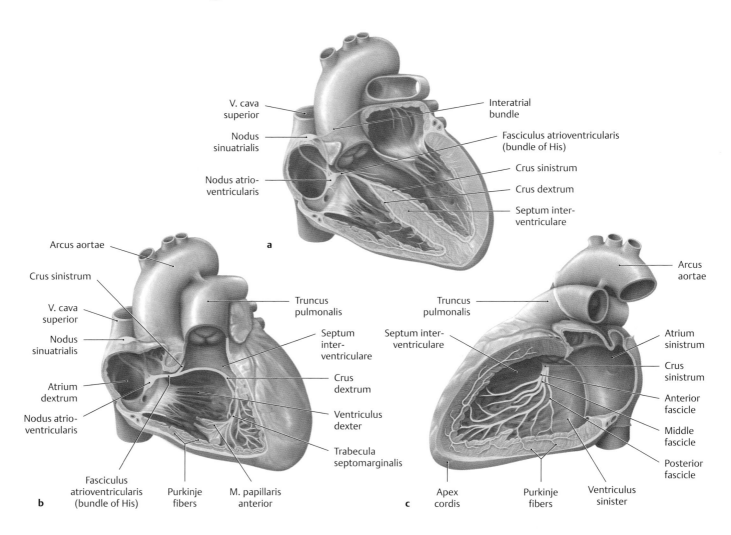

V. cava superior

Nodus sinuatrialis

Nodus atrio-ventricularis

Interatrial bundle

Fasciculus atrioventricularis (bundle of His)

Crus sinistrum

Crus dextrum

Septum inter-ventriculare

a

Arcus aortae

Crus sinistrum

V. cava superior

Nodus sinuatrialis

Atrium dextrum

Nodus atrio-ventricularis

Truncus pulmonalis

Septum inter-ventriculare

Crus dextrum

Ventriculus dexter

Trabecula septomarginalis

Fasciculus atrioventricularis (bundle of His)   Purkinje fibers   M. papillaris anterior

b

Truncus pulmonalis

Septum inter-ventriculare

Arcus aortae

Atrium sinistrum

Crus sinistrum

Anterior fascicle

Middle fascicle

Posterior fascicle

Apex cordis   Purkinje fibers   Ventriculus sinister

c

A Overview of cardiac impulse formation and conduction
Anterior view (**a**), right lateral view (**b**), left lateral view (**c**).
Even when the extrinsic nervous control of the cor is completely disrupted, it continues to beat. When supplied with oxygen and nutrients, it can even keep beating after it has been removed from the chest. This is made possible by an intrinsic, independent system that generates and conducts excitatory impulses in the cor. This system consists of specialized myocardial cells and has four main parts:

- Nodus sinuatrialis (SA node, sinus node)
- Nodus atrioventricularis (AV node)
- Fasciculus atrioventricularis (AV bundle, bundle of His)
- Crura dextrum and sinistrum

SA node (the "pacemaker" of the cor, approximately 1 cm long). The cardiac impulse begins in the SA node, a subepicardial node located on the posterior side of the atrium dextrum near the ostium venae cavae superioris. The SA node generates salvos of impulses which stimulate the atrial myocardium at a resting rate of 60–70 beats/min. The atrial impulses spread rapidly toward the ventriculi (particularly in the crista terminalis and internodal bundles between the SA and AV nodes, as shown by electrophysiologic studies). The impulses travel from the AV node to the fasciculus atrioventricularis, which distributes branches to the ventricular myocardium.(Direct impulse conduction from the atrium to the ventriculi is normally prevented by the insulating effect of the fibrous skeleton.)

AV node (approximately 5 mm long): located in the septum interatriale near the ostium sinus coronarii. This node delays impulse conduction to the ventriculi, allowing both atria to depolarize before ventricular contraction begins. It can also generate impulses spontaneously, but at a considerably lower rate than the SA node (approximately 40–50 depolarizations/min). Because of its slower rate, the AV node cannot act as a pacemaker for the cor when the SA node is intact.
Fasciculus atrioventricularis (bundle of His) (approximately 2 cm long). The fasciculus atrioventricularis is subendocardial while still in the atrium. It then passes through the trigonum fibrosum dextrum (see p. 107) to enter the septum interventriculare, where it divides (in the pars membranacea of the septum) into the crura dextrum and sinistrum. The AV bundle conducts impulses from the AV node to the ventriculi.
Crus sinistrum: branches to the left from the bundle of His and divides into three main fascicles (anterior, middle, and posterior).
Crus dextrum: initially continues in the septum interventriculare toward the apex cordis and is then distributed to the ventricular wall. The main trunk of the crus dextrum enters the trabecula septomarginalis, known also as the "moderator band." Finally the impulse is distributed throughout the ventricular myocardium by the Purkinje fibers.
Note: The Purkinje fibers stimulate the ventricular walls in a retrograde direction, proceeding from the apex cordis toward the atria. Thus the apical myocardium contracts first, pulling the apex cordis toward the plane of the valvae. The mm. papillares, which are stimulated by direct fibers from the crura, contract before the ventricular walls to ensure that the AV valves remain closed during ventricular systole.

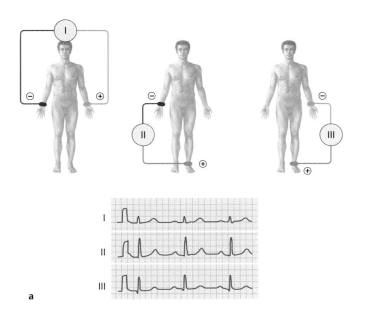

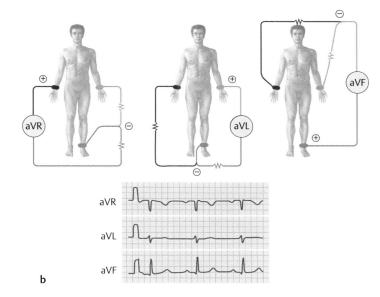

a

b

B Electrocardiogram (ECG): Standard leads
a Bipolar limb leads after Einthoven; **b** Unipolar limb leads after Goldberger; **c** Chest wall leads after Wilson.

Electrical impulses (called action potentials) generated by the SA node spread across the entire cor via its conduction system (see left page). The impulses produce an electric field, which is measurable on the body surface. Across this electric field, potential differences of up to 1 mV (1V = 1000 mV) occur between different points on the body surface (e.g., between right arm and left leg) during the spread of cardiac excitation and depolarization. Electrodes are used to record these potential differences on the body surface in the form of lines, spikes and curves (electrocardiogram). In a healthy cor, the spikes and waves show specific shapes and intervals between them, from which one can obtain information about heart rate (and thus cardiac rhythm), the electrical activity of the cor, and especially about the functioning or nonfunctioning of the impulse formation and conduction system of the cor. The standard surface ECG includes recordings from 12 leads: 6 limb leads (I, II, III, aVR, aVL, aVF) and 6 chest wall leads (V1–V6).

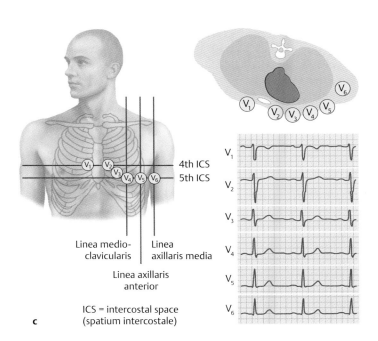

4th ICS
5th ICS

Linea medio-clavicularis | Linea axillaris media

Linea axillaris anterior

ICS = intercostal space (spatium intercostale)

c

C Names and definition of waves, spikes, and intervals in the ECG

Name	Definition
P wave	Atrial depolarization (< 0.1 s)
Q, R, and S wave (the QRS complex)	Beginning of ventricular excitation (< 0.1 s)
T wave	End of ventricular excitation
PQ interval	Onset of atrial excitation until the onset of ventricular excitation = conduction time = 0.1–0.2 s
QT interval	Q spike until the end of the T wave = time needed for both ventricles for de- and repolarization = 0.32–0.39 s. Varies based on the heart rate of the individual
Cardiac cycle	Interval between two R spikes
Heart rate	60 s/distance between R spikes (s) = beats/minute; e.g., 60/0.8 = 75

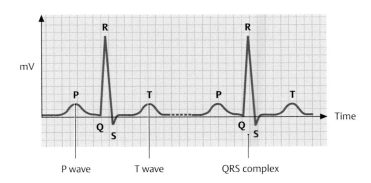

P wave   T wave   QRS complex

D ECG curve: Excitation cycle (recording of two heartbeats, after Wilson)
The ECG waveform has several spikes and waves, whose names and definitions are indicated in **C**.

3.12 Mechanical Action of the Cor

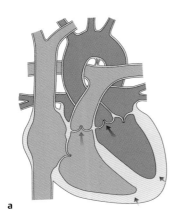

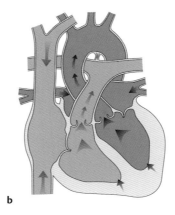

a

b

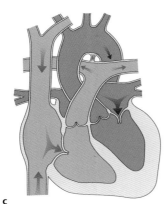

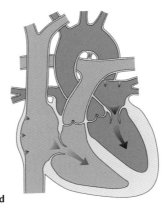

c

d

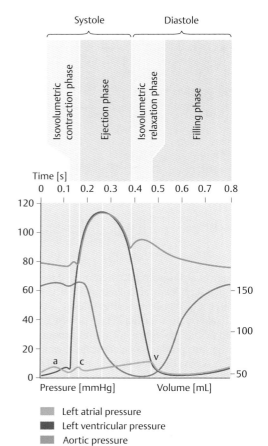

Systole   Diastole

Isovolumetric contraction phase | Ejection phase | Isovolumetric relaxation phase | Filling phase

Left atrial pressure
Left ventricular pressure
Aortic pressure
Left ventricular volume

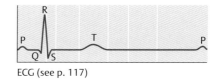

ECG (see p. 117)

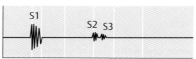

Heart sounds

S1 = first heart sound
(closure of the atrioventricular valves)

S2 = second heart sound
(closure of the semilunar valves)

S3 = split second heart sound) the valva
aortae (S2) closes before valva trunci
pulmonalis (S3)

e

A Phases of the heartbeat

a and **b** Ventricular systole: isovolumetric contraction (**a**) and ejection phase (**b**); **c** and **d** Ventricular diastole: isovolumetric relaxation (**c**) and filling phase (**d**); **e** Correlation between pressure, volume, ECG and heartbeats during systole and diastole. The heartbeat consists of two main phases: contraction (systole) and relaxation (diastole). A total of four phases are distinguished in the contraction and expansion of the ventriculi:

Ventricular systole:

- Isovolumetric contraction phase (**a**): The ventricular myocardium contracts and tightens around the blood column within the ventriculus. All valvae are closed, that is, the AV valves are *already* closed (ventricular pressure exceeds the atrial pressure), and the valvae aortae and trunci pulmonalis are *still* closed (ventricular pressure is still lower than the intra-arterial pressure). Isovolumetric contraction of the myocardium around the blood column produces a mechanical vibration that is audible as the first heart sound. In fact, it is the closure of the valvae atrioventriculares, that produces the first heart sound.
- Ejection phase (**b**): The AV valves remain closed and prevent the reflux of ventricular blood into the atria. As the intraventricular pressure exceeds the pressure in the

arteries, the valvae aortae and trunci pulmonalis, and blood flows into the aorta and truncus pulmonalis.

Ventricular diastole:

- Isovolumetric relaxation phase (**c**): The ventricular myocardium relaxes. All valvae are closed during this phase: The AV valves are *still* closed, and the valvae aortae and trunci pulmonalis are *already* closed (to prevent the reflux of ejected blood back into the ventriculi). Closure of the valvae aortae and trunci pulmonalis ("slamming doors") is audible as the second heart sound. Occasionally the arterial valvae close at slightly different times, producing a divided second heart sound.
- Filling phase (**d**): The intraventricular pressure is very low, and the arterial valvae remain closed. The AV valves open, and blood flows into the ventriculi. Ventricular filling results more from the movement of the valve plane than from atrial contraction: The valve plane moves toward the apex cordis during systole, and it returns very quickly to its initial position during diastole, "throwing itself" over the blood column.

Note: During both the isovolumetric contraction phase and the relaxation phase, there are periods in which all the valves are closed. By contrast, there is no point in the cardiac cycle when all valves are open.

Heart sounds are normal acoustical phenomena produced by the cor. Abnormal valvular heart sounds (murmurs) are described on p. 109. Although the first heart sound is generated by ventricular contraction itself, that first sound is clinically associated with closure of the valvae atrioventriculares.

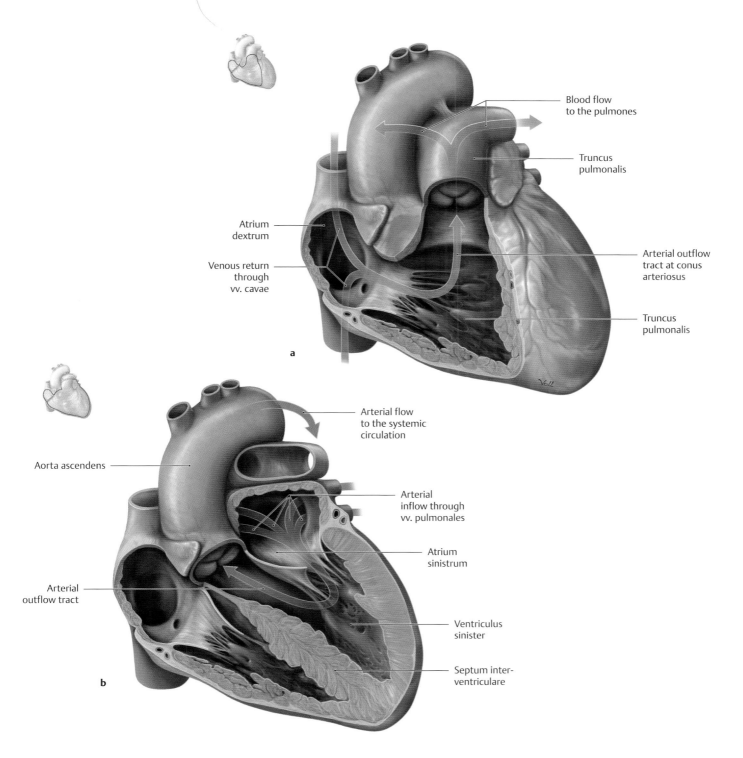

Blood flow
to the pulmones

Truncus
pulmonalis

Atrium
dextrum

Arterial outflow
tract at conus
arteriosus

Venous return
through
vv. cavae

Truncus
pulmonalis

a

Arterial flow
to the systemic
circulation

Aorta ascendens

Arterial
inflow through
vv. pulmonales

Atrium
sinistrum

Arterial
outflow tract

Ventriculus
sinister

Septum inter-
ventriculare

b

B Blood flow in the cor

The septa between the atria and ventriculi functionally divide the cor into two main parts: the right cor and left cor. The cardiac valvae define the direction of blood flow through both sides of the cor, enabling the right and left cor to function as finely coordinated tandem pumps.

Blood flow in the right cor (a): Anterior view with the atrium dextrum and ventriculus dexter cut open. Venous blood from the vv. cavae superior and inferior flows into the sinus venarum cavarum and enters the atrium dextrum. From there it flows across the open valva atrioventricularis dextra and passes through the ostium atrioventriculare dextrum along the inflow tract into the ventriculus dexter. Inside the ventriculus it is redirected into the outflow tract and pumped through the open valva trunci pulmonalis (shown closed here) and conus arteriosus into

the truncus pulmonalis. From there it flows through the aa. pulmonales into the pulmones, where it is oxygenated. The right cor pumps blood with a low oxygen tension.

Blood flow in the left cor (b): Left anterior view. All of the cardiac chambers have been cut open anteriorly. Oxygenated blood from the pulmone flows across the open valva atrioventricularis sinister and through the ostium atrioventriculare sinistrum along the inflow tract into the ventriculus sinister. There it is rerouted into the outflow tract and flows across the open valva aortae (shown closed here) through the ostium aortae into the aorta ascendens for distribution throughout the systemic circulation (after first perfusing the aa. coronariae). The left cor pumps blood with a high oxygen tension.

3.13 Arteriae Coronariae and Venae Cordis: Classification and Topography

A Arteriae coronariae and venae cordis

a Anterior view of the facies sternocostalis of the cor

b Posteroinferior view of the facies diaphragmatica of the cor

Because the cor functions continuously to pump blood, it has a high oxygen demand. This demand is met by the aa. coronariae dextra and sinistra—intrinsic cardiac vessels that have an extensive capillary network. The aa. coronariae spring from small dilations in the aorta (the sinus aortae) located just above the valva aortae. The main trunk of the a. coronaria sinistra, which is usually slightly larger, divides into

- R. circumflexus: runs in the sulcus coronarius (boundary between the atrium and ventriculus) around the *left* side of the cor to the posterior heart wall
- R. interventricularis anterior: runs in the sulcus interventricularis anterior (boundary between the ventriculi) to the apex cordis. Each of these vessels gives off smaller branches.

The a. coronaria dextra, usually smaller than the a. coronaria sinistra, runs in the sulcus coronarius around the *right* side of the cor to the posterior wall, where it forms the r. interventricularis posterior. It also gives off numerous branches (see p. 122).

Note: The aa. coronariae are functional end arteries because they form anastomoses that are not adequate for reciprocal blood flow. The aa. coronariae must efficiently deliver blood to an organ with constant high metabolic demand that is itself at elevated pressure, especially during systole. This difficult requirement is achieved in part by the anatomical relation between the valva aortae and the origin of the aa. coronariae, just superior to the valvulae. As the ventriculus sinister completes its contraction and the distended aorta begins to recoil, the valva aortae is forced closed by the backflow and a local surge in pressure (a pressure *hammer*) develops. This pressure hammer drives blood into the aa. coronariae. The cor is thus efficiently perfused at the maximum pressure that the cardiovascular system can reach.

The **vv. cardiacae** usually course with the aa. coronariae and consist of the vv. cardiacae magna, media, and parva. These veins open on the posterior heart wall into the *sinus coronarius*, which empties into the atrium dextrum. Additional smaller veins (vv. cardiacae minimae, not shown here, Thebesian veins) open directly into the cardiac chambers, mainly the atrium dextrum.

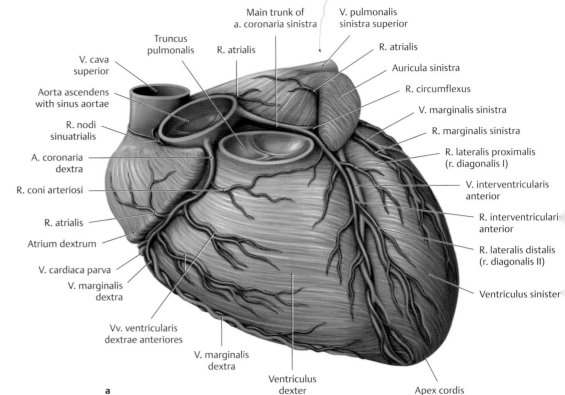

Main trunk of a. coronaria sinistra
V. pulmonalis sinistra superior
Truncus pulmonalis
R. atrialis
R. atrialis
V. cava superior
Auricula sinistra
Aorta ascendens with sinus aortae
R. circumflexus
R. nodi sinuatrialis
V. marginalis sinistra
A. coronaria dextra
R. marginalis sinistra
R. coni arteriosi
R. lateralis proximalis (r. diagonalis I)
R. atrialis
V. interventricularis anterior
Atrium dextrum
R. interventricularis anterior
V. cardiaca parva
R. lateralis distalis (r. diagonalis II)
V. marginalis dextra
Ventriculus sinister
Vv. ventricularis dextrae anteriores
V. marginalis dextra
Ventriculus dexter
Apex cordis

a

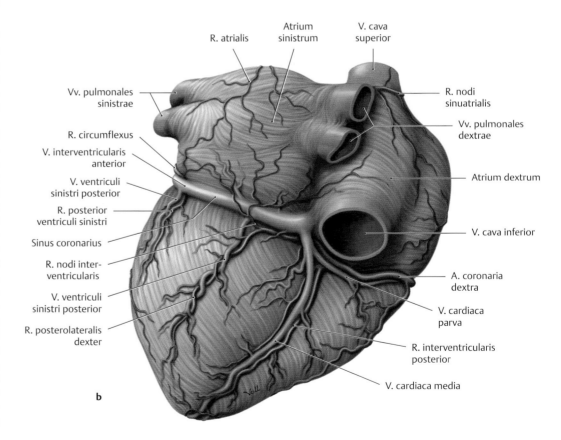

Atrium sinistrum
V. cava superior
R. atrialis
Vv. pulmonales sinistrae
R. nodi sinuatrialis
R. circumflexus
Vv. pulmonales dextrae
V. interventricularis anterior
Atrium dextrum
V. ventriculi sinistri posterior
R. posterior ventriculi sinistri
V. cava inferior
Sinus coronarius
R. nodi interventricularis
A. coronaria dextra
V. ventriculi sinistri posterior
V. cardiaca parva
R. posterolateralis dexter
R. interventricularis posterior
V. cardiaca media

b

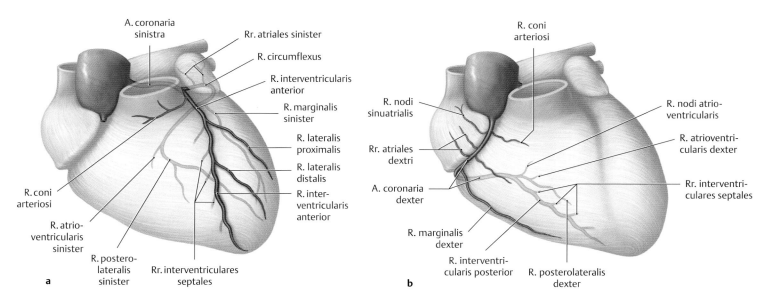

B Classification of the arteriae coronariae

a Branches of the a. coronaria sinistra; **b** Branches of the a. coronaria dextra (anterior views of the facies sternocostalis).

The diagram shows the normal or balanced circulation (70% of all cases). In the balanced type, the posterior wall of the cor (facies diaphragmatica; clinically: posterior wall) is supplied equally by the aa. coronariae sinistra and dextra (for details about right or left dominant coronary circulation, see pp. 122 and 123). Based on a recommendation by the American Heart Association, the individual aa. coronariae are divided into segments: a. coronaria dextra (segments 1–4); a. coronaria sinistra (segments 5–15). Segment 5 corresponds with the main trunk, segments 6–10 with the r. interventricularis anterior, and segments 11–15 with the r. circumflexus of the a. coronaria sinistra (see also p. 126).

C Branches of the arteriae coronariae*

Arteria coronaria sinistra (LCA)

R. circumflexus (LCX)
- Left rr. atriales
- R. marginalis sinister (LM)
- R. atrioventricularis sinister (LAV)
- R. posterolateralis sinister (LPL or PLA) or r. posterior ventriculi sinistri

R. interventricularis anterior (AIV or LAD, left anterior descending artery)
- R. coni arteriosi
- R. lateralis proximalis (r. diagonalis 1, D1)
- R. lateralis distalis (r. diagonalis 2, D2)
- Rr. interventriculares septales

Arteria coronaria dextra (RCA)
- R. nodi sinuatrialis (SAN)
- Right rr. atriales
- R. coni arteriosi
- R. nodi atrioventricularis (AVN)
- R. marginalis dexter (RM)
- R. interventricularis posterior (PIV or PDA, posterior descending artery)
- R. atrioventricularis dexter (RAV)
- Rr. interventriculares septales
- R. posterolateralis dexter (RPL or PLA)

*RCA, LCA, LCX and LAD are common medical abbreviations.

E Divisions of the venae cordis

Vena cardiaca magna
- V. marginalis sinistra
- V. interventricularis anterior
- V. ventriculi sinistri posterior

Vena cardiaca media (v. interventricularis posterior)

Vena cardiaca parva
- V. ventriculi dextri anterior
- V. marginalis dextra

Note: Venous blood collected by the vv. cardiacae is largely (75%) carried to the atrium dextrum via the sinus coronarius (coronary sinus system). Additionally, venous blood is drained via the transmural (superficial veins, which directly drain into the atrium) and endomural systems (veins from the inner layer of the myocardium, which directly empty into the lumen).

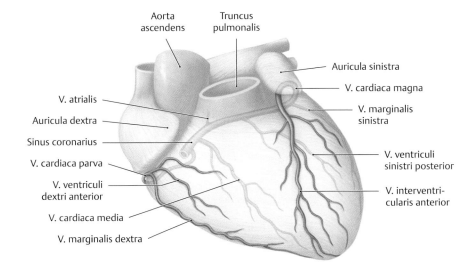

D Classification of venae cordis

Anterior view of the facies sternocostalis.

3.14 Arteriae Coronariae: Coronary Circulation

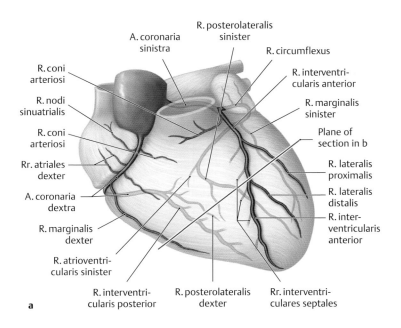

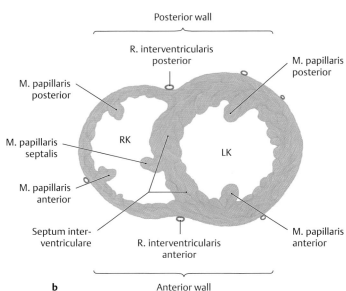

A Balanced (normal) coronary supply

a Course of the aa. coronariae dextra and sinistra (anterior view of the facies sternocostalis); **b** Cross-section of both ventriculi (area supplied by the a. coronaria dextra: colored in green, area supplied by the a. coronaria sinistra: colored in red).

In the balanced type of circulation (70%), the posterior wall of the cor is supplied equally by the aa. coronariae sinistra and dextra (the r. interventricularis posterior comes off the a. coronaria dextra). It is also referred to as codominant circulation supplying the posterior wall of the cor (facies diaphragmatica) (see **B**).

Note: Since the branches of the a. coronaria dextra also supply major centers of the conduction system (nodus sinuatrialis, nodus atrioventricularis, fasciculus atrioventricularis), a narrowing of the a. coronaria dextra often leads to arrhythmia.

B Distribution of the arteriae coronariae sinistra and dextra

Distribution	Arteria coronaria sinistra	Arteria coronaria dextra
Atrium sinistrum	Rr. atriales and a r. atrialis intermedius of the r. circumflexus	
Atrium dextrum		Rr. atriales and r. atrialis intermedius
Ventriculus sinister • Anterior wall • Lateral wall • Posterior wall	• R. interventricularis anterior and its proximal and distal rr. laterales (diagonal) • R. marginalis sinister of the r. circumflexus • Partly by the r. posterior ventriculi sinistri of the r. circumflexus	 • Partly by the r. posterolateralis dexter
Ventriculus dexter • Anterior wall • Lateral wall • Posterior wall	• Strip near the septum by the r. coni arteriosi and small twigs from the r. interventricularis anterior	• R. coni arteriosi with smaller twigs and the r. marginalis dexter • R. marginalis dexter • R. interventricularis posterior
Septum interventriculare	Rr. interventriculares septales (supply the larger anterior part of the septum)	Rr. interventriculares septales (supply the smaller posterior part of the septum)
Nodus sinuatrialis (sinus node)		R. nodi sinuatrialis
Nodus atrioventricularis (AV node)		R. nodi atrioventricularis

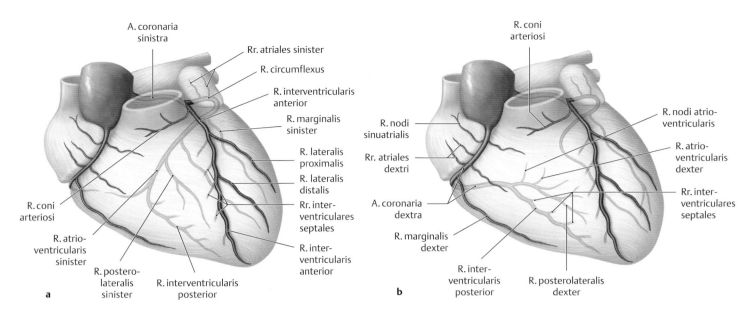

a

- A. coronaria sinistra
- Rr. atriales sinister
- R. circumflexus
- R. interventricularis anterior
- R. marginalis sinister
- R. lateralis proximalis
- R. lateralis distalis
- Rr. interventriculares septales
- R. interventricularis anterior
- R. coni arteriosi
- R. atrioventricularis sinister
- R. posterolateralis sinister
- R. interventricularis posterior

b

- R. coni arteriosi
- R. nodi sinuatrialis
- Rr. atriales dextri
- A. coronaria dextra
- R. marginalis dexter
- R. nodi atrioventricularis
- R. atrioventricularis dexter
- Rr. interventriculares septales
- R. interventricularis posterior
- R. posterolateralis dexter

C Left and right dominant coronary circulation
a Left dominant circulation; **b** Right dominant circulation.
Left and right dominant circulations each occur in 15% of corda. Both types of circulation differ in how the posterior wall of the cor is supplied:

- **Left dominant circulation (a)** is dominated by a strong r. circumflex, which ends as the r. interventricularis posterior at the posterior wall. In addition to the posterior parts of the septum interventriculare, it also supplies parts of the ventriculus dexter.
- **Right dominant circulation (b)** is dominated by the a. coronaria dextra, which in addition to the r. interventricularis posterior also

supplies the largest part of the posterior wall with the help of a strong r. posterolateralis dexter. The r. circumflexus of the a. coronaria sinistra is weakly developed (for details about the differences between the three types of circulation see also fig. **Da–c**)

Note: Because the r. interventricularis posterior is variable in its development and origin, there is also considerable variation in the supply to the ventriculi sinister and dexter and septum interventriculare by the aa. coronariae dextra and sinistra.

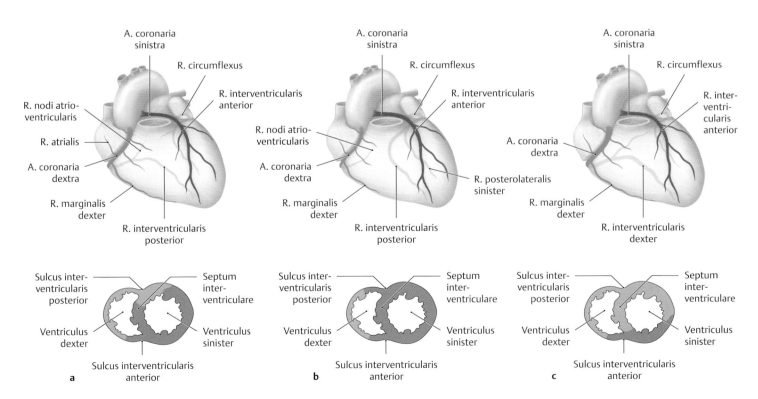

a

- A. coronaria sinistra
- R. circumflexus
- R. interventricularis anterior
- R. nodi atrioventricularis
- R. atrialis
- A. coronaria dextra
- R. marginalis dexter
- R. interventricularis posterior
- Sulcus interventricularis posterior
- Septum interventriculare
- Ventriculus dexter
- Ventriculus sinister
- Sulcus interventricularis anterior

b

- A. coronaria sinistra
- R. circumflexus
- R. interventricularis anterior
- R. nodi atrioventricularis
- A. coronaria dextra
- R. marginalis dexter
- R. posterolateralis sinister
- R. interventricularis posterior
- Sulcus interventricularis posterior
- Septum interventriculare
- Ventriculus dexter
- Ventriculus sinister
- Sulcus interventricularis anterior

c

- A. coronaria sinistra
- R. circumflexus
- R. interventricularis anterior
- A. coronaria dextra
- R. marginalis dexter
- R. interventricularis dexter
- Sulcus interventricularis posterior
- Septum interventriculare
- Ventriculus dexter
- Ventriculus sinister
- Sulcus interventricularis anterior

D Comparison of the types of coronary circulation
a Balanced circulation (in 70% of corda); **b** Left dominant circulation (in 15% of corda); **c** Right dominant circulation (in 15% of corda).

Diagrams each show a ventral view and a cross-section of both chambers, viewed from above; a. coronaria sinistra and area it supplies colored in red, a. coronaria dextra and area it supplies colored in green.

123

3.15 Coronary Heart Disease (CHD) and Heart Attack

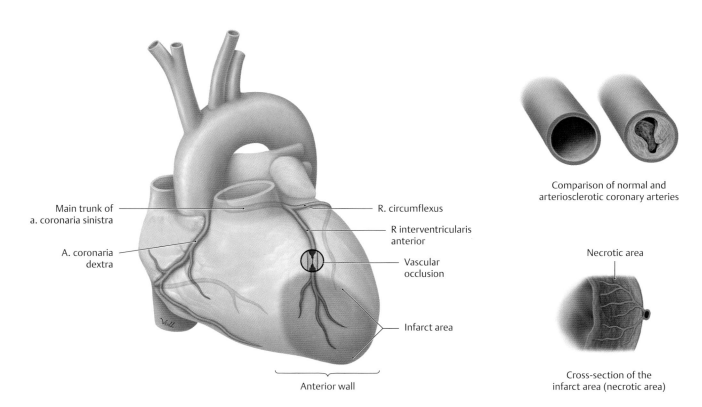

Main trunk of
a. coronaria sinistra

A. coronaria
dextra

R. circumflexus

R interventricularis
anterior

Vascular
occlusion

Infarct area

Anterior wall

Comparison of normal and
arteriosclerotic coronary arteries

Necrotic area

Cross-section of the
infarct area (necrotic area)

A Acute myocardial infarction

Acute myocardial infarction is characterized by necrosis of myocardial tissue as a result of total occlusion or subcritical impairment of coronary blood flow (incidence rate in Germany 330/100,000 population per year). Acute myocardial infarction is often the result of coronary heart disease (CHD see **C**). Acute myocardial necrosis (myocardial infarction) usually occurs when an arteriosclerotic plaque ruptures (see **D**) which leads to thrombotic occlusion of one or multiple branches of the aa. coronariae (known as one-, two-, or three-vessel disease). Myocardial ischemia lasting for 20–30 minutes results in tissue necrosis with the subendocardial layers of the myocardium being damaged first. They are the farthest away from the blood capillaries and have a high rate of oxygen consumption. The damage is the result of the myocardium switching to anaerobic glycolysis, which leads to a reduced ability to produce ATP. The increase in metabolic waste products also inhibits the production of glycolytic ATP. As a result, cells (in particular the cellular membrane, mitochondria, and sarcoplasmic reticulum) are irreversibly damaged. Subsequent intracellular calcium ion overload in turn leads to activation of membrane phospholipases and the formation of inflammatory mediators. As a result, granulocytes and macrophages migrate into the infarct area. The necrotic area is filled in by the formation of granulation tissue. If the patient survives the myocardial infarction, the repair of the necrotic area, in which necrotic tissue is replaced by scar tissue composed of collagen, is usually complete by six weeks.

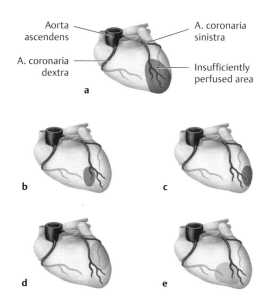

Aorta
ascendens

A. coronaria
dextra

A. coronaria
sinistra

Insufficiently
perfused area

a

b

c

d

e

B Infarct localizations and possible complications

The following infarct localizations are based on the location of a. coronaria stenosis:

a Anterior wall infarction
b Supra-apical anterior infarction
c Anterior lateral infarction
d Posterior lateral infarction
e Posterior infarction

Blockage of the a. coronaria dextra more frequently leads to arrhythmia because the a. coronaria dextra supplies the nodus sinuatrialis among other structures (see p. 122). Approximately 30% of all patients die within an hour of onset of acute myocardial infarction. The main causes of death include arrhythmia and the ensuing ventricular fibrillation (sudden cardiac death) as well as left ventricular insufficiency and cardiogenic shock. Additional complications include cardiac ruptures (particularly septal perforation) with ensuing pericardial tamponade, mitral insufficiency caused by m. papillarius rupture, and myocardial aneurysm.

C Overview of coronary heart disease (CHD) and myocardial ischemia

Definition: Stenosis of the aa. coronariae caused by arteriosclerosis (also known as coronary sclerosis) and the resulting reduced myocardial blood flow (ischemia).

Epidemiology: most common cause of death in Germany; incidence of CHD increases after age 50 (in women mainly after menopause), with men three times more likely to develop CHD than women.

Pathogenesis of myocardial ischemia When the aa. coronariae are stenosed as a result of arteriosclerosis (see **D**), they cannot spontaneously transport more blood. Yet this is necessary in order to rapidly supply the myocardium with more oxygen during physical exertion or psychological excitement. The increase in myocardial oxygen demand under stress is mainly due to an elevated heart rate and increased cardiac muscle contractility caused by activation of the sympathetic nervous system. A healthy heart responds by raising the diastolic blood pressure in the aorta and reducing coronary resistance to 20% of the resting value. It can thus increase coronary blood flow under stress to about 5 times the resting level; this is known as the coronary reserve. The ability of sclerotic aa. coronariae to dilate is reduced or minimal, leading to insufficient blood supply to the myocardium. The result is ischemia with too little oxygen being supplied to the respective area of the heart muscle. This eventually leads to myocardial tissue necrosis (see **A**). The arteriovenous oxygen difference cannot increase in the heart, because the heart's oxygen consumption from the aa. coronariae is maximal even in the resting state.

Clinical symptoms: Symptoms usually occur with a reduction in vascular lumen size of 75% or greater:

- Cardinal sign: (*angina pectoris*) squeezing, searing pain behind the breast bone (retrosternal), triggered by physical activity and/or psychological stress; pain often spreads to the left side of the thorax and the left arm, and sometimes to the neck, teeth, mouth, and jaw area as well as to the back.
- Accompanying symptoms: sweating, shortness of breath, reduced functional capacity
- Stable angina pectoris: pain vanishes when physical activity or stress has ended.
- Unstable angina pectoris: more frequent bouts of pain, which are more severe and last longer. They don't vanish once physical activity has ended or stress is over; significantly increased risk of heart attack.

Note: 25% of patients with stable angina pectoris will develop a myocardial infarction within 5 years, patients with unstable angina pectoris will suffer a myocardial infarction within 4 weeks. In more than half of all patients, sudden cardiac death or myocardial infarction are the first "signs" of CHD.

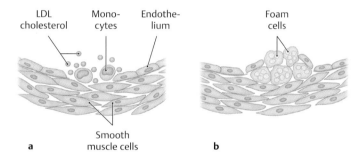

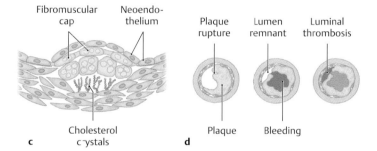

D Pathogenesis of arteriosclerotic changes in the arteriae coronariae (after Greten)

a Initial lesion; **b** Early lesion; **c** Late lesion; **d** Coronary occlusion.

Predilection sites of arteriosclerotic lesions are the proximal portions of the coronary vessels, particularly in the area where vessels divide as these areas are characterized by increased turbulent blood flow, which is a factor in initiating lesions. Coronary stenosis is caused initially by damage to the endothelium associated with certain risk factors (see **E**). With the help of adhesion proteins, monocytes attach to the sites of initial lesions and migrate as macrophages into the vessel wall. Through accumulation of lipids (mainly oxidized LDL cholesterol), macrophages transform into foam cells. These arteriosclerotic early lesions are also known as fatty streaks. Subsequently, additional cells migrate into the vessel wall. As a result, smooth muscle cells and fibroblasts proliferate forming a fibrous matrix composed of collagen, proteoglycans, calcium, and extracellular lipid deposits. The latter become confluent and are stored in a cavity covered by a fibrous cap and neoendothelium. In this way, complex lesions develop. These fibrous plaques increasingly lead to luminal stenosis. In the course of further progression, particularly lipid-rich plaques may rupture which can lead to intraplaque hemorrhage and formation of thromboses and subsequently to partial or complete coronary occlusion. These plaques, also known as vulnerable plaques, are characterized by high lipid accumulation, increased inflammatory cell activity (macrophages and T-lymphocytes) and high concentrations of tissue-resident coagulation factors.

E Cardiovascular risk factors for arteriosclerosis and CHD

Risk factors for CHD are conditions that occur more frequently in patients with CHD than in healthy subjects. It should be noted that not all cardiovascular events can be explained by the presence of these risk factors. The following risk factors promote arteriosclerosis and thus CHD:

- Arterial hypertension
- Being overweight (BMI > 25kg/m^2)
- Lack of exercise
- Hyperlipidemia (particularly lipid metabolic disorder with increased LDL levels and low HDL cholesterol)
- Tobacco abuse
- Diabetes mellitus
- Hereditary disposition

Note: The risk of developing CHD increases disproportionately if multiple risk factors are present.

3.16 Conventional Coronary Angiography (Heart Catheter Examination)

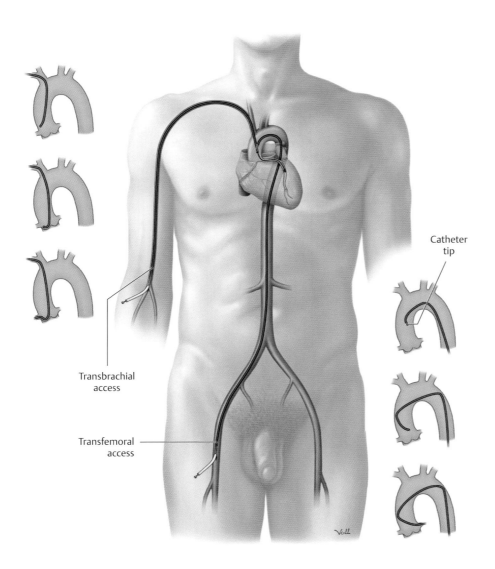

Transbrachial access

Transfemoral access

Catheter tip

A Heart catheter examination: Principle and execution

Conventional or selective coronary angiography (known as heart catheter examination) is an imaging technique, which uses X-rays and water-soluble iodinated contrast media to make the inside space, or lumen, of the aa. coronariae visible. It provides evidence for, or information about, the localization of coronary stenoses or occlusions. The heart catheter examination is an invasive procedure. It is done by performing left heart catheterization. A pre-shaped, stable catheter, through which X-ray dye is injected into the arteries, is advanced through the aorta. (*Note:* The aa. coronariae exit just above the valva aortae.) This is performed either via a trans*brachial* or more commonly via a trans*femoral* approach (right a. femoralis puncture). The angiogram begins with the injection of contrast agents. Arteria coronaria perfusion is documented with X-rays. If possible, every segment of the aa. coronariae should be displayed using two projections, which are perpendicular to each other (RAO and LAO projections, see **D** and **E**). Because it is an invasive procedure, conventional coronary angiography is not without risks (e.g., sensitivity to contrast agents, vascular damage, cardiac complications). However, in specialized centers, the incidence of severe complications is less than 1%.

Currently, selective coronary angiography is considered the gold standard for the diagnosis of a. coronaria disease (approx. 600,000 diagnostic and 200,000 interventional procedures per year in Germany). Other imaging technologies (MR and CT coronary angiography), which are less invasive and carry a very low risk, serve as an alternative. Both procedures allow for a detailed display of the aa. coronariae without invasive arterial puncture and sometimes even without using contrast agents (MR angiography).

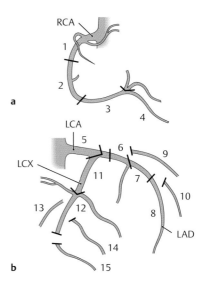

B Arteria coronaria segmentation
a A. coronaria dextra (RCA); **b** A. coronaria sinistra (LCA) and their individual segments (as suggested by the American Heart Association, AHA): a. coronaria dextra (segments 1-4); a. coronaria sinistra (segments 5-15).

RCA 1 = proximal portion; 2 = mid portion; 3 = distal portion; 4 = r. interventricularis posterior (PIV) and r. posterolateralis dexter (RPL)

LCA 5 = main trunk of the a. coronaria sinistra

LAD 6 = proximal portion; 7 = mid portion (distal to origin of first r. lateralis, D1); 8 = distal portion (distal to origin of second r. lateralis, D2); 9 = D1; 10 = D2

LCX 11 = proximal portion; 12 = distal portion (origin of r. marginalis sinister, LM); 13 = left r. atrioventricularis (LAV); 14 = r. posterior ventriculi sinistri; 15 = r. posterolateralis sinister (LPL)

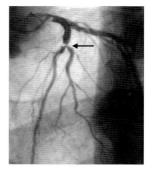

C Severe stenosis of the r. circumflexus
Selective coronary angiography in a 30 degree RAO projection. The arrow points to a severe stenosis in segment 11 (proximal portion) of the r. circumflexus (LCX) (from: Claussen, C.D. et al.: Pareto Reihe Radiologie. Herz/Pareto Series Radiology. Heart, Thieme, Stuttgart 2007).

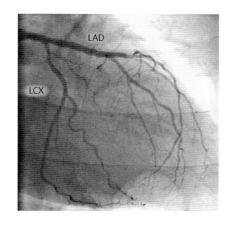

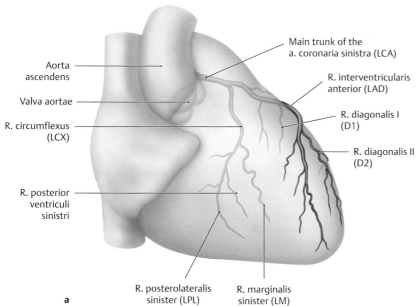

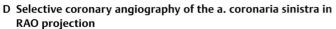

Aorta ascendens

Valva aortae

R. circumflexus (LCX)

R. posterior ventriculi sinistri

R. posterolateralis sinister (LPL)

R. marginalis sinister (LM)

Main trunk of the a. coronaria sinistra (LCA)

R. interventricularis anterior (LAD)

R. diagonalis I (D1)

R. diagonalis II (D2)

a

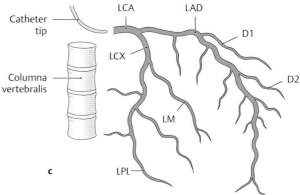

b

Catheter tip

Columna vertebralis

LCA   LAD

D1

LCX

D2

LM

LPL

c

D Selective coronary angiography of the a. coronaria sinistra in RAO projection

a Course of the a. coronaria sinistra (LCA); **b** Selective coronary angiography of the LCA; **c** Schematic representation of the individual branches.

Note: In RAO projections, the columna vertebralis is always projected to the left side.

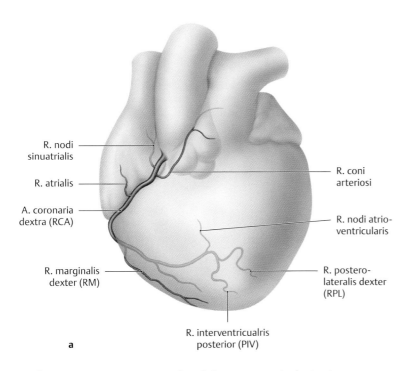

R. nodi sinuatrialis

R. atrialis

A. coronaria dextra (RCA)

R. marginalis dexter (RM)

R. coni arteriosi

R. nodi atrio-ventricularis

R. postero-lateralis dexter (RPL)

R. interventricualris posterior (PIV)

a

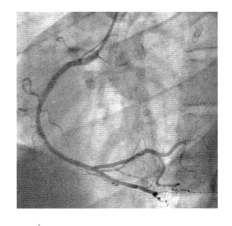

b

Catheter tip

Columna vertebralis

RCA

RM

RPL

PIV

c

E Selective coronary angiography of the a. coronaria dextra in LAO projection

a Course of the a. coronaria dextra (RCA); **b** Selective coronary angiography of the RCA; **c** Schematic representation of the individual branches.

Note: In LAO projections, the columna vertebralis is always projected to the right side.

(All angiographic images on this page are from Thelen, M. et al.: Bildge-bende Kardiodiagnostik/Cardiac Imaging Thieme, Stuttgart 2007.)

3.17 Multislice Spiral Computed Tomography (MSCT) Coronary Angiography

A Common cardiac imaging planes used in CT

a At the level of the truncus pulmonalis; **b** Display of the heart chambers; **c** At the level of the aortic root; **d** Below the atrium sinistrum (from Reiser, M. et al.: Radiologie [Duale Reihe] 2. Aufl./Radiology, 2nd edition Thieme, Stuttgart 2006).

Note: Because invasive *conventional* coronary angiography (see p. 126) is followed by a coronary intervention (balloon dilatation, stent, see p. 130) in only 30–40% of cases, less invasive procedures such as MSCT coronary angiography have become an increasingly important tool in the diagnosis of coronary heart disease (CHD, see p. 124). Nowadays, multislice spiral computed topography (MSCT) can answer almost all clinically relevant questions regarding diagnostic and interventional radiology. It is possible, for example, to create 0.5 mm thick slices or reconstruct three-dimensional images of the cor and coronary vessels with common 64-slice spiral computed tomography without motion artifacts (using ECG synchronization) (see fig. **Ea** and **b**).

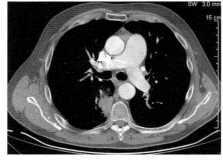

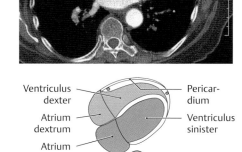

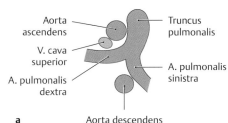

a

Aorta ascendens	Truncus pulmonalis
V. cava superior	
A. pulmonalis dextra	A. pulmonalis sinistra
	Aorta descendens

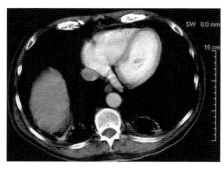

b

Ventriculus dexter	Pericardium
Atrium dextrum	Ventriculus sinister
Atrium sinistrum	
	Aorta descendens

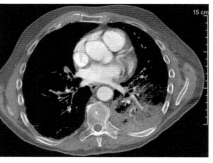

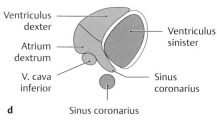

c

Atrium dextrum	Truncus pulmonalis
Aorta ascendens	A. coronaria sinistra
Atrium sinistrum	
	Aorta descendens

d

Ventriculus dexter	Ventriculus sinister
Atrium dextrum	
V. cava inferior	Sinus coronarius
	Sinus coronarius

B Representation of the origins of the arteriae coronariae

Schematic representation of an axial CT section just above the valva aortae (see also sectional plane of **Ac**). In this representation, the aortic root is surrounded by the two atria and the right outflow tract (truncus pulmonalis). The location of the ventriculus sinister between the branches of the main trunk of the a. coronaria sinistra is indicated.

Note: The valva aortae with its three pocket-like valvulae forms three recesses or sinuses, a left-, a right-, and a non-coronary sinus, which are each delimited by their corresponding valvula (valvulae semilunares sinistra, dextra, and non coronaria). The left a. coronaria sinistra arises from the left sinus coronarius, and the a. coronaria dextra from the right sinus coronarius. Coronary anomalies usually involve the origin of the aa. coronariae. However, they are rarely encountered in the general population.

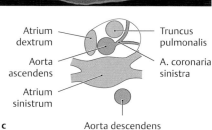

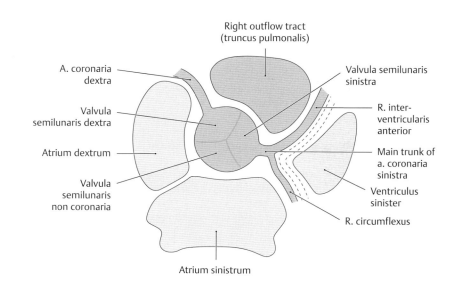

A. coronaria dextra
Valvula semilunaris dextra
Atrium dextrum
Valvula semilunaris non coronaria
Atrium sinistrum
Right outflow tract (truncus pulmonalis)
Valvula semilunaris sinistra
R. interventricularis anterior
Main trunk of a. coronaria sinistra
Ventriculus sinister
R. circumflexus

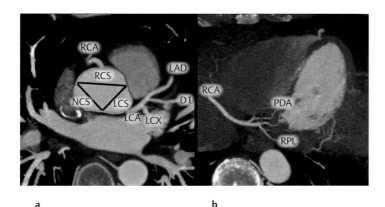

a   b

C CT anatomy of the origin of the arteriae coronariae

a Axial CT section at the level of the origin of the aa. coronariae:

LCS, RCS, NCS = left-, right-, and non-coronary sinus,
RCA = a. coronaria dextra,
LCA = main trunk of the a. coronaria sinistra,
LCX = r. circumflexus,
LAD, left anterior descending artery = r. interventricularis anterior,
D1 – diagonal branch 1;

b Course of the a. coronaria dextra (RCA) toward the posterior wall of the cor and branching into a r. interventricularis posterior (PDA, posterior descending artery) and a r. posterolateralis dexter (RPL).
(from Becker, C.: CT- Diagnostik der koronaren Herzkrankheit [Teil I: Indikation, Durchfuehrung und Normalbefundung der CT-Koronarography], Radiologie up2date1/CT diagnosis of coronary heart disease, Thieme, Stuttgart 2008.)

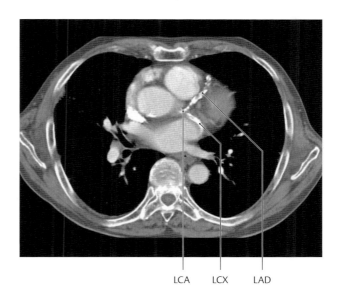

LCA   LCX   LAD

D CT anatomy of coronary sclerosis of the arteria coronaria sinistra

Transverse (axial) section at the level where the a. coronaria sinistra originates.
An important use of cardiac CT technology is in evaluating coronary calcium deposits in arteriosclerotic coronary arteries. This procedure does not require the use of contrast agents. The image shows a diffuse coronary sclerosis of the main trunk of the a. coronaria sinistra (LCA) as well as the r. circumflexus (LCX) and r. interventricularis anterior (LAD) (from: Claussen, C.D. et al.: Pareto Reihe Radiologie. Herz/Radiology. Heart, Thieme, Stuttgart 2007).

pRCA SAN LCX pLAD mLAD D1

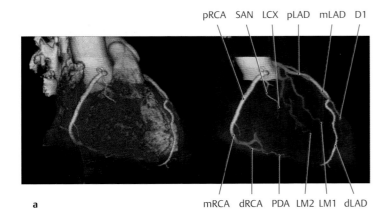

a   mRCA dRCA PDA LM2 LM1 dLAD

pRCA SAN mLAD LCA pLAD D1 LCX

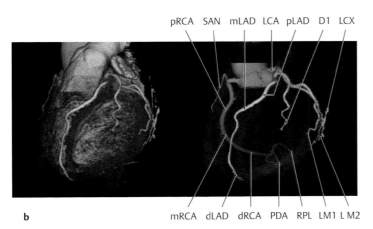

b   mRCA dLAD dRCA PDA RPL LM1 L M2

E Three-dimensional reconstruction of the cor using CT scan images

a CT anatomy of the cor in a 30-degree RAO projection; **b** Anatomy of the cor in a 60-degree LAO projection.
After the injection of contrast agent, the aa. coronariae (or rather the column of contrast medium) can be three-dimensionally reconstructed. Depending on which projection (RAO, right anterior oblique; LAO, left anterior oblique) and angulation was used (30 or 60 degrees), the clarity, with which the course of the aa. coronariae can be displayed, varies.

pRCA, mRCA, and dRCA = proximal, middle, and distal portion of the a. coronaria dextra
PDA, posterior descending artery = r. interventricularis posterior
RPL = r. posterolateralis dexter
SAN = n. nodi sinuatrialis
LCA = main trunk of the a. coronaria sinistra
pLAD, mLAD and dLAD, left anterior descending artery = proximal, middle and distal portion of the r. interventricularis anterior
LCX = r. circumflexus
D1 = r. diagonal 1
LM1 = rr. marginales sinistri
LM2 = rr. posterolaterales sinistri

(from Becker, C.: CT-Diagnostik der koronaren Herzkrankheit [Teil I: Indikation, Durchfuehrung und Normalbefundung der CT-Koronarography], Radiologie up2date1/CT diagnosis of coronary heart disease, Thieme, Stuttgart 2008.)

3.18 Balloon Dilatation, Aortocoronary Venous, and Arterial IMA Bypass

A Interventional and surgical options for treatment of coronary artery stenosis

The goal of coronary intervention is to improve the prognosis (*prognostic indicators*) and/or symptoms (*symptomatic indicators*) in patients with coronary heart disease (CHD). By restoring sufficient perfusion and oxygenation to the myocardium, myocardial performance is improved. Failure to achieve satisfactory results by treating CHD with drugs indicates the need for interventional (invasive procedure using a catheter advanced along the a. femoralis) or surgical treatments (surgery to open the thorax, etc.). Additionally, in cases of acute myocardial infarction, revascularization with aortocoronary bypasses becomes

an increasingly important tool. The following procedures are the most commonly performed:

- **Interventional techniques (PCI = percutaneous coronary intervention):**
  - percutaneous transluminal coronary angioplasty (PTCA)
  - percutaneous transluminal stent placement;

- **surgical coronary revascularization techniques:**
  - aortocoronary venous bypass (ACVB)
  - internal mammary artery bypass (IMA bypass).

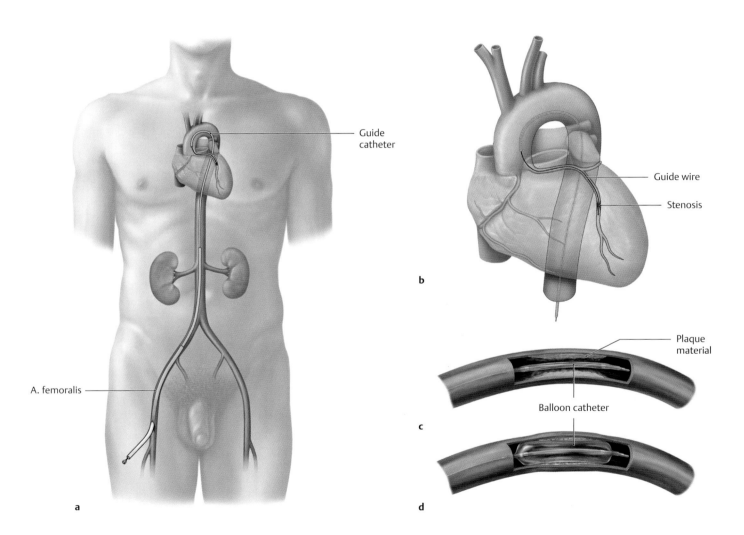

Guide catheter

Guide wire

Stenosis

A. femoralis

Plaque material

Balloon catheter

a

b

c

d

B Percutaneous transluminal coronary angioplasty (PTCA)
a Probing the a. coronaria using a guide catheter to insert a guide wire; **b** Passing the stenosis with a guide wire; **c** and **d** Placement of a balloon catheter over the guide wire and dilatation of the stenosis.

The PTCA procedure consists of balloon dilatation of narrowed aa. coronariae. The a. femoralis (**a**) is punctured and a guide wire is used to probe the affected a. coronaria. Via the guide wire, a balloon catheter is placed in the narrowed portion of the artery and then inflated in a controlled fashion to 8–20 atm (**c** and **d**), resulting in the compression of plaque material and dilatation of the lumen. Approximately 50–80%

of balloon dilatations are successful. However in 15–30% of all cases, a restenosis develops during the first year after the procedure. Contraindications include high-grade stenoses in areas where the aa. coronariae branch. Due to possible complications (risk of perforation or occlusion as a result of intimal dissection), coronary dilatations are always performed with cardiovascular surgeons on standby. Since the long-term results (one year post procedure) of dilatations are worse than with bypass surgeries, the use of dilatation methods is currently viewed very critically.

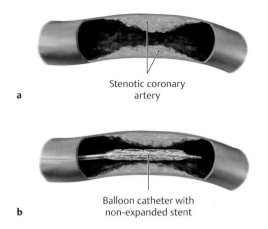

a   Stenotic coronary artery

b   Balloon catheter with non-expanded stent

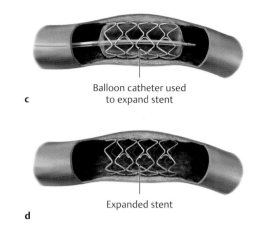

c   Balloon catheter used to expand stent

d   Expanded stent

C Stent placement

The placement of wire mesh stents is a standard procedure (80% of all interventions) in PCI. Using balloon catheters, the metal stents are positioned in the affected segment of the a. coronaria and expanded by inflation of the balloon catheter (at 12 atm). The dilated segment is supported by the stent and thus kept open. Compared to classic balloon dilatation, stent placement results in a considerably lower rate of restenosis (for example by causing less intimal hyperplasia).

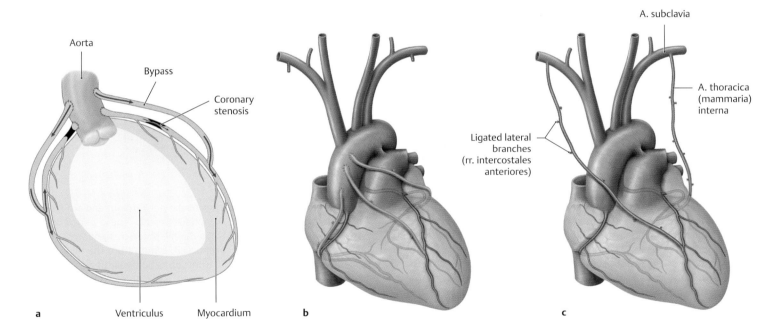

a   Aorta — Bypass — Coronary stenosis — Ventriculus — Myocardium

b

c   A. subclavia — A. thoracica (mammaria) interna — Ligated lateral branches (rr. intercostales anteriores)

D Surgical coronary revascularization

a Aortocoronary venous bypass (ACVB): In this type of surgical myocardial revascularization one or multiple venous grafts (usually from the v. saphena magna) are placed between the aorta ascendens and the post-stenotic segment of the a. coronaria. Thus, the grafted vessels bypass the occluded (right) or narrowed (left) segments of the affected arteries. Necessary requirements include a vessel that can be anastomosed post-stenosis and has a diameter of at least 1 mm, and adequate peripheral drainage and functional myocardium in the affected region of the heart. Revascularization with venous bypasses plays an important role in the treatment of acute myocardial infarction.

b Aortocoronary venous bypass in a patient with three vessel disease: In this case, venous grafts are anastomosed to the a. coronaria dextra, and to the rr. interventricularis anterior and circumflexus of the a. coronaria sinistra.

c Arterial IMA bypass (IMA = internal mammary artery): In addition to leg veins, arteries are increasingly being used for a. coronaria revascularization. Generally, the left and right internal mammary arteries (LIMA; RIMA; aa. thoracicae internae) are used as in situ grafts, or the a. radialis is used as a "free" graft. The distal a. thoracica interna is released from its vascular bed and its side branches tied off—up to where it branches from the a. subclavia. The artery is then anastomosed to the post-stenotic a. coronaria. The advantage of IMA bypasses over ACVB is a significantly lower occlusion rate. Compared with the patency rate for ACVB of 50% after ten years, 90% of arterial bypass grafts are patent after 10 years. Moreover, cardiac incidents (angina pectoris, myocardial infarction, sudden cardiac death) occur with less frequency following bypass surgery using IMA grafts than after venous bypass surgery.

3.19 Lymphatic Drainage of the Cor

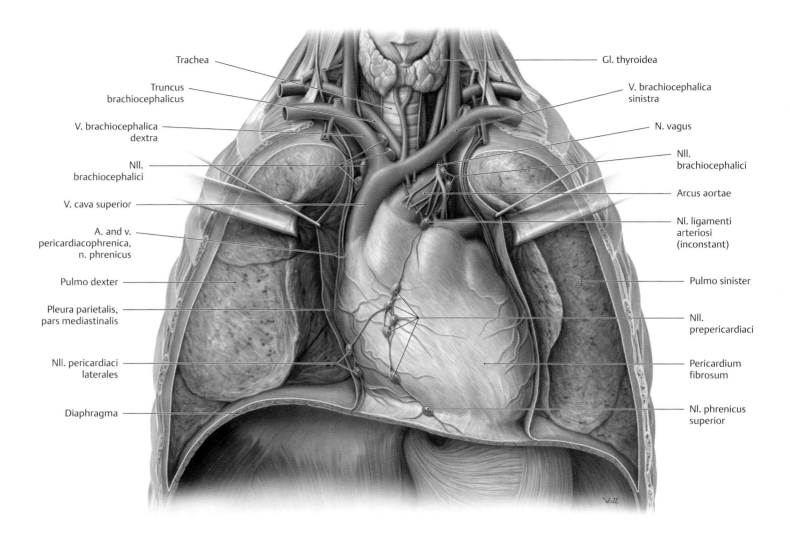

A Lymph nodes and lymphatic drainage of the pericardium
Anterior view of the opened thorax. The cavitates pleurales have been opened, and the pulmone and pleura have been retracted laterally. Due to the close topographical relationship between the cor and pericardium, the lymphatic drainage of the cor and pericardium is discussed together: Both pericardial and cardiac lymph is ultimately conveyed to the trunci bronchomediastinales, but through different primary nodi lymphoidei. Lymph node groups of varying size (nll. prepericardiaci and pericardiaci

laterales) lie anterior and adjacent to the pericardium and are interconnected by a network of fine lymphatic vessels. These pericardial nodi lymphoidei may drain inferiorly (to the nll. phrenici superiores) or cranially (usually to the nll. brachiocephalici). Lymph from the nll. pericardiaci is ultimately conveyed to the trunci bronchomediastinales (see p. 91), which open at the junction of the vv. subclaviae or internae jugulares dextrae and sinistrae.

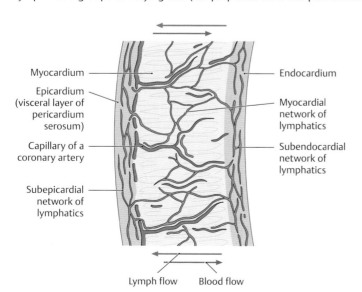

B Lymphatic drainage of the heart wall (after Földi and Kubik)
Section through the heart wall. There are three networks of densely interconnected vasa lymphatica, corresponding to the three layers of the heart wall:

- Epicardium (lamina visceralis of the pericardium serosum): A subepicardial network collects lymph from the epicardium and from the other two networks. The subepicardial network conveys the lymph to the collecting vessels and nodi lymphoidei of the cor.
- Myocardium: The very extensive myocardial network collects lymph from the myocardium and also from the subendocardial network. Vasa lymphatica of the myocardial network often follow the distribution of the vasa capillaria sanguinea that arise from the aa. coronariae. Thus the blood (red arrows) and lymph (green arrows) flow in opposite directions.
- Endocardium: A subendocardial network collects lymph from the endocardium and conveys it to the subepicardial network, either directly or via the myocardial network.

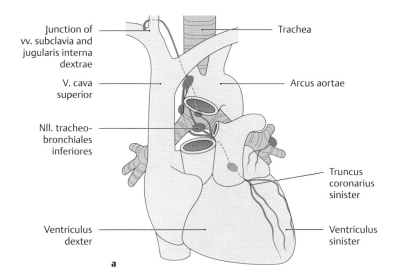

Junction of vv. subclavia and jugularis interna dextrae

V. cava superior

Nll. tracheo-bronchiales inferiores

Ventriculus dexter

Trachea

Arcus aortae

Truncus coronarius sinister

Ventriculus sinister

a

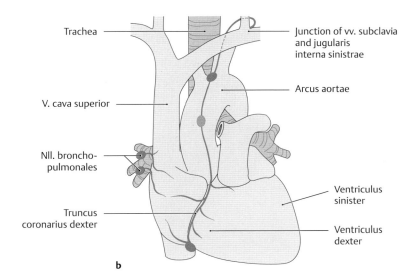

Trachea

V. cava superior

Nll. broncho-pulmonales

Truncus coronarius dexter

Junction of vv. subclavia and jugularis interna sinistrae

Arcus aortae

Ventriculus sinister

Ventriculus dexter

b

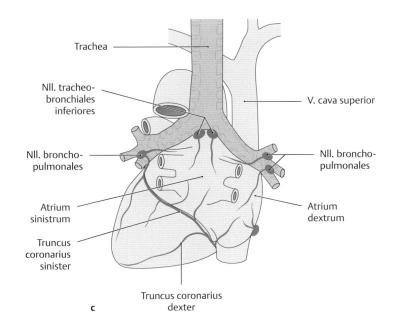

Trachea

Nll. tracheo-bronchiales inferiores

Nll. broncho-pulmonales

Atrium sinistrum

Truncus coronarius sinister

V. cava superior

Nll. broncho-pulmonales

Atrium dextrum

Truncus coronarius dexter

c

C Lymphatic drainage of the cor (after Földi and Kubik)

The cor viewed from the anterior aspect (**a, b**) and posterior aspect (**c**).

The lymphatic drainage of the ventriculi (and part of the atria) can be roughly divided into two regions (see **a** and **b**):

- The *left region* (**a**) encompasses the ventriculus sinister, a small strip of the ventriculus dexter, and portions of the atrium sinistrum. It conveys its lymph through a "left coronary trunk" to the nll. tracheobronchiales inferiores, which drain to the junction of the vv. subclavia and jugularis interna dextrae (directly or via the right truncus bronchomediastinalis).
- The *right region* (**b**) mainly encompasses the ventriculus dexter and portions of the atrium dextrum. It conveys its lymph through a "right coronary trunk" along the pars ascendens aortae and then to the junction of the vv. subclavia and jugularis interna sinistrae.

This arrangement creates two "crossed" pathways for lymphatic drainage:

- *Right region* → "right coronary trunk" → junction of the vv. subclavia and jugularis interna dextrae;
- *Left region* → "left coronary trunk" → junction of the vv. subclavia and jugularis interna sinistrae.

Lymphatic drainage of the rest of the atria: Portions of the atria that are outside the above regions drain to the nll. tracheobronchiales inferiores or to the ipsilateral nll. bronchopulmonales and thence to the trunci bronchomediastinales.

133

3.20 Innervation of the Cor

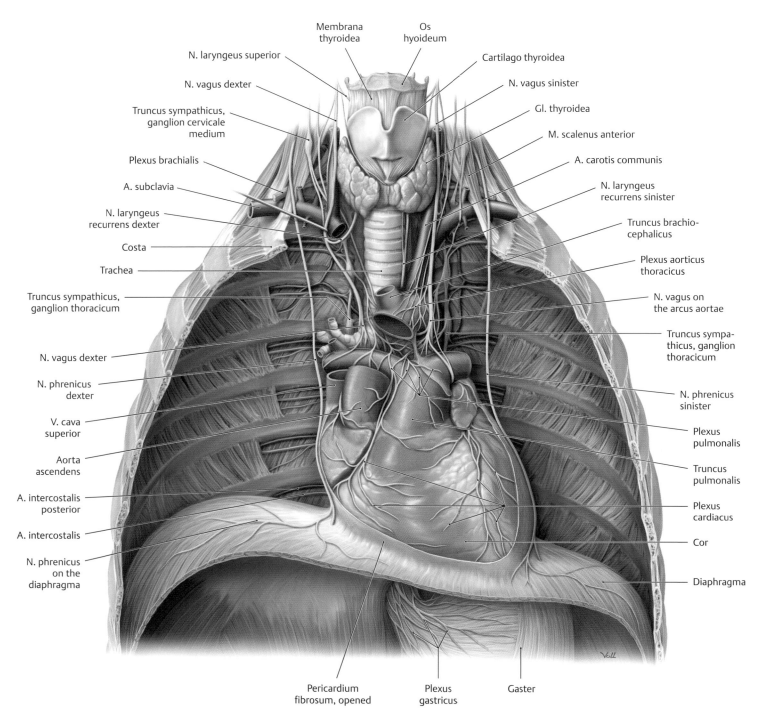

Membrana thyroidea
Os hyoideum
N. laryngeus superior
Cartilago thyroidea
N. vagus dexter
N. vagus sinister
Truncus sympathicus, ganglion cervicale medium
Gl. thyroidea
M. scalenus anterior
Plexus brachialis
A. carotis communis
A. subclavia
N. laryngeus recurrens sinister
N. laryngeus recurrens dexter
Costa
Truncus brachio-cephalicus
Trachea
Plexus aorticus thoracicus
Truncus sympathicus, ganglion thoracicum
N. vagus on the arcus aortae
Truncus sympa-thicus, ganglion thoracicum
N. vagus dexter
N. phrenicus sinister
N. phrenicus dexter
Plexus pulmonalis
V. cava superior
Truncus pulmonalis
Aorta ascendens
A. intercostalis posterior
Plexus cardiacus
A. intercostalis
Cor
N. phrenicus on the diaphragma
Diaphragma
Pericardium fibrosum, opened
Plexus gastricus
Gaster

A Autonomic nerves of the cor

Anterior view of the opened thorax with the pulmonales, pleura, and internal fasciae removed. The pericardium has been broadly opened anteriorly. The vessels surrounding the cor are intact except for a portion of the aorta ascendens, which has been removed to display the a. pulmonalis dextra. Part of the upper abdomen is also shown. The plexus cardiacus, plexus pulmonalis, and plexus aorticus thoracicus can be clearly identified on the cor and surrounding vessels. These plexuses receive fibers from the nn. vagi and truncus sympathica. The **nn. vagi dexter and sinister** initially run in the anterior part of the mediastinum superius. After giving off branches to the plexuses, they enter the mediastinum posterius (see **B**). **Sympathetic fibers** pass to the plexus cardiacus in the form of the nn. cardiaci cervicales (from the three ganglia cervicalia) and rr. cardiaci thoracici (from the ganglia thoracica) (see **B**). *Note:* Most of the autonomic fibers in the plexuses are extremely fine, but in this dissection they are shown larger for clarity. The n. phrenicus does not innervate the cor but does give off somatosensory branches to the pericardium (rr. pericardiaci, not shown here) in the mediastinum medium on its way to the diaphragma (see p. 99).

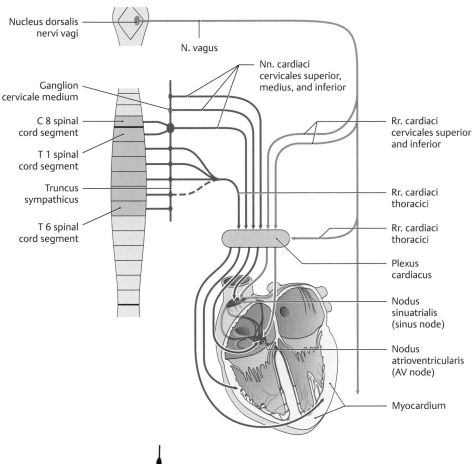

Nucleus dorsalis nervi vagi

N. vagus

Nn. cardiaci cervicales superior, medius, and inferior

Ganglion cervicale medium

C 8 spinal cord segment

T 1 spinal cord segment

Truncus sympathicus

T 6 spinal cord segment

Rr. cardiaci cervicales superior and inferior

Rr. cardiaci thoracici

Rr. cardiaci thoracici

Plexus cardiacus

Nodus sinuatrialis (sinus node)

Nodus atrioventricularis (AV node)

Myocardium

B Autonomic innervation of the cor

Parasympathetic: N. vagus fibers from the nucleus posterior nervi vagi give off the rr. cardiaci cervicales superiores and inferiores in the neck and the rr. cardiaci thoracici in the thorax. The rr. cardiaci pass to the plexus cardiacus.

Sympathetic: The three sympathetic ganglia cervicalia give off the nn. cardiaci superior, medius, and inferior, and the ganglia thoracica give off the rr. cardiaci thoracici. All of the rr. cardiaci radiate to the *plexus cardiacus*, which distributes fibers to the nodus sinuatrialis, nodus atrioventricularis, myocardium, and coronary vessels. The sympathetic axons, all postsynaptic, innervate all these targets directly, while the parasympathetic axons from the n. vagus synapse to the nodus sinuatrialis, nodus atrioventricularis, myocardium, and coronary vessels. The *pars sympathica* increases the rate and force of myocardial contractions and dilates the coronary vessels, while the *pars parasympathica* acts primarily to slow the heart rate. Drugs that act on both systems are used in the treatment of numerous diseases including hypertension, myocardial infarction, and cardiac arrhythmias.

Note: Since the cor has its own pacemaker (see p. 116), the autonomic nervous system does not generate the heartbeat, but instead acts on the SA node to regulate cor rate, and on other areas of the heart to modulate its function under different physiological loads.

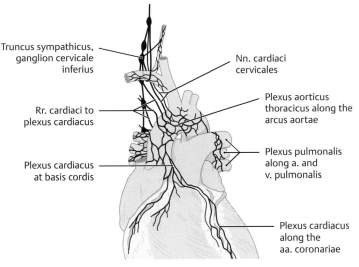

Truncus sympathicus, ganglion cervicale inferius

Nn. cardiaci cervicales

Rr. cardiaci to plexus cardiacus

Plexus aorticus thoracicus along the arcus aortae

Plexus cardiacus at basis cordis

Plexus pulmonalis along a. and v. pulmonalis

Plexus cardiacus along the aa. coronariae

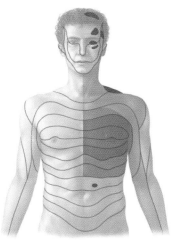

C Autonomic plexuses about the cor

Extensive autonomic nerve plexuses are formed on the cor and surrounding vessels. These plexuses receive fibers from the partes sympathica and parasympathica of the nervous systems (not shown here):

- Plexus cardiacus: located on the cor, especially prominent at the basis cordis and along the coronary vessels (cardiac innervation).
- Plexus aorticus thoracicus: located about the aorta thoracica (fibers to the cor and other plexuses: plexus pulmonalis, plexus oesophageus).
- Plexus pulmonalis: surrounding the aa. (and vv.) pulmonales and the bronchi. The plexus pulmonalis is consistently paired, the two parts being connected to each other and to the plexus cardiacus (supply the arbor bronchialis and intrapulmonary vessels).

D Referred pain and autonomic reactions associated with heart disease

In patients with heart disease, especially coronary occlusive disease (angina or infarction), the **pain** radiates to characteristic body regions:

- Left shoulder and left arm (particularly the inside of the left arm)
- Left half of the neck and head (jaw pain may present as a "toothache," cranial pain as a "headache")
- Left epigastric region.

Autonomic reactions may be noted in the dermatomes over the cor and in more distant dermatomes: a change in cutaneous blood flow, sweating, piloerection (body hairs "standing on end"), and occasional pupillary dilation (mydriasis) in the left eye.

4.1 Lungs: Location in the Thorax

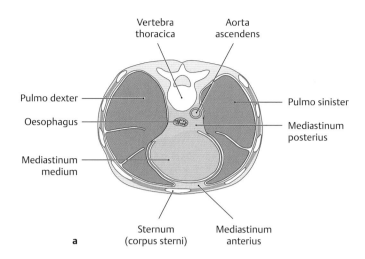

Vertebra thoracica — Aorta ascendens

Pulmo dexter

Oesophagus

Mediastinum medium

Pulmo sinister

Mediastinum posterius

Sternum (corpus sterni) — Mediastinum anterius

a

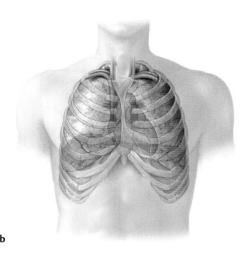

b

A Location of the lungs in the thorax: Topographical relations

a Transverse section through the thorax, superior view. The lungs completely occupy the cavitates pleurales sinistra and dextra flanking the mediastinum. Anteriorly, they approach each other in front of the pericardium and posteriorly they are located close to the columna vertebralis. Due to the asymmetrical position of the cor, the left lung is slightly smaller than the right lung (see **D**).

b Projections of the lungs onto the skeleton thoracis, anterior view. Superiorly, both lungs extend above the apertura thoracis superior; inferiorly, the undersurface of the lungs arches over the domes of the diaphragma. The distinct notch at the inferior medial border of the left lung is due to the heart, which is partially overlapped by the medial border of the lungs.

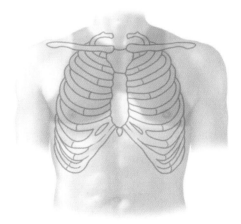

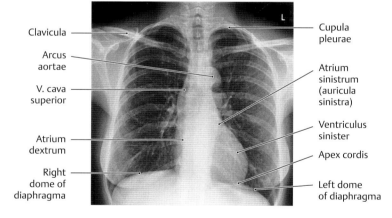

Clavicula — Cupula pleurae

Arcus aortae

V. cava superior — Atrium sinistrum (auricula sinistra)

Atrium dextrum — Ventriculus sinister

Right dome of diaphragma — Apex cordis

Left dome of diaphragma

B Percussion field of the lungs

Anterior view. The air-filled lungs constitute a resonant cavity that produces a *sonorous lung sound* on percussion of the chest. The sonorous lung field extends cranially, with attenuation, to the apices of the lungs at the apertura thoracis superior. It also extends to the front of the chest, again with attenuation, and closely approaches the anterior midline (recessus costomediastinalis with margo anterior pulmonis on deep inspiration, see pp. 138 and 141). The fluid-filled cor dampens the lung sounds, producing an area of cardiac dullness (see p. 97). A sharp transition from lung sound to liver sound is clearly audible at the margo inferior of the right lung, since the hepar is a solid organ with less resonance (medium-pitched, nonsonorous percussion sound).

Note: The lung percussion field does not precisely match the anatomical extent of the lungs because only well-aerated portions of the lung are sonorous to percussion. The anatomical extent of the lungs is greater than the percussion field.

C Radiographic appearance of the normal lungs

Anterior view. Different regions of the lungs show different degrees of lucency in the chest radiograph. The perihilar region of the lung (where the bronchi principales enter the lung and vessels enter and leave the lung) is less radiolucent than the peripheral region, which contains small-caliber vascular branches and bronchi segmentales. Additionally, the perihilar lung region is partly covered by the cor. These "shadows" appear as white or bright areas on the radiograph. The same effect is observed in diseased lung areas, which appear more opaque as a result of fluid infiltration (inflammation) or tissue proliferation (neoplasia). These opacities are easier to detect in the peripheral part of the lung, which is inherently more radiolucent than the perihilar lung.

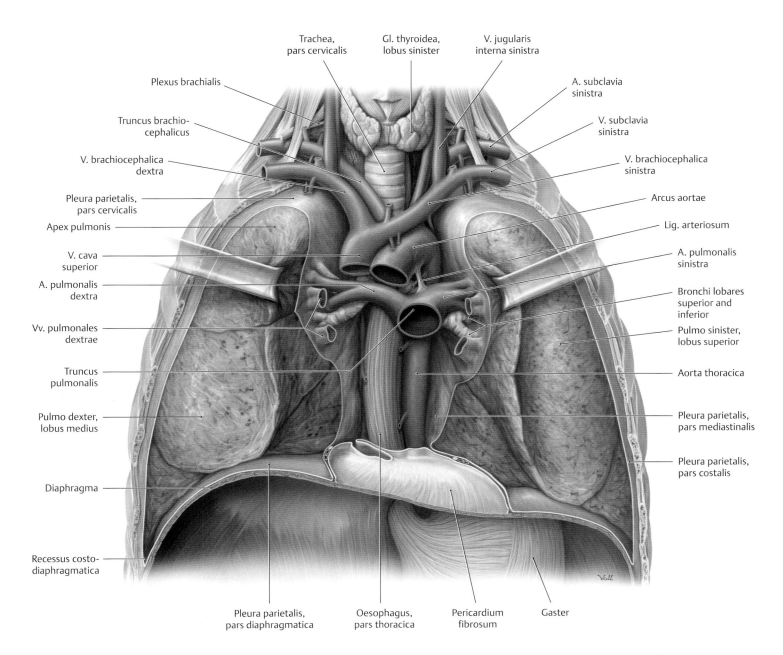

Trachea, pars cervicalis

Gl. thyroidea, lobus sinister

V. jugularis interna sinistra

Plexus brachialis

A. subclavia sinistra

Truncus brachio-cephalicus

V. subclavia sinistra

V. brachiocephalica dextra

V. brachiocephalica sinistra

Pleura parietalis, pars cervicalis

Arcus aortae

Apex pulmonis

Lig. arteriosum

V. cava superior

A. pulmonalis sinistra

A. pulmonalis dextra

Bronchi lobares superior and inferior

Vv. pulmonales dextrae

Pulmo sinister, lobus superior

Truncus pulmonalis

Aorta thoracica

Pulmo dexter, lobus medius

Pleura parietalis, pars mediastinalis

Pleura parietalis, pars costalis

Diaphragma

Recessus costo-diaphragmatica

Pleura parietalis, pars diaphragmatica

Oesophagus, pars thoracica

Pericardium fibrosum

Gaster

D The lungs in situ

Anterior view of the opened thorax (depiction simplified). The cor and pericardium have been removed. The vessels surrounding the cor have been transected, and all mediastinal connective tissues have been removed. The lungs have been retracted laterally to stretch and expose the bronchi principales. The cavitas abdominis has been opened and eviscerated, leaving only the gaster in place. The pars cervicalis of the trachea is still visible below the cartilago cricoidea. Shortly below its entry into the chest through the apertura thoracis superior, the trachea is almost completely obscured by the great vessels. The pars thoracica of the oesophagus can be seen below the bifurcatio tracheae, which lies directly behind the pars ascendens aortae. The lungs in the cavitates pleurales closely approach the columna vertebralis *posteriorly*,

while *anteriorly* they extend in front of the pericardium and narrow the mediastinum anterius. Percussion of the chest yields a "sonorous" lung sound (see **B**) which is dulled by the cor and pericardium. The extent of the lungs depends on the phase of respiration (see p. 159), but the apices pulmonum always extend into the apertura thoracis superior, which is closed by a condensation of loose connective tissue—the membrana suprapleuralis. The apical lung tissue is pictured here as soft and pliant, corresponding to its natural consistency. It should be noted that when the cavitates pleurales are opened at operation, the lungs tend to collapse toward the hilum owing to their elastic recoil; they do not completely fill the cavitates pleurales as shown here. (For clarity, the lungs are portrayed in an expanded state.)

4.2 Cavitates Pleurales

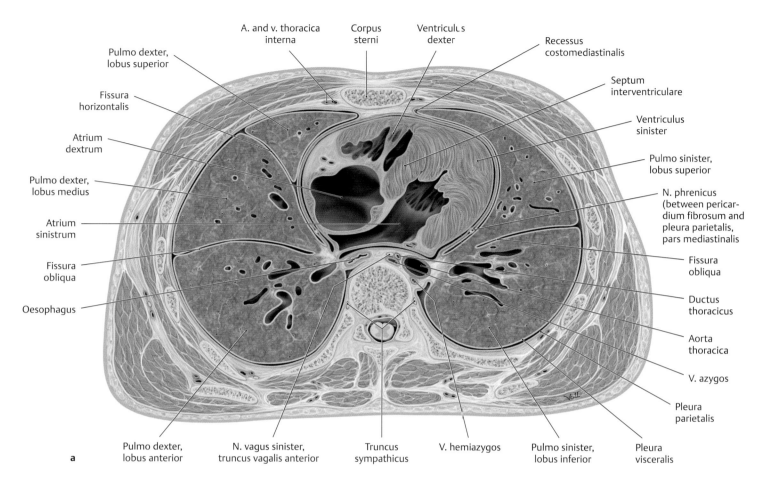

a

Labels (clockwise from top):
A. and v. thoracica interna — Corpus sterni — Ventriculus dexter — Recessus costomediastinalis — Septum interventriculare — Ventriculus sinister — Pulmo sinister, lobus superior — N. phrenicus (between pericardium fibrosum and pleura parietalis, pars mediastinalis) — Fissura obliqua — Ductus thoracicus — Aorta thoracica — V. azygos — Pleura parietalis — Pleura visceralis — Pulmo sinister, lobus inferior — V. hemiazygos — Truncus sympathicus — N. vagus sinister, truncus vagalis anterior — Pulmo dexter, lobus anterior — Oesophagus — Fissura obliqua — Atrium sinistrum — Pulmo dexter, lobus medius — Atrium dextrum — Fissura horizontalis — Pulmo dexter, lobus superior

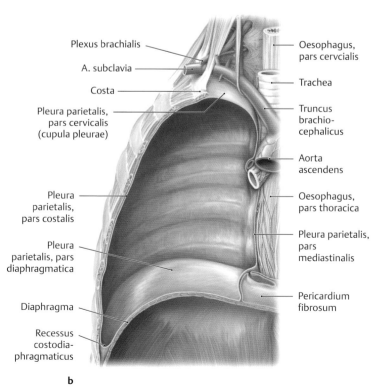

b

Labels: Plexus brachialis — A. subclavia — Costa — Pleura parietalis, pars cervicalis (cupula pleurae) — Pleura parietalis, pars costalis — Pleura parietalis, pars diaphragmatica — Diaphragma — Recessus costodiaphragmaticus — Oesophagus, pars cervicalis — Trachea — Truncus brachiocephalicus — Aorta ascendens — Oesophagus, pars thoracica — Pleura parietalis, pars mediastinalis — Pericardium fibrosum

A Pleura and cavitates pleurales: Structure and topography

a Transverse section through the thorax, inferior view; **b** Anterior view of the right cavitas pleuralis, which has been opened.

The cavitates pleurales are paired like the lungs they enclose, which is one reason they have a greater extent than the lungs:

- anteriorly, they extend past the pericardium to just behind the sternum, and in the dorsomedial direction up to the columna vertebralis (**a**);
- due to the arching of the dome of the diaphragma, the inferior margin of the cavitates pleurales extends downward and overlaps with the cavitas abdominis (**b**);
- due to the asymmetrical position of the cor in the mediastinum, the left cavitas pleuralis is slightly smaller than the right cavitas pleuralis (**a**);
- because the cavitates pleurales have a greater extent than the lungs, recesses develop in them (see also p. 141).

Completely analogous to the cavitates peritonealis and pericardialis, each cavitas pleuralis is composed of two serous layers: the pleura visceralis (pleura pulmonalis attached to the surface of the lung) and the pleura parietalis (attached to the fascia endothoracica). As a result of the attachment to the thorax, the pleura and thus the lungs (which adhere to the walls of the cavitates pleurales through capillary forces) automatically follow the movements of the chest wall. The line of junction between the tunicae serosae pleurae visceralis and parietalis occurs along at the medial surface of the lungs (see p. 36). The capillary fissure-like space between the pleurae visceralis and parietalis contains a small amount of clear serous fluid. This fluid layer allows both layers of the pleura to glide past each other and at the same time serves to hold the pleural layers together by capillary forces. For more about the topographical parts of the pleural layers see **C**.

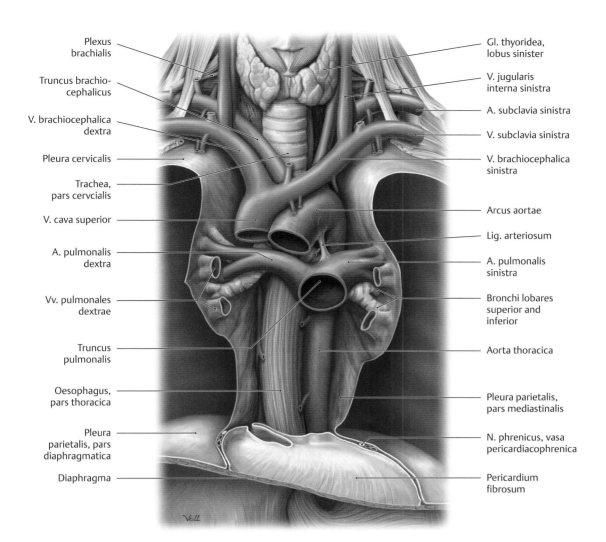

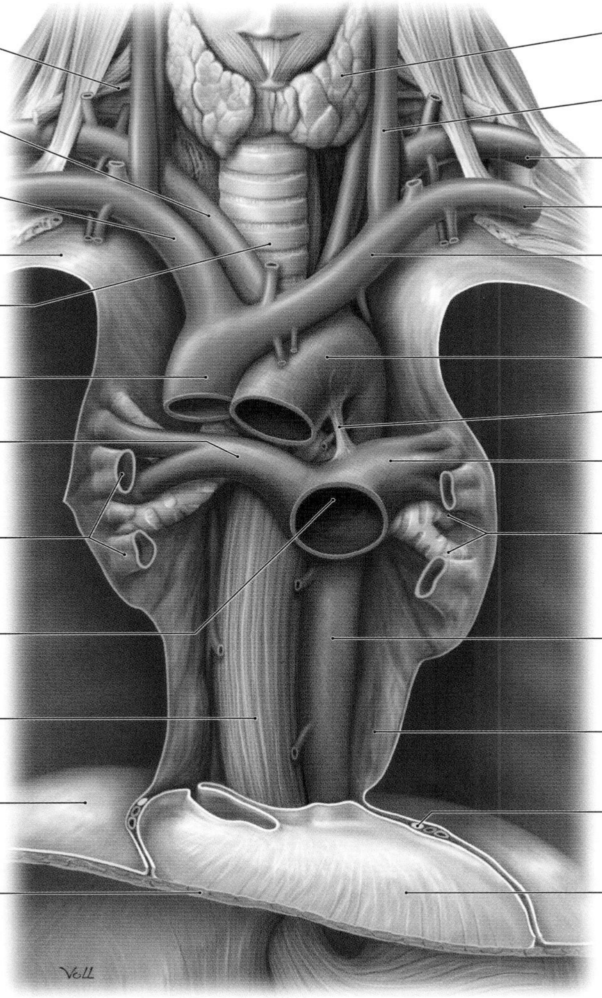
Plexus brachialis
Truncus brachio-cephalicus
V. brachiocephalica dextra
Pleura cervicalis
Trachea, pars cervcialis
V. cava superior
A. pulmonalis dextra
Vv. pulmonales dextrae
Truncus pulmonalis
Oesophagus, pars thoracica
Pleura parietalis, pars diaphragmatica
Diaphragma
Gl. thyoridea, lobus sinister
V. jugularis interna sinistra
A. subclavia sinistra
V. subclavia sinistra
V. brachiocephalica sinistra
Arcus aortae
Lig. arteriosum
A. pulmonalis sinistra
Bronchi lobares superior and inferior
Aorta thoracica
Pleura parietalis, pars mediastinalis
N. phrenicus, vasa pericardiacophrenica
Pericardium fibrosum

B Pars mediastinalis of the pleura and the mediastinum

The mediastinum is bounded on either side by the cavitates pleurales from which it is separated by the pars mediastinalis of the pleura parietalis. The pars mediastinalis pleurae is in direct contact with the mediastinal connective tissue. All neurovascular structures running between mediastinum and lungs (e.g., bronchi, aa. pulmonales, vv. pulmonales) are wrapped in pars mediastinalis pleurae, which fuses with the outer layer of the connective tissues of these neurovascular structures. The nn. phrenici and aa./vv. pericardiophrenicae, which are only just visible at the bottom of the diagram, pass between the pars mediastinalis pleurae and pericardium.

C Portions of the pleura parietalis

Portion	Location	Adjacent layer of connective tissue
Pars costalis	Inner chest wall	Fascia endothoracica
Pars diaphragmatica	Surface of the diaphragma	Fascia phrenicopleuralis
Pars mediastinalis	Lateral to mediastinum	Unnamed, direct transition to the connective tissue of the mediastinum
Cupula pleurae	Apical, above the apertura thoracis superior	Membrana suprapleuralis (Sibson's fascia)

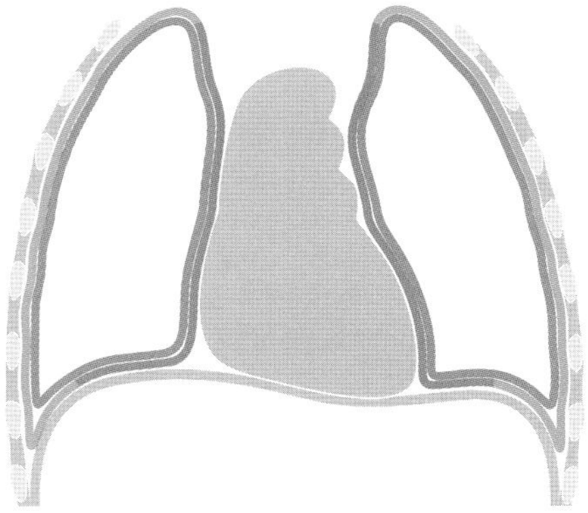

Pleura parietalis innervated by nn. intercostales
Pleura parietalisa innervated by nn. phrenici
Pleura visceralis innervated by the autonomic nervous system

D Innervation of the pleura

The *pleura parietalis*, as part of the trunk wall, is innervated by somatic sensory nerves: The pars mediastinalis and the largest part of the pars diaphragmatica are supplied by the nn. phrenici. A small part of the pars diaphragmatica located close to the ribs is also supplied by nn. intercostales. The pars costalis is innervated by nn. intercostales. The *pleura visceralis* is the organ-related layer and as such receives a sparse innervation by visceral sensory fibers, probably from the pars sympathica of the nervous system. The corresponding neuronal perikarya are located in ganglia sensoria nervorum spinalium—their branching axons pass through the ganglion sympathicum without terminating.

4.3 Boundaries of the Lungs and Pleura Parietalis

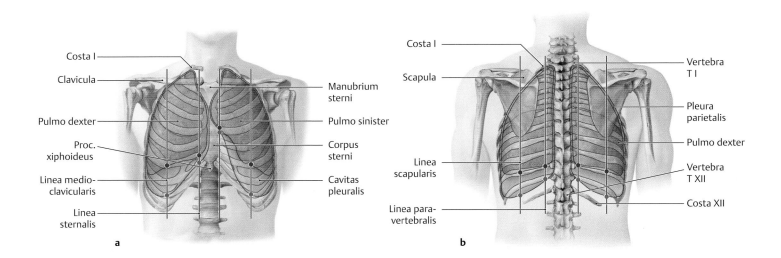

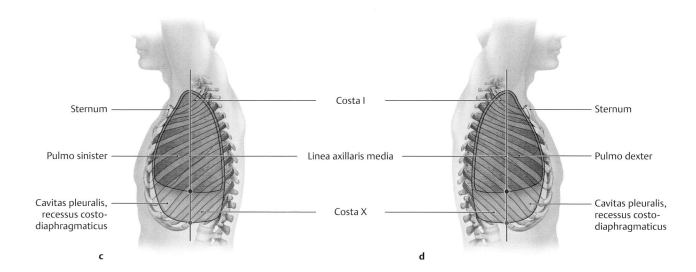

A Projections of the boundaries of the lungs and pleura parietalis onto the skeleton thoracis

Anterior view (**a**), posterior view (**b**), view from the left and right sides (**c** and **d**). The diagrams show the boundaries of the pleura parietalis and lungs. The table (see **B**) summarizes some of the projection sites of the pleura and lungs onto the anterior, posterior, and lateral thoracic wall. The pleura parietalis lines the inner surface of the skeleton thoracis and projects itself onto palpable or visible bony landmarks.

The connection between these landmarks forms the boundaries of the pleura parietalis (important in cases of pleural inflammations with effusion – visible on radiographs).
Note: The asymmetrical position of the cor makes the cavitas pleuralis slightly smaller on the left side than on the right side. This causes the boundaries of the pleura parietalis on the left side at the level of the cor to shift more laterally than on the right side.

B Relations of the lungs and pleural boundaries to landmarks on the skeleton thoracis

Reference line	Pulmo dexter	Right pleura parietalis	Pulmo sinister	Left pleura parietalis
Linea sternalis	Intersects costa VI	Intersects costa VII	Intersects costa IV	Intersects costa IV
Linea medioclavicularis	Runs parallel to costa VI	Runs parallel to costa VII	Intersects costa VI	Intersects costa VII
Linea axillaris media	Intersects costa VIII	Intersects costa IX	Same as pulmo dexter	Same as right side
Linea scapularis	Intersects costa X	Intersects costa XI	Same as pulmo dexter	Same as right side
Linea paravertebralis	Intersects costa XI	Extends to the T 12 vertebra	Same as pulmo dexter	Same as right side

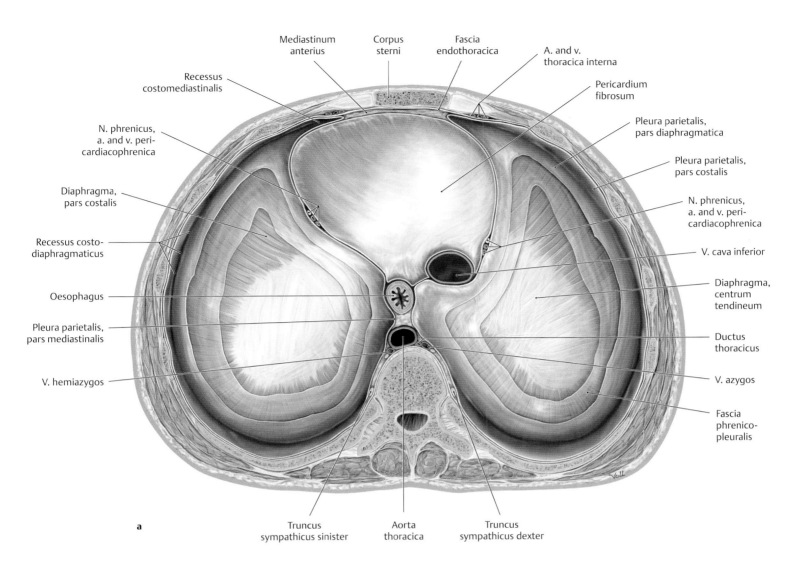

Mediastinum anterius

Recessus costomediastinalis

Corpus sterni

Fascia endothoracica

A. and v. thoracica interna

Pericardium fibrosum

N. phrenicus, a. and v. pericardiacophrenica

Pleura parietalis, pars diaphragmatica

Pleura parietalis, pars costalis

Diaphragma, pars costalis

N. phrenicus, a. and v. pericardiacophrenica

Recessus costodiaphragmaticus

V. cava inferior

Oesophagus

Diaphragma, centrum tendineum

Pleura parietalis, pars mediastinalis

Ductus thoracicus

V. hemiazygos

V. azygos

Fascia phrenicopleuralis

a

Truncus sympathicus sinister

Aorta thoracica

Truncus sympathicus dexter

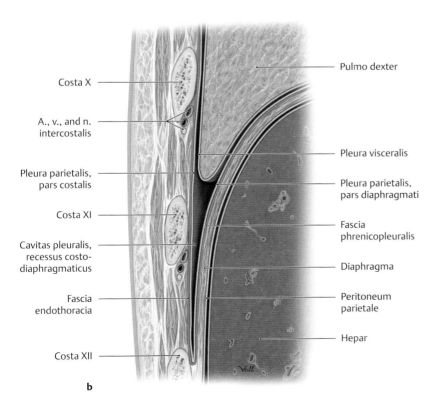

Costa X

A., v., and n. intercostalis

Pleura parietalis, pars costalis

Costa XI

Cavitas pleuralis, recessus costodiaphragmaticus

Fascia endothoracica

Costa XII

Pulmo dexter

Pleura visceralis

Pleura parietalis, pars diaphragmati

Fascia phrenicopleuralis

Diaphragma

Peritoneum parietale

Hepar

b

C Recesses of the pleura parietalis

a Superior view, the cor and lungs have been removed, the pleura parietalis has been removed over a large area of the diaphragma; **b** Detail from a parasagittal section through the right side of the thorax and abdomen, viewed from the lateral side.

The extent of the pleura *visceralis*, which directly invests the lung, is identical to that of the lung. However, the pleura *parietalis*, which completely lines the inner surface of the chest wall, has a greater extent than the lungs. This arrangement creates two major recesses within the cavitas pleuralis:

- The *recessus costodiaphragmaticus*, located on each side of the domes of the diaphragma, facing the ribs (**b**), which is lined by the partes costalis and diaphragmatica of the pleura parietalis, and
- The *recessus costomediastinalis*, located anterior to the pericardium, on the left and right sides of the mediastinum anterius (**a**), which is lined by the partes costalis and mediastinalis of the pleura parietalis.

For more about the function of the recessus pleurales, see p. 159.

4.4 Trachea

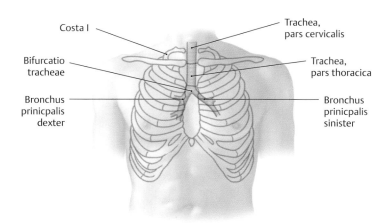

A The trachea projected onto the neck and thorax

The trachea is located in the mediastinum and lies precisely in the median plane. The initial part (pars cervicalis) of the trachea begins just below the larynx, and its pars thoracica ends at the bifurcatio tracheae. The trachea expands during inspiration and contracts during expiration. The projection in the figure shows the appearance of the trachea at functional residual capacity (relaxed end-expiration).

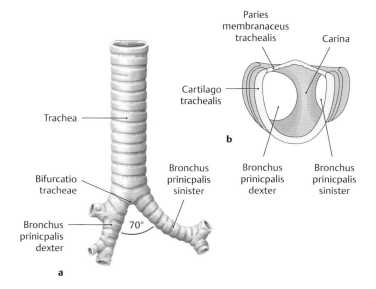

B Shape of the trachea

a Anterior view; **b** Superior view of the bifurcatio tracheae.

The trachea is a flexible air-conducting tube 10 to 12 cm long. At the approximate level of the corpora vertebrae T3–T4, it bifurcates into the bronchi principales sinister and dexter, which form an angle of approximately 55–70°. Viewed from the anterior side, the bifurcatio tracheae lies just below the junction of the manubrium and corpus sterni.

Note: The bronchus principalis dexter is more vertical than the bronchus principalis sinister, and therefore it is more common for aspirated foreign bodies to enter the bronchus principalis dexter than the sinister. This also makes it easier to view the interior of the bronchus principalis dexter with an endoscope. Owing to the asymmetry of the cor and the associated asymmetrical position of the lungs, the bronchus principalis sinister is slightly longer than the dexter.

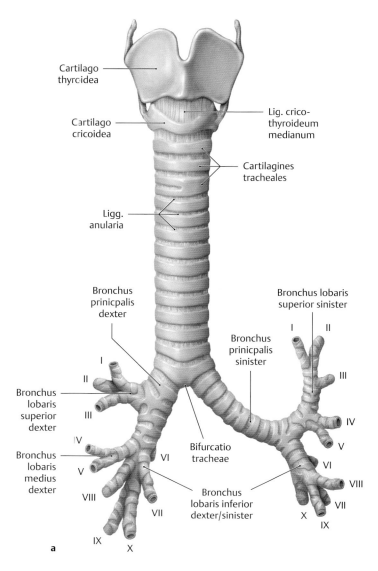

C Structure of the trachea and arbor bronchialis

a Anterior view; **b** Posterior view with opened posterior wall.

The trachea consists of 16–20 horseshoe-shaped rings composed of hyaline cartilage (the cartilagines tracheales) and a posterior paries membranaceus composed of connective tissue and m. trachealis (not shown here). The cartilagines tracheales are interconnected longitudinally by collagenous connective tissue (ligg. anularia). The two parts of the trachea are clearly distinguishable:

- Pars cervicalis: extends from the first cartilago trachealis below the cartilago cricoidea of the larynx at the level of the C6/C7 vertebrae to the apertura thoracis superior (see **A**);
- Pars thoracica: extends from the apertura thoracis superior to the bifurcatio tracheae, where the trachea divides into the bronchi principales dexter and sinister at the level of the T4 vertebra. A cartilaginous spur (carina, see **Bb**) at the bifurcatio tracheae projects upward into the tracheal lumen.

The bronchi principales sinister and dexter divide into two or three bronchi lobares, respectively, which subsequently branch into bronchi segmentales (see **D**).

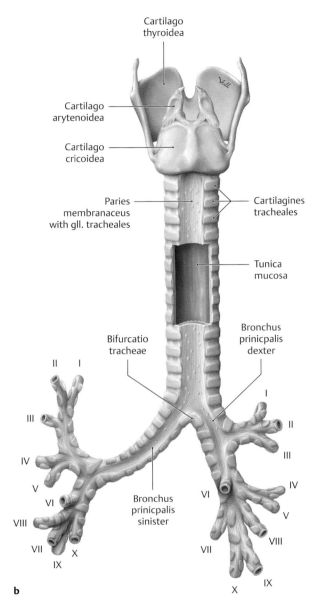

b

D Divisions of the trachea and arbor bronchialis

Bronchus principalis dexter	Bronchus principalis sinister
Bronchus lobaris superior dexter	*Bronchus lobaris superior sinister*
Bronchus segmentalis apicalis (I)	Bronchus segmentalis
Bronchus segmentalis posterior (II)	apicoposterior (I, II)
Bronchus segmentalis anterior (III)	Bronchus segmentalis anterior (III)
Bronchus lobaris medius	
Bronchus segmentalis lateralis (IV)	Bronchus lingularis superior (IV)
Bronchus segmentalis medialis (V)	Bronchus lingularis inferior (V)
Bronchus lobaris inferior dexter	*Bronchus lobaris inferior sinister*
Bronchus segmentalis superior (VI)	Bronchus segmentalis superior (VI)
Bronchus segmentalis basalis medialis (VII)	Bronchus segmentalis basalis medialis (VII)
Bronchus segmentalis basalis anterior (VIII)	Bronchus segmentalis basalis anterior (VIII)
Bronchus segmentalis basalis lateralis (IX)	Bronchus segmentalis basalis lateralis (IX)
Bronchus segmentalis basalis posterior (X)	Bronchus segmentalis basalis posterior (X)

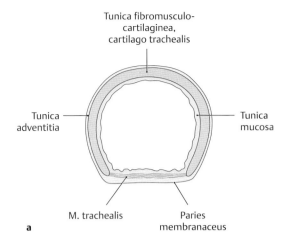

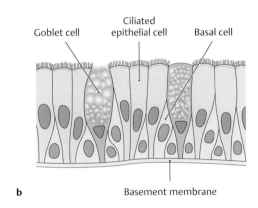

E Wall structure of the trachea and bronchi principales

a Wall structure (for the ultrastructure of the bronchial tree see p. 148f and 154f):

- Tunica mucosa with an epithelial layer and a lamina propria: The lamina propria contains glandulae seromucosae (gll. tracheales) which secrete a mucous film on the surface (for the epithelium see below).
- Tunica fibromusculocartilaginea: This contains the C-shaped rings of cartilago hyalina and, on the posterior tracheal wall, the smooth muscle of the trachealis and abundant connective tissue.
- Adventitial sheath of connective tissue: This integrates the trachea into the adjacent connective tissue of the neck and mediastinum and allows mobility.

Note: The epithelium of the carina, unlike that of the rest of the trachea, consists of nonkeratinized squamous epithelium.

b Structure of the epithelium: The mucosa of the trachea and bronchi contains a pseudostratified columnar respiratory epithelium. All cells contact the basement membrane, but not all cells extend to the surface of the lumen. The cells in contact with the surface are ciliated. These hairlike structures propel small foreign bodies that have been inhaled toward the larynx. Smoking tobacco decreases the flow of secretions, compromising airway clearance. Mucus secreting goblet cells without cilia are interspersed among the epithelial cells.

4.5 Lungs: Shape and Structure

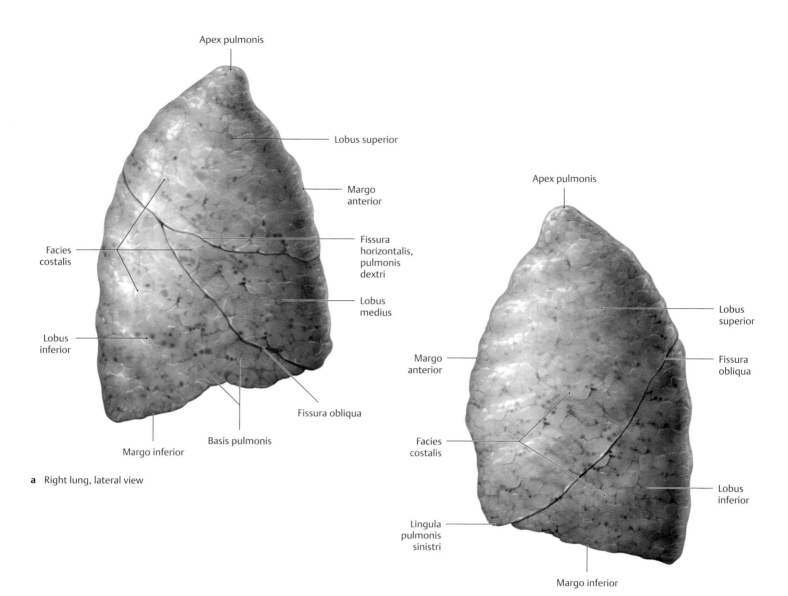

a Right lung, lateral view

b Left lung, lateral view

A Gross anatomy of the left and right lung

a, b Lateral view. **c, d** Medial view.

The color of the healthy lung ranges from gray to bluish-pink. Grayish-black particles are often visible beneath the pleural surface (as shown here) and are found even in nonsmokers. They do not necessarily have pathological significance, consisting of dust or carbonaceous particles that have been inhaled and deposited in the lung. A lung that has not been chemically fixed has a soft, spongy texture and collapses when taken from the chest. The shape shown above is the in vivo shape of the dynamically expanded lung (see p. 159). The right lung, with a volume of approximately 1500 cm, is slightly larger than the left lung, which has a volume of approximately 1400 cm (due to the inclination of the cor to the left side). Each of the lungs is divided into *lobi* by one or more inter-lobar *fissures:*

- The left lung is divided into two lobes (lobi superior and inferior) by one fissura obliqua.

- The right lung consists of three lobes (lobi superior, medius, and inferior) separated by one fissura *obliqua* and one fissura *horizontalis*. The pulmonary fissures are completely lined by pleura visceralis.

Note: Owing to the steep angle of the fissura obliqua in the left lung, the lingula of the lobus superior forms part of the basis pulmonis sinistri. The smallest morphologically distinct and autonomous structural unit of the lung is the *lobulus*, which is aerated by a bronchiolus. The pulmonary lobuli are separated from one another by (often incomplete) fibrous interlobular septa, demarcating numerous polyhedral areas that may be visible on the lung surface.

Aside from the differences noted above, both lungs have the same basic parts:

- The apex pulmonis, which extends into the apertura thoracis superior
- The basis pulmonis, which rests on the diaphragma

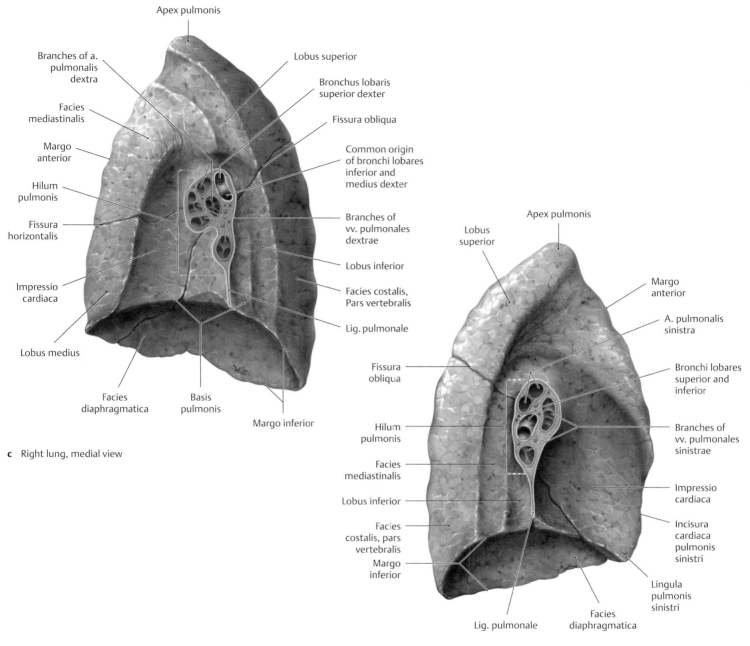

c Right lung, medial view

d Left lung, medial view

- Surfaces of the lung:
  - Facies costalis: relates laterally and posteriorly to the ribs. The pars vertebralis of the facies costalis faces the columna vertebralis (see **c, d**);
  - Facies mediastinalis: relates medially to the mediastinum.
  - Facies diaphragmatica (see **c, d**): relates inferiorly to the diaphragma.
  - Facies interlobares. In the chemically fixed specimen, impressions from the ribs are visible on the facies costalis, an impressio cardiaca on the facies mediastinalis, and an impression from the diaphragma leaflet on the facies diaphragmatica. The left lung additionally has a distinct *incisura* cardiaca in its margo anterior.
- Borders of the lung:
  - Margo anterior: sharp, thin border located at the junction of the facies costalis and mediastinalis (inserts into the recessus costomediastinalis).

  - Margo inferior: located at the junction of the facies diaphragmatica and facies costalis or mediastinalis, sharp at the facies costalis (inserts into the recessus costodiaphragmaticus) and blunt at the facies mediastinalis.
- Hilum: area where bronchi and neurovascular structures enter and leave the facies mediastinalis. The *radix* pulmonis comprises all of the blood vessels, lymphatics, bronchi, and nerves that enter and emerge at the hilum. Elements of the arbor bronchialis are generally located in the posterior part of the hilum. Pulmonary venous branches are anterior and inferior, and pulmonary arterial branches are found mainly in the upper part of the hilum.

Both lungs are invested by a serous membrane, the *pleura visceralis* (pulmonary pleura), which is reflected at the mediastinal surface to continue as the pleura parietalis. This pleural fold is ruptured when the lung is removed, appearing as the *lig. pulmonale*.

145

4.6 Lungs: Segmentation

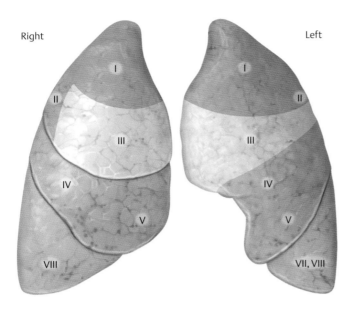

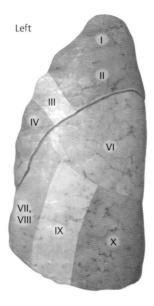

a Lungs, anterior view

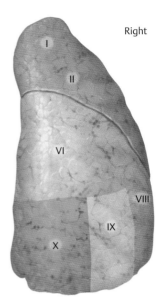

b Lungs, posterior view

A Segmental architecture of the lungs

Anterior view (**a**) and posterior view (**b**) of the left and right lung (lateral and medial views are shown in **C**).

The segmental architecture of the lung relates directly to the branching pattern of the arbor bronchialis (see p. 143). The basic structural unit of the lung is the *lobus*, whose boundaries are clearly defined on the surface of the lung by the interlobar fissurae. Each lobus is further subdivided into *segmenta*—wedge-shaped functional units whose apex points toward the pulmonary hilum. The pulmonary segmenta are incompletely separated from one another by thin connective tissue and are not discernible as separate units on the lung surface. Passing to the center of each segment are a bronchus segmentalis and an *a. segmentalis*, constituting the "bronchopulmonary segment" or segmentum

bronchopulmonale. The segmenta, in turn, consist of subsegments defined by the further branching pattern of the bronchi segmentales. Each lung consists basically of ten segmenta. Due to the presence of the cardiac notch in the *left* lung (see p. 147 **Da**), however, segment VII of that lung is often so small that it is not considered a separate segmentum but part of segmentum VIII. As noted above, the segmental boundaries are not visible on the surface of the lung. For partial resections of the lung (see **D**), the targeted segmenta are identified by clamping off the a. segmentalis. As the devascularized segmentum blanches, it contrasts sharply with the surrounding tissues that are still perfused. Intrasegmental blood flow can also be demonstrated by ultrasound scanning. The pulmonary segmenta are named and numbered as shown in table **B**.

B Segmental architecture of the lungs

Pulmo dexter	Pulmo sinister
Lobus superior	*Lobus superior*
Segmentum apicale (I)	Segmentum apicoposterius (I+II)
Segmentum posterius (II)	
Segmentum anterius (III)	Segmentum anterius (III)
Lobus medius	
Segmentum laterale (IV)	Segmentum lingulare superius (IV)
Segmentum mediale (V)	Segmentum lingulare inferius (V)
Lobus inferior	*Lobus inferior*
Segmentum superius (VI)	Segmentum superius (VI)
Segmentum basale mediale (VII)	Segmentum basale mediale (VII)
Segmentum basale anterius (VIII)	Segmentum basale anterius (VIII)
Segmentum basale laterale (IX)	Segmentum basale laterale (IX)
Segmentum basale posterius (X)	Segmentum basale posterius (X)

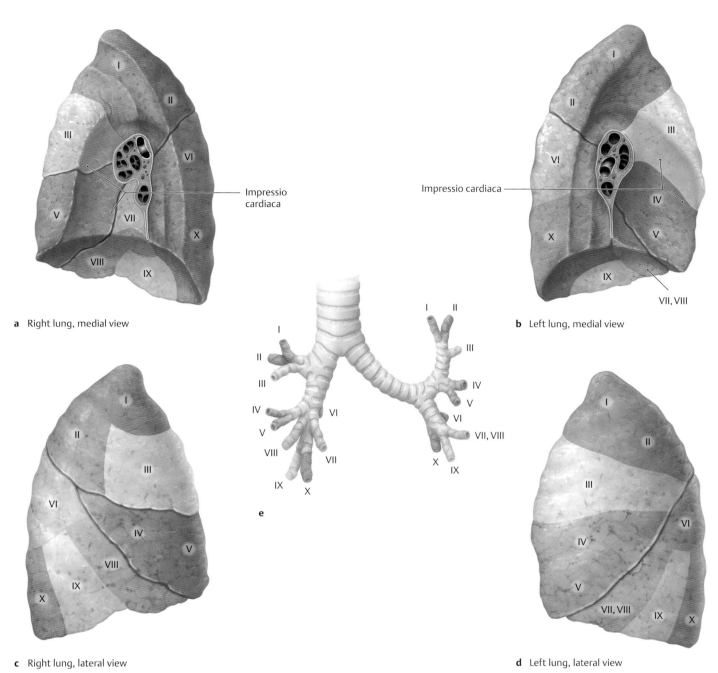

a Right lung, medial view

Impressio cardiaca

Impressio cardiaca

b Left lung, medial view

e

c Right lung, lateral view

d Left lung, lateral view

C Segmental architecture of the lungs: Segmenta bronchopulmonalia
Lateral and medial views of the right (**a, c**) and left (**b, d**) lung.

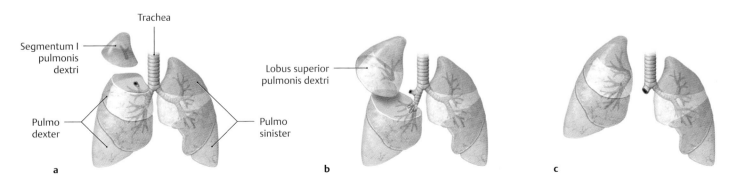

Trachea

Segmentum I
pulmonis
dextri

Pulmo
dexter

Pulmo
sinister

Lobus superior
pulmonis dextri

a

b

c

D Partial lung resections
The anatomical subdivision of the lungs into lobi and segmenta (see **B**) is exploited in partial lung resections:

- Segmentectomy (wedge resection): (**a**) Removal of one or more segmenta
- Lobectomy: (**b**) Removal of an entire lobus or (**c**) the complete resection of a lung (pneumonectomy).

4.7 Functional Structure of the Arbor Bronchialis

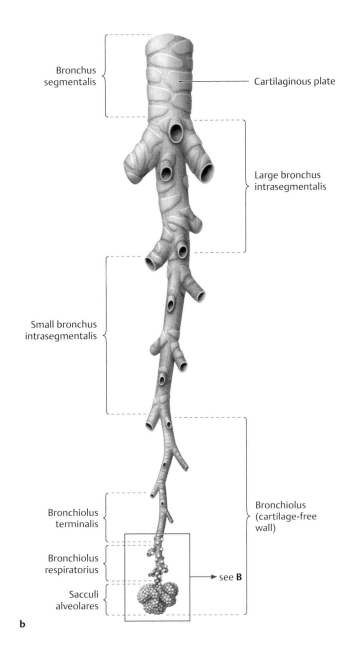

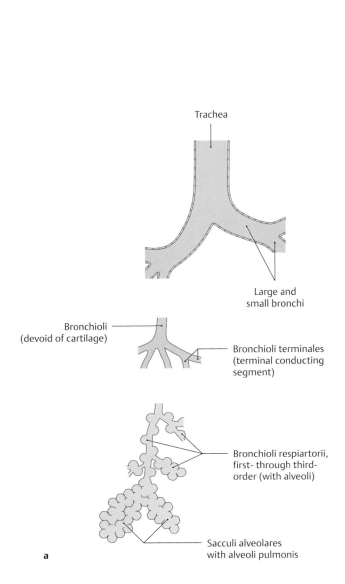

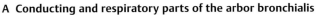

A Conducting and respiratory parts of the arbor bronchialis

The structure of the lung is organized to maximize the surface area available for gas exchange, and the arbor bronchialis is arranged to deliver the gases, in warmed and humidified (saturated with water vapor) air, to that specialized surface area. The exchange takes place mostly in *alveoli pulmonales*, microscopic pouches approximately 200–250 μm in diameter. The adult lungs contain about 300 million alveoli with a total surface area of nearly 150 m². From the trachea, the arbor bronchialis branches into successively finer divisions (22 "dichotomous" divisions, in which each passage divides into two smaller passages). The parts of the arbor bronchialis are classified functionally as *conducting* or *respiratory:*

- Conducting part (blue): bronchi principales, bronchi lobares, bronchi segmentales and intrasegmentales, bronchioli, and bronchioli terminales
- Respiratory part (red): bronchioli respiratorii, ductuli alveolares (not visible), and sacculi alveolares.

The arbor bronchialis presents a uniform structure of a specialized air-conduction tube out to the level of the bronchi segmentales. The bronchial wall is reinforced by cartilage rings or plates and is lined internally by a pseudostratified columnar, ciliated epithelium (with goblet cells; see p. 143). The walls of the *smaller* bronchi do not have cartilage reinforcement. The concentric musculature of these bronchi acquires a lattice-like structure (see **B**), and the pseudostratified epithelium is replaced by a single layer of prismatic, ciliated epithelial cells. Goblet cells become less numerous and are no longer present past the level of the bronchiolus terminalis. The bronchiolus terminalis is the final segment of the air-conducting portion of the arbor bronchialis. Each bronchiolus terminalis aerates one *acinus pulmonalis*. A group of three to five acini whose bronchioli terminales arise near one another on the arbor bronchialis forms a lobulus, which is the smallest morphologically distinct structural unit of the lung.

Note: Although the vascular tree and arbor bronchialis are closely related functionally, the vascular tree (see p. 154) is discussed following the sections about the pulmonary and bronchial vessels. Since the vascular tree is composed of the terminal branches of the pulmonary and bronchial vessels, knowledge of these vessels is essential for understanding the structure of the vascular tree.

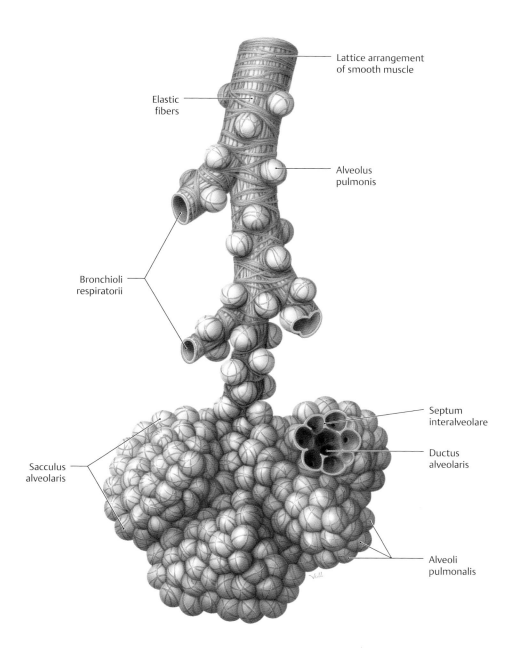

Lattice arrangement of smooth muscle

Elastic fibers

Alveolus pulmonis

Bronchioli respiratorii

Septum interalveolare

Ductus alveolaris

Sacculus alveolaris

Alveoli pulmonalis

B Structure of a bronchiolus respiratorius

The bronchioli respiratorii dichotomously divide into first- through third-order bronchioli respiratorii, the thinnest of which is less than 0.5 mm in diameter. Alveoli begin to appear on the first-order bronchioli respiratorii, marking the start of the respiratory portion of the lung. The alveoli are isolated initially, then become more numerous and are collected into saculi. Each saculus has a central open space, a ductus alveolaris, that is continuous with the lumen of its bronchiolus respiratorius. The alveolar walls are composed of thin squamous epithelium and are in direct contact with the vasa capillaria sanguinea to allow for gas exchange. Adjacent alveoli are separated from one another by a porous septum interalveolare. Connective tissue with abundant elastic fibers is interposed between the branches of the arbor bronchialis and the alveoli. When these elastic fibers are stretched during inspiration, they store energy and provide the mechanism for the elastic recoil of the lung during expiration.

In patients with bronchial asthma the bronchioli are hypersensitive, and constriction of the smooth muscle in the bronchiolar walls can be triggered by allergens (e.g., pollen) or by stimuli like cold that are trivial to non-asthmatics. Since these walls are not cartilage-reinforced, the bronchioli narrow and restrict the passage of air to the alveoli (obstructive ventilatory impairment), causing dyspnea (respiratory distress).

4.8 Arteriae and Venae Pulmonales

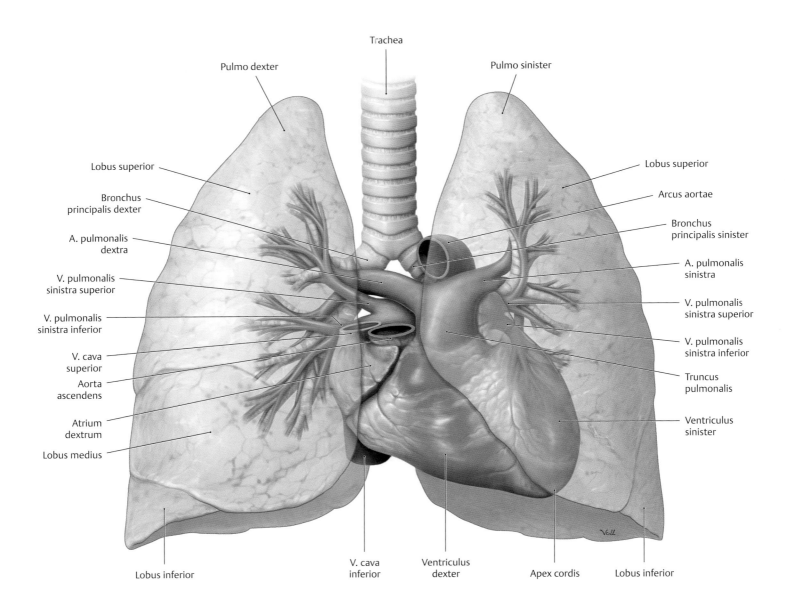

A Overview of the pulmonary vessels
Anterior view of a "heart-lung **preparation**."
The vv. cavae have been cut close to the heart, and a segment has been removed from the aorta ascendens and arcus aortae to display the division of the truncus pulmonalis, which is inferior to the arcus aortae, and the origin of the a. pulmonalis dexter. The lungs and heart are shown partially transparent. The arteries and veins that pass to the lung are divided into two groups:

- *Aa. and vv. pulmonales,* which carry blood to the lungs and back for gas exchange (O_2, CO_2)
- *Aa. and vv. bronchiales* (not shown here), which *supply blood* to parts of the lungs themselves (see p. 152)

The **divisions of the aa. pulmonales** basically follow the branching pattern of the arbor bronchialis (see p. 142). Two or three arterial branches, called aa. lobares, accompany the two (left) or three (right) bronchi lobares into the lung. (The aa. lobares are larger than the bronchi

lobares.) As the arbor bronchialis branches into *bronchi segmentales,* the arteries similarly divide into *aa. segmentales.* The artery and its associated bronchus are always placed at the center of the structural lung unit, first occupying the center of a lobus, then the center of a *segmentum bronchopulmonale* (see p. 146).

The **divisions of the vv. pulmonales** do not follow the branching pattern of the arbor bronchialis, instead coursing between pulmonary segmenta to collect blood from within (partes intrasegmentales) and among (partes intersegmentales) adjacent segments. Thus vv. pulmonales are named differently than aa. pulmonales (see **C** and **D**). In cases of left ventricular insufficiency, blood backs up in the vv. pulmonales. As a result, the boundaries of the pulmonary segmenta become visible on radiographs.

Note: The aa. pulmonales carry deoxygenated blood to the lungs, and the vv. pulmonales carry oxygenated blood from the lungs to the cor. In order to ensure a consistent presentation throughout this atlas, the arteries are still colored red and the veins are colored blue.

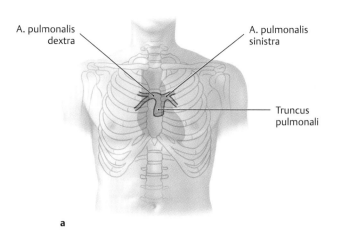

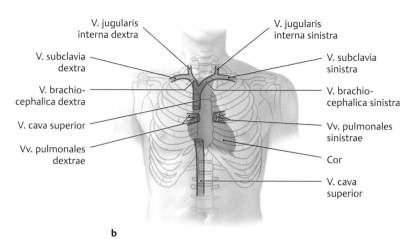

a

b

B Projection of the arteriae and venae pulmonales onto the chest wall
Anterior view.

a Projection of the arteriae pulmonales onto the chest wall: The truncus pulmonalis arises from the ventriculus dexter, which is anterior owing to the slightly rotated position of the cor, and divides into aa. pulmonales sinistra and dexter, one for each lung. The truncus pulmonalis appears on chest radiographs as a knob-like shadow on the left cardiac border above the ventriculi.

Note: The truncus pulmonalis lies to the left of the midline in the chest. As a result, the a. pulmonalis dextra (length approximately 2–3 cm) is longer than the a. pulmonalis sinistra.

b Projection of the venae pulmonales onto the chest wall: Normally, a pair of vv. pulmonales open into the atrium sinistrum on each side. Taken together, the vv. pulmonales dextra and sinistra and both vv. cavae form an asymmetrical cruciform pattern on the chest radiograph.

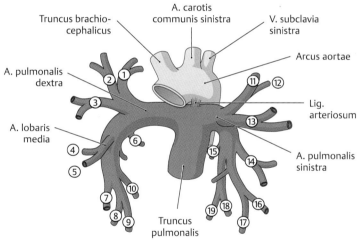

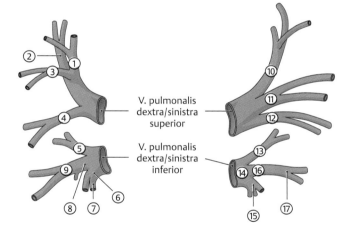

C The arteriae pulmonales and their branches

Pulmo dexter Arteria pulmonalis dextra	Pulmo sinister Arteria pulmonalis sinistra
Aa. lobares superiores ① A. segmentalis apicalis ② A. segmentalis posterior ③ A. segmentalis anterior	*Aa. lobares superiores* ⑪ A. segmentalis apicalis ⑫ A. segmentalis posterior ⑬ A. segmentalis anterior
A. lobaris media ④ A. segmentalis lateralis ⑤ A. segmentalis medialis	⑭ A. lingularis
Aa. lobares inferiores ⑥ A. segmentalis superior ⑦ A. segmentalis basalis anterior ⑧ A. segmentalis basalis lateralis ⑨ A. segmentalis basalis posterior ⑩ A. segmentalis basalis medialis	*Aa. lobares inferiores* ⑮ A. segmentalis superior ⑯ A. segmentalis basalis anterior ⑰ A. segmentalis basalis lateralis ⑱ A. segmentalis basalis posterior ⑲ A. segmentalis basalis medialis

D The venae pulmonales and their tributaries

Pulmo dexter Venae pulmonales dextrae	Pulmo sinister Venae pulmonales sinistrae
V. pulmonalis dextra superior ① V. apicalis ② V. posterior ③ V. anterior ④ V. lobi medii	*V. pulmonalis sinistra superior* ⑩ V. apicoposterior ⑪ V. anterior ⑫ V. lingularis
V. pulmonalis dextra inferior ⑤ V. superior ⑥ V. basalis communis ⑦ V. basalis inferior ⑧ V. basalis superior ⑨ V. basalis anterior	*V. pulmonalis sinistra inferior* ⑬ V. superior ⑭ V. basalis communis ⑮ V. basalis inferior ⑯ V. basalis superior ⑰ V. basalis anterior

151

4.9 Rami and Venae Bronchiales

A Rami and venae bronchiales

Anterior view. The trachea and bronchi are shown partially transparent.

a Arterial supply of the bronchi: The bronchi derive their blood supply from the aorta thoracica via rr. bronchiales that follow the divisions of the bronchi principales. It is not uncommon for one of the rr. bronchiales to arise from an a. intercostalis posterior (usually on the right side), rather than directly from the aorta. Given the relationship of the bronchi to the pars thoracica aortae, the rr. bronchiales usually enter the bronchi from the posterior side. The blood pressure within these arteries is equal to the systemic pressure, not the pulmonary pressure (as is the case in the aa. pulmonales).

Note: The trachea is supplied with arterial blood by small rr. tracheales (not shown here) that may arise from the pars thoracica aortae, the a. thoracica interna, or the truncus thyrocervicalis, depending on the level of the trachea that is supplied.

b Venous drainage of the bronchi: The bronchi are drained by vv. bronchiales, which usually open into the v. hemiazygos accessoria on the left side. On the right side, the veins may drain via collaterals into the v. azygos, but may also empty into the vv. pulmonales, causing a small amount of deoxygenated bronchial blood to be mixed with the much larger outflow of pulmonary blood on its way to the left atrium. Small vv. tracheales (not shown here) empty into the v. cava superior, left v. brachiocephalica, or v. thoracica interna at different levels of the trachea.

Note: A pulmonary embolism occurs when a blood clot forms in a vein (usually a leg or pelvic vein) and is carried into one of the aa. pulmonales. Depending on its size, the clot blocks one of the branches of the a. pulmonalis and in extreme cases the entire artery. The mechanical blockage of a large artery to the lungs leads to acute increased pressure in the ventriculus dexter of the cor, which can result in acute right-sided heart failure. Large pulmonary emboli are often fatal. If, however, a pulmonary embolism occludes a small-caliber vessel, the mechanical blockage and increased pressure on the cor are considerably less severe and the cor compensates for it without any significant problems. Arterial occlusion usually does not result in necrosis of lung tissue as the rr. bronchiales ensure delivery of nutrients and oxygen to the tissues of the lungs.

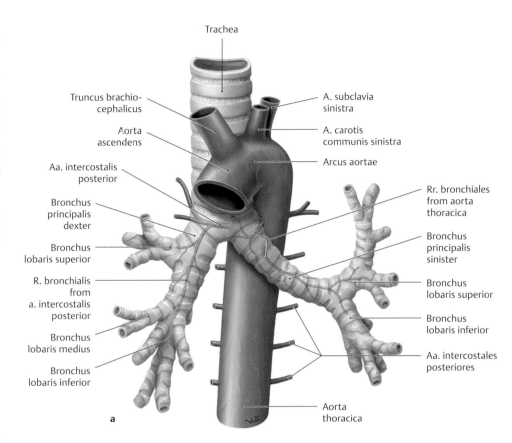

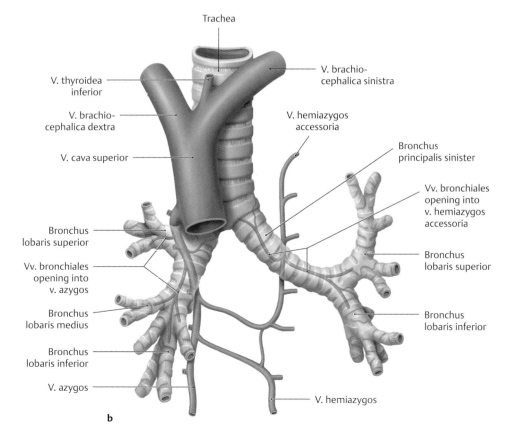

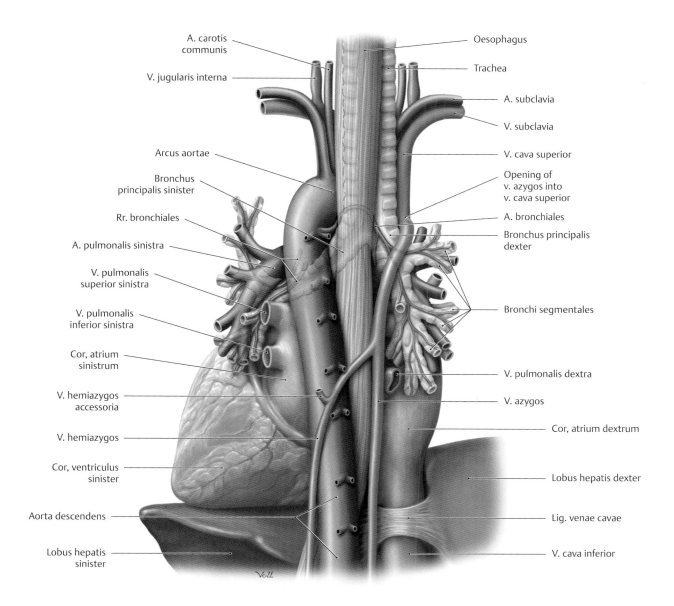

A. carotis communis

V. jugularis interna

Arcus aortae

Bronchus principalis sinister

Rr. bronchiales

A. pulmonalis sinistra

V. pulmonalis superior sinistra

V. pulmonalis inferior sinistra

Cor, atrium sinistrum

V. hemiazygos accessoria

V. hemiazygos

Cor, ventriculus sinister

Aorta descendens

Lobus hepatis sinister

Oesophagus

Trachea

A. subclavia

V. subclavia

V. cava superior

Opening of v. azygos into v. cava superior

A. bronchiales

Bronchus principalis dexter

Bronchi segmentales

V. pulmonalis dextra

V. azygos

Cor, atrium dextrum

Lobus hepatis dexter

Lig. venae cavae

V. cava inferior

B Rami bronchiales and their topographical relation to the arteriae pulmonales
Isolated organ group composed of cor, major vessels, trachea, oesophagus, and hepar, posterior view.

Note: The rr. bronchiales originate from the proximal portion of the aorta descendens.

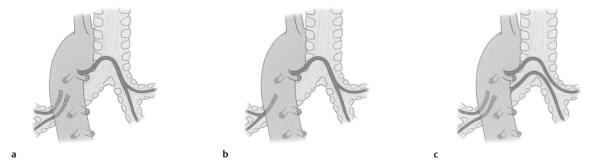

a

b

c

C Origin of the rami bronchiales from the aorta: Normal anatomy and variations (after Platzer)
Posterior view.

a Normal anatomical case (40 % of cases): on the right side of the aorta arise a r. bronchialis and an a. intercostalis posterior, on the left side arise two rr. bronchiales;

b Variation 1 (15–30 % of cases): only *one* r. bronchialis arises from the left and the right sides of the aorta;

c Variation 2 (12–23 %): *two* rr. bronchiales arise from the left and the right sides of the aorta.

4.10 Functional Structure of the Vascular Tree

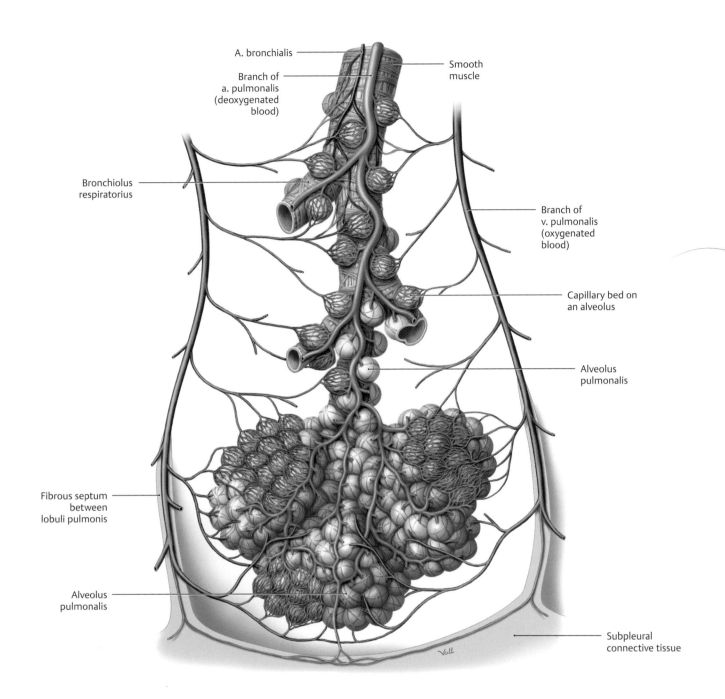

A. bronchialis

Smooth muscle

Branch of a. pulmonalis (deoxygenated blood)

Bronchiolus respiratorius

Branch of v. pulmonalis (oxygenated blood)

Capillary bed on an alveolus

Alveolus pulmonalis

Fibrous septum between lobuli pulmonis

Alveolus pulmonalis

Subpleural connective tissue

A Overview of vascular tree structure

Note: In previous sections, arteries have been colored in red and veins have been colored in blue. However, since this paragraph discusses in particular the functional structure of the vascular tree, this standard convention of coloring is not followed here. Instead, branches of the a. pulmonalis (arterial side of circulation) are colored in blue, because of low oxygen levels, and branches of the vv. pulmonales (venous side of circulation) are colored in red because of high oxygen levels.

The vascular tree is made up of the finest terminal branches of the aa. and vv. pulmonales as well as the rr. and vv. bronchiales. These branches of the vasa publica (aa. and vv. pulmonales) and vasa privata (rr. and vv. bronchiales) are analogous to those of the arbor bronchialis (see p. 152). Because of this arrangement, gas exchange can occur between air in the alveoli (in the finest branches of the arbor bronchialis) and blood (in the finest branches of the pulmonary vessels).

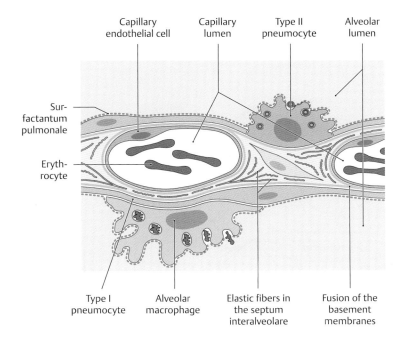

Labels for the cellular diagram (top to bottom, clockwise):
Capillary endothelial cell · Capillary lumen · Type II pneumocyte · Alveolar lumen · Surfactantum pulmonale · Erythrocyte · Type I pneumocyte · Alveolar macrophage · Elastic fibers in the septum interalveolare · Fusion of the basement membranes

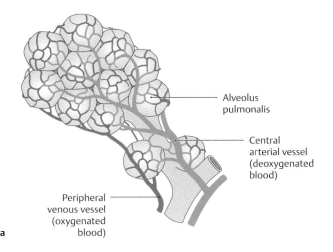

a

Labels: Alveolus pulmonalis · Central arterial vessel (deoxygenated blood) · Peripheral venous vessel (oxygenated blood)

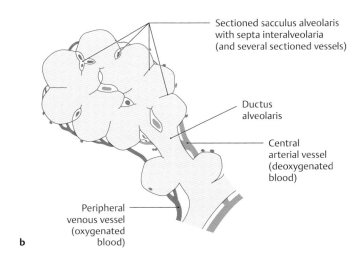

b

Labels: Sectioned sacculus alveolaris with septa interalveolaria (and several sectioned vessels) · Ductus alveolaris · Central arterial vessel (deoxygenated blood) · Peripheral venous vessel (oxygenated blood)

B Epithelial lining of the alveoli

The alveoli are lined by two types of alveolar epithelial cells (pneumocyti):

- Pneumocyti typi I: They cover approximately 90 % of the alveolar surface, are spread out flat and form a continuous layer (cap cells). They are closely interconnected by tight junctions.
- Pneumocyti typi II: Relative to total number, they are as common as pneumocyti typi I. However, because of their rounded shape they cover only 10 % of the alveolar surface. They are found among pneumocyti typi I, often at alveolar-septal junctions, and thus they are also referred to as niche cells. They produce and secrete a protein-phospholipid film called surfactantum pulmonale, which is distributed over the entire alveolar surface and lowers the surface tension of the alveoli, making it easier for the lung to expand. The immature lung of the preterm infant often fails to produce sufficient surfactantum. Thus, preterm infants often suffer from respiratory problems. Pneumocyti typi II continuously produce and reabsorb surfactantum so that a large amount of surfactantum is reused. Only a fraction is cleared by alveolar macrophages.

At the sites where type I alveolar epithelial cells come into contact with the capillary endothelial cells, their basement membranes are fused together. The anatomical distance from the alveolar lumen to the capillary lumen, over which gaseous diffusion takes place, measures only 0.5 μm at that location.

Note: All diseases which

- increase the diffusion distance between the alveolar lumen and capillary lumen (edematous fluid collection or inflammation),
- decrease the aeration of the lung (alveolar destruction due to emphysema, for example) or decrease lung perfusion (capillary obliteration), or
- cause fluid infiltration of the alveoli (pneumonia)
- will decrease the efficiency of alveolar–capillary gas exchange, leading to respiratory compromise.

C Relationship between the sacculus alveolaris and pulmonary vessels

In **a**, a branch of the a. pulmonalis carrying oxygen-depleted blood from the ventriculus dexter is depicted in blue. A corresponding branch of the pulmonary venous system is shown in red, carrying oxygen-enriched blood back to the left cor. Pulmonary arterial branches are intimately apposed to, and follow closely the course of, the respiratory bronchiolus branches, sending capillaries over the sacculi alveolares and invading the alveolar septa. The sectioned sacculus alveolaris (**b**) clearly shows that the vessels not only surround the alveoli on the outer surface of the sacculus but also penetrate the septa interalveolaria, enabling the capillaries to undergo gas exchange with multiple adjacent alveoli.

Note: In most of the circulatory system, small arterial and corresponding venous branches tend to follow parallel courses, but this is not true in the pulmonary circulation. While pulmonary arterial branches follow the same segmental and lobular branching pattern as the arbor bronchialis, the vv. pulmonales have a more independent course, not closely apposed to the bronchioli, remaining on the periphery of lobuli and segments, and often crossing lobular boundaries. This difference in conformation between aa. and vv. pulmonales is demonstrated dramatically in **A**.

4.11 Innervation and Lymphatic Drainage of the Trachea, Arbor Bronchialis, and Lungs

A Autonomic innervation of the trachea and arbor bronchialis

Parasympathetic: Branches from both nn. vagi are distributed to the pars cervicalis of the trachea, mostly via the nn. laryngei recurrentes. At the thoracic level they form rr. tracheales that enter the plexus pulmonalis, which is heavily branched at the hilum pulmonis.

Sympathetic: Few postsynaptic fibers are distributed to the trachea; numerous rr. pulmonales thoracici (postsynaptic branches of the ganglia thoracica) pass into the plexus pulmonalis.

The plexus pulmonalis regulates the caliber and secretory activity of the bronchi and influences the caliber of the pulmonary vessels. Activation of the pars parasympathica of the nervous system causes the bronchi to constrict (as in bronchial asthma), while activation of the pars sympathica causes bronchial dilation. Thus, drugs that activate the pars sympathica of the nervous system cause bronchial dilation and may be useful in the treatment of acute bronchial asthma. The autonomic effects on the pulmonary vessels provide a means of varying the perfusion to different areas of the lung by controlling vascular calibers. For example, the autonomic system can greatly reduce the blood flow to poorly ventilated lung areas during shallow respiration.

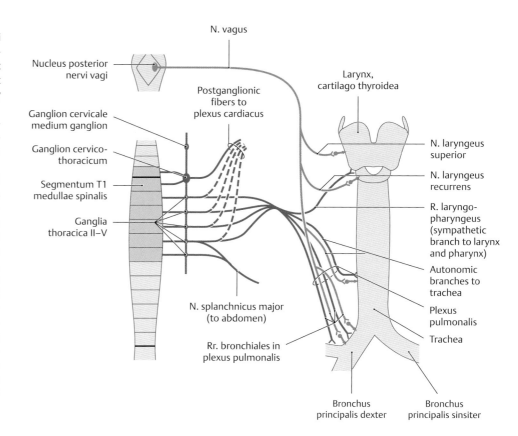

B Nodi lymphoidei of the trachea, bronchi, and lungs

Anterior view. The following nodi lymphoidei can be distinguished inside and outside the lungs, listed in order from deep to superficial (see **C**):

- Inside the lung: nodi intrapulmonales in the lung tissue and at the divisions of the bronchi segmentales; nodi bronchopulmonales at the division of the bronchi lobares.
- Outside the lung: nodi tracheobronchiales inferiores and superiores at the bifurcatio tracheae and on both bronchi principales; nodi paratracheales along both sides of the trachea.

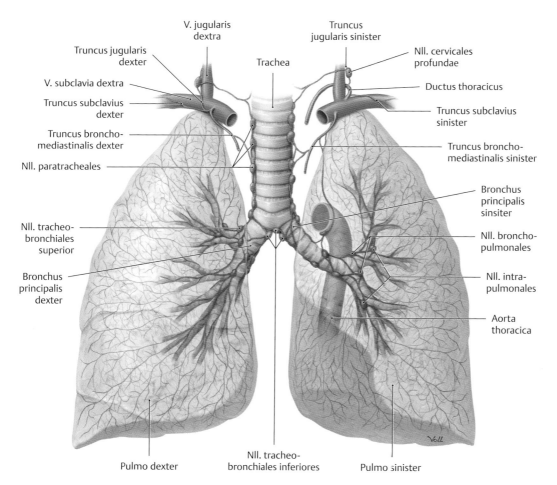

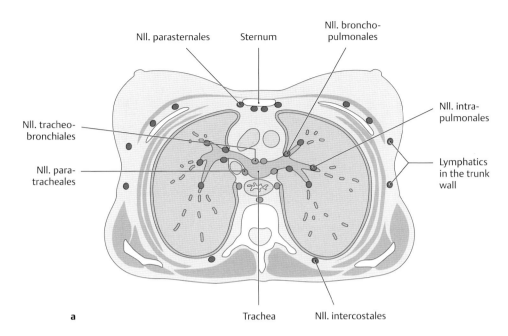

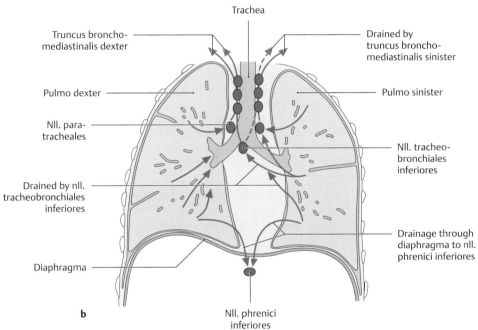

C Lymphatic drainage of the lungs, arbor bronchialis, and trachea
a, **b** Transverse and coronal sections viewed from above (**a**) and from the front (**b**). The lymphatic drainage of the lungs and bronchi is handled by two separate networks of delicate vasa lymphatica (see **b**):

- The *peribronchial network* follows the branching pattern of the arbor bronchialis (see p. 143) and collects lymph from the bronchi and most of the lungs.
- The *subpleural network* (smaller) bordering the lungs collects lymph from peripheral lung areas and from the pleura *visceralis*. The pleura parietalis (part of the chest wall) is drained by the nll. intercostales and nll. parasternales of the chest wall.

These two networks communicate at the hilum pulmonis and convey lymph *cranially*, ultimately to the nodi tracheobronchiales (deep tissue areas may drain to the nll. intrapulmonales or bronchopulmonales, but the lung as a whole is drained by the nll. tracheobronchiales). Lymph flows from the nll. tracheobronchiales to the nll. paratracheales and trunci bronchomediastinales, which terminate at the junction of the vv. subclaviae and jugulares internae independently or after joining the ductus thoracicus or ductus lymphaticus dexter.

Note: Lymph from the *left* lobus inferior may also drain to the right truncus bronchomediastinalis via (inferior) nll. tracheobronchiales. The lobi inferiores of *both* pulmonales may drain cranially, but they may also drain inferiorly to the nll. phrenici superioris or may drain through the diaphragma to the nll. phrenici inferiores.

The **trachea** drains to the nll. paratracheales, which may empty directly into the truncus jugularis or indirectly via the nll. bronchomediastinales.
Note: Nll. tracheobronchiales that lie very close to the hilum pulmonis are known in clinical parlance as the "hilar lymph nodes." Their enlargement in response to pathological processes may be detectable by imaging studies.

4.12 Respiratory Mechanics

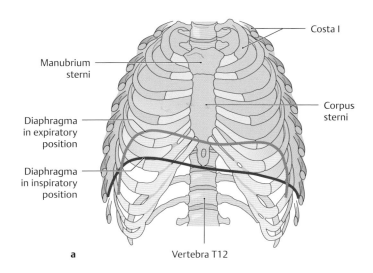

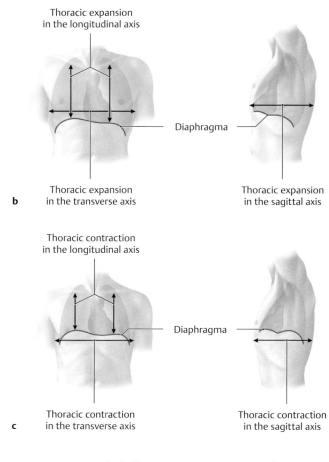

A Basic principles of respiratory mechanics

The mechanics of external respiration (as opposed to the internal respiration of cells and tissues) are based on a rhythmical increase and decrease in the thoracic volume, with an associated expansion and contraction of the lungs. As the lung expands, the pressure within the lung falls and air is drawn into the lung (inspiration). As the lung contracts, the pulmonary pressure rises and air is expelled from the lungs (expiration). Thus, contrary to a common misconception, air is not pumped into the lungs during respiration but is sucked into the lungs by the "bellows effect," a negative intrapulmonary pressure. The ribs, the thoracic muscles (especially the mm. intercostales), and the elastic fibers in the lung interact as follows during respiration:

- When the diaphragma moves to the **inspiratory position** (red), the ribs are elevated by the mm. intercostales (chiefly the mm. intercostales externi) and the mm. scaleni. Because the ribs are curved and are directed obliquely downward, elevation of the ribs expands the chest transversely (toward the flanks) and anteriorly. Meanwhile the diaphragma leaflets are lowered by muscular contraction (red outline in **a**), causing the chest to expand inferiorly. The epigastric angle is also increased (see **d**). These processes result in an overall expansion of the thoracic volume.
- When the diaphragma moves to the **expiratory position** (blue), the chest becomes smaller in all dimensions and the thoracic volume is decreased. This process does not require additional muscular energy. The muscles that are active during inspiration are relaxed, and the lung contracts as the myriad elastic fibers in the lung tissue that were stretched on inspiration release their stored energy, causing an elastic recoil. For forcible expiration, however, the muscles that assist expiration (mainly the mm. intercostales interni) can actively lower the rib cage more rapidly and to a greater extent than is possible by passive elastic recoil alone.

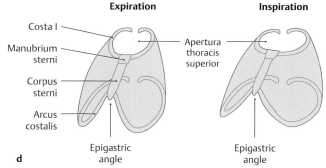

B Respiratory muscles

Active during inspiration	Active during expiration
Mm. scaleni	Mm. intercostales interni
Mm. intercostales externi	M. transversus thoracis
Mm. intercartilaginei	Mm. subcostales
Mm. serrati posteriores superior and inferior	
Diaphragma	

When the upper limb is fixed (e.g., by bracing the arm on a table), the muscles of the shoulder girdle, whose primary action is to move the shoulder girdle, can elevate and expand the thorax, to which they are attached. They can also function as auxiliary respiratory muscles during forced respiration, when breathing is made difficult (dyspnea) by disease.

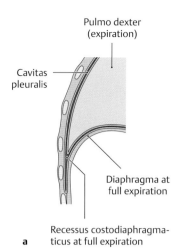

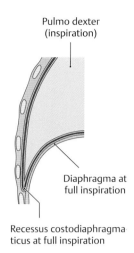

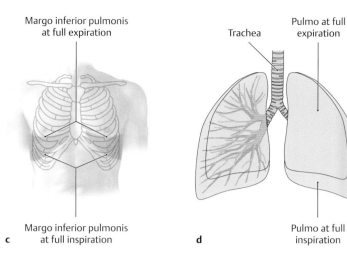

a Pulmo dexter (expiration) — Cavitas pleuralis — Diaphragma at full expiration — Recessus costodiaphragmaticus at full expiration

b Pulmo dexter (inspiration) — Diaphragma at full inspiration — Recessus costodiaphragma ticus at full inspiration

c Margo inferior pulmonis at full expiration — Margo inferior pulmonis at full inspiration

d Trachea — Pulmo at full expiration — Pulmo at full inspiration

C Respiratory changes in lung volume

a–c Respiratory contraction and expansion of the lung. Capillary forces in the pleural space cause the lung to "stick" to the wall of the cavitas pleuralis, forcing the lung to follow changes in the thoracic volume. This is particularly evident in the recessus pleurales—sites where the lung does not fully occupy the cavitas pleuralis at functional residual capacity (the resting position between inspiration and expiration, see p. 141). As the dome of the diaphragma flattens during inspiration (see **A**), the recessus costodiaphragmaticus expands and the lung is "sucked" into the resulting space, though it does not

fill it completely. During expiration, the lung retracts from the recess somewhat. The respiratory changes in the volume of the recessus costodiaphragmaticus lead to considerable displacement of the margines inferiores pulmonum (**c**).

d Respiratory movements of the arbor bronchialis. As the thoracic volume changes during respiration, the entire arbor bronchialis moves within the lung. These structural movements are more pronounced in portions of the arbor bronchialis that are more distant from the hilum pulmonis.

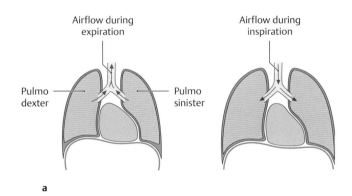

a Pulmo dexter — Airflow during expiration — Airflow during inspiration — Pulmo sinister

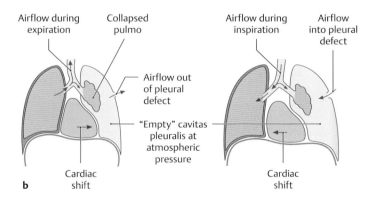

b Airflow during expiration — Collapsed pulmo — Airflow out of pleural defect — "Empty" cavitas pleuralis at atmospheric pressure — Cardiac shift — Airflow during inspiration — Airflow into pleural defect — Cardiac shift

D Change in respiratory mechanics due to pneumothorax

a Normal respiratory mechanics: The cavitas pleuralis is hermetically sealed on all sides.

b Pneumothorax: With injury to the left pleura parietalis, outside air can enter the cavitas pleuralis. The mechanical effect of the capillary pleural space (see **C**) is lost, and the left lung collapses from the inherent elasticity of its connective tissue. It no longer participates in respiration. The right cavitas pleuralis is intact and can function independently. Air is sucked into the opened cavitas pleuralis during inspiration and is expelled during expiration. Because normal respiratory pressure variations still prevail in the right cavitas pleuralis but are absent on the left side due to the pleural defect, the mediastinum shifts toward the normal side during expiration and returns toward the midline during inspiration ("mediastinal flutter").

c Tension pneumothorax (valve pneumothorax): Tissue that has been traumatically detached and displaced covers the defect in the cavitas pleuralis from the inside like a mobile flap, preventing the expulsion of air. Air passes through the defect in one direction only: from outside to inside. Because of this check-valve mechanism, a small amount of air enters the cavitas pleuralis with each breath

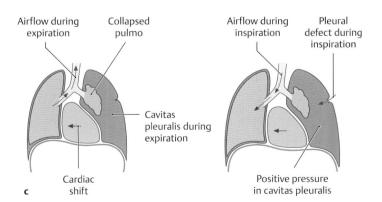

c Airflow during expiration — Collapsed pulmo — Cavitas pleuralis during expiration — Cardiac shift — Airflow during inspiration — Pleural defect during inspiration — Positive pressure in cavitas pleuralis

but cannot escape, similar to air being pumped into a bicycle tire. The mediastinum is gradually shifted toward the normal side (mediastinal shift), which may cause kinking of the vessels around the cor. Without treatment, tension pneumothorax is invariably fatal.

159

4.13 Radiological Anatomy of the Lungs and Vascular System

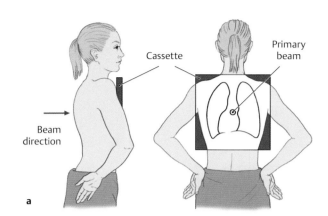

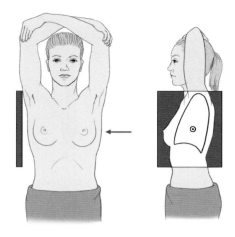

Beam direction

Cassette

Primary beam

a

a

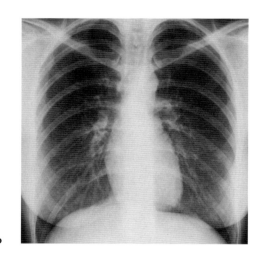

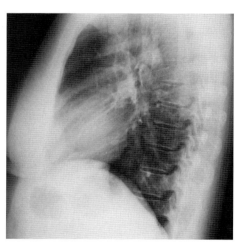

b

b

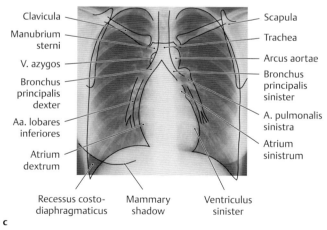

Clavicula

Manubrium sterni

V. azygos

Bronchus principalis dexter

Aa. lobares inferiores

Atrium dextrum

Scapula

Trachea

Arcus aortae

Bronchus principalis sinister

A. pulmonalis sinistra

Atrium sinistrum

Recessus costo-diaphragmaticus

Mammary shadow

Ventriculus sinister

c

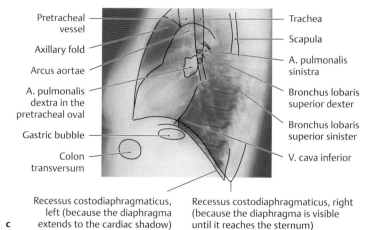

Pretracheal vessel

Axillary fold

Arcus aortae

A. pulmonalis dextra in the pretracheal oval

Gastric bubble

Colon transversum

Trachea

Scapula

A. pulmonalis sinistra

Bronchus lobaris superior dexter

Bronchus lobaris superior sinister

V. cava inferior

Recessus costodiaphragmaticus, left (because the diaphragma extends to the cardiac shadow)

Recessus costodiaphragmaticus, right (because the diaphragma is visible until it reaches the sternum)

c

A Posterior-anterior (PA) chest radiograph (from Lange, S. Radiologische Diagnostik der Thoraxerkrankungen, 3. Aufl./ Diagnostic Thoracic Radiology, 3rd edition, Thieme, Stuttgart 2005)

a The patient stands with the anterior chest wall on the cassette (the beam "passes" through the patient in a posterior-to-anterior direction with the central beam targeted at the level of the 6th vertebra thoracica). The radiographs are taken with the patient keeping the mouth open, breathing in and holding the breath. The back of the hands are placed on the hips with the elbows turned forward;

b Posterior-anterior chest radiograph (PA radiograph; viewed from an anterior to posterior direction);

c Explanation of the visible structures.

B Lateral chest radiograph (from Lange, S. Radiologische Diagnostik der Thoraxerkrankungen, 3. Aufl./Diagnostic Thoracic Radiology, 3rd edition, Thieme, Stuttgart 2005)

a The patient is standing with the left or right side against the cassette, with both arms raised above the head. The central beam is targeted a hand's width below the left (right) axilla;

b Lateral chest radiograph;

c Explanation of the visible structures.

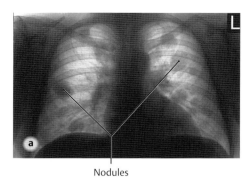

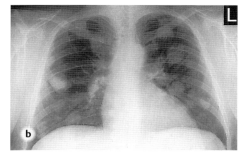

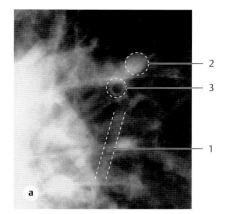

Nodules

C Terminology to describe conventional radiographic findings (from Reiser, M. et al.: Radiologie [Duale Reihe], 2. Aufl./ Radiology, 2nd edition, Thieme, Stuttgart 2006)

The terminology used to describe conventional radiographic findings dates back to the era of *photofluorography*. On the fluorescent screens that were used back then, radiopaque areas, such as the cor and bones, but also lung metastases (also known as nodules), appear as shadows because they show weaker light emission (**a**). Compared with the fluorescent screen, modern radiographs (**b**) produce inverted images (negative images): The low absorption areas (radiolucent areas) appear as dark areas and the opacities (radiopaque areas) as bright areas.

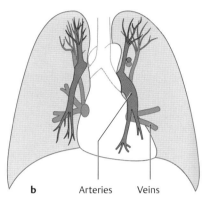

Arteries Veins

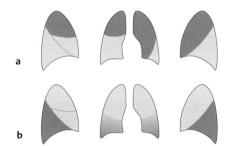

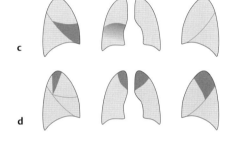

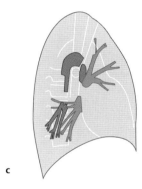

D Opacity in lung diseases

Lateral and anterior views of the right and left lung.

a Opacity of both lobi superiores; **b** Opacity of both lobi inferiores; **c** Opacity of the lobus medius (pulmonis dextri); **d** Opacity of segmentum apicale on both sides.

In most cases, opacities that follow the lines of segmental lung boundaries are almost always due to inflammation of the lungs.

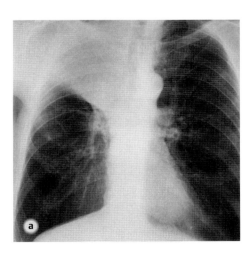

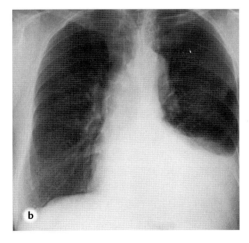

E Pulmonary opacities on an AP chest radiograph (from Lange, S.: Radiologische Diagnostic der Thoraxerkrankungen, 3. Aufl./Diagnostic Thoracic Radiology, 3rd edition, Thieme, Stuttgart 2005)

a Right superior lobe atelectasis due to damage to the bronchus lobaris superior dexter caused by a central carcinoma. This resulted in reduced ventilation of the affected lobus superior and subsequent collapse of lung tissue;

b Left basal pleural effusion causing complete opacification of the lateral recessus costodiaphragmaticus. Opacity is higher laterally, concave to the lung and does not follow lobar boundaries.

F Radiographic appearance of pulmonary vessels (from Reiser, M. et al.: Radiologie [Duale Reihe], 2. Aufl./Radiology, 2nd edition, Thieme, Stuttgart 2006)

a Detail from AP chest radiograph close to the hilum pulmonis: The image shows a longitudinal view of a vessel (1), an oblique view of a vessel (2), and an oblique view of a bronchus (3). Farther out in the periphery, opacities are usually not detectable.

b Schematic view of the vascular bundle in an AP projection.
Note: Arteries always run adjacent to the bronchi; arteries to the lobi superiores run medial to the veins, and lobus inferior veins run horizontally and cross the lobus inferior arteries.

c Schematic view of the vascular bundle, lateral view.
Note: In the retrocardiac vascular bundle, the veins descend more anteriorly than the arteries.

161

4.14 Computed Tomography of the Lungs

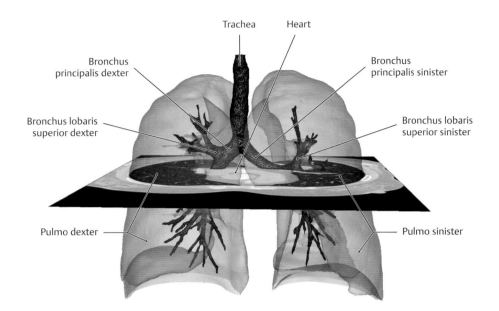

Trachea | Heart

Bronchus principalis dexter

Bronchus principalis sinister

Bronchus lobaris superior dexter

Bronchus lobaris superior sinister

Pulmo dexter

Pulmo sinister

A Reconstruction of the arbor bronchialis from cross-sectional images

Anterior view. Three-dimensional reconstruction of the bronchial tree from individual CT scans. The result is a high resolution, three-dimensional display. For orientation purposes, a CT section displaying the thorax with part of the cor and lungs is shown. Unlike the older technique of bronchography (radiographic contrast examination of the bronchi), this procedure is less debilitating for patients. Because of the high resolution of the scan, even small changes in the arbor bronchialis can be detected and accurately localized. Using this technique, a bronchial carcinoma, an often malignant tumor that is particularly common in smokers, can be precisely localized.

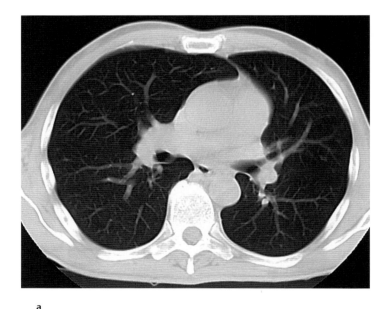

a

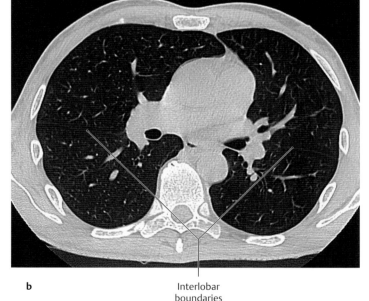

b

Interlobar boundaries

B CT scans of the lungs using a lung window thickness that is dependent on the layer to be examined (from Lange, S.: Radiologische Diagnostic der Thoraxerkrankungen, 3. Aufl./ Diagnostic Thoracic Radiology, 3rd edition, Thieme, Stuttgart 2005)
Computed tomography allows for a view of the lungs, mediastinum, pleura, and chest wall in an axial layer without any overlapping structures, and with the bronchi serving as an anatomical landmark (see also **C**). In conventional chest CT scans, 8–10 mm thick slices are routinely examined (**a**), because they allow for a better evaluation of the vascular and arbor bronchialis in their entirety. HR-CT (high resolution CT) uses a slice thickness of 1–3 mm (**b**). The higher resolution makes both the interlobar boundaries and the secondary pulmonary lobuli, the smallest functional units of the lung parenchyma, visible. Usually, this technique is used to diagnose cavea thoracis abnormalities, areas of emphysema and bronchiectasis.
Note: Transverse (axial) CT images are evaluated from a inferior view.

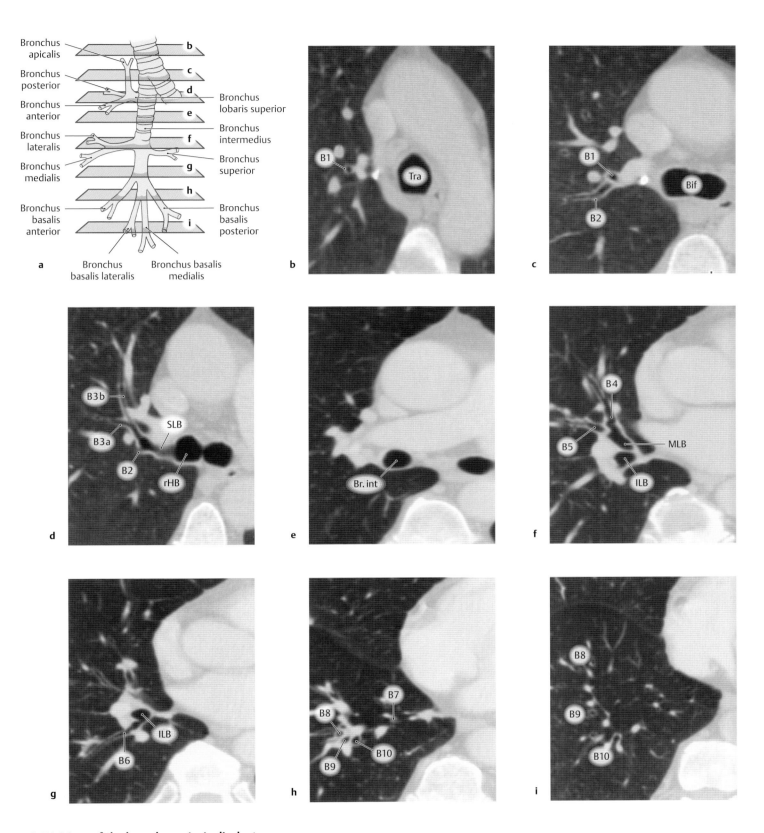

Bronchus apicalis — b
Bronchus posterior — c
— d — Bronchus lobaris superior
Bronchus anterior — e
— Bronchus intermedius
Bronchus lateralis — f
— Bronchus superior
Bronchus medialis — g
— h
Bronchus basalis anterior — — Bronchus basalis posterior
— i
a
Bronchus basalis lateralis   Bronchus basalis medialis

C Divisions of the bronchus principalis dexter

Tra	Trachea	
Bif	Bifurcatio tracheae	
rHB	Bronchus principalis dexter	
Br. int	Bronchus intermedius	
SLB	Bronchus lobaris superior	
MLB	Bronchus lobaris medius	
ILB	Bronchus lobaris inferior	

B1	Bronchus segmentalis apicalis
B2	Bronchus segmentalis posterior bronchus
B3	Bronchus segmentalis anterior
B4	Bronchus segmentalis lateralis

B5	Bronchus segmentalis medialis
B6	Bronchus segmentalis superior
B7	Bronchus segmentalis basalis medialis

B8	Bronchus segmentalis basalis anterior
B9	Bronchus segmentalis basalis lateralis
B10	Bronchus segmentalis basalis posterior

(from: Lange, S Radiologische Diagnostic der Thoraxerkrankungen, 3. Aufl./Diagnostic Thoracic Radiology, 3rd edition Thieme, Stuttgart 2005).

163

5.1 Oesophagus: Location and Divisions

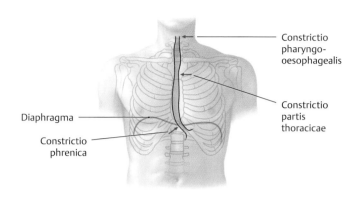

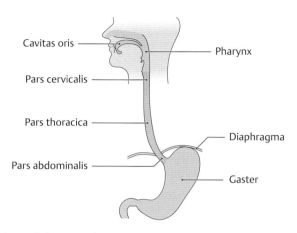

A Projection onto the skeleton thoracis

Anterior view. The oesophagus is located slightly to the right of the midline, especially in its course through the thorax, where it descends along the right side of the aorta. It pierces the diaphragma just below the processus xiphoideus of the sternum. The arrows mark the sites of the three normal anatomical constrictions of the oesophagus (see **C**).

B Divisions of the oesophagus

Anterior view with the head turned to the right. The oesophagus is approximately 23–27 cm long, 1–2 cm in diameter, and is divided into three parts:

- Pars cervicalis: just anterior to the columna vertebralis in the neck, extends from C6 to T1.
- Pars thoracica: the longest part, located in the mediastinum superius and posterius, extends from T1 to the hiatus oesophageus of the diaphragma (at approximately T11).
- Pars abdominalis: the shortest part, located in the cavitas peritonei, extends from the diaphragma to the ostium cardiacum of the gaster.

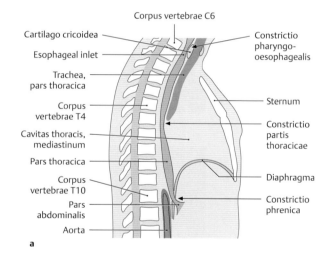

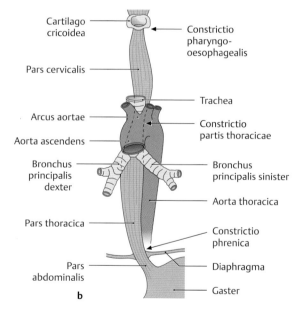

C Constrictions and curves of the oesophagus

Right lateral view (**a**), anterior view (**b**).
The oesophagus has three normal anatomical constrictions, which are projected at the levels of specific vertebrae (**a**). The constrictions are caused by adjacent structures that indent the oesophagus and by functional closure mechanisms (constrictio phrenica, see p. 167). These constrictions are visible during gastroscopy, and the scope must be carefully maneuvered past them (normal width of the oesophagus is approximately 20 mm):

- Upper constriction (constrictio pharyngooesophagealis, 14–16 cm from the incisor teeth), corresponds to the esophageal inlet in the pars cervicalis of the oesophagus (see p. 166). It is located where the oesophagus passes behind the cartilago cricoidea (C6) and has a maximum width of approximately 14 mm.
- Middle constriction (constrictio partis thoracicae, 25–27 cm from the incisors), located where the oesophagus passes to the right of the arcus aortae and aorta thoracica (at T4/T5). Maximum width is 14 mm.

- Lower constriction (constrictio phrenica, 36–38 cm from the incisors), located at the start of the pars abdominalis of the oesophagus, where it pierces the diaphragma (T10/T11). Functional closure of the oesophagus by muscles and veins of the esophageal wall. The pars abdominalis is normally occluded except during swallowing (see p. 167). Maximum width is 14 mm.

Besides its constrictions, the oesophagus also presents characteristic **curves** (**b**): an upper curve to the left (in the pars cervicalis), a mid-level curve to the right (in the pars thoracica, caused by the adjacent pars thoracica aortae), and a lower curve to the left (in the pars abdominalis). Additionally, the oesophagus is slightly concave anteriorly in the sagittal plane, following the curvature of the columna vertebralis (kyphosis thoracica, **a**).

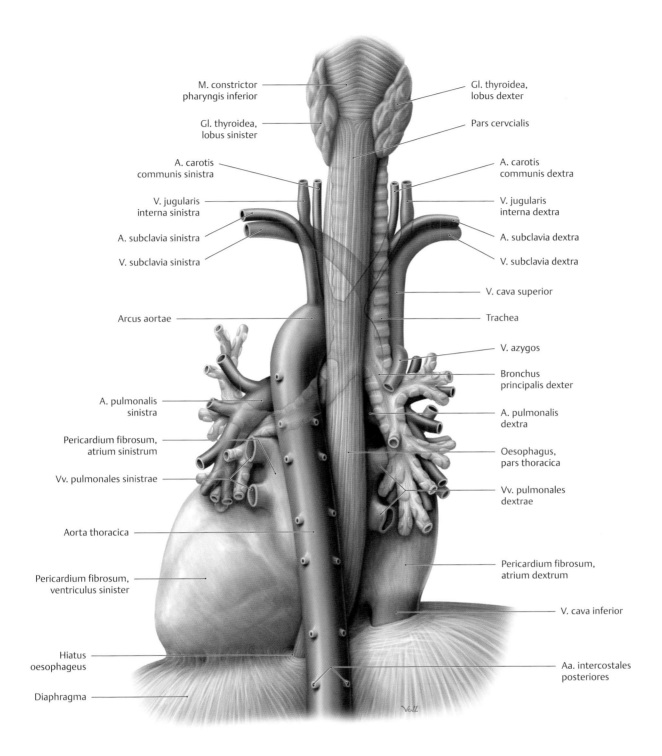

M. constrictor pharyngis inferior

Gl. thyroidea, lobus sinister

A. carotis communis sinistra

V. jugularis interna sinistra

A. subclavia sinistra

V. subclavia sinistra

Arcus aortae

A. pulmonalis sinistra

Pericardium fibrosum, atrium sinistrum

Vv. pulmonales sinistrae

Aorta thoracica

Pericardium fibrosum, ventriculus sinister

Hiatus oesophageus

Diaphragma

Gl. thyroidea, lobus dexter

Pars cervcialis

A. carotis communis dextra

V. jugularis interna dextra

A. subclavia dextra

V. subclavia dextra

V. cava superior

Trachea

V. azygos

Bronchus principalis dexter

A. pulmonalis dextra

Oesophagus, pars thoracica

Vv. pulmonales dextrae

Pericardium fibrosum, atrium dextrum

V. cava inferior

Aa. intercostales posteriores

D Topographical relations of the oesophagus, posterior view
The relations of the oesophagus to the pericardium, great vessels, and trachea are depicted here. The close proximity of the oesophagus to the atrium sinistrum and pars thoracica aortae can be seen. Due to the asymmetrical position of the cor in the thorax, the vv. pulmonales dextrae are closer to the oesophagus than the vv. pulmonales sinistrae. The oesophagus initially descends to the right of the aorta, but just above the diaphragma it crosses in front of the aorta before piercing the diaphragma to enter the cavitas abdominis (see **C**). The oesophagus is loosely attached by its own connective tissue (tunica adventitia) to the connective tissue of the mediastinum (important for swallowing). It is stabilized somewhat by the attachment of its anterior wall to the back of the trachea, again by numerous slips of connective tissue.
Note: The trachea develops as an outgrowth from the oesophagus during early embryonic development, at which time a communication exists between the two structures. Normally this communication closes, but its persistence results in a tracheoesophageal fistula, which may allow food to enter the trachea and reach the lung, causing recurrent episodes of pneumonia.

5.2 Oesophagus: Inlet and Outlet, Opening and Closure

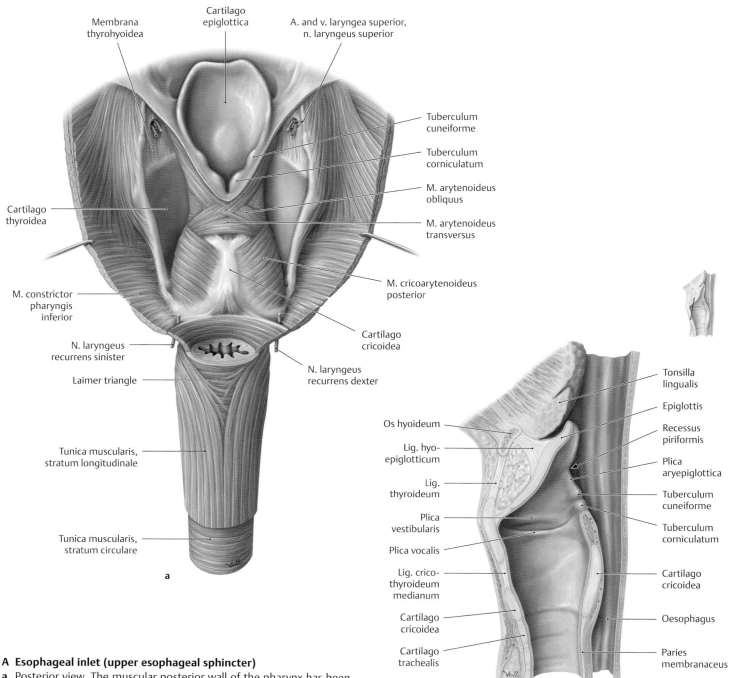

Cartilago epiglottica

Membrana thyrohyoidea

A. and v. laryngea superior, n. laryngeus superior

Tuberculum cuneiforme

Tuberculum corniculatum

M. arytenoideus obliquus

M. arytenoideus transversus

Cartilago thyroidea

M. cricoarytenoideus posterior

M. constrictor pharyngis inferior

Cartilago cricoidea

N. laryngeus recurrens sinister

N. laryngeus recurrens dexter

Laimer triangle

Tunica muscularis, stratum longitudinale

Tunica muscularis, stratum circulare

a

Os hyoideum

Lig. hyo-epiglotticum

Lig. thyroideum

Plica vestibularis

Plica vocalis

Lig. crico-thyroideum medianum

Cartilago cricoidea

Cartilago trachealis

Tonsilla lingualis

Epiglottis

Recessus piriformis

Plica aryepiglottica

Tuberculum cuneiforme

Tuberculum corniculatum

Cartilago cricoidea

Oesophagus

Paries membranaceus

b

A Esophageal inlet (upper esophageal sphincter)

a Posterior view. The muscular posterior wall of the pharynx has been divided and reflected laterally, and the uppermost esophageal segment has been opened posteriorly. At the posterior junction of the longitudinal esophageal musculature with the pharyngeal musculature, the longitudinal muscles are thin and do not span the full circumference of the oesophagus. This area of muscular weakness ("Laimer triangle") is a site of vulnerability for the development of diverticula (see p. 169). This diagram shows the oesophagus with an expanded, stellate lumen near the esophageal inlet, as it would appear during swallowing. While in the resting state, the esophageal inlet usually has the form of a transverse slit. The musculature of the upper oesophagus is a continuation of the (skeletal) musculi

pharyngis and consists of striated fibers that give way distally to smooth muscle (not shown here).

b Midsagittal section, viewed from the left side. In the lateral view, both the tunica muscularis oesophagi and tunica mucosa oesophagi are visible. Additionally, the diagram shows the posterior dilation of the oesophagus, and thus the size of the oesophagus relative to the larynx. The constrictio pharyngooesophagealis, located behind the cartilago cricoidea, is also clearly visible.

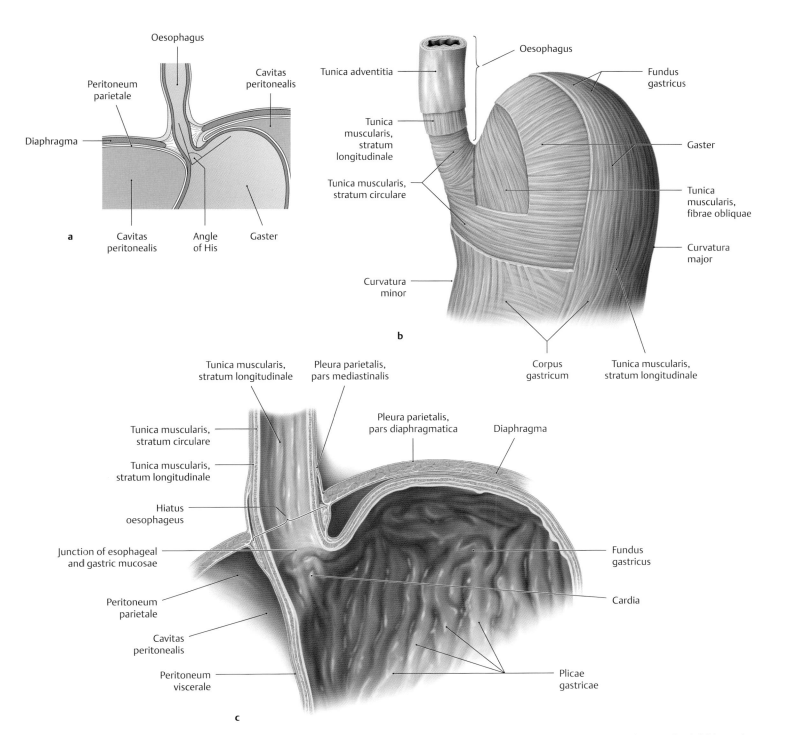

B Esophageal outlet and esophageal closure

Functional closure of the esophageal outlet is an important mechanism for preventing the backflow of gastric contents, especially hydrochloric acid, into the distal oesophagus (gastroesophageal reflux). This mechanism is essential because the tunica mucosa oesophagi, unlike the tunica mucosa gastris, is vulnerable to corrosive injury by stomach acid. As a result, repeated exposure to hydrochloric acid can cause esophageal inflammation (reflux esophagitis). Early, relatively mild forms of this reflux ("heartburn") are often manifested by a burning retrosternal pain that is most pronounced in the supine position (at night). Effective closure of the oesophagus is based on several factors:

- Narrowing of the esophageal outlet by
  - the circular muscles of the oesophagus (see **b**) and

- submucous venous plexuses, which raise longitudinal folds in the tunica mucosa oesophagi (see **c**). These prominent veins function as portosystemic collaterals in response to an obstruction of portal venous blood flow (see p. 171). Together, the esophageal circular muscles and venous plexuses provide "angiomuscular closure" at the esophagogastric junction;
- The structurally narrow muscular hiatus oesophageus in the diaphragm (see **c**);
- Connective tissue and fat surrounding the esophagogastric junction (**c**);
- Continuity of the esophageal and gastric musculature (**b**), and the oblique angle at which the oesophagus joins the gaster just below the diaphragma (the angle of His, see **a**).

167

5.3 Oesophagus: Wall Structure and Weaknesses

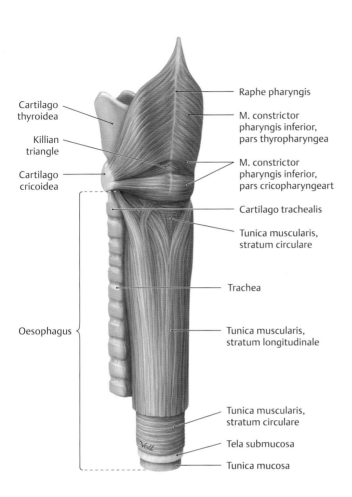

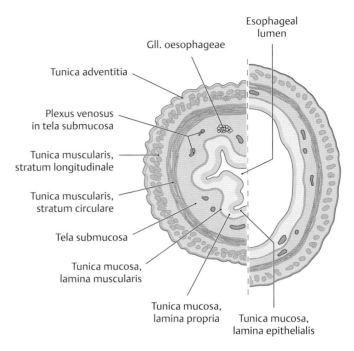

B Microscopic structure of the esophageal wall

Transverse section through an oesophagus in the contracted (left) and relaxed state (right). The layers of the esophageal wall are typical of a hollow viscus in the digestive tract:

- The *tunica mucosa*, which consists of an epithelial layer, lamina propria, and lamina muscularis. The epithelial layer is composed of stratified, nonkeratinized squamous epithelium (for mechanical resistance to food passage).
- The *tela submucosa*, a loose layer of connective tissue that contains numerous glands (gll. oesophageae) whose secretions lubricate the tunica mucosa to facilitate food passage. Particularly in the lower oesophagus, the tela submucosa contains numerous veins that participate in the closure of the esophageal outlet (see p. 167).
- The *tunica muscularis*, consisting of an inner layer of circular muscle and an outer layer of longitudinal muscle. Smooth-muscle contractions aid in the peristaltic propulsion of food.
- The *tunica adventitia*, a layer of loose connective tissue that tethers the oesophagus to the mediastinal connective tissue and is firmly attached to the connective tissue of the posterior tracheal wall.

A Structure of the esophageal wall

Posterior view. Portions of the pharynx, larynx, and trachea are also shown; and the outermost layer (tunica adventitia, see **B**) has been removed. The esophageal wall has been telescoped to display both layers of the tunica muscularis (the strata circulare and longitudinale). They are connected to the mm. pharyngis at the esophageal inlet (hidden here by the pharynx). The muscles of the oesophagus can generate powerful peristaltic movements directed toward the gaster (actively propelling a food bolus to the stomach in 5–8 seconds), and they can reverse the direction of these movements during vomiting (antiperistalsis).

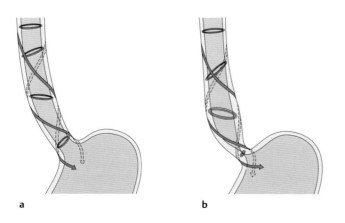

C Functional architecture of the esophageal muscles

During the act of swallowing, the esophageal outlet at the cardiac end of the gaster opens (**a**) and then immediately closes (**b**). The strata longitudinale and circulare of the tunica muscularis of the oesophagus (see **A**) contain numerous fibers that wind *obliquely* around the organ (see the circles in the figure). The musculature is additionally "twisted" due to the embryonic rotation of the gut (see p. 43). Owing to the presence of longitudinal, circular, and oblique fibers, the oesophagus can be narrowed and closed as needed (by the action of the circular fibers) at its inlet and outlet (see p. 167), but it can also be simultaneously narrowed and shortened by the combined action of the longitudinal, circular and oblique fibers to generate peristaltic motion toward the gaster during swallowing.

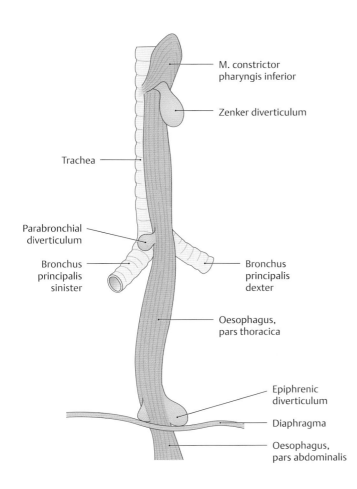

M. constrictor
pharyngis inferior

Zenker diverticulum

Trachea

Parabronchial
diverticulum

Bronchus
principalis
sinister

Bronchus
principalis
dexter

Oesophagus,
pars thoracica

Epiphrenic
diverticulum

Diaphragma

Oesophagus,
pars abdominalis

D Development of esophageal diverticula

Esophageal *diverticula* (abnormal outpouchings or sacs) most commonly develop at a weak spot like that located above the hiatus oesophageus of the diaphragma (parahiatal or epiphrenic diverticulum, 10% of cases). These are "false" *pulsion diverticula* in which the tunica mucosa and tela submucosa herniate through weak spots in the tunica muscularis due to a rise of pressure in the oesophagus (e.g., during normal swallowing). A Zenker diverticulum, often described as the most common esophageal diverticulum (70% of cases), is actually a *hypopharyngeal* diverticulum occurring at the junction of the pharynx and oesophagus (the "Killian triangle"). This wall protrusion is also called a pharyngoesophageal diverticulum. The remaining 20% of esophageal diverticula do not occur at typical weak spots and are characterized by the protrusion of all wall layers ("true" diverticula, *traction diverticula*). They usually result from an inflammatory process such as lymphangitis, in which case they occur at the site where the oesophagus closely approaches the bronchi and nll. tracheobronchiales (thoracic or parabronchial diverticulum).

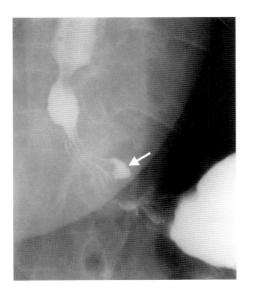

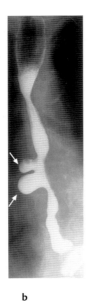

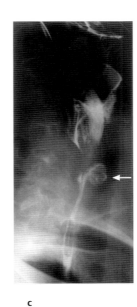

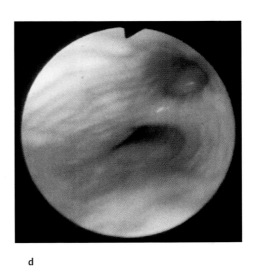

a b c d

E Barium swallow (a-c) and endoscopy (d) used to diagnose diverticula (from: Reiser, M et al.: Radiologie [Duale Reihe], 2 Aufl./ Radiology, 2nd edition. Thieme, Stuttgart 2006)

a Epiphrenic diverticulum with small pooling of contrast medium (arrow) directly above the diaphragma;

b Traction diverticulum (double-contrast view, arrows) at the level of the bifurcatio tracheae;

c Zenker diverticulum directly below the cartilago cricoidea, pooling of contrast material detected (arrow);

d Endoscopic view, the esophageal diverticulum is recognizable through an additional orifice in the esophageal wall.

5.4 Arteries and Veins of the Oesophagus

A Blood vessels of the oesophagus

a Arteries, **b** veins.

Posterior wall of the thorax and upper abdomen, viewed from the anterior aspect. All of the thoracic organs have been removed except for the oesophagus and part of the trachea. The proximal portion of the gaster has been left in the abdomen.

Note: The oesophagus is supplied by three groups of arteries, consistent with its division into three parts (see p. 164), and it is likewise drained by three venous groups (see **B**).

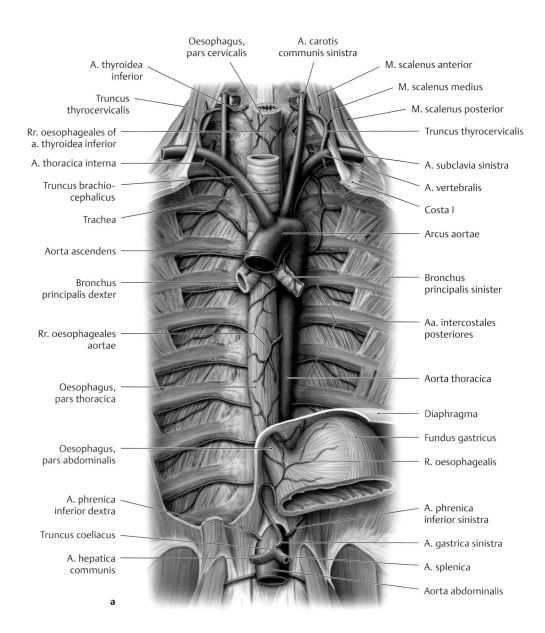

Oesophagus, pars cervicalis · A. carotis communis sinistra · A. thyroidea inferior · M. scalenus anterior · M. scalenus medius · Truncus thyrocervicalis · M. scalenus posterior · Rr. oesophageales of a. thyroidea inferior · Truncus thyrocervicalis · A. thoracica interna · A. subclavia sinistra · Truncus brachiocephalicus · A. vertebralis · Costa I · Trachea · Aorta ascendens · Arcus aortae · Bronchus principalis dexter · Bronchus principalis sinister · Rr. oesophageales aortae · Aa. intercostales posteriores · Oesophagus, pars thoracica · Aorta thoracica · Diaphragma · Fundus gastricus · Oesophagus, pars abdominalis · R. oesophagealis · A. phrenica inferior dextra · A. phrenica inferior sinistra · Truncus coeliacus · A. gastrica sinistra · A. hepatica communis · A. splenica · Aorta abdominalis

a

B Arterial supply and venous drainage of the oesophagus

Part of oesophagus	Arterial supply	Venous drainage (see Ab)

• Pars cervicalis	• Rr. oesophageales
	  – Usually from the a. thyroidea inferior or
	  – Direct branches (rare, not shown here) from the truncus thyrocervicalis or a. carotis communis
		• Esophageal veins
		  – Drain to v. thyroidea inferior or
		  – Left v. brachiocephalica

• Pars thoracica	• Rr. oesophageales from the aorta thoracica, distributed to the anterior and posterior sides of the oesophagus	• Vv. oesophageales
		  – Drain at upper left into the v. hemiazygos accessoria or left v. brachiocephalica
		  – Drain at lower left into the v. hemiazygos
		  – Drain into the v. azygos on the right side

• Pars abdominalis (smallest arteries and veins serving the oesophagus)	• R. oesophagealis of the a. gastrica sinistra	• Vv. oesophageales draining into the v. gastrica sinistra

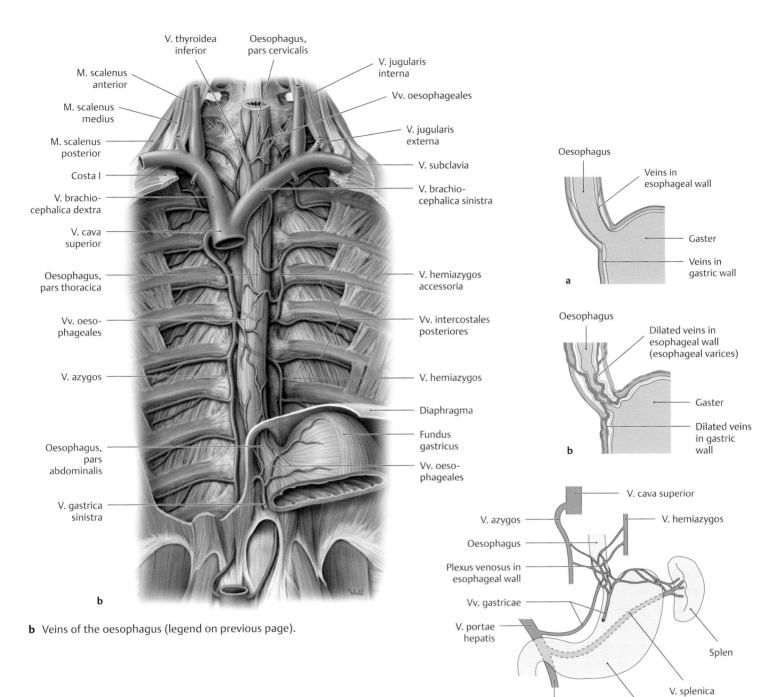

b Veins of the oesophagus (legend on previous page).

C Submucous venous plexuses and venous collaterals

a, b Submucous venous plexuses and varices in the oesophagus
(after Stelzner): The smallest tributaries of the vv. oesophageales
pass through all layers of the esophageal wall, accompanied by arterial branches, to the lamina propria of the tunica mucosa. In the adjacent, thicker tela submucosa they form an extensive plexus that
contributes to functional closure of the oesophagus at the junction of
its partes thoracica and abdominalis (see p. 167). This venous plexus
is continuous with an analogous plexus at the gastric inlet. With any
obstruction of portal venous flow to the hepar (as in cirrhosis associated with chronic alcoholism), these anastomoses provide a collateral pathway by which the venous blood flow may be diverted into
the submucous venous plexuses of the oesophagus, causing them to
undergo varicose dilation (esophageal varices, see **b**). There may be
associated abnormal dilation of the gastric veins.

c Esophageal venous collaterals (after Strohmeyer and Dölle):
Venous anastomoses provide two routes for draining the veins at the
junction of the partes thoracica and abdominalis of the oesophagus:

1. Via the vv. azygos or hemiazygos to the v. cava superior (thoracic
   route)
2. Via the v. gastrica sinistra to the v. portae hepatis (abdominal
   route)

Thus, when portal venous flow becomes obstructed in the hepar (cirrhosis), blood may be diverted through the vv. oesophageales to the
v. cava superior (portosystemic collaterals, see p. 219)

5.5 Lymphatic Drainage of the Oesophagus

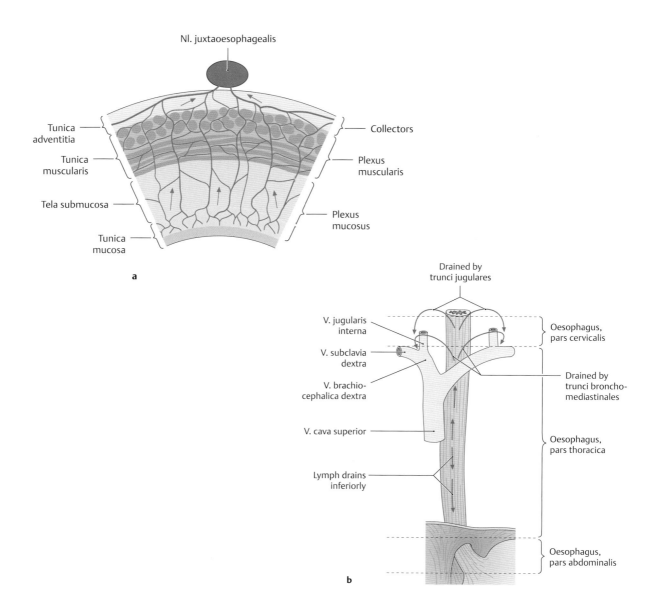

A Lymphatic drainage of the oesophagus

a Lymphatic drainage of the esophageal wall, **b** lymphatic drainage at different levels of the oesophagus.

Lymph from the oesophagus flows from inside to outside through the various wall layers (**a**), draining initially to the nodi lymphoidei that are distributed along the esophageal wall (nodi juxtaoesophageales, see **B**). There are three principal directions of lymphatic drainage, which correspond roughly to the three divisions of the oesophagus (**b**):

- The *pars cervicalis* of the oesophagus drains cranially, mainly to the nll. profundi cervicales laterales and then to the truncus jugularis.
- The *pars thoracica* of the oesophagus drains in two principal directions:
  - Cranially to the trunci bronchomediastinales (upper half).
  - Inferiorly (partly via the nll. phrenici *superiores*) to the trunci bronchomediastinales (lower half). Fine vasa lymphatica may convey

a small amount of lymph through the hiatus oesophageus into the upper abdomen to the pars abdominalis of the oesophagus (lymph may drain to the nll. phrenici *inferiores* as well as the nll. coeliaci). The "watershed" area for these two flow directions lies at the approximate midpoint of the pars thoracica oesophagi, whose upper part may also drain to nodi paratracheales.

- The *pars abdominalis* of the oesophagus, like the gaster, drains to the nll. coeliaci (not shown here). Thus, when the flow direction in these lowest esophageal nodi lymphoidei is reversed (a simple change of body posture or intracavitary pressure change due to breathing or bearing down can alter the direction of lymph flow), lymph from the gaster (which may bear malignant cells from gastric carcinoma) can reflux across the diaphragma and enter the nll. thoracis.

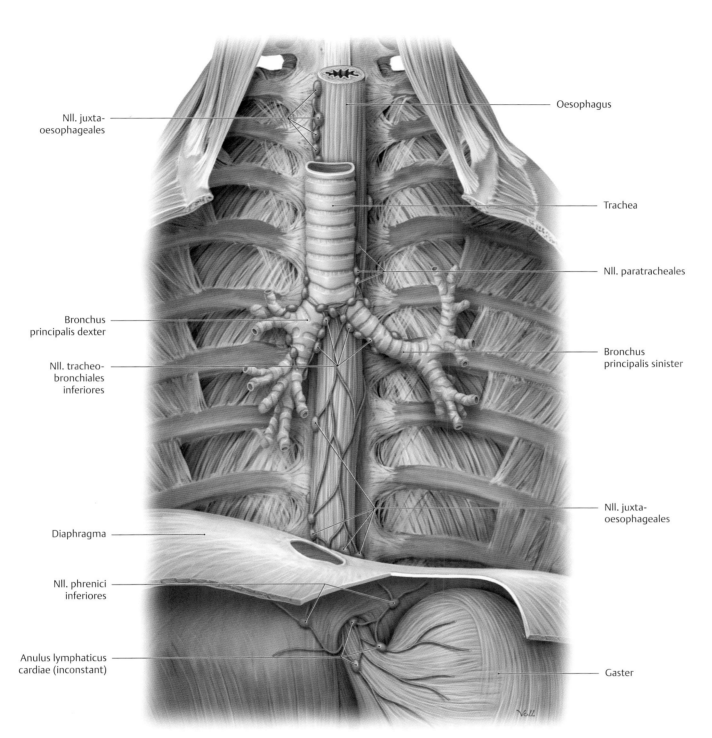

Nll. juxta-
oesophageales

Oesophagus

Trachea

Nll. paratracheales

Bronchus
principalis dexter

Nll. tracheo-
bronchiales
inferiores

Bronchus
principalis sinister

Nll. juxta-
oesophageales

Diaphragma

Nll. phrenici
inferiores

Anulus lymphaticus
cardiae (inconstant)

Gaster

B Nodi lymphoidei of the oesophagus

Anterior view of the opened thorax. All thoracic organs, with the exception of a portion of the trachea, the bronchi principales, and the oesophagus have been removed. Part of the abdomen is shown, and the gaster has been retracted slightly downward. A portion of the diaphragma has been excised to display the hiatus oesophageus. The oesophagus is covered by a network of fine vasa lymphatica that carry lymph to the nll. juxtaoesophageales. Lymph from the nll. juxtaoesophageales drains to collecting nodes or directly into the truncus jugularis or the right and left trunci bronchomediastinales (see **A**). Esophageal lymphatics near the bifurcatio tracheae also communicate with the nodi tracheobronchiales (inferiores). Vasa lymphatica descend with the oesophagus through the hiatus oesophageus, and they may connect at the abdominal level with the inconstant anulus lymphaticus cardiae that surrounds the ostium cardiacum of the gaster (drains to the nodi coeliaci). The esophageal nodi lymphoidei at this level may also connect with the nodi lymphatici on the inferior surface of the diaphragma (nodi phrenici *inferiores*).

Note: The nll. juxtaoesophageales are classified as a subgroup of the mediastinal nodi lymphoidei (see also p. 91).

5.6 Innervation of the Oesophagus

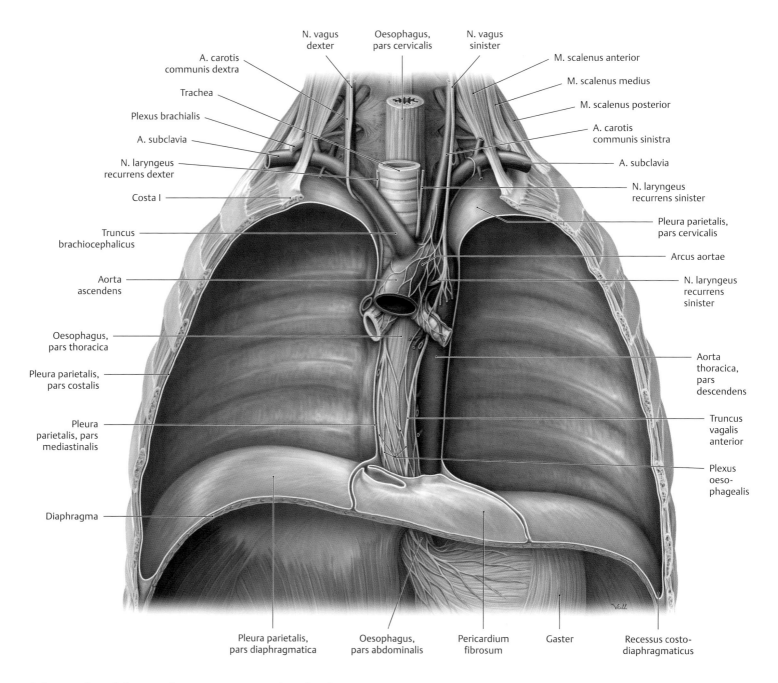

A Innervation of the oesophagus. Overview

Anterior view with the thorax opened. All organs except for the trachea and oesophagus have been removed. The left and right nn. vagi give off branches to the oesophagus. These branches form the plexus oesophageus. The plexus, located on the anterior and posterior esophageal walls, further descends and enters the abdomen as the trunci vagales anterior and posterior. The plexus oesophageus also receives fibers from the sympathetic chain.

B Effects of the partes sympathica and parasympathica of the nervous system on the oesophagus

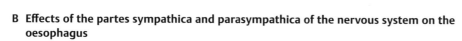

Pars sympathica	Pars parasympathica
• Decreases peristalsis	• Increases peristalsis
• Decreases gl. oesophagea secretions	• Increases gl. oesophagea secretions

C Referred pain from the oesophagus

Anterior view. As with other visceral structures, pain in the oesophagus may not be localized to the organ itself, but may instead seem to originate elsewhere. Esophageal pain may be referred to cutaneous areas over the sternum. The phenomenon is called "referred pain."

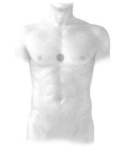

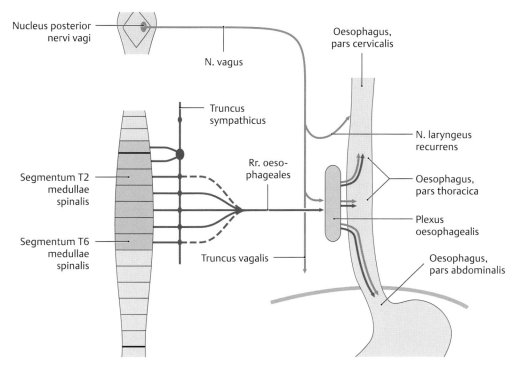

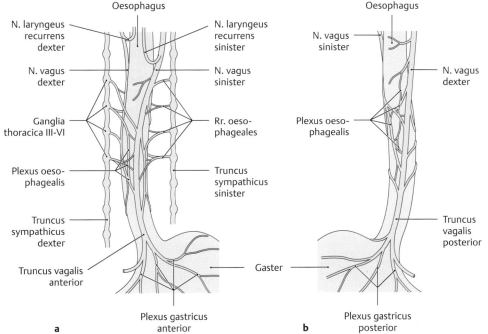

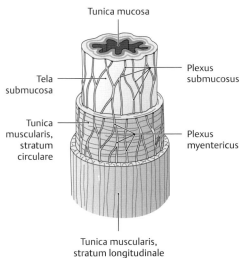

D Autonomic innervation of the oesophagus

Parasympathetic fibers arise from the nuclei posteriores nervorum vagorum and enter the nn. vagi. The n. vagus gives off parasympathetic motor fibers to the pars cervicalis of the oesophagus via the n. laryngeus recurrens. Other vagal axons form an extensive plexus oesophageus, which extends to abdominal levels of the oesophagus. These presynaptic fibers synapse on scattered parasympathetic ganglion cells (not depicted here) in the esophageal wall. The embedded ganglion cells in turn innervate esophageal smooth muscle and glands.

Note: The n. vagus also conveys direct motor innervation, without an intervening local synapse, from the nucleus ambiguus in the truncus encephali (not shown here) to striated muscle in the pars cervicalis oesophagi via the n. laryngeus recurrens.

Sympathetic fibers are contributed mostly by the second through sixth thoracic ganglia trunci sympathici. These postsynaptic axons enter the plexus oesophageus but directly innervate the oesophagus. The ganglion sympathicum cervicale medium contributes innervation to the pars cervicalis of the oesophagus. On the whole, sympathetic innervation is much less extensive than the parasympathetic supply to the oesophagus.

E Formation of the plexus oesophageus

The oesophagus and part of the gaster, viewed from the anterior side (**a**) and posterior side (**b**).

Initially the nn. vagi descend a short distance on the left and right sides of the oesophagus as the left and right nn. vagi, but then they turn anteriorly and posteriorly owing to the 90° clockwise rotation of the oesophagus (viewed from above) that occurs during embryonic development. The left n. vagus now becomes the truncus vagalis anterior, and the right n. vagus becomes the truncus vagalis posterior. Both trunks exchange a considerable number of fibers, however, so that the truncus vagalis anterior (actually a derivative of the left n. vagus) also contains fibers from the right n. vagus, and vice versa. Both nn. vagi and both trunci vagales distribute numerous fibers to the oesophagus, which form the anterior and posterior plexus oesophagei. The plexus oesophageus is continuous inferiorly with the plexus gastricus. The pars cervicalis of the oesophagus is supplied by the nn. laryngei recurrentes, which arise from the nn. vagi. The postganglionic sympathetic fibers enter the plexus oesophageus, which thus contains both parasympathetic and sympathetic fibers. On the whole, however, the parasympathetic innervation of the oesophagus is greater than its sympathetic innervation.

F Autonomic nerve plexuses in the esophageal wall

Oblique view of the oesophagus, dissected to show the different wall layers. Like all hollow organs in the gastrointestinal tract, the oesophagus has its own autonomous intramural nervous system. This system consists mainly of two plexuses, which are located in the tela submucosa (plexus submucosus) and in the tunica muscularis (plexus myentericus). These plexuses are composed of intramural ganglion cells that are interconnected by an extensive network and control the muscular functions of the oesophagus (e.g., peristalsis). The activity of this autonomous network is modulated by the partes sympathica and parasympathica of the nervous systems (see **B**).

5.7 Thymus

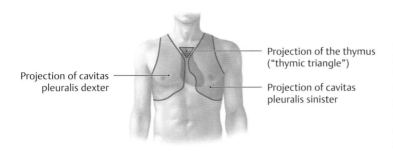

Projection of the thymus ("thymic triangle")

Projection of cavitas pleuralis dexter

Projection of cavitas pleuralis sinister

A Projection of the thymus onto the chest wall

For clarity, the cavitates pleurales have also been projected onto the chest wall. The thymus lies in the mediastinum superius and extends down into the mediastinum anterius, where it is anterior to the corand great vessels and posterior to the sternum. The area in which the thymus projects onto the chest wall is sometimes called the "thymic triangle." On the chest radiograph of a very small child, the large thymus may appear to broaden the silhouette of the cardiac base.

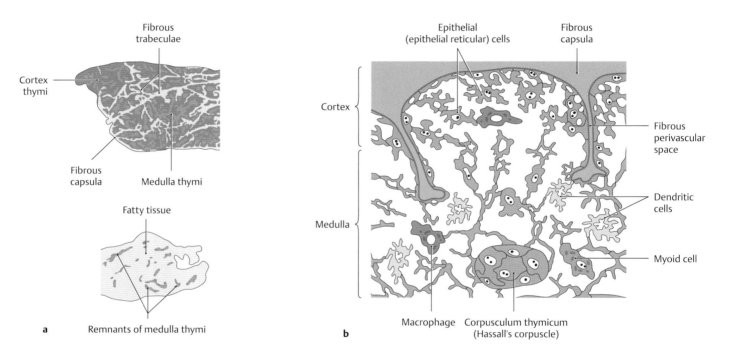

a   Remnants of medulla thymi

b   Macrophage   Corpusculum thymicum (Hassall's corpuscle)

B Histological structure of the thymus

a Structure of the thymus in adolescence (above) and old age (below). The thymus is a primary lymphatic (lymphoepithelial) organ that has a predominantly endodermal origin (saccus pharyngeus tertius) but also contains ectodermal elements. It plays a central role in the maturation of T (thymus) lymphocytes and their differentiation into immunologically competent cells. Additionally, immune-modulating hormones (thymosin, thymopoietin, thymulin) are produced in the thymus. Congenital absence of the thymus results in severe immunodeficiency. The thymus consists of a cortex and medulla. The cortex thymi appears much darker-staining due to the predominance of thymocytes (precursors to T-lymphocytes). The inner medulla thymi appears lighter-staining as a result of fewer thymocytes and an increase in the number of epithelial cells. Fine, vascularized trabeculae extend from the delicate fibrous capsule of the thymus into the parenchyma, subdividing the organ into numerous lobuli.

b Functional architecture (as described by Lüllmann Rauch). The thymus consists of a basic epithelial framework (lymphoepithelial organ). During embryonic development, the precursors of T-lymphocytes migrate into the thymus and mature (under the control of the epithelial cells) into immunocompetent T-lymphocytes. The

epithelial cells form a densely packed, subcapsular layer that creates a boundary between the interior of the thymus and the cortical capillaries in the fibrous trabeculae (the "blood-thymus barrier," not shown here). Epithelial (epithelial reticular) cells with long processes join together in the cortex and medulla thymi to form a three-dimensional network that encloses the thymocytes. (Thymocytes are not shown here in order to display other cell types clearly.) Epithelial cells in the medulla aggregate to form the corpuscula thymica (Hassall's corpuscles). The innermost cells in large corpuscula thymica often degenerate into a homogeneous mass. The function of the corpuscula thymica is not yet fully understood. The thymus contains several other cell types as well:

• Macrophages (phagocytosis of thymocytes)
• Dendritic cells (antigen presentation)
• Myoid cells (function unclear)

Maturation of the thymocytes occurs during their migration from the cortex to the medulla. A mature T-lymphocyte can recognize foreign antigens and differentiate them from endogenous cells ("autotolerance").

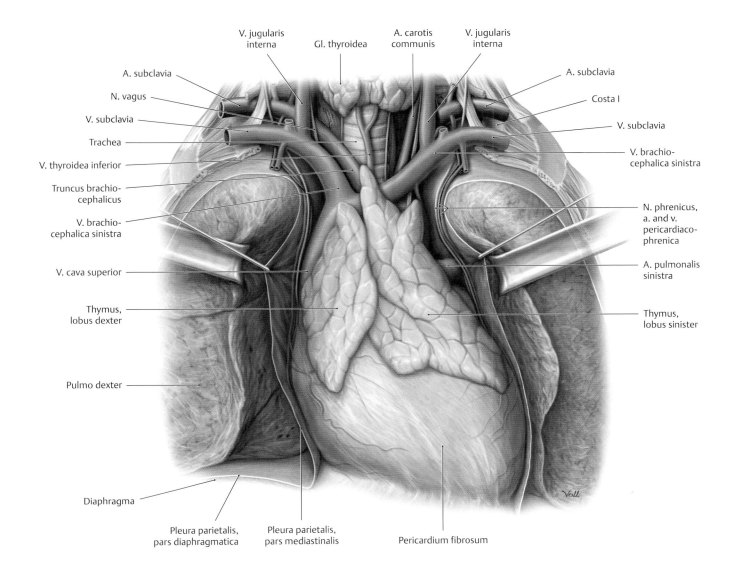

V. jugularis interna

Gl. thyroidea

A. carotis communis

V. jugularis interna

A. subclavia

N. vagus

V. subclavia

Trachea

V. thyroidea inferior

Truncus brachio-cephalicus

V. brachio-cephalica sinistra

V. cava superior

Thymus, lobus dexter

Pulmo dexter

Diaphragma

A. subclavia

Costa I

V. subclavia

V. brachio-cephalica sinistra

N. phrenicus, a. and v. pericardiaco-phrenica

A. pulmonalis sinistra

Thymus, lobus sinister

Pleura parietalis, pars diaphragmatica

Pleura parietalis, pars mediastinalis

Pericardium fibrosum

C Size and shape of the thymus

Anterior view into the mediastinum superius of a 2-year-old child. The thymus is still well developed at this age, consisting of two prominent lobi (right and left) that are subdivided by fibrous septa into numerous lobuli. Usually the thymus is apposed to the anterior surface of the pericardium and lies anterior to the v. cava superior, vv. brachiocephalicae, and aorta. In a small child, the thymus may extend up into the neck almost to the level of the gl. thyroidea, lying posterior to the lamina pretrachealis of the fascia cervicalis. When the thymus reaches its greatest size during puberty, it has a maximum weight of 20–50 g.

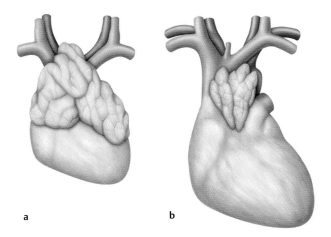

a   b

D Size of the thymus in newborns (a) and in adults (b)

In adults, the thymus is smaller than in newborns and lies in the mediastinum superius. In newborns, the thymus extends down into the mediastinum inferius.

6.1 Surface Anatomy, Topographical Regions, and Palpable Bony Landmarks

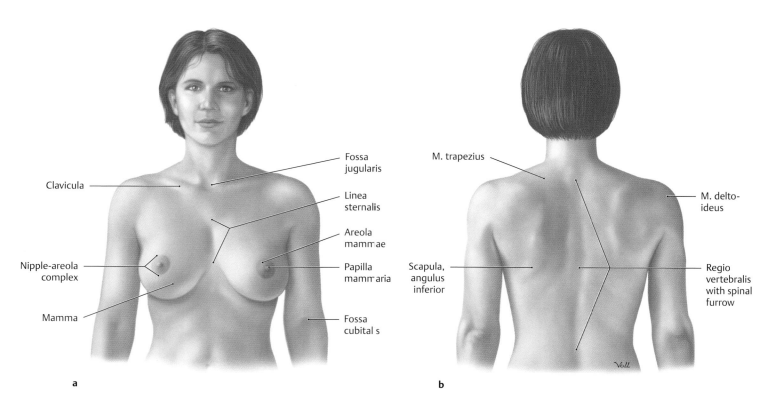

a

b

A Surface of the female thorax
a Anterior view; **b** Posterior view.

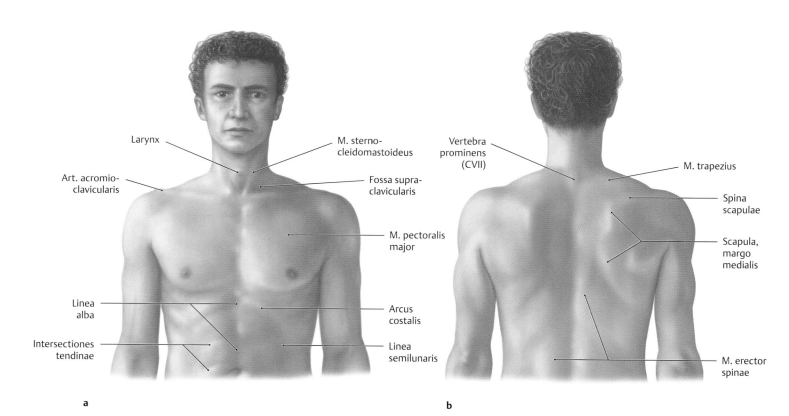

a

b

B Surface of the male thorax
a Anterior view; **b** Posterior view.

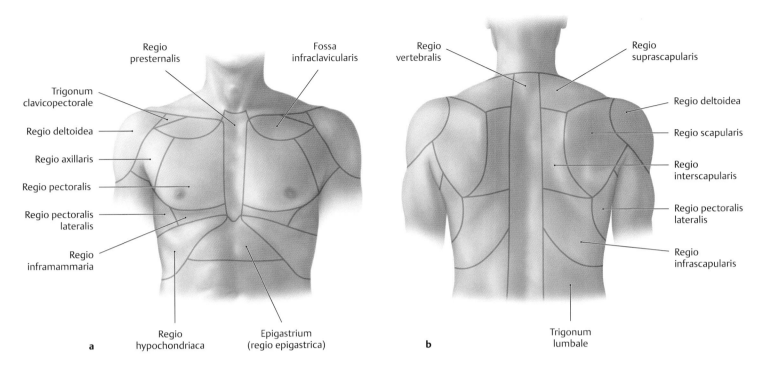

C Topographical anatomy of the male thorax
a Anterior view; **b** Posterior view.

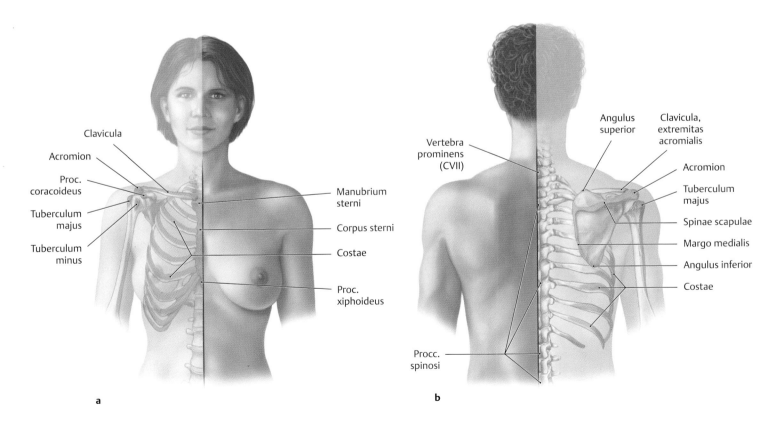

D Surface anatomy and palpable bony landmarks in the thoracic region
a Anterior view; **b** Posterior view.

6.2 Anatomical Landmarks of the Skeleton Thoracis (Projection of Organs)

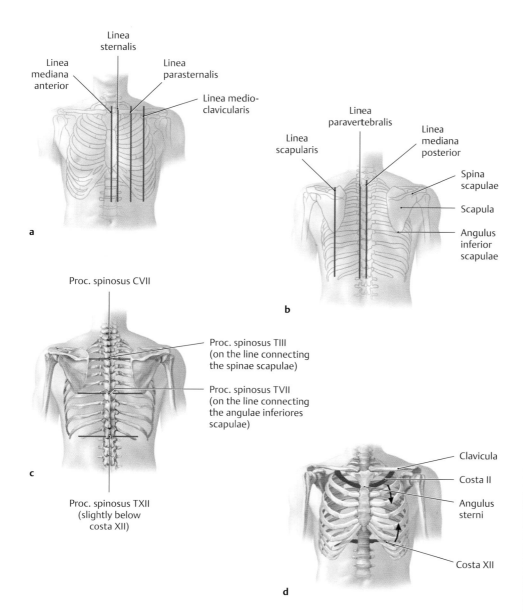

B Projection of anatomical structures onto the vertebrae thoracicae

T I	Margo superior of the scapula
T II/III	Incisura jugularis of the sternum
T III	• Medial border of the spina scapulae • Posterior end of the pulmonary fissura obliqua
T III/IV	• Bifurcatio tracheae • Root of the arcus aortae
T III–IV	Manubrium sterni
T IV	End of the arcus aortae
T IV/V	Angulus sterni
T V	Ductus thoracicus crosses the midline
T V–VIII	Sternum
T VII	• Angulus inferior scapulae • V. hemiazygos accessoria crosses the midline to the right and opens into the v. azygos

T VIII	• Foramen venae cavae of the diaphragma
	  – V. cava inferior
	  – Right n. phrenicus
	• Left n. phrenicus pierces the diaphragma to the left of the centrum tendineum
	• V. hemiazygos crosses the midline to the right and opens into the v. azygos

T VIII/IX	• Symphysis xiphosternalis • Aa. and vv. epigastricae superiores pass through the diaphragma • Processus xiphoideus
T VIII–X	Superior border of the hepar (moves with respiration)

T X	• Hiatus oesophageus of the diaphragma:
	  – Oesophagus
	  – Truncus vagalis anterior
	  – Truncus vagalis posterior

T XII	• Hiatus aorticus of the diaphragma:
	  – Aorta
	  – Vv. azygos and hemiazygos
	  – Ductus thoracicus
	• Origin of the truncus coeliacus (inferior border of T XII)
	• Nn. splanchnici pass through the crura of the diaphragma
	• Truncus sympathicus passes below the lig. arcuatum mediale: planum transpyloricum (line in abdomen, see p. 228)

A Anatomical landmarks of the skeleton thoracis

The skeleton thoracis presents a number of visible and palpable landmarks that are accessible to physical and radiographic examination (see **B**). These landmarks can be used to define reference lines for describing and evaluating the location and extent of organs based on their relationship to the lines:

- Longitudinal reference lines (**a, b**) are defined by visible or palpable anterior (**a**) and posterior (**b**) bony structures and provide information on the location and extent of specific thoracic organs (e.g., the topical heartbeat is palpable in the left mid-clavicular line).
- Most horizontal reference lines (**c**) are defined by the position of specific vertebrae thoracicae. The seventh vertebra cervicalis

(C VII) is easily identified by palpating its very prominent processus spinosus. It provides a starting point from which the examiner can locate all 12 vertebrae thoracicae (T I–T XII). The levels of the T III and T VII vertebrae correspond respectively to the medial end of the spina scapulae and the angulus inferior of the scapula.

- The ribs as anatomical landmarks (**d**). The levels of intrathoracic organs also correlate with specific ribs and spatia intercostalia, particularly on the anterior side. The costa prima is usually difficult to palpate because it is behind the clavicula. The costa secunda, however, is attached to the palpable angulus sterni (where the corpus and manubrium sterni join). Past the costa secunda, the examiner should have no difficulty counting down the remaining ribs.

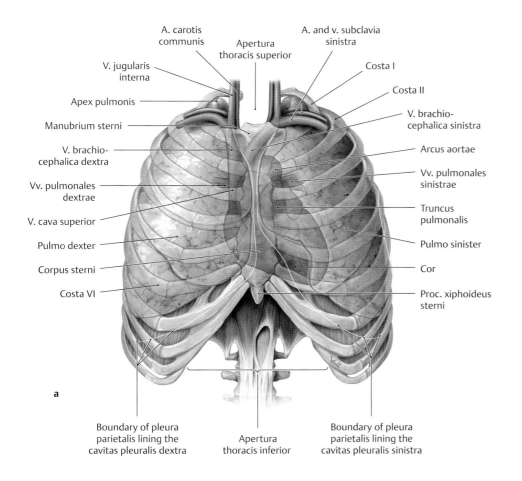

A. carotis communis
Apertura thoracis superior
A. and v. subclavia sinistra
V. jugularis interna
Costa I
Costa II
Apex pulmonis
Manubrium sterni
V. brachio-cephalica sinistra
V. brachio-cephalica dextra
Arcus aortae
Vv. pulmonales dextrae
Vv. pulmonales sinistrae
V. cava superior
Truncus pulmonalis
Pulmo dexter
Pulmo sinister
Corpus sterni
Cor
Costa VI
Proc. xiphoideus sterni

a

Boundary of pleura parietalis lining the cavitas pleuralis dextra
Apertura thoracis inferior
Boundary of pleura parietalis lining the cavitas pleuralis sinistra

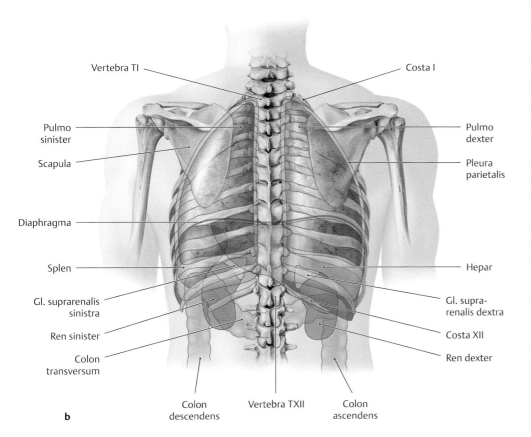

Vertebra TI
Costa I
Pulmo sinister
Pulmo dexter
Scapula
Pleura parietalis
Diaphragma
Splen
Hepar
Gl. suprarenalis sinistra
Gl. supra-renalis dextra
Ren sinister
Costa XII
Colon transversum
Ren dexter

b

Colon descendens
Vertebra TXII
Colon ascendens

C Overview of the thorax

a Anterior view. The mm. intercostales, fasciae, and abdominal organs have been removed. **b** Simplified schematic view from the posterior side. The scapulae and several abdominal organs have been outlined for clarity. The cavitas thoracis is one of the three main body cavities, along with the cavitates abdominis and pelvis. The wall surrounding the cavitas thoracis consists of

- bones: 12 vertebrae thoracicae, 12 pairs of costae, and the sternum
- connective tissue: internal fasciae of the thorax, muscle fasciae
- muscles: chiefly the mm. intercostales, internal muscles, and diaphragma

The cavitas thoracis is divided into the centrally located unpaired mediastinum, which contains the mediastinal organs, and the paired cavitates pleurales. The mediastinum contains the central motor of the circulatory system, the heart, and the thoracic part of the digestive system, the oesophagus. The cavitates pleurales enclose the major organs of respiration, the pulmones. Also, a number of neurovascular structures pass through or terminate within the thorax.

The bony cavea thoracis is open at its apex at the apertura thoracis superior (thoracic inlet), which is closely bounded and protected by muscles and connective tissue but communicates structures from the neck. The apertura thoracis inferior (thoracic outlet) is almost completely sealed from the cavitas abdominis by the diaphragma and its fasciae (shown most clearly in **a**).

Note: The diaphragma is normally in the shape of a high dome, with a substantial superior convexity that places part of the cavitas abdominis above the apertura thoracis inferior (see the abdominal organs shadowed in **b**). A perforating injury perpendicular to the trunk wall, as from a gunshot or stab wound, may thus simultaneously breach both the cavitates abdominis and thoracis ("multicavity injury").

6.3 Structure of the Anterior Thoracic Wall and its Neurovascular Structures

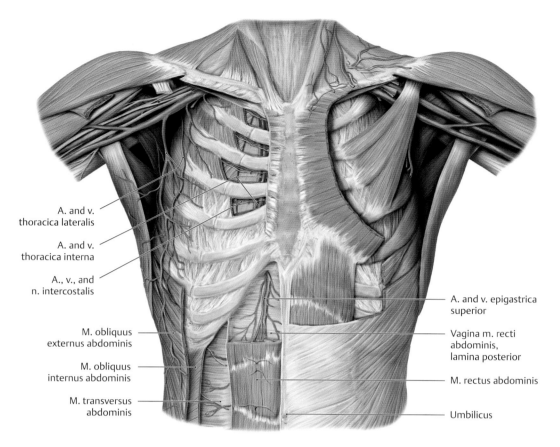

A. and v. thoracica lateralis

A. and v. thoracica interna

A., v., and n. intercostalis

M. obliquus externus abdominis

M. obliquus internus abdominis

M. transversus abdominis

A. and v. epigastrica superior

Vagina m. recti abdominis, lamina posterior

M. rectus abdominis

Umbilicus

A Neurovascular structures of the anterior trunk wall
Anterior view. On the right side of the trunk, the mm. pectorales major and minor have been completely removed and the mm. obliqui externus and internus abdominis have been partially removed to display both epifascial (subcutaneous) and deep (subfascial) neurovascular structures. For the depiction of the a. and vv. epigastricae superiores the superior part of the right m. rectus abdominis has been removed or rendered transparent. In order to illustrate the course of the aa. and vv. intercostales, the spatia intercostalia have been exposed.

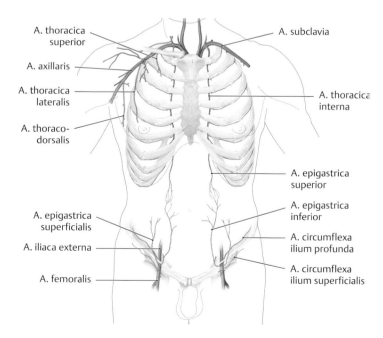

A. thoracica superior

A. subclavia

A. axillaris

A. thoracica lateralis

A. thoracico-dorsalis

A. thoracica interna

A. epigastrica superior

A. epigastrica inferior

A. epigastrica superficialis

A. iliaca externa

A. circumflexa ilium profunda

A. circumflexa ilium superficialis

A. femoralis

B The arterial supply of the anterior trunk wall
Anterior view. The anterior trunk wall receives its blood supply from two main sources: the a. thoracica interna, which arises from the a. subclavia, and the a. epigastrica inferior, which arises from the a. iliaca externa. It is also supplied by smaller vessels arising from the a. axillaris (a. thoracica superior, a. thoracodorsalis, and a. thoracica lateralis) and from the a. femoralis (a. epigastrica superficialis and a. circumflexa ilium superficialis).

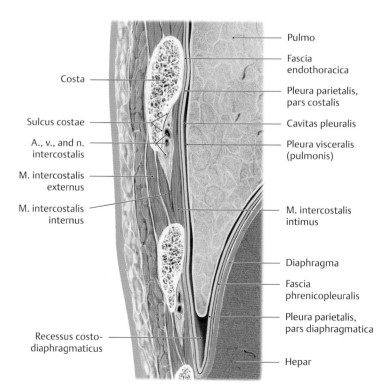

Costa

Sulcus costae

A., v., and n. intercostalis

M. intercostalis externus

M. intercostalis internus

Pulmo

Fascia endothoracica

Pleura parietalis, pars costalis

Cavitas pleuralis

Pleura visceralis (pulmonis)

M. intercostalis intimus

Diaphragma

Fascia phrenicopleuralis

Pleura parietalis, pars diaphragmatica

Recessus costo-diaphragmaticus

Hepar

C Structure of the lateral thoracic wall
Coronal section through the lateral thoracic wall and recessus costodiaphragmaticus.

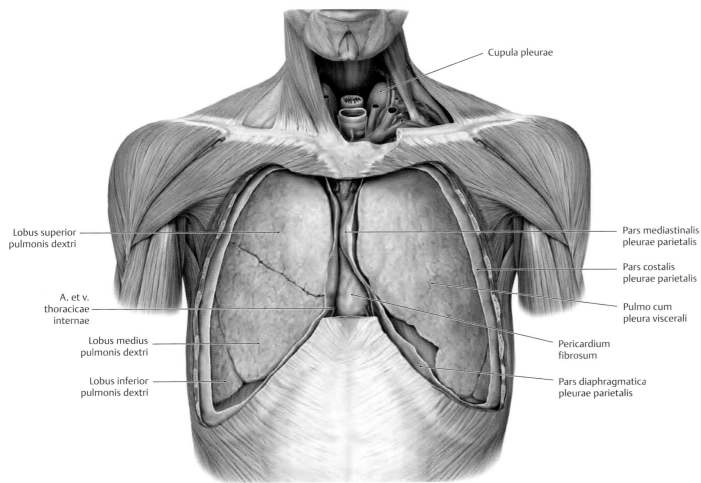

Cupula pleurae

Lobus superior pulmonis dextri

A. et v. thoracicae internae

Lobus medius pulmonis dextri

Lobus inferior pulmonis dextri

Pars mediastinalis pleurae parietalis

Pars costalis pleurae parietalis

Pulmo cum pleura viscerali

Pericardium fibrosum

Pars diaphragmatica pleurae parietalis

D Thorax, cavitates pleurales have been opened
Anterior view.

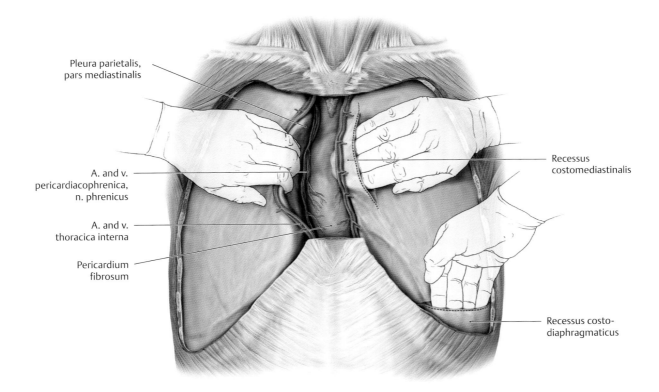

Pleura parietalis, pars mediastinalis

A. and v. pericardiacophrenica, n. phrenicus

A. and v. thoracica interna

Pericardium fibrosum

Recessus costomediastinalis

Recessus costo-diaphragmaticus

E Recessus costomediastinalis and costodiaphragmaticus
On the left side, the pleura parietalis has been slit open parasternally and above the 9th rib so that the recessus costomediastinalis and costodiaphragmaticus can be located with the fingertips. On the right side, the pulmo together with its pars mediastinalis pleurae has been carefully loosened from the pericardium in order to display the a. and v. pericardiacophrenica and n. phrenicus.

183

6.4 Thoracic Organs in situ: Anterior, Lateral, and Inferior Views

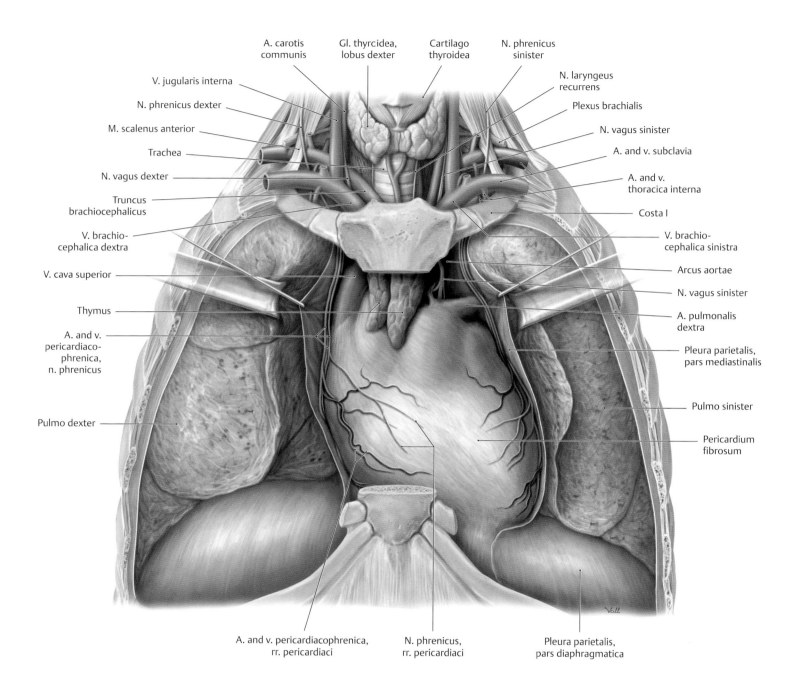

A. carotis communis — Gl. thyrcidea, lobus dexter — Cartilago thyroidea — N. phrenicus sinister

V. jugularis interna — N. laryngeus recurrens

N. phrenicus dexter — Plexus brachialis

M. scalenus anterior — N. vagus sinister

Trachea — A. and v. subclavia

N. vagus dexter — A. and v. thoracica interna

Truncus brachiocephalicus — Costa I

V. brachio-cephalica dextra — V. brachio-cephalica sinistra

V. cava superior — Arcus aortae

Thymus — N. vagus sinister

A. and v. pericardiaco-phrenica, n. phrenicus — A. pulmonalis dextra

Pleura parietalis, pars mediastinalis

Pulmo sinister

Pulmo dexter — Pericardium fibrosum

A. and v. pericardiacophrenica, rr. pericardiaci — N. phrenicus, rr. pericardiaci — Pleura parietalis, pars diaphragmatica

A Mediastinum, anterior view with the anterior thoracic wall removed

Coronal section through the thorax. All connective tissue has been removed from the mediastinum anterius. This dissection displays a prominent thymus, occupying the mediastinum superius and extending inferiorly into the mediastinum anterius. Visible structures that are continued from the mediastinum superius into the neck or upper limb include branches of the arcus aortae, the v. cava superior, and the trachea, although the latter is mostly obscured by the vessels surrounding the heart. The mediastinum medium, visible in this coronal section, is dominated by the heart and pericardium (fused to the diaphragma) and the associated neurovascular structures—the n. phrenicus and a. and v. pericardiacophrenica. These vessels descend along the pericardium toward the diaphragma while giving off rr. pericardiaci.

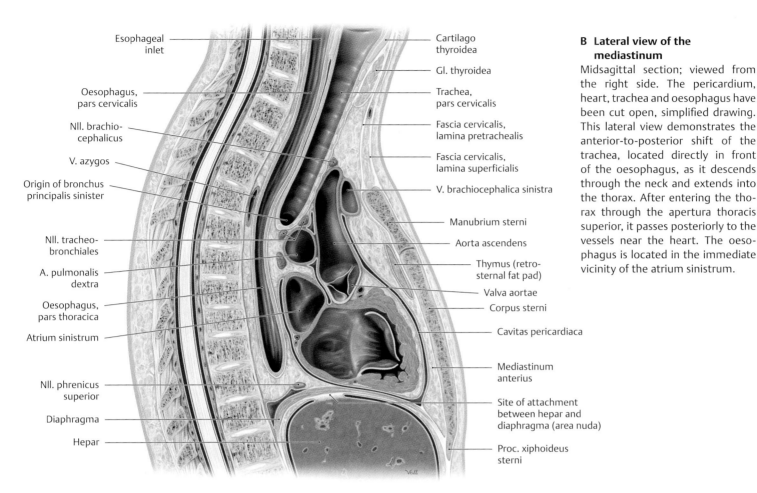

Esophageal inlet

Oesophagus, pars cervicalis

Nll. brachio-cephalicus

V. azygos

Origin of bronchus principalis sinister

Nll. tracheo-bronchiales

A. pulmonalis dextra

Oesophagus, pars thoracica

Atrium sinistrum

Nll. phrenicus superior

Diaphragma

Hepar

Cartilago thyroidea

Gl. thyroidea

Trachea, pars cervicalis

Fascia cervicalis, lamina pretrachealis

Fascia cervicalis, lamina superficialis

V. brachiocephalica sinistra

Manubrium sterni

Aorta ascendens

Thymus (retro-sternal fat pad)

Valva aortae

Corpus sterni

Cavitas pericardiaca

Mediastinum anterius

Site of attachment between hepar and diaphragma (area nuda)

Proc. xiphoideus sterni

B Lateral view of the mediastinum

Midsagittal section; viewed from the right side. The pericardium, heart, trachea and oesophagus have been cut open, simplified drawing. This lateral view demonstrates the anterior-to-posterior shift of the trachea, located directly in front of the oesophagus, as it descends through the neck and extends into the thorax. After entering the thorax through the apertura thoracis superior, it passes posteriorly to the vessels near the heart. The oesophagus is located in the immediate vicinity of the atrium sinistrum.

A. and v. thoracica interna

Corpus sterni

Recessus costomediastinalis

Pulmo dexter, lobus superior

Fissura horizontalis

Atrium dextrum

Pulmo dexter, lobus medius

Atrium sinistrum

Fissura obliqua

Oesophagus

N. vagus sinister (truncus vagalis anterior)

V. azygos

Ventriculus dexter

Septum interventriculare

Ventriculus dexter

Pulmo sinister, lobus superior

N. phrenicus sinister

Fissura obliqua

Pericardium fibrosum et pars mediastinalis pleurae parietalis

Aorta thoracica

Pleura parietalis

Pleura parietalis

Pleura visceralis

Pulmo dexter, lobus inferior

Truncus sympathicus

V. hemiazygos

Pulmo sinister, lobus inferior

C Inferior view of the mediastinum

Transverse section at the level of the 8th vertebra thoracis.
This diagram clearly shows the asymmetrical position of the heart in the thorax (see also p. 97). From both sides, the recessus costomediastinales extend between the heart and sternum (see p. 183).

185

6.5 Thoracic Organs in situ: Posterior Views

A Posterior view of the mediastinum (after Platzer)
The vertebrae thoracicae have been removed, and parts of the posterior thoracic wall and left pleura parietalis have been removed, in order to display the pulmones.
Note the course of the ductus thoracicus between the aorta thoracica and oesophagus.

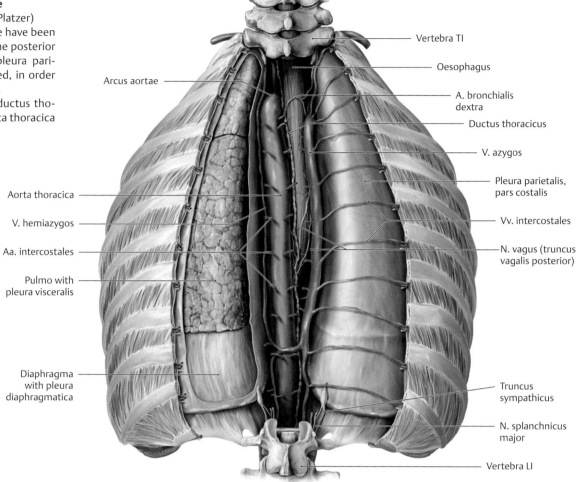

- Vertebra TI
- Oesophagus
- A. bronchialis dextra
- Ductus thoracicus
- V. azygos
- Pleura parietalis, pars costalis
- Vv. intercostales
- N. vagus (truncus vagalis posterior)
- Truncus sympathicus
- N. splanchnicus major
- Vertebra LI

- Arcus aortae
- Aorta thoracica
- V. hemiazygos
- Aa. intercostales
- Pulmo with pleura visceralis
- Diaphragma with pleura diaphragmatica

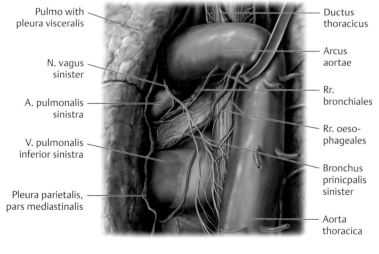

- Pulmo with pleura visceralis
- N. vagus sinister
- A. pulmonalis sinistra
- V. pulmonalis inferior sinistra
- Pleura parietalis, pars mediastinalis
- Ductus thoracicus
- Arcus aortae
- Rr. bronchiales
- Rr. oesophageales
- Bronchus prinicpalis sinister
- Aorta thoracica

a

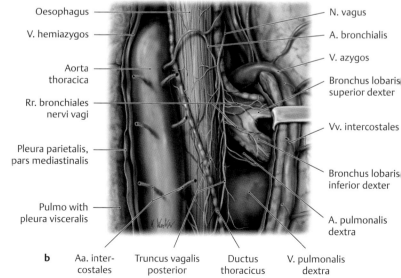

- Oesophagus
- V. hemiazygos
- Aorta thoracica
- Rr. bronchiales nervi vagi
- Pleura parietalis, pars mediastinalis
- Pulmo with pleura visceralis
- N. vagus
- A. bronchialis
- V. azygos
- Bronchus lobaris superior dexter
- Vv. intercostales
- Bronchus lobaris inferior dexter
- A. pulmonalis dextra

b   Aa. inter-   Truncus vagalis   Ductus   V. pulmonalis
costales   posterior   thoracicus   dextra

B Hilum of the pulmo sinister (a) and dexter (b), posterior view (after Platzer)
In order to show the hilum pulmonis sinistri, the aorta at the junction of the arcus aortae and aorta thoracica has been retracted laterally in (**a**). In (**b**), the v. azygos has been retracted laterally to display the hilum pulmonis dextri.

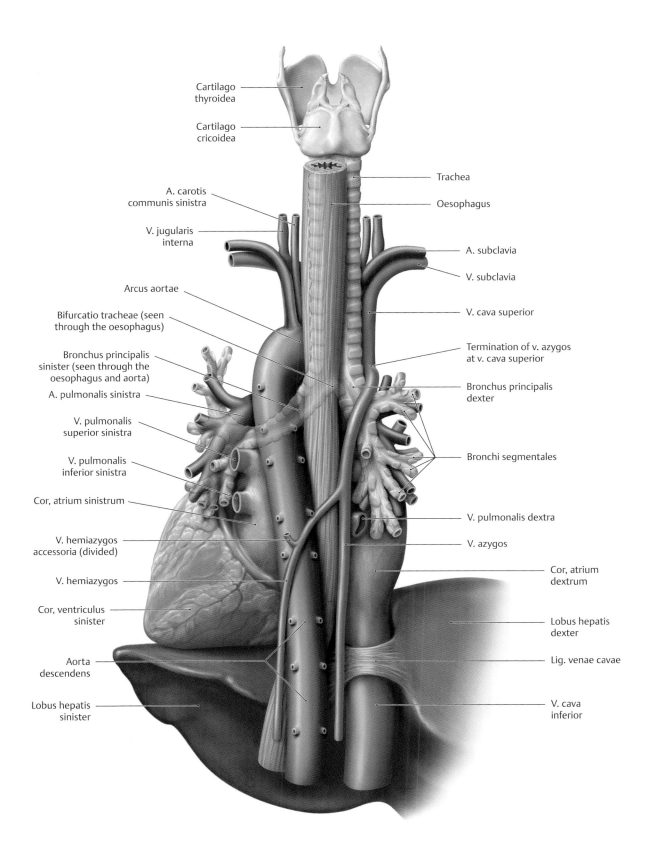

Cartilago thyroidea

Cartilago cricoidea

Trachea

Oesophagus

A. carotis communis sinistra

V. jugularis interna

A. subclavia

V. subclavia

Arcus aortae

V. cava superior

Bifurcatio tracheae (seen through the oesophagus)

Termination of v. azygos at v. cava superior

Bronchus principalis sinister (seen through the oesophagus and aorta)

Bronchus principalis dexter

A. pulmonalis sinistra

V. pulmonalis superior sinistra

Bronchi segmentales

V. pulmonalis inferior sinistra

Cor, atrium sinistrum

V. pulmonalis dextra

V. hemiazygos accessoria (divided)

V. azygos

V. hemiazygos

Cor, atrium dextrum

Cor, ventriculus sinister

Lobus hepatis dexter

Aorta descendens

Lig. venae cavae

Lobus hepatis sinister

V. cava inferior

C Contents of the mediastinum, posterior view
The structures in the mediastinum posterius are depicted in this view. Note particularly the course of the aorta descendens, the vv. azygos and hemiazygos, and the oesophagus, which is posterior to the trachea and partially obscures it. (An anterior view of the mediastinum posterius is shown on p. 192.) The topographical relations of the aorta change several times along its course. The proximal part of the aorta ascends in the mediastinum medium, which is a subdivision of the mediastinum inferius. At that level the aorta lies anterior to the trachea and oesophagus.

It then ascends into the mediastinum superius, where it curves posteriorly and to the left to form the arcus aortae. This curve lies to the left of the oesophagus and trachea, and it arches over the bronchus principalis sinister (the aorta "rides" upon that bronchus). In its further course the aorta turns back slightly medially and posteriorly and descends behind the oesophagus in the mediastinum posterius, where it is closely related to the vv. azygos and hemiazygos. Note also the very close proximity of the hepar to the right side of the heart.

6.6 Heart (Cor): Cavitas Pericardiaca

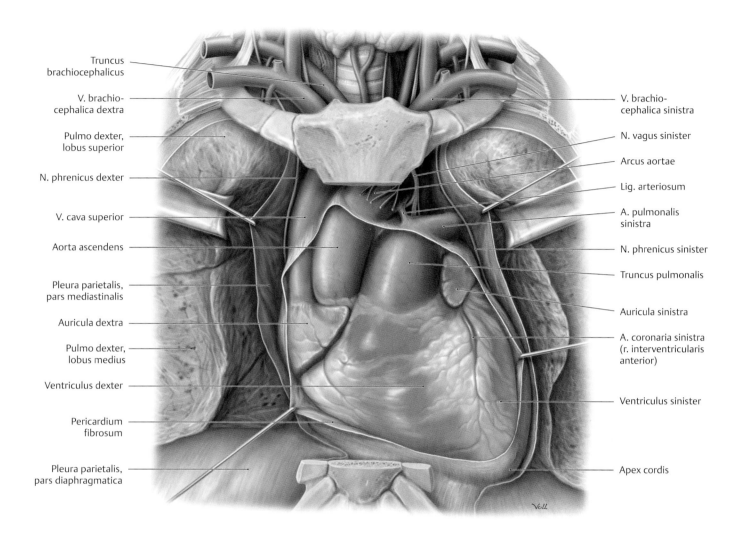

Truncus brachiocephalicus

V. brachio-cephalica dextra

Pulmo dexter, lobus superior

N. phrenicus dexter

V. cava superior

Aorta ascendens

Pleura parietalis, pars mediastinalis

Auricula dextra

Pulmo dexter, lobus medius

Ventriculus dexter

Pericardium fibrosum

Pleura parietalis, pars diaphragmatica

V. brachio-cephalica sinistra

N. vagus sinister

Arcus aortae

Lig. arteriosum

A. pulmonalis sinistra

N. phrenicus sinister

Truncus pulmonalis

Auricula sinistra

A. coronaria sinistra (r. interventricularis anterior)

Ventriculus sinister

Apex cordis

A **The cavitas pericardiaca has been opened to display the facies sternocostalis of the heart**

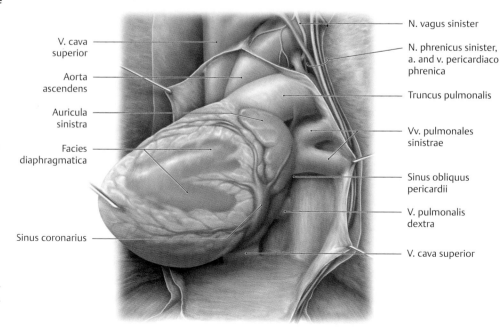

V. cava superior

Aorta ascendens

Auricula sinistra

Facies diaphragmatica

Sinus coronarius

N. vagus sinister

N. phrenicus sinister, a. and v. pericardiaco phrenica

Truncus pulmonalis

Vv. pulmonales sinistrae

Sinus obliquus pericardii

V. pulmonalis dextra

V. cava superior

B **Facies diaphragmatica of the heart (also known as posterior wall of the heart)**
After lifting the heart, the facies diaphragmatica of the heart and the sinus obliquus pericardii become visible.

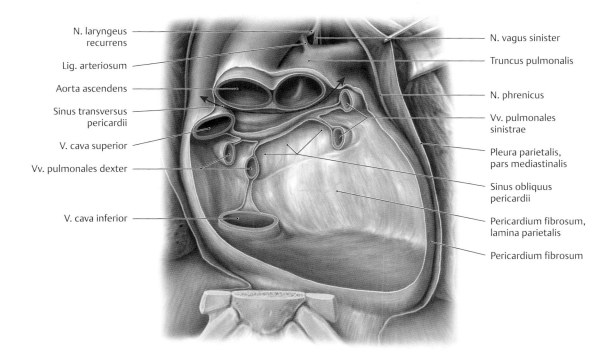

N. laryngeus recurrens

Lig. arteriosum

Aorta ascendens

Sinus transversus pericardii

V. cava superior

Vv. pulmonales dexter

V. cava inferior

N. vagus sinister

Truncus pulmonalis

N. phrenicus

Vv. pulmonales sinistrae

Pleura parietalis, pars mediastinalis

Sinus obliquus pericardii

Pericardium fibrosum, lamina parietalis

Pericardium fibrosum

C Cavitas pericardiaca after the heart has been removed
Note the location where the lamina parietalis is folded back onto the lamina visceralis, and the attachment between the pericardium and diaphragma.

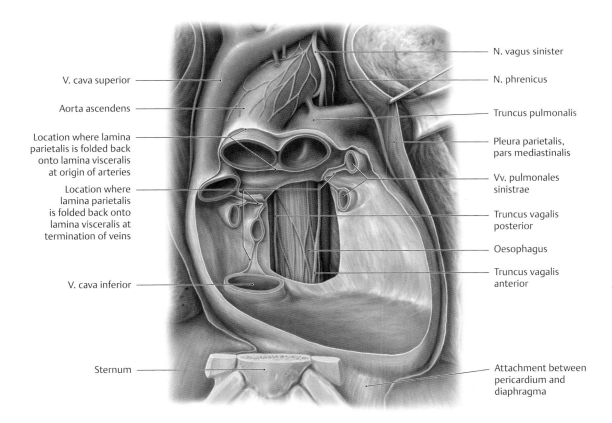

V. cava superior

Aorta ascendens

Location where lamina parietalis is folded back onto lamina visceralis at origin of arteries

Location where lamina parietalis is folded back onto lamina visceralis at termination of veins

V. cava inferior

Sternum

N. vagus sinister

N. phrenicus

Truncus pulmonalis

Pleura parietalis, pars mediastinalis

Vv. pulmonales sinistrae

Truncus vagalis posterior

Oesophagus

Truncus vagalis anterior

Attachment between pericardium and diaphragma

D Course of the oesophagus along the posterior aspect of the atrium sinistrum
After a window is cut in the pericardium in the area of the sinus obliquus pericardii, the oesophagus, which courses in the immediate vicinity, and the truncus vagalis anterior become visible.

6.7 Overview of the Mediastinum

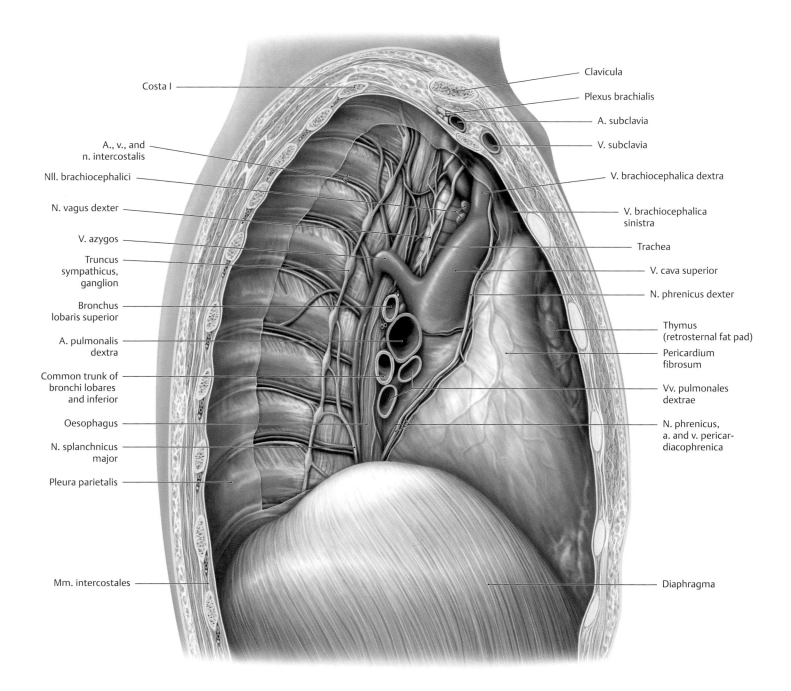

A Mediastinum viewed from the right side

Parasagittal section. The entire right lung and most of the wall of the pleural cavity have been removed (parietal pleura, see p. 192) to display the structures of the *posterior mediastinum* adjacent to the vertebrae, most notably the sympathetic trunk, and the azygos vein opening into the superior vena cava. In the *middle mediastinum*, the (right) phrenic nerve and the (right) pericardiacophrenic artery and vein are visible on the pericardium. The (right) vagus nerve is directly visible on the lateral wall of the esophagus. The trachea, which lies on the median plane, is partially obscured by other structures (n. vagus, v. azygos, nodi lymphoidei). The transected superior lobar bronchus and truncus communis bronchorum lobarium medii et inferioris are clearly visible. Coming from the mediastinum, these bronchi lie superior and inferior to the a. pulmonalis and extend into the right lung. The thymus, relatively prominent here, is large in early postnatal life (see p. 177), but regresses in adulthood, eventually replaced in old age by a small retrosternal fat pad (involuted thymus).

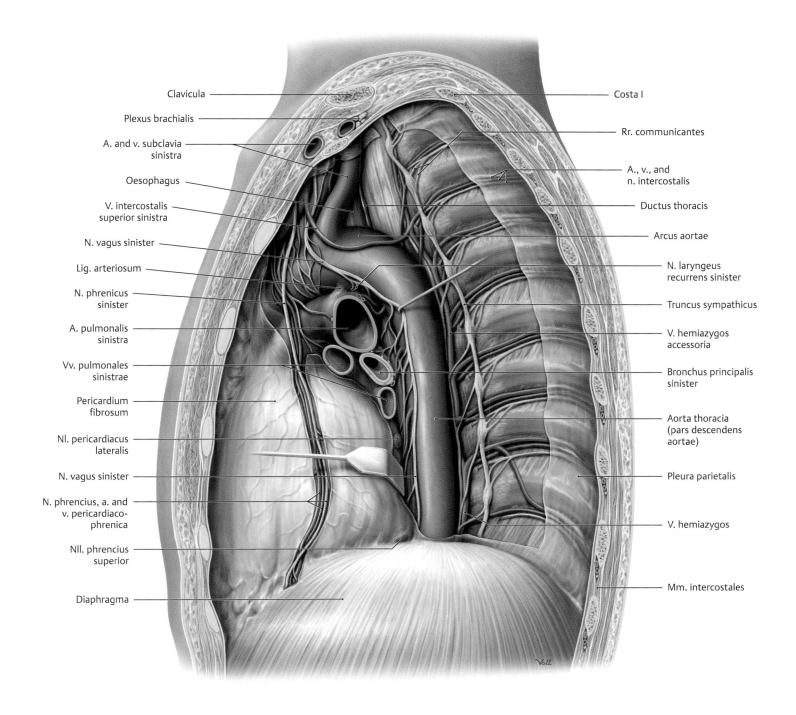

Clavicula

Plexus brachialis

A. and v. subclavia sinistra

Oesophagus

V. intercostalis superior sinistra

N. vagus sinister

Lig. arteriosum

N. phrenicus sinister

A. pulmonalis sinistra

Vv. pulmonales sinistrae

Pericardium fibrosum

Nl. pericardiacus lateralis

N. vagus sinister

N. phrencius, a. and v. pericardiaco-phrenica

Nll. phrencius superior

Diaphragma

Costa I

Rr. communicantes

A., v., and n. intercostalis

Ductus thoracis

Arcus aortae

N. laryngeus recurrens sinister

Truncus sympathicus

V. hemiazygos accessoria

Bronchus principalis sinister

Aorta thoracia (pars descendens aortae)

Pleura parietalis

V. hemiazygos

Mm. intercostales

B Mediastinum viewed from the left side
Parasagittal section. The entire left lung and most of the parietal pleura of the left pleural cavity have been removed, but the pericardium remains intact. The left-sided elements of paired mediastinal structures (sympathetic trunk, vagus nerve, phrenic nerve, pericardiacophrenic vessels) can be identified. Visible unpaired structures include the hemiazygos vein and the (inconstant) accessory hemiazygos vein. The dominant vessel in this field is the aorta, of which the aortic arch and descending aorta can be seen anterior and lateral to the esophagus. Both left pulmonary veins have been transected near their terminations in the left atrium of the heart, again demonstrating the close topographical relationship between the left atrium and esophagus. The trachea is almost entirely obscured in a left paramedian section. Only the transected bronchus principalis sinister is clearly visible between the vv. pulmonales dextrae.

6.8 Mediastinum Posterius

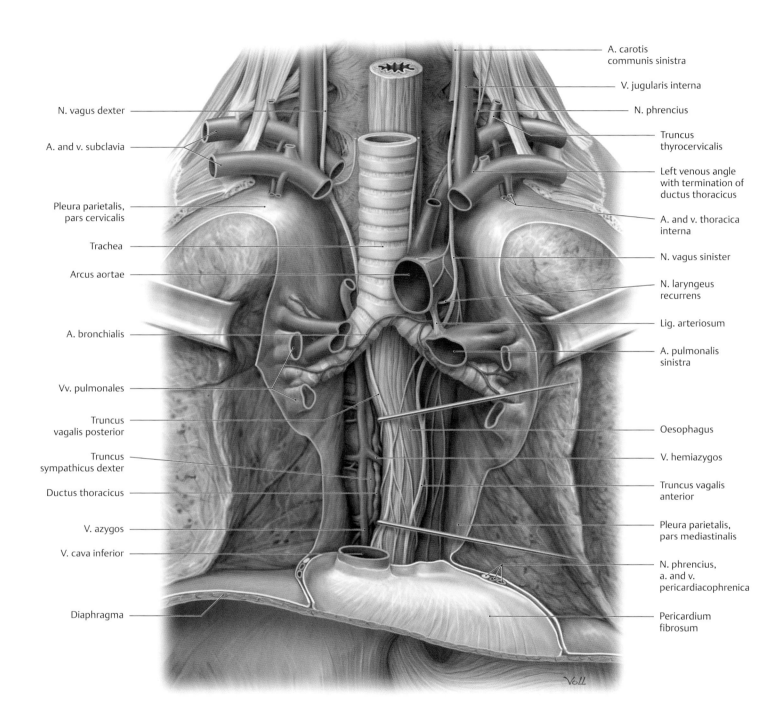

N. vagus dexter

A. and v. subclavia

Pleura parietalis,
pars cervicalis

Trachea

Arcus aortae

A. bronchialis

Vv. pulmonales

Truncus
vagalis posterior

Truncus
sympathicus dexter

Ductus thoracicus

V. azygos

V. cava inferior

Diaphragma

A. carotis
communis sinistra

V. jugularis interna

N. phrencius

Truncus
thyrocervicalis

Left venous angle
with termination of
ductus thoracicus

A. and v. thoracica
interna

N. vagus sinister

N. laryngeus
recurrens

Lig. arteriosum

A. pulmonalis
sinistra

Oesophagus

V. hemiazygos

Truncus vagalis
anterior

Pleura parietalis,
pars mediastinalis

N. phrencius,
a. and v.
pericardiacophrenica

Pericardium
fibrosum

A Mediastinum posterius, anterior view
The heart has been removed, and the oesophagus has been slightly
retracted laterally. The major structures of the mediastinum posterius are visible: oesophagus, nn. vagi, pars thoracica aortae, aa. and
vv. intercostales, vv. azygos, and hemiazygos and truncus sympathicus.

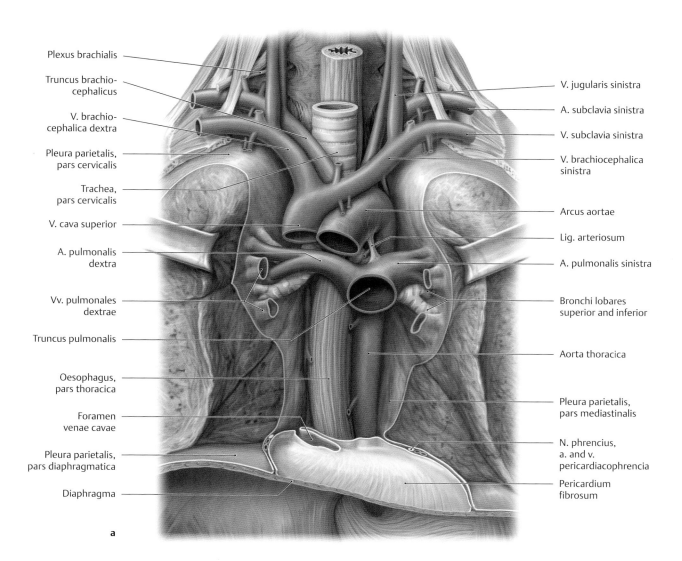

Plexus brachialis

Truncus brachio-
cephalicus

V. brachio-
cephalica dextra

Pleura parietalis,
pars cervicalis

Trachea,
pars cervicalis

V. cava superior

A. pulmonalis
dextra

Vv. pulmonales
dextrae

Truncus pulmonalis

Oesophagus,
pars thoracica

Foramen
venae cavae

Pleura parietalis,
pars diaphragmatica

Diaphragma

V. jugularis sinistra

A. subclavia sinistra

V. subclavia sinistra

V. brachiocephalica
sinistra

Arcus aortae

Lig. arteriosum

A. pulmonalis sinistra

Bronchi lobares
superior and inferior

Aorta thoracica

Pleura parietalis,
pars mediastinalis

N. phrencius,
a. and v.
pericardiacophrencia

Pericardium
fibrosum

a

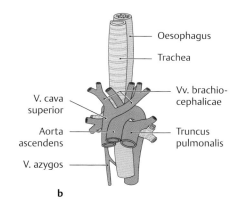

Oesophagus

Trachea

V. cava
superior

Vv. brachio-
cephalicae

Aorta
ascendens

Truncus
pulmonalis

V. azygos

b

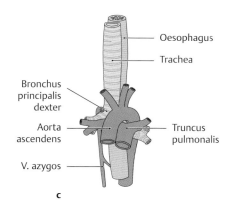

Oesophagus

Trachea

Bronchus
principalis
dexter

Aorta
ascendens

Truncus
pulmonalis

V. azygos

c

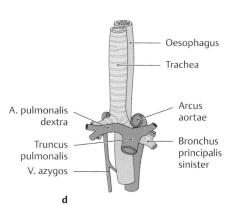

Oesophagus

Trachea

A. pulmonalis
dextra

Arcus
aortae

Truncus
pulmonalis

Bronchus
principalis
sinister

V. azygos

d

B Topographical relations (after Agur)
a Anterior view; the heart has been removed;
b–**e** In the drawings above, structures are progressively removed to obtain greater exposure of the trachea and bronchi:

b situs similar to **a.** With all structures intact, the trachea can be seen anterior to the oesophagus. The bifurcatio tracheae is covered by the arcus aorticus and a. pulmonalis;

c with the v. cava superior and vv. brachiocephalicae removed, the bronchus principalis dexter is just visible and the v. azygos is seen "riding" on the right bronchus lobaris superior;

d the aorta ascendens and much of the arcus aortae have been removed, exposing the bifurcatio tracheae and aa. pulmonales;

e with the truncus pulmonalis removed, the aorta "rides" upon the bronchus principalis sinister.

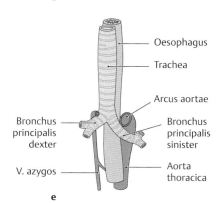

Oesophagus

Trachea

Arcus aortae

Bronchus
principalis
dexter

Bronchus
principalis
sinister

V. azygos

Aorta
thoracica

e

193

6.9 Mediastinum Superius

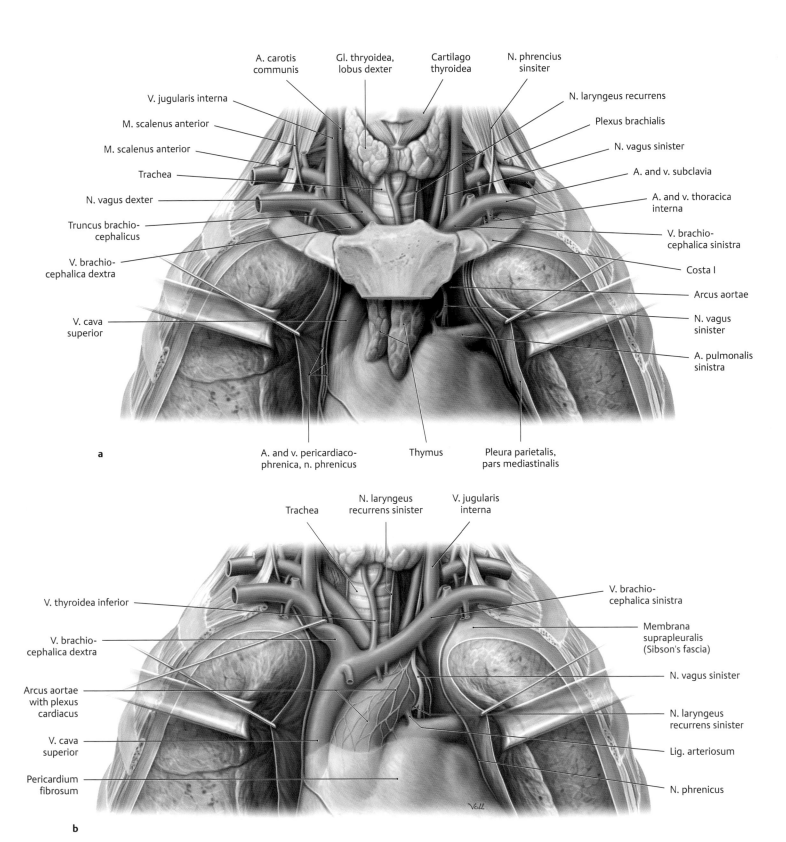

A carotis communis | Gl. thryoidea, lobus dexter | Cartilago thyroidea | N. phrencius sinister

V. jugularis interna
M. scalenus anterior
M. scalenus anterior
Trachea
N. vagus dexter
Truncus brachio-cephalicus
V. brachio-cephalica dextra
V. cava superior

N. laryngeus recurrens
Plexus brachialis
N. vagus sinister
A. and v. subclavia
A. and v. thoracica interna
V. brachio-cephalica sinistra
Costa I
Arcus aortae
N. vagus sinister
A. pulmonalis sinistra

A. and v. pericardiaco-phrenica, n. phrenicus | Thymus | Pleura parietalis, pars mediastinalis

a

N. laryngeus recurrens sinister | V. jugularis interna
Trachea

V. thyroidea inferior
V. brachio-cephalica dextra
Arcus aortae with plexus cardiacus
V. cava superior
Pericardium fibrosum

V. brachio-cephalica sinistra
Membrana suprapleuralis (Sibson's fascia)
N. vagus sinister
N. laryngeus recurrens sinister
Lig. arteriosum
N. phrenicus

b

A View of the apertura thoracis superior and the mediastinum superius

a The corpus sterni and adjacent ribs have been removed; at the level of the apertura thoracis superior, the mediastinum superius borders the neck; the actual structures of the mediastinum superius become visible only after removal of the manubrium sterni (see **b**);

b The mediastinum superius is exposed: the manubrium sterni, and the thymus or thymus remnants (retrosternal fat pad) have been removed.

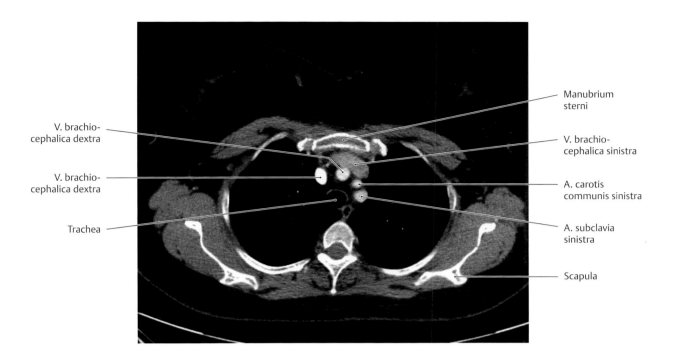

V. brachio-
cephalica dextra

V. brachio-
cephalica dextra

Trachea

Manubrium
sterni

V. brachio-
cephalica sinistra

A. carotis
communis sinistra

A. subclavia
sinistra

Scapula

B Cross-sectional anatomy of the superior thoracic aperture
Transverse (axial) CT scan (soft-tissue window) at the level of the aper-
tura thoracis superior (manubrium sterni or T 3), inferior view (original
C Transverse section at the level of the apertura thoracis superior

Inferior view. figure Prof. Dr. med. S. Müller-Hülsbeck, Diagnostic and
Interventional Radiology/Neuroradiology, Ev. Luth. Diakonissenanstalt,
Flensburg).

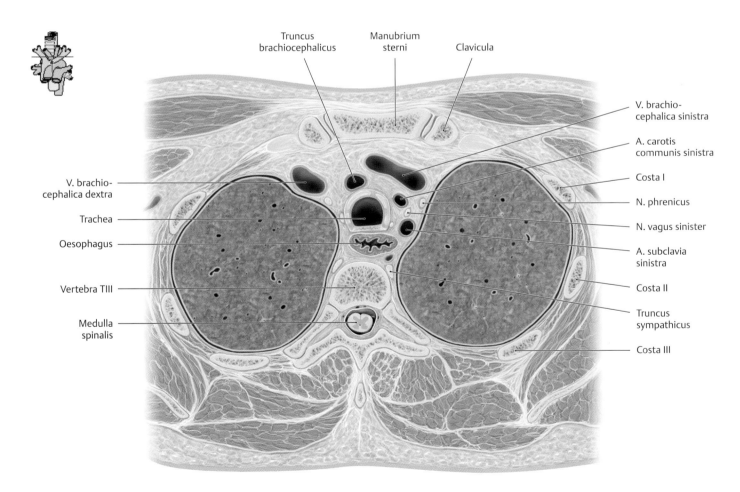

Truncus
brachiocephalicus

Manubrium
sterni

Clavicula

V. brachio-
cephalica sinistra

A. carotis
communis sinistra

Costa I

N. phrenicus

N. vagus sinister

A. subclavia
sinistra

Costa II

Truncus
sympathicus

Costa III

V. brachio-
cephalica dextra

Trachea

Oesophagus

Vertebra TIII

Medulla
spinalis

C Transverse section at the level of the apertura thoracis superior
Inferior view.

6.10 Arcus Aortae and Apertura Thoracis Superior

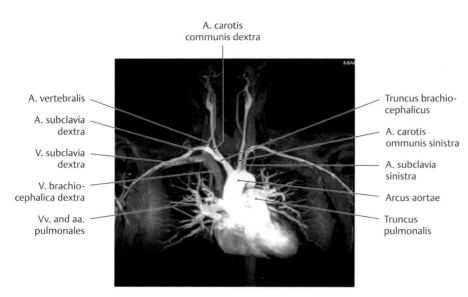

A Contrast-enhanced MR angiography of the vessels near the heart

The image shows an MR angiogram of the normal anatomy of the vessels near the heart (contrast agent administered intravenously via the fossa cubitalis). The image was generated using the MIP (maximum intensity projection) technique. It uses 3D fast gradient echo sequences, measured at the identical location before and after administration of contrast agent. The subsequent subtraction of images generates 3D data, which includes only vessel information. Using this technique, images from a dynamic series (e.g., pulmonary circulation) can be obtained within a few seconds (original figure Prof. Dr. med. S. Müller-Hülsbeck, Diagnostic and Interventional Radiology/Neuroradiology, Ev. Luth. Diakonis-senanstalt, Flensburg).

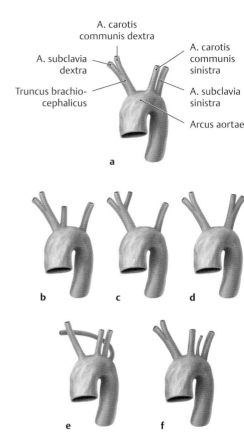

C Origin of the branches of the arcus aortae: common pattern and variations (after Lippert and Pabst)
Anterior view.

a Common pattern (70% of cases): The right a. subclavia and right a. carotis communis arise together from the truncus brachiocephalicus, which arises from the arcus aortae; however, the left a. carotis communis and left a. subclavia arise directly from the arcus aortae.

b Variation 1 (13% of cases): The truncus brachiocephalicus (with its two branches, the right a. subclavia and the right a. carotis communis) and left a. carotis communis arise together from the arcus aortae.

c Variation 2 (9% of cases): In addition to the right a. subclavia and right a. carotis communis, the left a. carotis communis also arises from the truncus brachiocephalicus.

d Variation 3 (1% of cases): There are two trunci brachiocephalici: one divides into the right a. subclavia and right a. carotis communis, the other divides into the left a. subclavia and left a. carotis communis.

e Variation 4 (1% of cases): The right a. subclavia is the last branch to arise from the arcus aortae. This is called arteria lusoria (from lat. lusorius = play).

f Variation 5 (1% of cases): The left a. vertebralis arises directly from the arcus aortae.

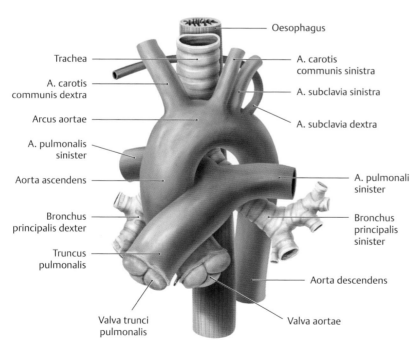

B Congenital anomalies of the arcus aortae: Aberrant arcus aortae (arteria lusoria)

If the right a. subclavia arises as the last vessel from the arcus aortae distal to the left a. subclavia and then courses behind the trachea and oesophagus it may produce a condition called aberrant a. subclavia (arteria lusoria) (see also **C**). Indications for surgery exist only if the patient presents with clinical symptoms (dysphagia, dyspnea, and stridor).

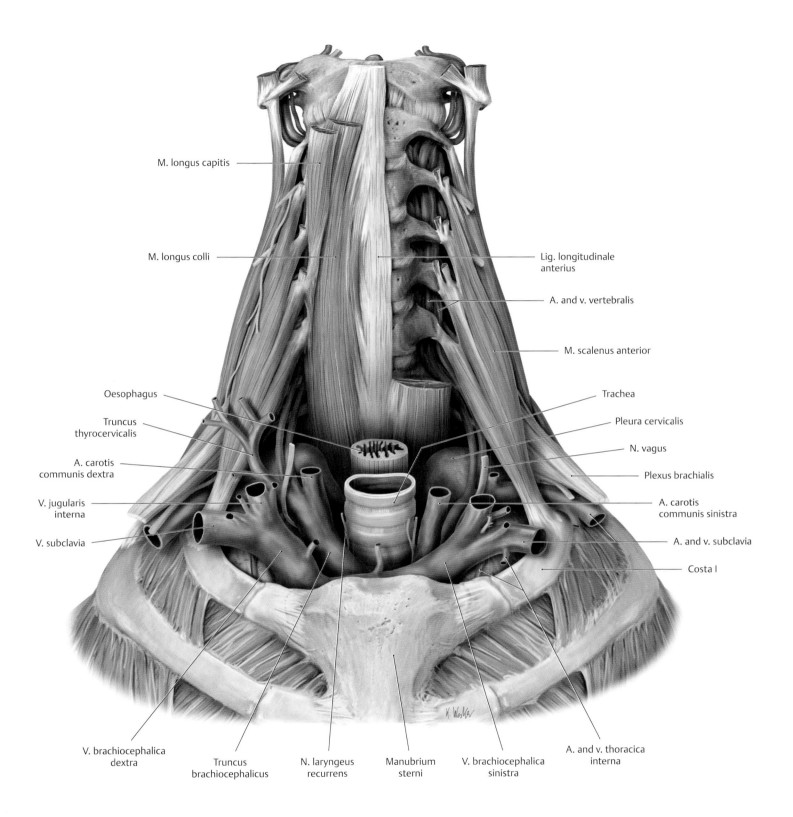

M. longus capitis

M. longus colli

Lig. longitudinale anterius

A. and v. vertebralis

M. scalenus anterior

Oesophagus

Truncus thyrocervicalis

A. carotis communis dextra

V. jugularis interna

V. subclavia

Trachea

Pleura cervicalis

N. vagus

Plexus brachialis

A. carotis communis sinistra

A. and v. subclavia

Costa I

V. brachiocephalica dextra

Truncus brachiocephalicus

N. laryngeus recurrens

Manubrium sterni

V. brachiocephalica sinistra

A. and v. thoracica interna

D Topography of the branches of the arcus aortae in the apertura thoracis superior

Anterior view after the cervical viscera have been removed. Parts of the prevertebral muscles (mm. longus capitis and longus colli) have also been removed to display the course of the left a. vertebralis.

6.11 Clinical Aspects: Coarctation of the Aorta

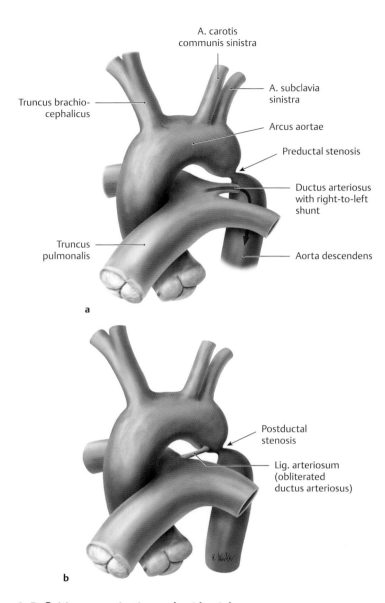

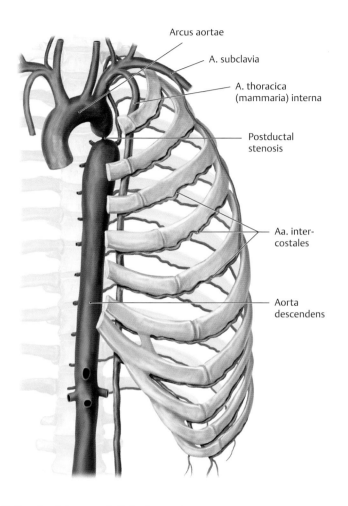

A Definition, organization and epidemiology

a Preductal aortic isthmus stenosis; **b** Postductal aortic isthmus stenosis.

Aortic isthmus stenosis (coarctation of the aorta) is characterized by a localized narrowing between the arcus aortae and the aorta descendens (the isthmus aortae). Thus, it is distal to the origin of the left a. subclavia, approximately at the level of the lig. arteriosum (the obliterated ductus arteriosus). Corresponding with the topographical relation to the lig. arteriosum, the two types are classified as preductal and postductal forms:

- preductal form: the narrowing is proximal to the patent ductus arteriosus, and
- postductal form: the narrowing is distal to the obliterated ductus arteriosus (lig. arteriosum).

Because preductal coarctation leads to symptoms in the first few years of life, it is also called the "infantile form." The postductal form, which usually develops after the child has reached adolescence, is also known as the "adult form." A narrowing of the arcus aortae in the isthmus aortae is a relatively common anomaly (5–7 % of all congenital cardiac and vascular malformations; boy:girl ratio is 3:1). Because clinical symptoms don't always occur (see **B**), the clinical presentation is rare.

B Pathophysiology and clinical symptoms

Coarctation of the aorta leads to a characteristic increase in blood pressure (hypertension) in the upper systemic circulation while at the same time blood pressure in the lower half of the body drops (hypotension). Cardinal signs include the difference in arterial pressure between upper and lower limbs (weak or absent femoral pulses) as well as cold feet and intermittent claudication caused by insufficient supply of blood.

- Low blood pressure in the lower body caused by **preductal stenosis** with a patent ductus arteriosus results in a right-to-left shunt accompanied by cyanosis of the lower body and right ventricular loading (dyspnea, tachypnea). This condition can lead to a life-threatening emergency in infants that requires surgery to correct (resection of the stenotic segment and end-to-end anastomosis).
- **Postductal stenosis** with an obliterated ductus arteriosus (shown here) results in the development of collateral circulation between the partes thoracica and abdominalis aortae (via the a. subclavia, a. thoracica interna and/or aa. intercostales). Depending on how well-functioning the collateral circulation is, patients may experience few or no symptoms at all. If patients do suffer from symptoms, the cardinal sign is often treatment-resistant hypertension, which early in life is often accompanied by headaches, ringing in the ear, dizziness, and nosebleeds. Complications of chronic hypertension in the upper body (left ventricular hypertrophy, coronary heart disease, cerebral hemorrhage) develop only later in life.

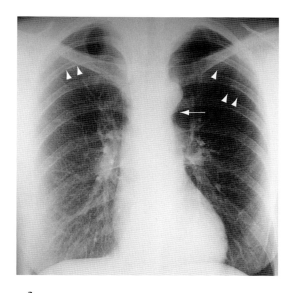
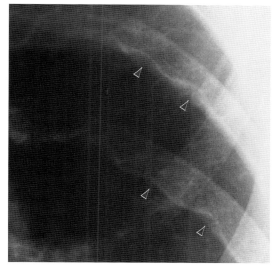

a

b

C Conventional diagnostic radiology

a and **b** Postductal aortic isthmus stenosis in an anterior-posterior projection (from Reiser, M. et al.: Radiologie [Duale Reihe], 2. Aufl./Radiology, 2nd edition, Thieme, Stuttgart 2006).

The aorta thoracica shows mild changes in aortic contour. The post-stenotic aorta descendens is dilated, the arcus aortae is narrowed and the outer outline of the aorta shows a visible indentation at the level of the stenotic segment (arrow). Rib notching (enlarged detail in b, red arrowheads) refers to bone changes around the sulcus costae caused by dilation and elongation of the enlarged aa. intercostales. It is typically visible at the inferior edges of the ribs.

The extent and localization of the stenosis is best displayed in an angiographic projection using either MRI or spiral CT including three-dimensional reconstruction (see p. 162).

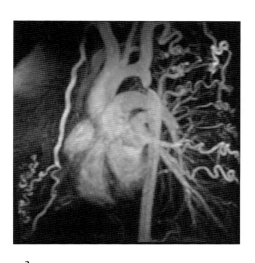
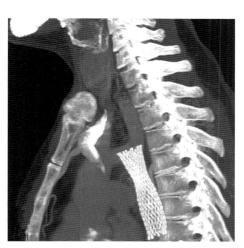
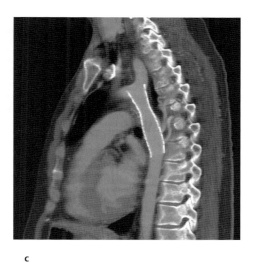

a

b

c

D Interventional therapy of aortic isthmus stenosis

Unlike surgical treatment of aortic isthmus stenosis in infants, over the past few years aortic isthmus stenosis in adults has been increasingly treated with minimally invasive, interventional techniques (balloon dilatation and/or stent placement).

a MR angiography of aortic isthmus stenosis in an adult, with severe stenosis and pronounced collaterals; **b** CT after balloon dilatation and placement of a self-expanding nitinol stent; **c** control CT scan 22 months after stent placement (from Schneider et al.: Kardiologie up-2date 4/2008, DOI 10.1055/s-2007-995625, Thieme, Stuttgart).

6.12 Clinical Aspects: Aortic Aneurysm

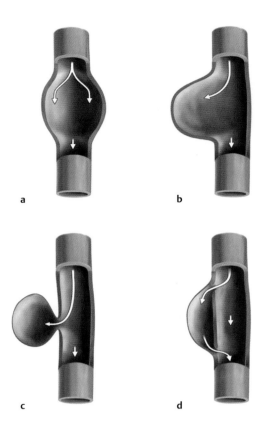

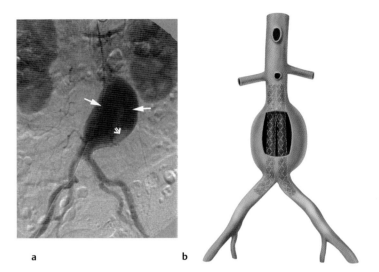

B Infrarenal aortic aneurysm: Symptoms, diagnosis, and treatment

a Evidence of a saccular infrarenal aortic aneurysm without involvement of the aa. renales or pelvic arteries, obtained from digital subtraction angiography (DSA). Thrombotic deposits on the wall of the aneurysm are visible (Reiser, M. et al.: Radiologie [Duale Reihe], 2. Aufl./Radiology, 2nd edition, Thieme, Stuttgart 2006);

b Schematic representation of a vascular prosthesis for bypassing infrarenal aortic aneurysms (an aortoiliac bifurcation prosthesis).

Symptoms: abdominal aneurysms cause symptoms when the enlarged vessel compresses other structures (neighboring vertebrae) or organs (ureter, nerves, etc.) (Symptoms are typically thoracic or abdominal pain as well as back pain radiating in a belt-like fashion). Parietal thromboses can lead to embolisms with acute peripheral ischemia. However, a ruptured aneurysm manifests itself as constant severe pain (acute abdominal) and signs of shock.

Note: A ruptured aortic aneurysm is a severe and acute life-threatening emergency. Only immediate surgery can save the patient's life (surgical death rate between 30 and 50 %).

Diagnosis: Most aortic aneurysms are diagnosed with the help of ultrasound examinations. This least invasive technique usually ensures a reliable assessment regarding localization and extent of the aneurysm. CT examination with contrast media is the preferred technique when assessing the size (relative to the perfused lumen and wall thrombosis) and relative anatomical positions of thoracic and abdominal aneurysms. Transarterial digital subtraction angiography (usually DSA) provides information about the vascular branches, particularly the aa. renales.

Treatment: The indication for treatment is based on the risk of rupture. Characteristic symptoms, distinct patterns of asymmetry (as shown here) as well as a diameter of more than 5 cm and rapid growth (more than 1 cm per year), are considered an absolute indication for surgery. The surgical procedure consists of resection of the aortic aneurysm and graft replacement. Nowadays, interventional therapy is often used to treat infrarenal aortic aneurysms. Using a femoral approach a catheter is placed into the aorta. With the help of the catheter a covered, fixed plastic prosthetic stent is positioned (endoluminal stent placement).

A Definition and classification

An aneurysm is an abnormal enlargement of an artery, usually caused by atherosclerosis. An aneurysm can develop in any artery but usually occurs in the infrarenal aorta abdominalis (90 % of cases); peripheral aneurysms are predominantly found in the aa. popliteae. Aneurysms are classified as follows:

- **True aneurysms (a, b):** enlargement of the vascular lumen involving all layers of the arterial wall with the vascular wall remaining intact. A morphologic distinction exists between spindle-shaped (fusiform) aneurysms involving the entire circumference of the vascular wall and saccular (*sacciform*) aneurysms, which involve only part of the circumference.
- **False aneurysms (pseudoaneurysms) (c):** a perivascular hematoma, which often develops following perforation of the vascular wall (e.g., arterial puncture) or at anastomotic sites after vascular surgery. If the vessel fails to occlude, blood escapes into the perivascular connective tissue leading to the formation of an aneurysmal cavity lined with thrombotic material.
- **Dissecting aneurysms (d):** a tear of the tunica intima/media and subsequent dilatation of the tunica media/adventitia leads to the formation of a second "false" lumen in the vascular wall. This leads to development of a vessel with two channels, one non-perfused and the other perfused. Depending on the location of the intimal tear, also known as the entry site, the entire aorta or only the aorta abdominalis can be affected. As the disease progresses, external perforation (rupture with subsequent bleeding) or perforation of the dissected membrane back into the perfused lumen (called reentry) can occur, see **C**.

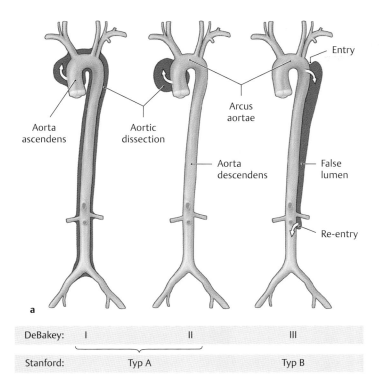

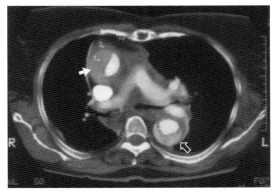

DeBakey:	I		II		III
Stanford:		Typ A			Typ B

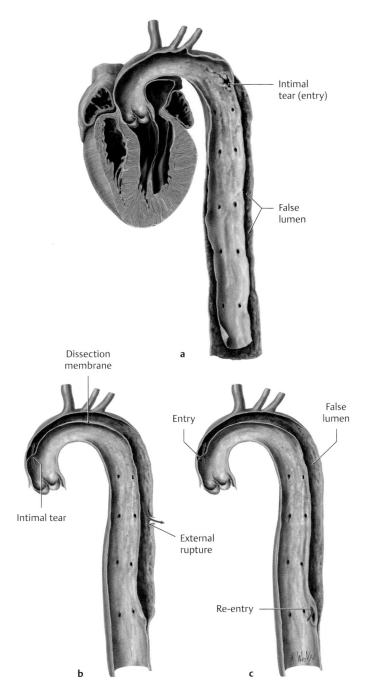

C Aortic dissection: Classification based on anatomica location

a Aortic dissections can be classified according to anatomical location in the Stanford or DeBakey systems. The most common is the **Stanford classification**, which is based on the location of the entry site of the dissection:

- Dissections involving the pars ascendens aortae (Stanford type A, approximately 80 % of cases)
- Dissections involving the pars descendens aortae (Stanford type B, approximately 20 % of cases).

The **DeBakey classification** further differentiates Stanford type A:

- DeBakey type I (involves the whole aorta) and
- DeBakey type II (involves the ascending aorta);
- DeBakey type III equals Stanford type B (dissection involves the descending aortae).

b Axial computed tomography (inferior view) of an aortic dissection type I according to DeBakey (Stanford type A) demonstrating the partes ascendens (white arrow) and descendens (open arrow) aortae: Delayed filling of the false lumen shows up as a lower density than the true lumen (from: Reiser, M. et al.: Radiologie [Duale Reihe], 2. Aufl./Radiology, 2nd edition, Thieme, Stuttgart 2006).

D Pathophysiology of aortic dissection

a Aortic dissection with intimal tear and false lumen; **b** Aortic dissection with intimal tear and rupture through outside wall; **c** Aortic dissection with intimal tear (entry) and re-entry tear.

In a classic aortic dissection (incidence of 2.6–3.5/100,000 population), arterial hypertension initially leads to degenerative changes in the layers of the aortic wall, which results in an intimal tear and a partial media tear. The aortic wall splits producing false and true lumens, which are separated by the dissection membrane. Depending on the loca-tion of the initial intimal tear, the whole aorta (intimal tear at the level of the pars thoracica aortae) or only the pars abdominalis aortae is involved. Protrusion of the dissection membrane may lead to secondary occlusion of visceral branches resulting in ischemic syndromes. As the disease progresses, a perforation through the outside wall of the aorta (rupture and hemorrhage) or back into the true lumen (prognostically beneficial re-entry) may occur.

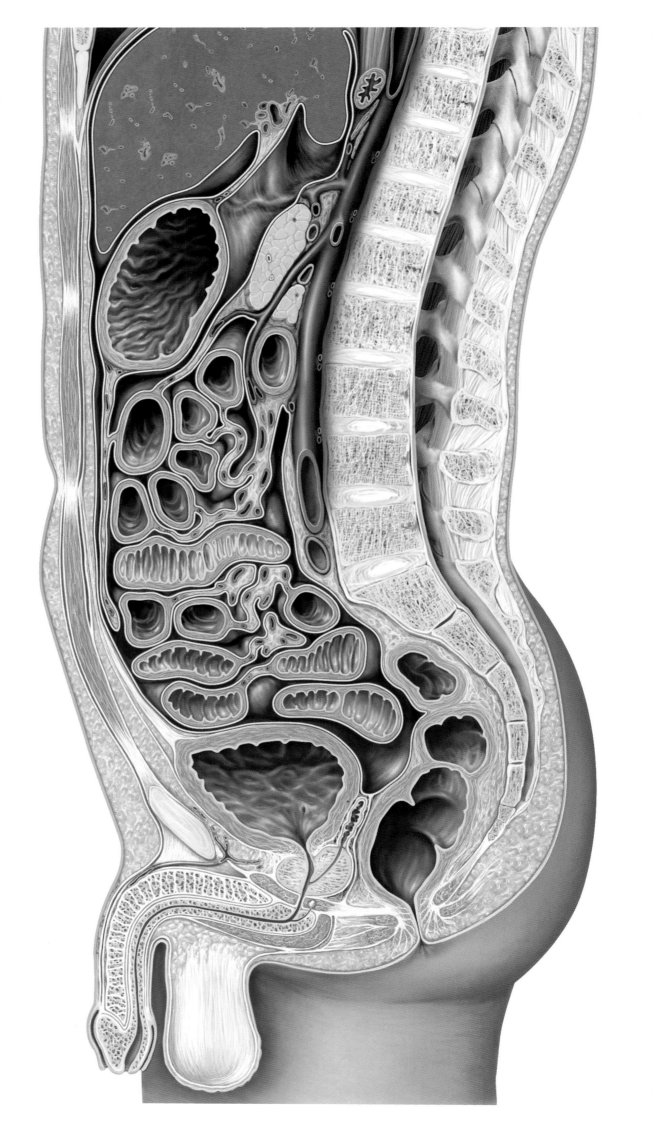

C Abdomen and Pelvis

1.1 Architecture, Wall Structure, and Functional Aspects

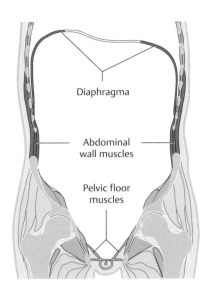

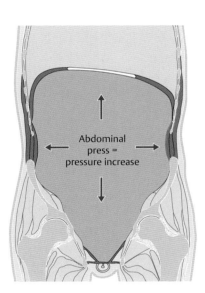

a

A Architecture and wall structure of the cavitas abdominis and cavitas pelvis

Whereas the cavitas thoracica and cavitas abdominis are separated by the diaphragma, the cavitas abdominis and cavitas pelvis are continuous with each other. They are divided topographically by the linea terminalis. Thus, they form a single functional unit (see p. 2). Bones (columna vertebralis, cavea thoracis, and pelvis) as well as muscles (diaphragma, abdominal wall, and diaphragma pelvis muscles) along with their fasciae and aponeuroses form the walls of this space. It is bounded by the following structures:

- Superiorly (see **Ca**): diaphragma with right and left domes and centrum tendineum
- Inferiorly (see **Cb**): bony pelvis, muscles of the pelvic wall (m. iliacus, m. obturator internus, m. piriformis, and m. coccygeus), and mm. diaphragmatis pelvis (mainly the m. levator ani forming most of the diaphragma pelvis)
- Posteriorly (see **Cc**): lumbar columna vertebralis, deep muscles of the abdominal wall (m. quadratus lumborum and m. psoas major), and mm. dorsi proprii
- Anteriorly and laterally (see **Cd**): anterior and lateral muscles of the abdominal wall together with their aponeuroses (m. rectus abdominis and m. transversus abdominis as well as mm. obliqui internus and externus abdominis)

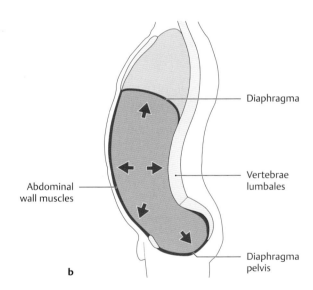

b

B Functional aspects of abdominal and pelvic wall structure: Abdominal press

Abdominal press is made possible by the structure of the abdominal and pelvic walls, which plays an important role in their elastic properties. "Abdominal press" describes the voluntary contraction of the diaphragma, and abdominal and pelvic muscles. When the muscles contract they reduce the volume of the cavitas abdominis thereby significantly raising the intra-abdominal pressure: pressure in the standing position is approximately 1.7 kPa (2.75 mmHg), when lying down it is approximately 0.2 kPa (1.5 mmHg), and under strain including coughing or squeezing it is 10–20 kPa (75–150 mmHg).

Abdominal press is important in

- Emptying of the rectum (defecation), of the bladder (micturition), and of the stomach (vomiting),
- Uterine contractions during the expulsive phase of labor ("expulsive pains"),
- Stabilizing the columna vertebralis (mainly the lumbar spine) and the trunk (the wall stiffens like the wall of an inflated ball), for example

when lifting heavy loads, but also in the standing posture (hydrostatic effect of abdominal press).

Hernias occur when the pressure load is greater than the strength of the complex myofascial network. They develop either in the anterior abdominal wall or more commonly in the groin region because the weight of the pelvic and abdominal organs puts increasing strain on the wall structures, which increases from superior to inferior. Additionally, the diaphragma pelvis muscles in particular are much less able to withstand the increased abdominal pressure than the abdominal wall muscles or the diaphragma. During abdominal press, closure of the glottis and the retaining of air in the lungs gives support to the diaphragma; there is no such compensatory mechanism in the diaphragma pelvis muscles making it a characteristic weak spot. After excessive stretching (e.g., caused by vaginal delivery) the diaphragma pelvis is unable to maintain the pelvic organs in their normal position (pelvic floor descent) and provides inadequate support for the abdominal press. The results are urinary and fecal incontinence.

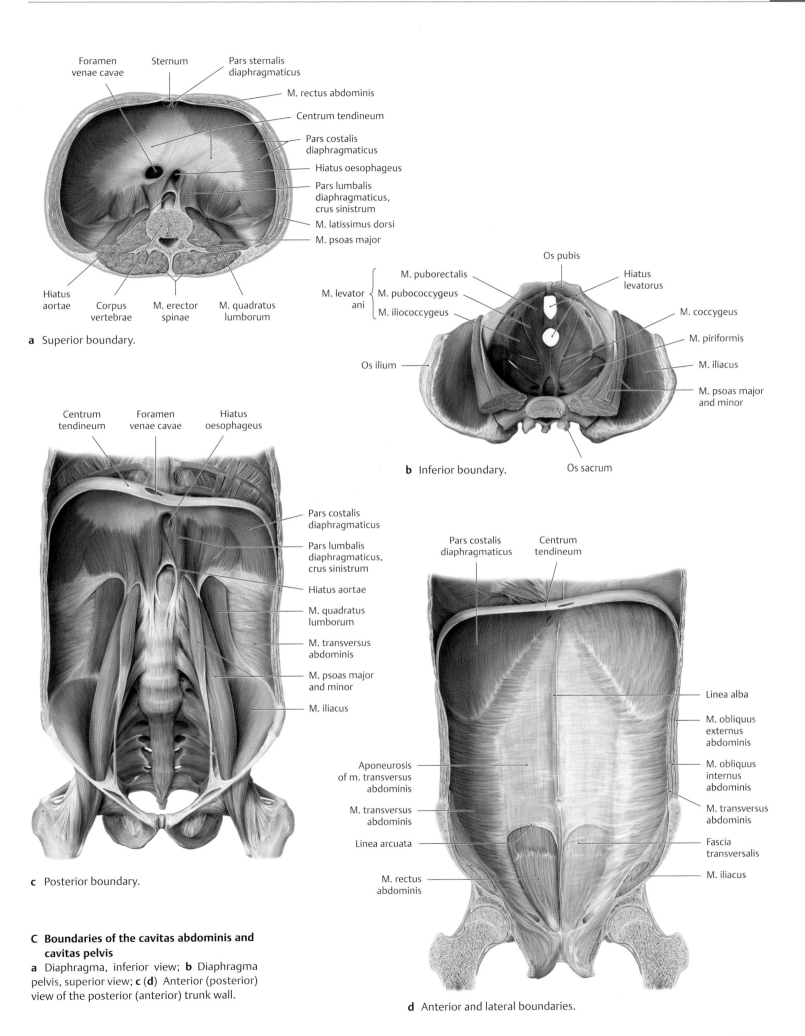

Foramen venae cavae

Sternum

Pars sternalis diaphragmaticus

M. rectus abdominis

Centrum tendineum

Pars costalis diaphragmaticus

Hiatus oesophageus

Pars lumbalis diaphragmaticus, crus sinistrum

M. latissimus dorsi

M. psoas major

Hiatus aortae

Corpus vertebrae

M. erector spinae

M. quadratus lumborum

a Superior boundary.

Os pubis

M. levator ani
{ M. puborectalis
M. pubococcygeus
M. iliococcygeus

Hiatus levatorus

M. coccygeus

M. piriformis

Os ilium

M. iliacus

M. psoas major and minor

b Inferior boundary.

Os sacrum

Centrum tendineum

Foramen venae cavae

Hiatus oesophageus

Pars costalis diaphragmaticus

Pars lumbalis diaphragmaticus, crus sinistrum

Hiatus aortae

M. quadratus lumborum

M. transversus abdominis

M. psoas major and minor

M. iliacus

Pars costalis diaphragmaticus

Centrum tendineum

Linea alba

M. obliquus externus abdominis

M. obliquus internus abdominis

Aponeurosis of m. transversus abdominis

M. transversus abdominis

M. transversus abdominis

Fascia transversalis

Linea arcuata

M. iliacus

M. rectus abdominis

c Posterior boundary.

d Anterior and lateral boundaries.

C Boundaries of the cavitas abdominis and cavitas pelvis
a Diaphragma, inferior view; **b** Diaphragma pelvis, superior view; **c** (**d**) Anterior (posterior) view of the posterior (anterior) trunk wall.

1.2 Divisions of the Cavitas Abdominis and Cavitas Pelvis

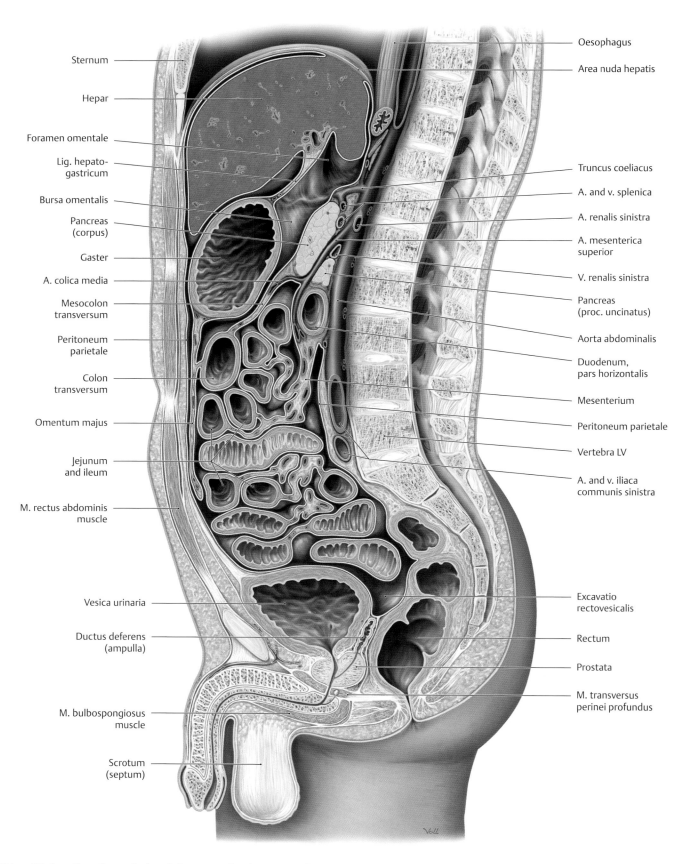

Sternum

Hepar

Foramen omentale

Lig. hepato-
gastricum

Bursa omentalis

Pancreas
(corpus)

Gaster

A. colica media

Mesocolon
transversum

Peritoneum
parietale

Colon
transversum

Omentum majus

Jejunum
and ileum

M. rectus abdominis
muscle

Vesica urinaria

Ductus deferens
(ampulla)

M. bulbospongiosus
muscle

Scrotum
(septum)

Oesophagus

Area nuda hepatis

Truncus coeliacus

A. and v. splenica

A. renalis sinistra

A. mesenterica
superior

V. renalis sinistra

Pancreas
(proc. uncinatus)

Aorta abdominalis

Duodenum,
pars horizontalis

Mesenterium

Peritoneum parietale

Vertebra LV

A. and v. iliaca
communis sinistra

Excavatio
rectovesicalis

Rectum

Prostata

M. transversus
perinei profundus

A Midsagittal section through the abdomen and pelvis, viewed from the left side

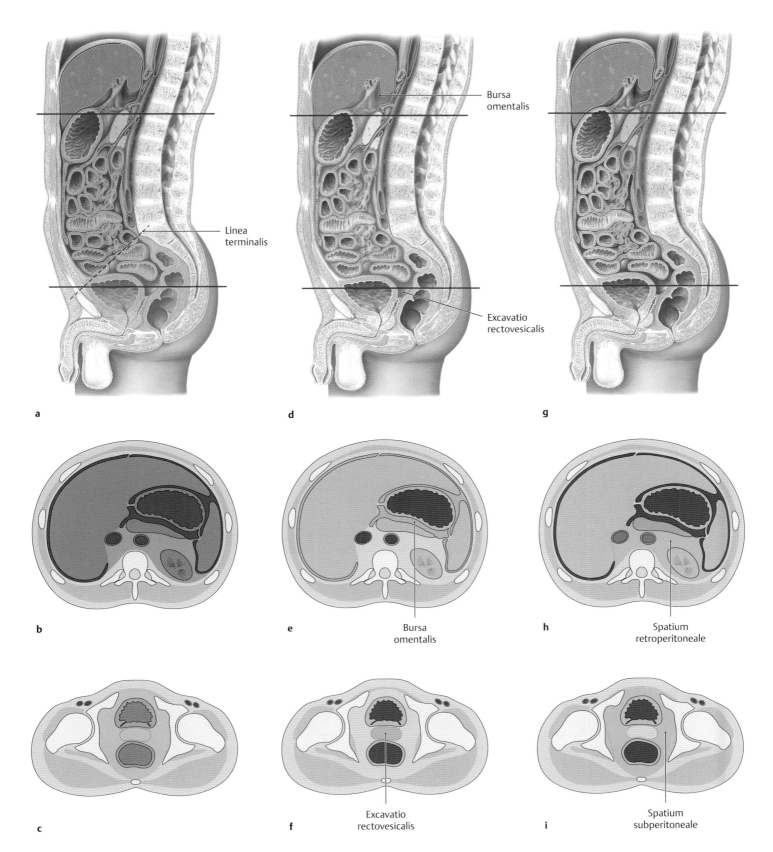

B Divisions of the cavitas abdominis and cavitas pelvis

Each column of diagrams shows a midsagittal section viewed from the left side, as well as two axial sections, one at the L1 level and the other at the lower part of the os sacrum, both viewed from below.

a–c Topography of body cavities: cavitas abdominis and cavitas pelvis (imaginary line separating the two cavities is the linea terminalis);

d–f Serous cavities (peritoneal spaces): abdominal cavitas peritonealis and pelvic cavitas peritonealis;

g–i Connective tissue spaces (spatia extraperitonealia): spatium retroperitoneale and spatium subperitoneale; serous cavities and spatia extraperitonealia are separated by peritoneum (see p. 209).

1.3 Classification of Internal Organs Based on their Relationship to the Cavitas Abdominis and Cavitas Pelvis

The organs of the abdomen and pelvis can be classified according to various topographical criteria:

- By layers in the anteroposterior direction (**A**)
- By levels in the craniocaudal direction (**B**)
- As intra- or extraperitoneal based on their peritoneal investment (**C, D**)

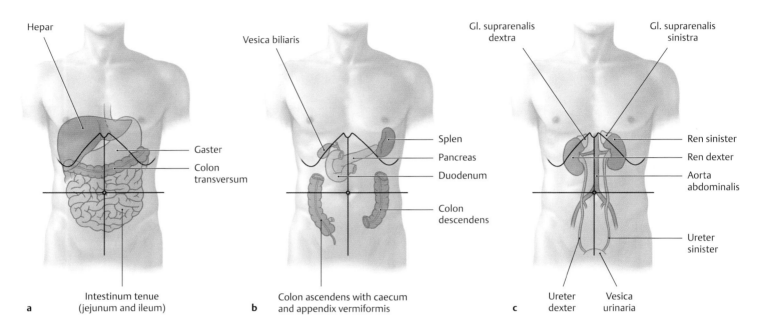

a   Intestinum tenue (jejunum and ileum)

b   Colon ascendens with caecum and appendix vermiformis

c   Ureter dexter   Vesica urinaria

A Classification of the abdominal and pelvic organs by layers
The abdominal and pelvic organs can be roughly divided into three layers in the anteroposterior direction. This classification is particularly useful from a surgical standpoint.
Note: Larger organs may occupy more than one layer (see p. 206).

a   Anterior layer: hepar, gaster, colon transversum, jejunum, ileum, and vesica urinaria (for clarity not shown here, but shown with the other urinary organs in **c**);

b   Middle layer: hepar, duodenum, pancreas, splen, colon ascendens and descendens, and uterus (not shown for clarity, extends into the anterior layer);

c   Posterior layer: great vessels, renes, ureteres, and gll. suprarenales (for clarity, the vesica urinaria is shown in its relationship to the other urinary organs, see **a**).

B Classification of the abdominal and pelvic organs by levels
In this classification the organs are roughly assigned to craniocaudal levels based on their relationship to the mesocolon transversum (upper and lower abdominal organs) and pelvis minor (pelvic organs). Because the kidneys and gll. suprarenales are retroperitoneal, they are not listed in the table. When the kidney is projected onto the abdominal wall, its inferior pole extends into the lower abdomen.

Level	Organs located there
• **Upper abdomen** (above the mesocolon transversum)	• Gaster • Duodenum • Hepar • Vesica biliaris and biliary tract • Splen • Pancreas
• **Lower abdomen** (between the mesocolon transversum and apertura pelvis superior)	• Jejunum and ileum • Caecum and parts of the colon *Note:* The colon transversum, while located in the upper abdomen, is classified functionally as part of the lower abdomen.
• **Pelvis minor**	• Vesica biliaris • Terminal portion of ureter • Rectum • Uterus, tuba uterina, ovarium, and vagina • Portions of the ductus deferens, prostata, and gl. vesiculosa (the testis and epididymis are outside the cavitas pelvis)

C Location of intraperitoneal and extraperitoneal organs in the abdomen and pelvis

Midsagittal section (renes outside the sectional plane) viewed from the left side.

The cavitas peritonealis is a closed cavity that is lined by **peritoneum** and surrounded on all sides by the spatium extraperitoneale. Laterally, anteriorly, and superiorly, the spatium extraperitoneale appears like a very narrow slit (see p. 207). Only its posterior portion (spatium retroperitoneale) and inferior portion (spatium extraperitoneale of the pelvis) are true spaces that contain organs. Because peritoneum covers the organs (peritoneum viscerale) and walls (peritoneum parietale), the intraperitoneal organs can easily glide upon one another. The extraperitoneal organs, such as the vesica urinaria or rectum are not, or are only partially, covered by peritoneum. The vesica urinaria is covered by peritoneum only on one side (on its superior surface), which enables it to expand upward as it becomes distended with urine. This part of the peritoneum, which in females also covers large parts of the uterus, is known as peritoneum urogenitale.

The **mesenterium** is a band of connective tissue (a suspensory ligament also referred to as "meso"), which is also covered by peritoneum– by peritoneum parietale near where the mesenterium is attached to the body wall and by peritoneum viscerale near where it is attached to the organs. The mesenterium contains the neurovascular structures of the intraperitoneal organs that are "suspended" from it. This suspensory ligament allows the intraperitoneal organs to have greater mobility than extraperitoneal organs, which are embedded in the connective tissue of the wall of the cavitas peritonealis, either primarily because they were retroperitoneal when they formed or secondarily because they "migrated" behind the peritoneum during the course of embryonic development (see **D** and p. 47).

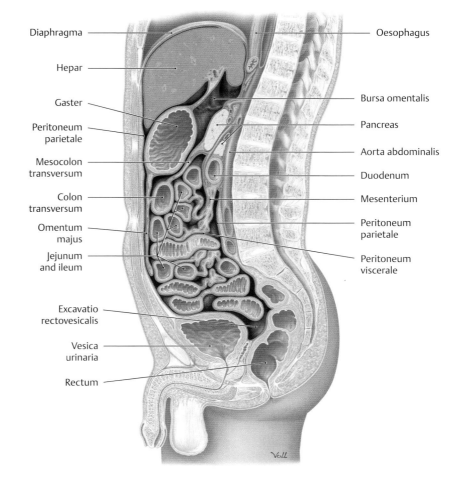

Labels (clockwise): Diaphragma, Oesophagus, Hepar, Bursa omentalis, Gaster, Pancreas, Peritoneum parietale, Aorta abdominalis, Mesocolon transversum, Duodenum, Colon transversum, Mesenterium, Omentum majus, Peritoneum parietale, Jejunum and ileum, Peritoneum viscerale, Excavatio rectovesicalis, Vesica urinaria, Rectum

D Intra- and extraperitoneal organs of the abdomen and pelvis

Location in relation to the peritoneum	Organs
Intraperitoneal (Organs are completely covered by peritoneum and are suspended by mesenterium)	
• In the abdominal cavitas peritonealis	• Gaster, splen, hepar and vesica biliaris, intestinum tenue (parts of the partes superior and ascendens of the duodenum plus jejunum and ileum), colon transversum and sigmoideum, caecum (portions of variable size may be extraperitoneal, see below)
• In the pelvic cavitas peritonealis	• Fundus and corpus uteri, the ovaria, and the tubae uterinae and possibly the superior portion of the rectum
Extraperitoneal (Organs without a mesenterium; their neurovascular structures are located in the extraperitoneal connective tissue)	
Primarily extraperitoneal (extraperitoneal from the outset)	
• Behind the abdominal or pelvic cavitas peritonealis, thus retroperitoneal • Below the pelvic cavitas peritonealis, thus infra- or subperitoneal	• Renes, gll. suprarenales, ureteres • Vesica urinaria, prostata, vesicula seminalis, cervix uteri, vagina, and rectum past the flexura sacralis (the vesica urinaria is covered by peritoneum superiorly [peritoneum urogenitale])
Secondarily extraperitoneal (become extraperitoneal during the course of embryonic development; the organs are covered by peritoneum anteriorly)	
• Behind the abdominal or pelvic cavitates peritoneales, thus retroperitoneal	• Intestinum tenue (duodenum: partes descendens, horizontalis, and part of the pars ascendens), pancreas, colon ascendens and descendens, parts of the caecum (see above), rectum up to the flexura sacralis

209

2.1 Branches of the Aorta Abdominalis: Overview and Paired Branches

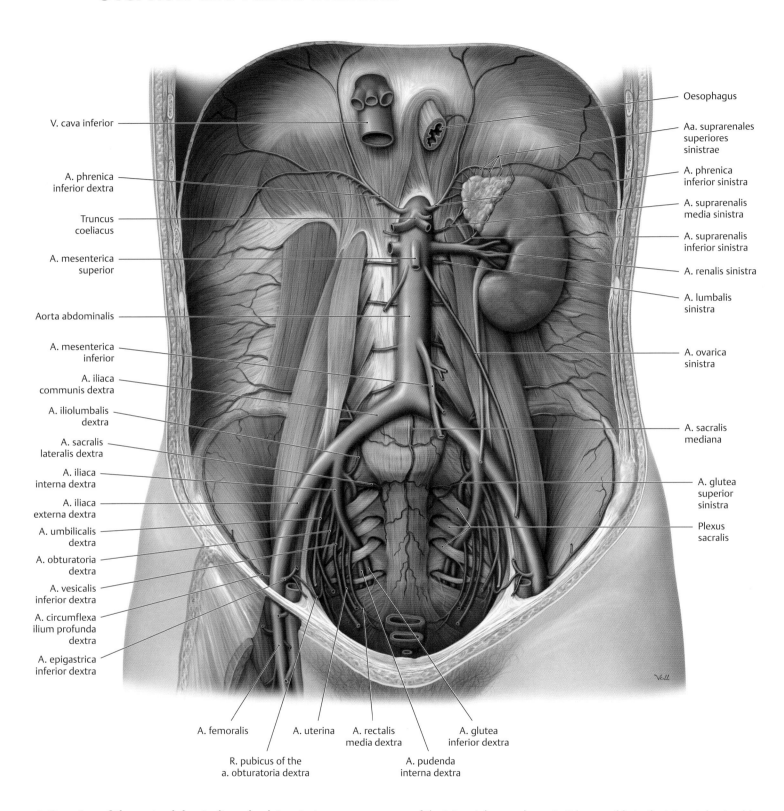

V. cava inferior

A. phrenica inferior dextra

Truncus coeliacus

A. mesenterica superior

Aorta abdominalis

A. mesenterica inferior

A. iliaca communis dextra

A. iliolumbalis dextra

A. sacralis lateralis dextra

A. iliaca interna dextra

A. iliaca externa dextra

A. umbilicalis dextra

A. obturatoria dextra

A. vesicalis inferior dextra

A. circumflexa ilium profunda dextra

A. epigastrica inferior dextra

Oesophagus

Aa. suprarenales superiores sinistrae

A. phrenica inferior sinistra

A. suprarenalis media sinistra

A. suprarenalis inferior sinistra

A. renalis sinistra

A. lumbalis sinistra

A. ovarica sinistra

A. sacralis mediana

A. glutea superior sinistra

Plexus sacralis

A. femoralis   A. uterina   A. rectalis media dextra   A. glutea inferior dextra

R. pubicus of the a. obturatoria dextra   A. pudenda interna dextra

A Overview of the aorta abdominalis and pelvic arteries (abdominal organs removed)

Anterior view (female pelvis). The oesophagus has been pulled slightly inferiorly, and the peritoneum has been completely removed.
The aorta abdominalis is the distal continuation of the aorta thoracica. It descends slightly to the left of the midline to approximately the level of the L4 vertebra, as shown in **B** (or possibly to the L5 vertebra in older individuals). There it divides into the paired aa. iliacae communes (bifurcatio aortae). The aa. iliacae communes divide further into the aa. iliacae internae and externae. The aorta abdominalis (see **C**) and its major branches give origin to various "subbranches" that supply the abdomen and pelvis (see **D**).

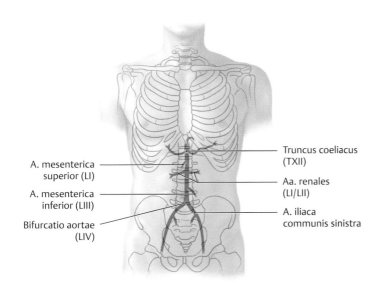

A. mesenterica superior (LI)

A. mesenterica inferior (LIII)

Bifurcatio aortae (LIV)

Truncus coeliacus (TXII)

Aa. renales (LI/LII)

A. iliaca communis sinistra

B Projection of the aorta abdominalis and its major branches onto the columna vertebralis and pelvis

Anterior view of the five major arterial trunks. The major branches of the aorta abdominalis can be identified in imaging studies based on their relationship to the vertebrae.

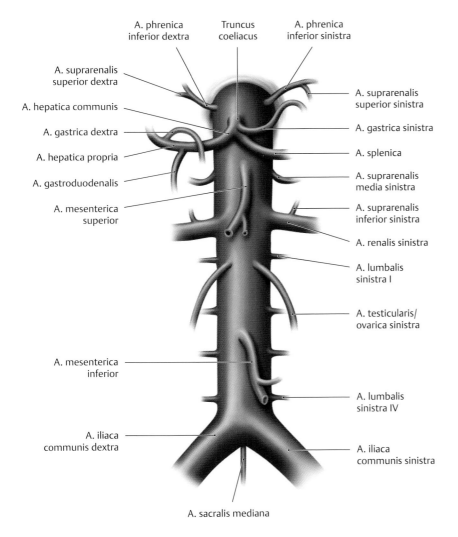

A. phrenica inferior dextra
Truncus coeliacus
A. phrenica inferior sinistra

A. suprarenalis superior dextra

A. hepatica communis

A. gastrica dextra

A. hepatica propria

A. gastroduodenalis

A. mesenterica superior

A. mesenterica inferior

A. iliaca communis dextra

A. suprarenalis superior sinistra

A. gastrica sinistra

A. splenica

A. suprarenalis media sinistra

A. suprarenalis inferior sinistra

A. renalis sinistra

A. lumbalis sinistra I

A. testicularis/ ovarica sinistra

A. lumbalis sinistra IV

A. iliaca communis sinistra

A. sacralis mediana

C Sequence of branches from the aorta abdominalis

D Functional groups of arteries that supply the abdomen and pelvis

The branches of the aorta abdominalis and pelvic arteries can be divided into five broad functional groups (→ = give rise to). For details about the areas supplied by the unpaired branches see p. 213.

Paired branches (and one unpaired branch) that supply the diaphragma, renes, gll. suprarenales, posterior abdominal wall, columna vertebralis, and gonadae (see C)
• Aa. phrenicae inferiores dextra et sinistra → Aa. suprarenales superiores dextra et sinistra • Aa. suprarenales mediae dextra et sinistra • Aa. renales dextra et sinistra → Aa. suprarenales inferiores dextra et sinistra • Aa. testiculares (ovaricae) dextra et sinistra • Aa. lumbales dextrae et sinistrae (first through fourth) • A. sacralis mediana (with lowest lumbar arteries)
One unpaired trunk that supplies the hepar, vesica biliaris, pancreas, splen, gaster, and duodenum (see C, pp. 213 and 265)
• Truncus coeliacus with – A. gastrica sinistra – A. splenica – A. hepatica communis
One unpaired trunk that supplies the intestinum tenue and intestinum crassum as far as the flexura coli sinistra (see C, pp. 213 and 269)
• A. mesenterica superior
One unpaired trunk that supplies the intestinum crassum from the flexura coli sinistra (see C, p. 213)
• A. mesenterica inferior
One indirect (see below) paired trunk that supplies the pelvis (see A, p. 213)
• A. iliaca interna (from the a. iliaca communis, not directly from the aorta, hence an "indirect paired trunk")

211

2.2 Branches of the Aorta Abdominalis: Unpaired and Indirect Paired Branches

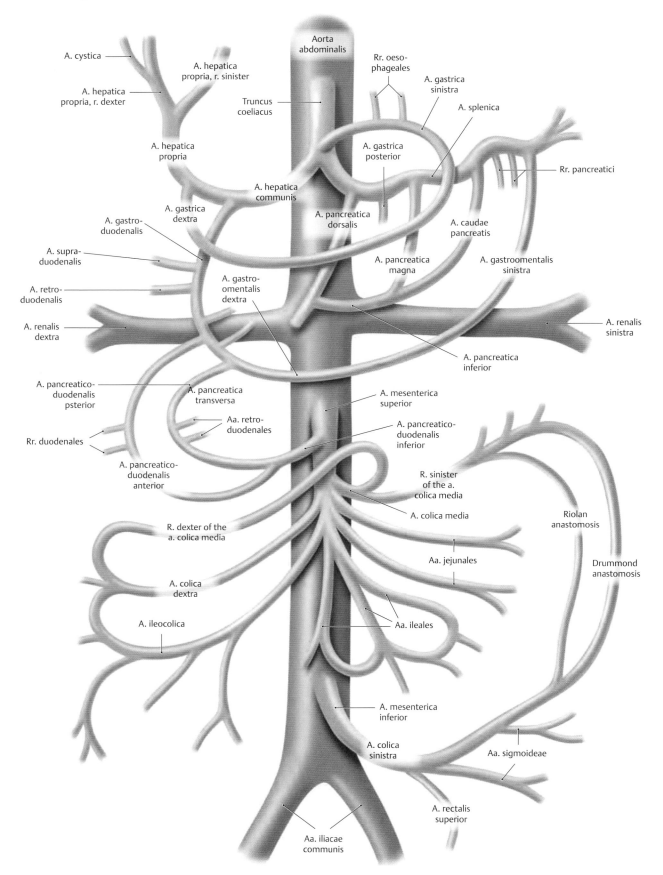

A Classification of arteries supplying the abdomen and pelvis

Red: Branches of the truncus coeliacus. These supply the proximal bowel segments from the abdominal part of the oesophagus to the pancreas and duodenum.

Green: Branches of the a. mesenterica superior. These supply the middle bowel segments from the pancreas and duodenum to the flexura coli sinistra.

Blue: Branches of the a. mesenterica inferior. These supply the distal bowel segments from the flexura coli sinistra to the rectum.

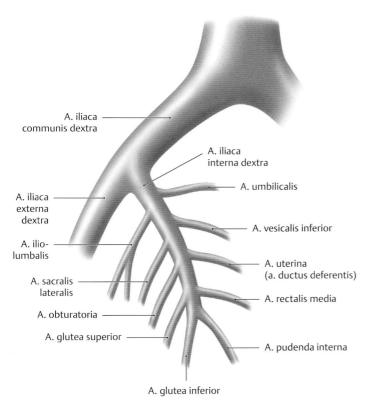

A. iliaca communis dextra

A. iliaca interna dextra

A. umbilicalis

A. iliaca externa dextra

A. vesicalis inferior

A. ilio-lumbalis

A. uterina (a. ductus deferentis)

A. sacralis lateralis

A. rectalis media

A. obturatoria

A. glutea superior

A. pudenda interna

A. glutea inferior

B Right a. iliaca communis with subbranches

The bifurcatio aortae is the point where the aorta abdominalis bifurcates into the two aa. iliacae communes, which give off multiple subbranches that supply the viscera and pelvic walls (see **D**).

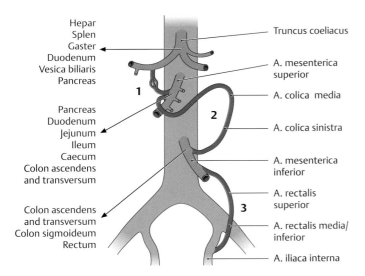

Hepar
Splen
Gaster
Duodenum
Vesica biliaris
Pancreas

Truncus coeliacus

A. mesenterica superior

A. colica media

1

Pancreas
Duodenum
Jejunum
Ileum
Caecum
Colon ascendens
and transversum

2

A. colica sinistra

A. mesenterica inferior

A. rectalis superior

Colon ascendens
and transversum
Colon sigmoideum
Rectum

3

A. rectalis media/ inferior

A. iliaca interna

C Abdominal arterial anastomoses

1 Between the truncus coeliacus and a. mesenterica superior via the aa. pancreaticoduodenales
2 Between the aa. mesentericae superior and inferior (aa. colicae media and sinistra; Riolan and Drummond anastomoses, see **A**)
3 Between the a. mesenterica inferior and a. iliaca interna (a. rectalis superior and a. rectalis media or inferior)

These anastomoses are important in that they can function as collaterals, delivering blood to intestinal areas that have been deprived of their normal blood supply.

D Classification of the arteries supplying the abdomen and pelvis

The branches of the pars abdominalis aortae and the pelvic arteries can be divided into the five major areas they supply. For details about the area supplied by the paired branches see p. 211.

Note the anastomoses particularly between the unpaired trunks (see Fig. **A** and **C**).

One unpaired trunk that supplies the hepar, vesica biliaris, pancreas, splen, gaster, and duodenum (see **A**)

- Truncus coeliacus with
  - A. splenica
    - → A. gastroomentalis sinistra
    - → A. gastrica posterior (and aa. gastricae breves)
    - → Rr. pancreatici
    - → A. caudae pancreatis
    - → A. pancreatica magna
    - → A. pancreatica dorsalis
    - → A. pancreatica inferior
    - → A. transversa pancreatis
  - A. gastrica sinistra → Rr. oesophageales
  - A. hepatica communis
    - → A. gastroduodenalis
      - → A. supraduodenalis (inconstant branch of the a. gastroduodenalis)
      - → A. retroduodenalis
      - → A. gastroomentalis dextra
      - → A. pancreaticoduodenalis superior anterior vel posterior
      - → Rr. duodenales
    - → A. gastrica dextra
    - → A. hepatica propria
      - → A. cystica

One unpaired trunk that supplies the intestinum tenue and intestinum crassum as far as the flexura coli sinistra (see **A**)

- A. mesenterica superior
  - → A. pancreaticoduodenalis inferior
  - → Aa. jejunales et ileales
  - → A. ileocolica
  - → A. colica dextra
  - → A. colica media

One unpaired trunk that supplies the intestinum crassum from the flexura coli sinistra (see **A**)

- A. mesenterica inferior
  - → A. colica sinistra
  - → Aa. sigmoideae
  - → A. rectalis superior

One indirect (see below) paired trunk that supplies the pelvis (see **B**)

- A. iliaca interna (from the a. iliaca communis, not directly from the aorta, hence an "indirect paired trunk") with branches that supply
  - → A. umbilicalis
    - → A. vesicalis superior
    - → A. ductus deferentis ♂
  - → A. vesicalis inferior
  - → A. uterina (A. ductus deferentis)
  - → A. rectalis media
  - → A. pudenda interna

The pelvic walls (parietal branches)
  - → A. iliolumbalis
  - → Aa. sacrales laterales
  - → A. obturatoria
  - → Aa. gluteae superior and inferior

2.3 Inferior Vena Caval System

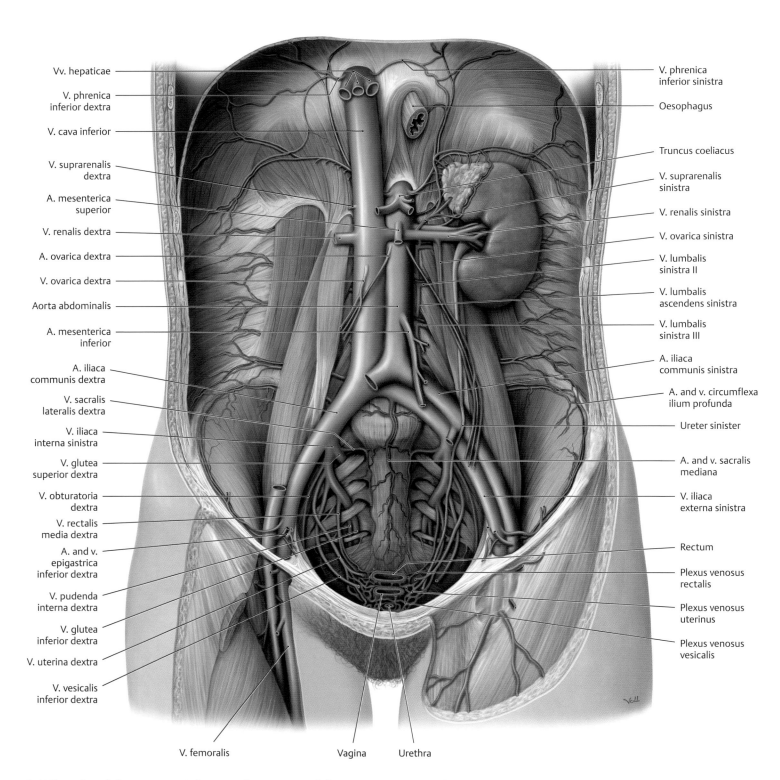

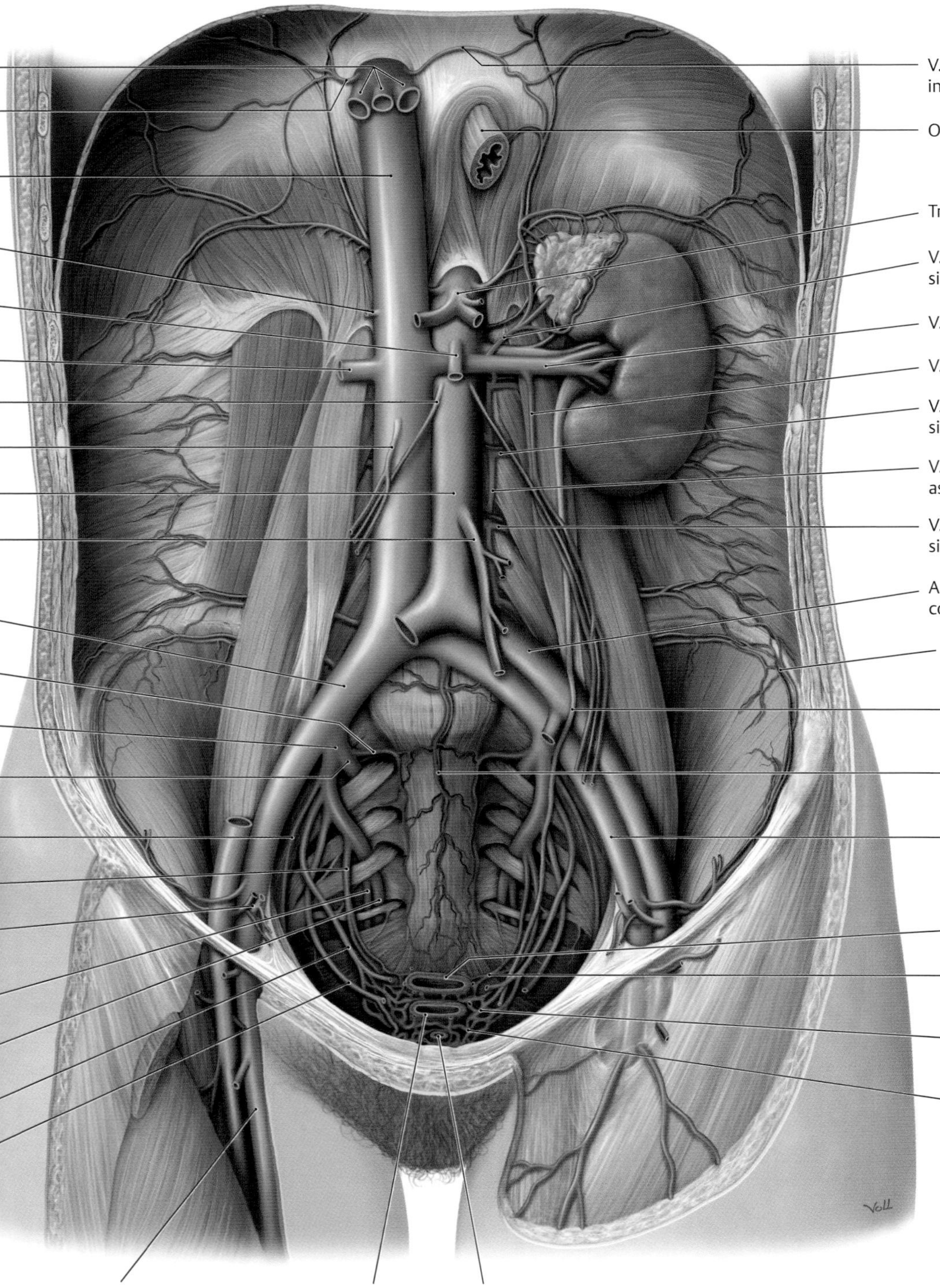
Vv. hepaticae
V. phrenica inferior dextra
V. cava inferior
V. suprarenalis dextra
A. mesenterica superior
V. renalis dextra
A. ovarica dextra
V. ovarica dextra
Aorta abdominalis
A. mesenterica inferior
A. iliaca communis dextra
V. sacralis lateralis dextra
V. iliaca interna sinistra
V. glutea superior dextra
V. obturatoria dextra
V. rectalis media dextra
A. and v. epigastrica inferior dextra
V. pudenda interna dextra
V. glutea inferior dextra
V. uterina dextra
V. vesicalis inferior dextra
V. femoralis
Vagina
Urethra
V. phrenica inferior sinistra
Oesophagus
Truncus coeliacus
V. suprarenalis sinistra
V. renalis sinistra
V. ovarica sinistra
V. lumbalis sinistra II
V. lumbalis ascendens sinistra
V. lumbalis sinistra III
A. iliaca communis sinistra
A. and v. circumflexa ilium profunda
Ureter sinister
A. and v. sacralis mediana
V. iliaca externa sinistra
Rectum
Plexus venosus rectalis
Plexus venosus uterinus
Plexus venosus vesicalis

A Tributaries of the vena cava inferior in the posterior abdomen and pelvis

Anterior view of an opened female abdomen. All organs but the left ren and gl. suprarenalis have been removed, and the oesophagus has been pulled slightly inferiorly.

The v. cava inferior receives numerous tributaries that return venous blood from the abdomen and pelvis (and, of course, from the lower limbs), analogous to the distribution of the paired abdominal aortic branches in this region. The v. cava inferior is formed by the union of the two vv. iliacae communes at the approximate level of the LV vertebra (see **C**), behind and slightly inferior to the bifurcatio aortae.

Note the special location of the left v. renalis and its risk of compression by the a. mesenterica superior (see p. 269): The left v. renalis passes in front of the aorta abdominalis but behind the a. mesenterica superior. Veins in the male pelvis are described on p. 347.

The veins in the pelvis have numerous variants. For example, the tributaries of the v. iliaca interna are frequently multiple (unlike those shown above) but unite to form a single trunk before entering the v. iliaca (see also p. 349).

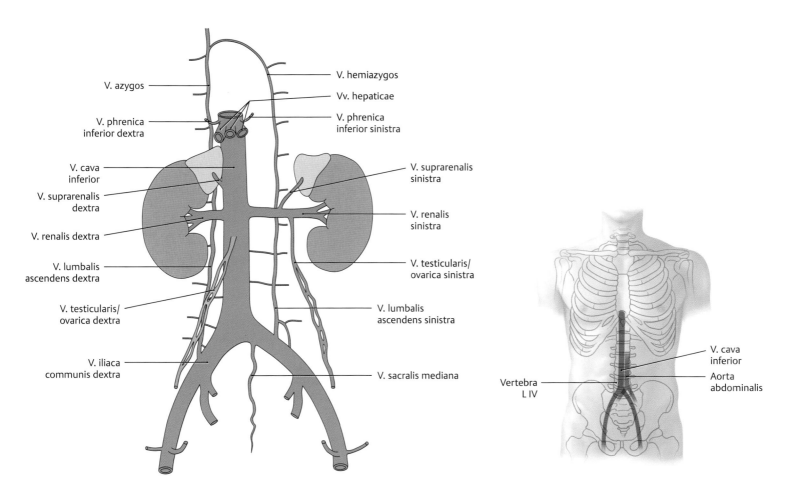

B Tributaries of the vena cava inferior
The difference in the venous drainage of the right and left renes is displayed more clearly here than in **A**. The continuity of the right v. lumbalis ascendens with the v. azygos is also shown.

Direct tributaries return venous blood directly to the v. cava inferior without passing through an intervening capillary bed. Direct tributaries drain the following organs:

- The diaphragma, abdominal wall, renes, gll. suprarenales, testes/ovaria, and hepar
- For the *pelvis* (via the v. iliaca communis) from the pelvic wall and floor, uterus, tubae uterinae, vesica urinaria, ureteres, accessory sex glands, lower rectum, and lower limb.

Indirect tributaries return blood that has passed through the capillary bed of the hepar via the hepatic portal system (see p. 217). The following organs have indirect tributaries:

- The splen
- The organs of the digestive tract: pancreas, duodenum, jejunum, ileum, caecum, colon, and upper rectum

Note: Venous blood from the v. cava inferior may drain through the vv. lumbales ascendentes into the v. azygos or hemiazygos and thence to the v. cava superior. Thus a connection between the two vv. cavae exists on the posterior wall of the abdomen and thorax: a cavocaval or intercaval anastomosis. The location and significance of cavocaval anastomoses are discussed on p. 218. Frequently an anastomosis exists between the v. suprarenalis and v. phrenica inferior (not shown here, see **A**) on the left side of the body.

C Projection of the vena cava inferior onto the columna vertebralis
The v. cava inferior ascends on the right side of the aorta abdominalis and pierces the diaphragma at the foramen venae cavae located at the T VIII level. The vv. iliacae communes unite at the L V level to form the v. cava inferior (see also **A**).

D Direct tributaries of the vena cava inferior

- Right and left vv. phrenicae inferiores
- Vv. hepaticae
- V. suprarenalis dextra
- Right and left vv. renales at the L I/L II level (the v. testicularis/ovarica sinistra and v. suprarenalis sinistra terminate in the left v. renalis)
- Vv. lumbales
- V. testicularis/ovarica dextra
- Vv. iliacae communes (L V level)
- V. sacralis mediana (often terminates in the left v. iliaca communis)

215

2.4 Portal Venous System (Vena Portae Hepatis)

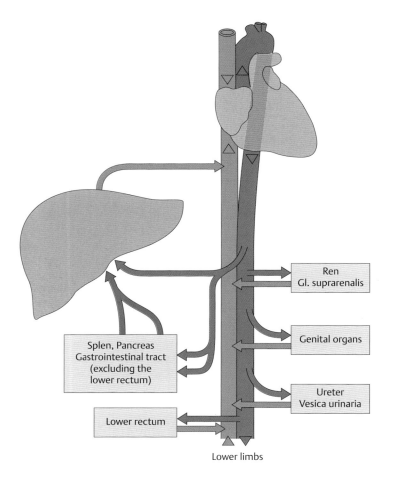

Lower limbs

A The portal venous system in the abdomen

The arterial blood supply and venous drainage of the abdominal and pelvic organs differ in their functional organization: While they derive their arterial blood supply entirely from the aorta abdominalis or one of its major branches, *venous drainage* is accomplished by one of two *different venous systems:*

1. Organ veins that drain directly or indirectly (via the vv. iliacae) into the v. cava inferior, which then returns the blood to the right heart (see also p. 214);
2. Organ veins that first drain directly or indirectly (via the vv. mesentericae or v. splenica) *into the v. portae hepatis*—and thus to the hepar—before the blood enters the v. cava inferior and returns to the ventriculus dexter cordis.

The *first pathway* serves the urinary organs, gll. suprarenales, genital organs, and the walls of the abdomen and pelvis. The *second pathway* serves the organs of the digestive system (hollow organs of the gastrointestinal tract, pancreas, vesica biliaris) and the splen (see **D**). Only the lower portions of the rectum are exempt from this pathway and drain directly through the vv. iliacae to the v. cava inferior. This (re)routing of venous blood through the hepatic portal system ensures that the organs of the digestive tract deliver their nutrient-rich blood to the liver for metabolic processing before it is returned to the heart. It also provides a route by which elements of degenerated red blood cells can be conveyed from the splen to the liver. Thus, the v. portae hepatis functions to deliver blood to the liver to support metabolism. This contrasts with the a. hepatica propria, which supplies the liver with oxygen and other nutrients. Anastomoses may develop between the portal venous system and vena caval system (portacaval anastomosis) and function as collateral pathways in certain diseases (see p. 218).

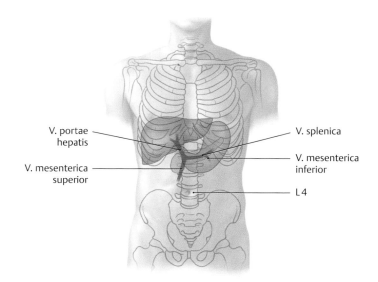

B Projection of the vena portae hepatis and its two major tributaries onto the columna vertebralis

The v. portae hepatis is formed by the union of the v. mesenterica *superior* and v. splenica to the right of the midline at the L 1 level. The v. mesenterica *inferior* typically opens into the splenic vein, also conveying its blood to the v. mesenterica inferior via this route.
Note the relationship of the v. portae hepatis to the liver, stomach, and pancreas.

C Tributaries of the vena portae hepatis

- **Vena mesenterica superior** (see p. 276) with its tributaries:
  – Vv. pancreaticoduodenales
  – Vv. pancreaticae
  – V. gastroomentalis dextra
  – Vv. jejunales
  – Vv. ileales
  – V. ileocolica
  – V. colica dextra
  – V. colica media
- **Vena mesenterica inferior** (see p. 277) with its tributaries:
  – V. colica sinistra
  – Vv. sigmoideae
  – V. rectalis superior
- **Vena splenica** (see p. 275) with its tributaries:
  – V. gastroomentalis sinistra
  – Vv. pancreaticae
  – Vv. gastricae breves
- **Direct tributaries** (see p. 275)
  – V. cystica
  – V. gastrica sinistra with vv. oesophageales
  – V. gastrica dextra
  – V. pancreaticoduodenalis superior posterior
  – V. prepylorica
  – Vv. paraumbilicales

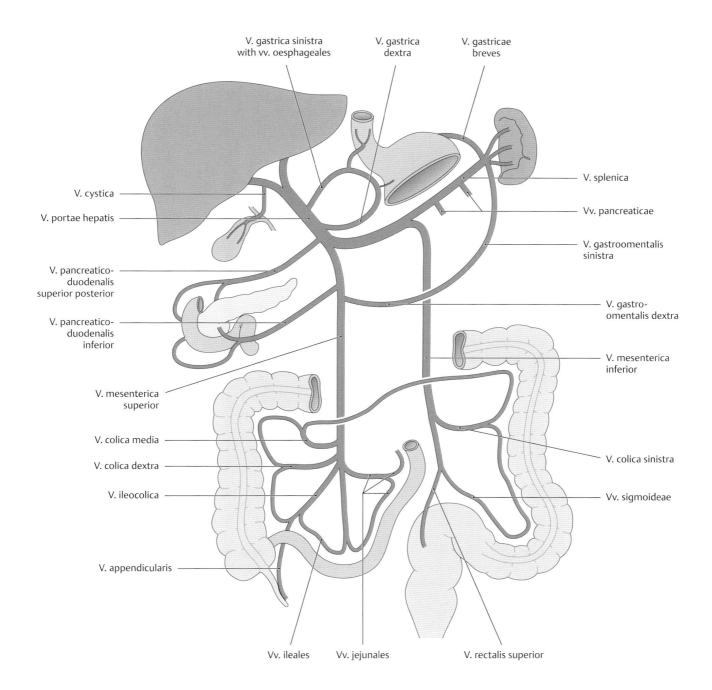

V. gastrica sinistra with vv. oesphageales

V. gastrica dextra

V. gastricae breves

V. cystica

V. portae hepatis

V. pancreatico-duodenalis superior posterior

V. pancreatico-duodenalis inferior

V. mesenterica superior

V. colica media

V. colica dextra

V. ileocolica

V. appendicularis

V. splenica

Vv. pancreaticae

V. gastroomentalis sinistra

V. gastro-omentalis dextra

V. mesenterica inferior

V. colica sinistra

Vv. sigmoideae

Vv. ileales

Vv. jejunales

V. rectalis superior

D Distribution of the vena portae hepatis (see also **C**)

The v. portae hepatis is a short vessel (total length 6–12 cm) with a large caliber. On entering the liver, it divides into two main branches, one for each of the lobi hepatis. The region drained by the v. portae hepatis corresponds to the region supplied by the truncus coeliacus and the aa. mesentericae superior and inferior. The v. portae hepatis receives venous blood from the hollow organs of the gastrointestinal tract (excluding the lower rectum) and from the pancreas, vesica biliaris, and splen. Some of this blood flows directly to the v. portae hepatis through the corresponding organ veins, and the rest reaches the vv. portae hepatis indirectly by way of the vv. mesentericae or v. splenica.

2.5 Venous Anastomoses in the Abdomen and Pelvis

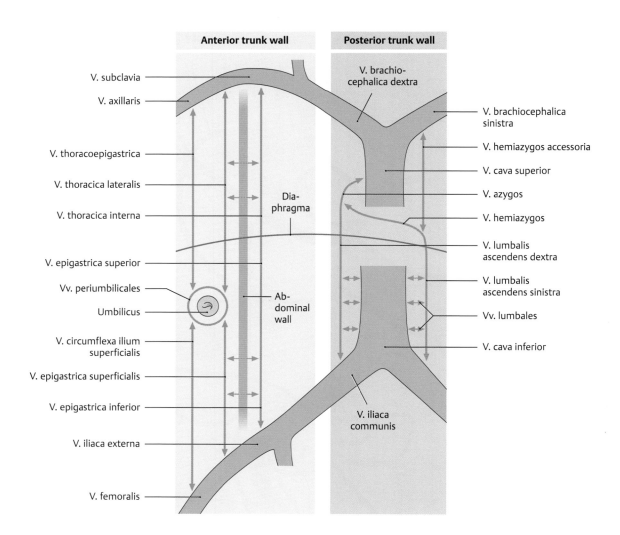

A Cavocaval (intercaval) anastomoses

Large venous anastomoses are present between the vv. cavae inferior and superior on the anterior and posterior trunk walls. Known as *cavocaval* or *intercaval anastomoses*, they provide collateral pathways for returning venous blood to the v. cava *superior* and right heart in patients with outflow obstructions affecting the v. cava *inferior* in the abdomen or the vv. iliacae communes in the pelvis. Veins of the chest wall form the cranial portion of this collateral network. The veins of the *anterior* abdominal wall provide both a *superficial* pathway (anterior to the m. rectus abdominis) and a *deep* pathway (posterior to the m. rectus abdominis). (In the chest, these pathways lie outside or inside the skeleton thoracis.)

Note: On the *anterior* trunk wall, the vv. paraumbilicales (see **B**) establish a collateral pathway between the v. portae hepatis and drainage to the vv. cavae. This portosystemic (portacaval) pathway is important in patients with obstructed portal venous flow and may affect the superficial and deep anterior pathways.

- Anastomoses on the *posterior wall* of the abdomen. They utilize the connection between the v. lumbalis ascendens and the v. azygos/hemiazygos. Two pathways are available:

  1. A *direct* pathway between the v. lumbalis ascendens and v. azygos/hemiazygos:
     V. cava inferior → (possibly via the v. iliaca communis) v. lumbalis ascendens → v. azygos/hemiazygos → **v. cava superior**.

  2. An *indirect* pathway between the v. lumbalis ascendens and v. azygos/hemiazygos by way of horizontal trunk wall veins (vv. intercostales and lumbales, mediated by venous plexuses on the columna vertebralis; for clarity, not shown here):
     V. cava inferior → (possibly via the v. iliacus communis) v. lumbalis ascendens → vv. lumbales → plexus venosus vertebralis → vv. intercostales posteriores → v. azygos/hemiazygos → **v. cava superior**.

- Anastomoses on the *anterior* wall of the abdomen. They utilize superficial and deep cutaneous veins, which may exchange blood between them. Two pathways are available:

  1. Deep pathway (posterior to the m. rectus abdominis):
     V. cava inferior → v. iliaca communis → v. iliaca externa → v. epigastrica inferior → v. epigastrica superior → v. thoracica interna → v. subclavia → v. brachiocephalica → **v. cava superior**.

  2. Superficial pathway (anterior to the m. rectus abdominis):
     V. cava inferior → v. iliaca communis → v. iliaca externa → v. femoralis → v. epigastrica superficialis/v. circumflexa ilium superficialis → v. thoracoepigastrica/v. thoracica lateralis → v. axillaris → v. subclavia → v. brachiocephalica → **v. cava superior**.

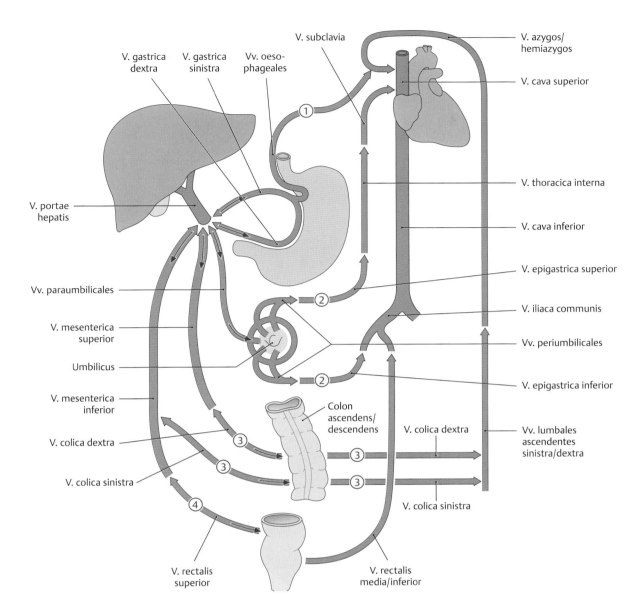

V. subclavia
V. azygos/hemiazygos
V. gastrica dextra
V. gastrica sinistra
Vv. oeso-phageales
V. cava superior
V. portae hepatis
V. thoracica interna
V. cava inferior
Vv. paraumbilicales
V. epigastrica superior
V. mesenterica superior
V. iliaca communis
Umbilicus
Vv. periumbilicales
V. mesenterica inferior
V. epigastrica inferior
V. colica dextra
Colon ascendens/descendens
V. colica dextra
Vv. lumbales ascendentes sinistra/dextra
V. colica sinistra
V. rectalis superior
V. colica sinistra
V. rectalis media/inferior

B Schematic of collateral pathways for the vena portae hepatis (porto-systemic collaterals)

Venous collateral pathways are also available between the portal venous system and the vv. cavae inferior and superior. These *portosystemic* collaterals are physiological pathways that can develop in response to (1) overlapping venous territories in organs (plexus venosi in the oesophagus, colon, rectum) or (2) the persistence of patent blood vessels that are normally obliterated after birth (v. umbilicalis, vv. paraumbilicae). These collateral pathways become clinically significant when the portal system is compromised (as in hepatic cirrhosis, for example). As venous pressure increases, the v. portae hepatis can divert blood away from the hepar and return it to the supplying vessels. Thus, veins that are normally *afferent* vessels for the hepar undergo a *flow reversal* (see red arrows) and transport blood back through the v. cava inferior or superior and and back to the cor. Portosystemic shunts can be life-saving, but nevertheless cause significant additional problems, because some of the vessels in the shunt pathways (in the oesophagus and rectum, specifically) are barely capable of handling the significant redirected blood flow, with consequent rise of pressure in the system, and are thus liable to rupture. The following four **collateral pathways** are of key importance:

① Through veins of the gaster and distal oesophagus (dilation of these veins may lead to esophageal varices, with risk of life-threatening hemorrhage):
V. portae hepatis ← vv. gastricae ← *vv. oesophageales* → v. azygos/hemiazygos → **v. cava superior**.

② Through veins of the anterior abdominal wall:
V. portae hepatis ← v. umbilicalis (pars patens) ← *vv. paraumbilicales* → v. epigastrica superior → v. thoracica interna → v. subclavia → **v. cava superior** *or*
V. porta hepatis ← v. umbilicalis (pars patens) → *vv. paraumbilicales* → v. epigastrica inferior → v. iliaca externa → **v. cava inferior**.
Note: Drainage from vv. paraumbilicales into the superficial veins (rare) of the anterior abdominal wall (vv. thoracoepigastricae, v. thoracica lateralis, v. epigastrica superficialis, see **A**) leads to dilation of these tortuous veins (Medusa head, caput medusae).

③ Through veins of the posterior abdominal wall:
V. portae hepatis ← v. mesenterica superior and v. mesenterica inferior ← vv. colicae sinistra et dextra → vv. lumbales ascendentes sinistra et dextra → v. azygos/v. hemiazygos → **vena cava superior**. The vv. lumbales ascendentes may also divert blood to the vena cava inferior.

④ Through the plexus venosus rectalis (with dilation):
V. portae hepatis ← v. mesenterica inferior ← v. rectalis superior ← vv. rectales mediae/*inferiores* → v. iliaca interna → **v. cava inferior**.

219

2.6 Trunci Lymphatici and Nodi Lymphoidei

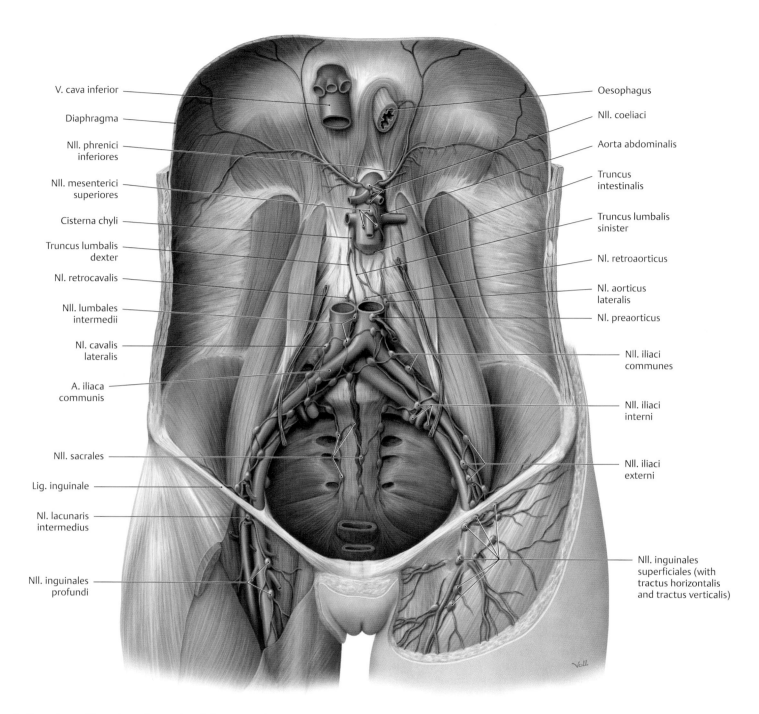

V. cava inferior

Diaphragma

Nll. phrenici
inferiores

Nll. mesenterici
superiores

Cisterna chyli

Truncus lumbalis
dexter

Nl. retrocavalis

Nll. lumbales
intermedii

Nl. cavalis
lateralis

A. iliaca
communis

Nll. sacrales

Lig. inguinale

Nl. lacunaris
intermedius

Nll. inguinales
profundi

Oesophagus

Nll. coeliaci

Aorta abdominalis

Truncus
intestinalis

Truncus lumbalis
sinister

Nl. retroaorticus

Nl. aorticus
lateralis

Nl. preaorticus

Nll. iliaci
communes

Nll. iliaci
interni

Nll. iliaci
externi

Nll. inguinales
superficiales (with
tractus horizontalis
and tractus verticalis)

A Overview of lymph nodes in the abdomen and pelvis

Anterior view of an opened female abdomen. All visceral structures have been removed except for major vessels, and the vasa lymphatica are shown larger for clarity. Size disparities between the nodi lymphoidei (1 mm to over 1 cm) and actual numbers (several hundred) are ignored. Nodi lymphoidei regionales (see **C**) may be arranged so densely that individual groups can scarcely be identified. Lymph nodes in the abdomen and pelvis are classified by their location as *parietal* or *visceral*. Nodi lymphoidei parietales are located *near* the *trunk wall* (often distributed along blood vessels), while nodi lymphoidei viscerales are located *near organs* in the connective tissue of the spatium extraperitoneale or in the mesenterium attached to an organ. A large percentage of nodi lymphoidei parietales are located on the posterior wall of the abdomen and pelvis: they are clustered around the large vessels that course on the posterior abdominal and pelvic walls, such as the aorta abdominalis and v. cava inferior in the abdomen and the aa. and vv. iliacae and their branches in the pelvis. Only a few nodi lymphoidei are located on the anterior wall, such as the nodi lymphoidei inguinales and the nodes around the a. iliaca externa (nodi iliaci). The lymph nodes and lymphatic vessels are arranged in an intricate network in the abdomen and pelvis, as they generally are elsewhere in the body. As a result, lymphatic drainage tends to follow multiple regional patterns of flow rather than a single well-defined pathway (see p. 222). Potential drainage routes are particularly numerous for the organs of the pelvis, where several organs may share lymphatic pathways. For example, certain lymph nodes are utilized (with varying degrees of preference) by the vesica urinaria, genital organs, and rectum.

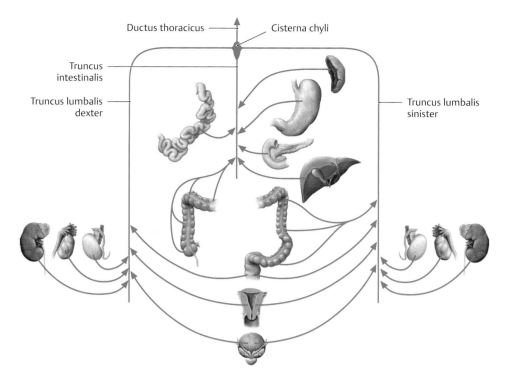

Ductus thoracicus — Cisterna chyli
Truncus intestinalis
Truncus lumbalis dexter
Truncus lumbalis sinister

B Trunci lymphatici in the abdomen and pelvis

Lymph from the abdominal and pelvic organs drains to the trunci lumbalis and intestinalis (see p. 222) after first passing through one or more lymph node groups (see **C**). An expansion, the cisterna chyli, is frequently present at the union of these trunks. Lymph from the cisterna chyli drains through the ductus thoracicus to the junction of the left vv. subclavia and jugularis interna. The ductus thoracicus is the principal lymphatic trunk that returns lymph to the venous system.

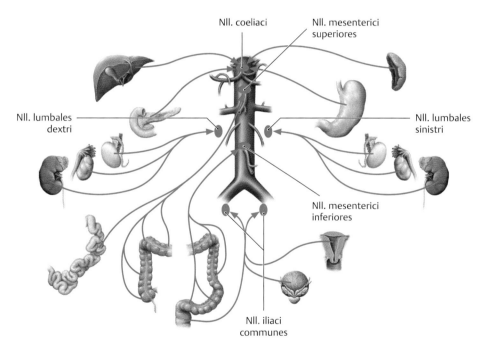

Nll. coeliaci
Nll. mesenterici superiores
Nll. lumbales dextri
Nll. lumbales sinistri
Nll. mesenterici inferiores
Nll. iliaci communes

C Nodus lymphoideus groups in the abdomen and pelvis

Before lymph from the organs of the abdomen and pelvis enters the trunci lymphatici, it is filtered by **lymph nodes** that collect the lymph from a particular organ (or region). After leaving the nodi regionales, the lymph drains to **collecting lymph nodes**. These are the nodes that collect lymph from several nodus lymphoideus groups and carry it to the trunci lymphatici. In the abdomen and pelvis, these are the trunci lumbalis and intestinalis.

Note: One nodus lymphoideus may function as a *nodus lymphoideus regionalis* for *various* organs, but at the same time it may collect lymph from several nodi regionales, functioning also as a *collecting nodus lymphoideus*. This principle is illustrated in the abdomen and pelvis by the nodi lymphoidei lumbales: They function as nodi lymphoidei regionales for the renes, gll. suprarenales, gonadae, and adnexa (see p. 314) and as collecting lymph nodes for the nodi iliaces.

D Nodus lymphoideus groups and tributary regions

Nodus lymphoideus groups and collecting lymph nodes	Location (see **C**)	Organs or organ segments that drain to these nodus lymphoideus groups (tributary regions)
Nll. coeliaci	Around the truncus coeliacus	Distal third of oesophagus, gaster, omentum majus, duodenum (partes superior and descendens), pancreas, splen, hepar, and vesica biliaris
Nll. mesenterici superiores	At the origin of the a. mesenterica superior	Second through fourth parts of duodenum, jejunum and ileum, caecum with appendix vermiformis, colon ascendens, colon transversum (proximal two-thirds)
Nll. mesenterici inferiores	At the origin of the a. mesenterica inferior	Colon transversum (distal third), colon descendens, colon sigmoideum, rectum (proximal part)
Nll. lumbales (dextri, intermedi, sinistri)	Around the pars abdominalis aortae and v. cava inferior	Diaphragma (abdominal side), renes, gll. suprarenales, testis and epididymis, ovarium, tuba uterina, fundus uteri, ureteres, retroperitoneum
Nll. iliaci	Around the aa. and vv. iliacae	Rectum (anal end), vesica urinaria and urethra, uterus (corpus and cervix), ductus deferens, vesica seminalis, prostata, external genitalia (via nll. inguinales)

2.7 Overview of the Lymphatic Drainage of Abdominal and Pelvic Organs

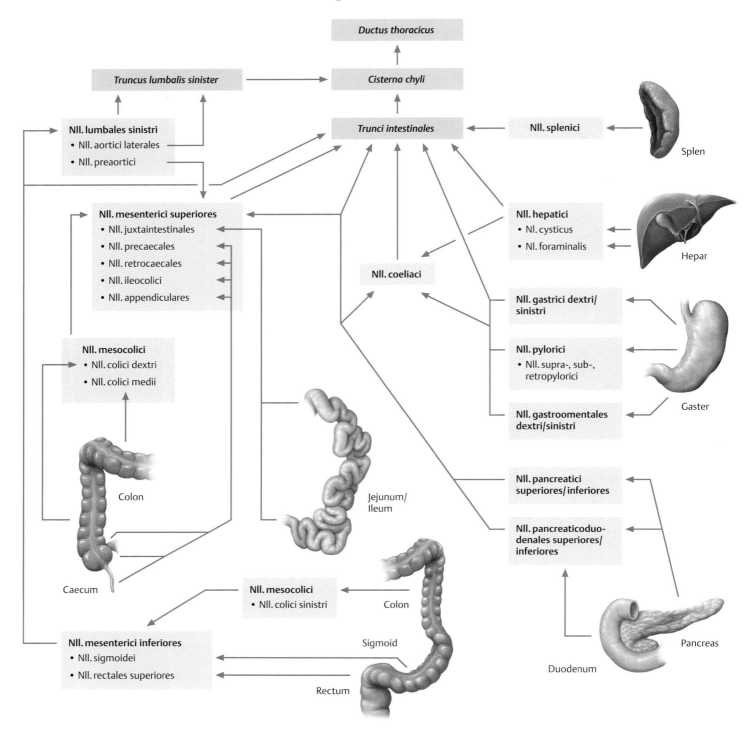

A Principal lymphatic pathways draining the digestive organs and splen

Lymph from the splen and most of the digestive organs drains directly from regional lymph nodes or through intervening collecting lymph nodes to the *trunci intestinales*. Exceptions are the colon descendens, colon sigmoideum, and the upper part of the rectum, which are drained by the *left truncus lumbalis*. The organs and nodi lymphoidei viscerales in the above schematic are served mainly by three large collecting stations (individual lymph nodes see p. 280 ff):

• Nll. coeliaci: collect lymph from the gaster, duodenum, pancreas, splen, and hepar. Topographically and at dissection, they are often indistinguishable from the nodi lymphoidei regionales of nearby upper abdominal organs.

• Nll. mesenterici superiores: collect lymph from the jejunum, ileum, colon ascendens, and colon transversum.

• Nll. mesenterici inferiores: collect lymph from the colon descendens, colon sigmoideum, and rectum.

These collecting lymph nodes drain *principally* through the trunci intestinales to the cisterna chyli. There is also an *accessory* drainage route to the cisterna chyli by way of the nll. lumbales sinistri.

The lymphatic drainage of the rectum is described on p. 283.

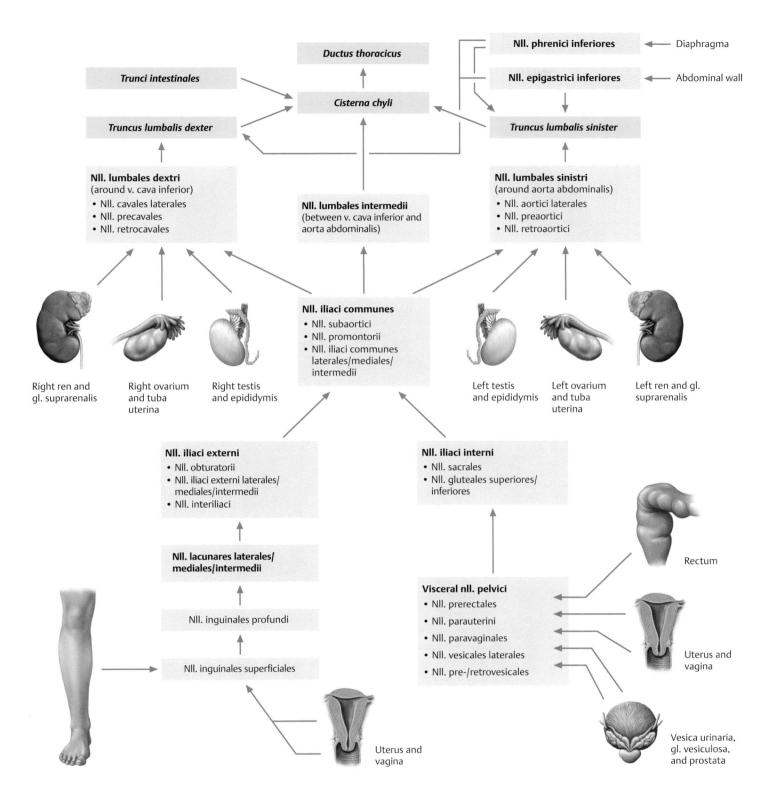

B Principal lymphatic pathways draining the organs of the retroperitoneum and pelvis (and lower limb)

Lymph from these organs drains principally to the right and left trunci lumbales. The following are important nodus lymphoideus groups for the organs of the retroperitoneum and pelvis (and lower limb):

- Nll. iliaci communes: collect lymph from the pelvic organs and lower limb.
- Nll. lumbales dextri and sinistri: collecting nodi for the nodi iliaci communes, also nodi lymphoidei regionales for the organs of the retroperitoneum *and* the gonadae, although the latter are located in the pelvis or scrotum. As the gonadae undergo their developmental descent, they maintain their lymphatic connection to the nodi lumbales (analogous to their blood supply, see p. 350). As a result, when tumors of the testis (or ovarium), for example, undergo lymphogenous spread, they tend to metastasize directly to the abdomen rather than to the pelvis.

Both the nll. iliaci and the nll. lumbales are classified as nodi lymphoidei *parietales*, a category that includes the nll. phrenici and epigastrici inferiores. Lymph nodes such as the nll. pararectales and nll. parauterini are classified as nodi lymphoidei *viscerales*.

2.8 Autonomic Ganglia and Plexuses

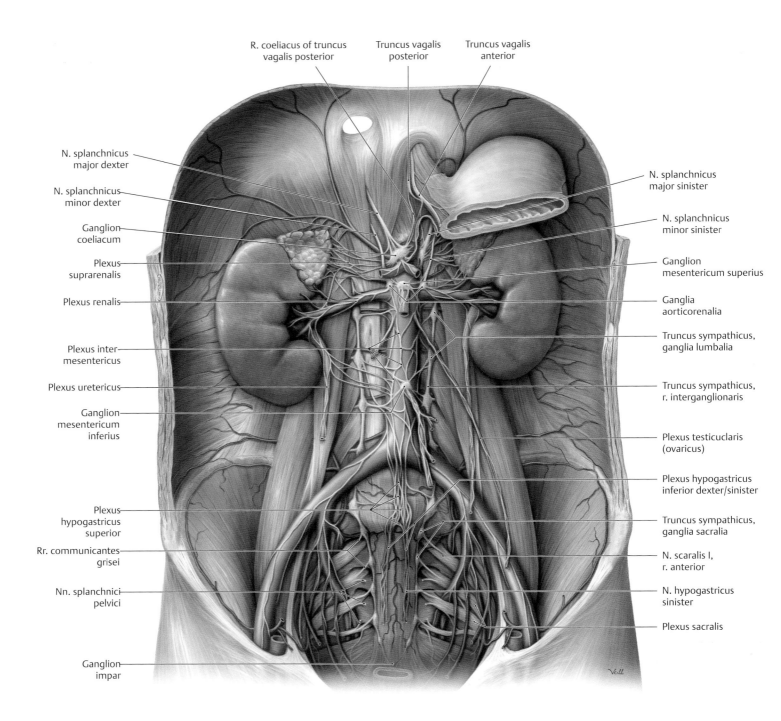

R. coeliacus of truncus vagalis posterior

Truncus vagalis posterior

Truncus vagalis anterior

N. splanchnicus major dexter

N. splanchnicus minor dexter

Ganglion coeliacum

Plexus suprarenalis

Plexus renalis

Plexus intermesentericus

Plexus uretericus

Ganglion mesentericum inferius

Plexus hypogastricus superior

Rr. communicantes grisei

Nn. splanchnici pelvici

Ganglion impar

N. splanchnicus major sinister

N. splanchnicus minor sinister

Ganglion mesentericum superius

Ganglia aorticorenalia

Truncus sympathicus, ganglia lumbalia

Truncus sympathicus, r. interganglionaris

Plexus testicuclaris (ovaricus)

Plexus hypogastricus inferior dexter/sinister

Truncus sympathicus, ganglia sacralia

N. scaralis I, r. anterior

N. hypogastricus sinister

Plexus sacralis

A Overview of ganglia autonomica and plexus autonomici in the abdomen and pelvis

Anterior view of an opened male abdomen and pelvis with all of the peritoneum removed. Almost all of the gaster has been removed, and the gastric stump and oesophagus have been pulled slightly inferior. The pelvic organs have been removed except for a rectal stump. The autonomic nervous system forms extensive *plexuses* and a number of *ganglia* around the aorta abdominalis and within the pelvis, the ganglia marking the sites where the first presynaptic neuron synapses with the second postsynaptic neuron. All of the plexus autonomici in front of and alongside the pars abdominalis aortae are collectively termed the *plexus aorticus abdominalis*. This structure also includes the individual plexuses located at the origins of the paired and unpaired branches of

the aorta abdominalis (see **B**). As a general rule, sympathetic and parasympathetic nerve fibers come together in the plexuses on their way to the target organ.

Note: The left and right nn. vagi are organized around the oesophagus to form the trunci vagales anterior and posterior. Both trunci contain fibers from both nn. vagi, the truncus vagalis *anterior* containing more fibers from the left n. vagus, the truncus vagalis *posterior* containing more fibers from the right n. vagus. While the truncus vagalis anterior generally terminates at the gaster, the truncus vagalis posterior goes on to supply the entire intestinum tenue and the intestinum crassum approximately to the junction of the middle and distal thirds of the colon transversum.

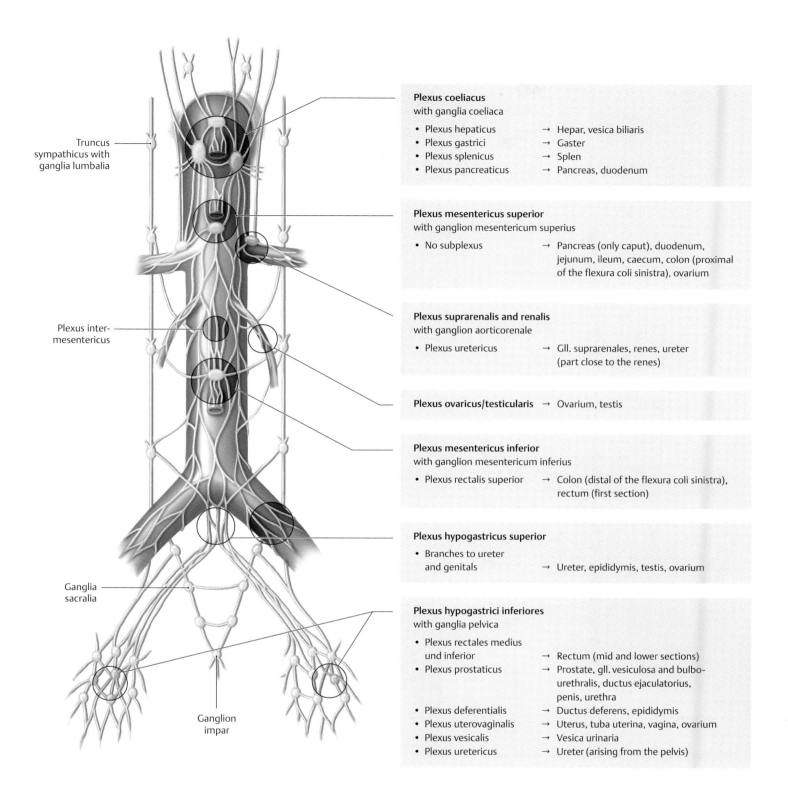

Plexus coeliacus
with ganglia coeliaca

- Plexus hepaticus → Hepar, vesica biliaris
- Plexus gastrici → Gaster
- Plexus splenicus → Splen
- Plexus pancreaticus → Pancreas, duodenum

Plexus mesentericus superior
with ganglion mesentericum superius

- No subplexus → Pancreas (only caput), duodenum, jejunum, ileum, caecum, colon (proximal of the flexura coli sinistra), ovarium

Plexus suprarenalis and renalis
with ganglion aorticorenale

- Plexus uretericus → Gll. suprarenales, renes, ureter (part close to the renes)

Plexus ovaricus/testicularis → Ovarium, testis

Plexus mesentericus inferior
with ganglion mesentericum inferius

- Plexus rectalis superior → Colon (distal of the flexura coli sinistra), rectum (first section)

Plexus hypogastricus superior

- Branches to ureter and genitals → Ureter, epididymis, testis, ovarium

Plexus hypogastrici inferiores
with ganglia pelvica

- Plexus rectales medius und inferior → Rectum (mid and lower sections)
- Plexus prostaticus → Prostate, gll. vesiculosa and bulbo-urethralis, ductus ejaculatorius, penis, urethra
- Plexus deferentialis → Ductus deferens, epididymis
- Plexus uterovaginalis → Uterus, tuba uterina, vagina, ovarium
- Plexus vesicalis → Vesica urinaria
- Plexus uretericus → Ureter (arising from the pelvis)

Truncus sympathicus with ganglia lumbalia

Plexus inter-mesentericus

Ganglia sacralia

Ganglion impar

B Organization of ganglia autonomica and plexus autonomici in the abdomen and pelvis

The ganglia and plexuses of the autonomic nervous system are named for the arteries that they accompany or around which they are distributed (e.g., the ganglion coeliacum and plexus mesentericus). In the pars *sympathica* of the nervous system, the presynaptic neuron synapses with the postsynaptic neuron in ganglia *distant* from the organs (or ganglion cells in a plexus distant from the organs); in the pars *parasympathica* of the nervous system, this synapse occurs in ganglia *near* the organs (or ganglion cells in a plexus near the organs). Thus, the ganglia parasympathica are usually located on the target organ or in its wall, where they receive branches from the trunci vagales or nn. splanchnici pelvici. *Note:* Even plexuses may contain aggregations of ganglion cells, sometimes very small. An example is the plexus renalis, which contains the ganglia renalia (too small to be shown in the drawing).

The plexus autonomici contain efferent (visceromotor) fibers as well as numerous afferent (viscerosensory) fibers for both their sympathetic and parasympathetic components.

2.9 Organization of the Partes Sympathica and Parasympathica of the Nervous System

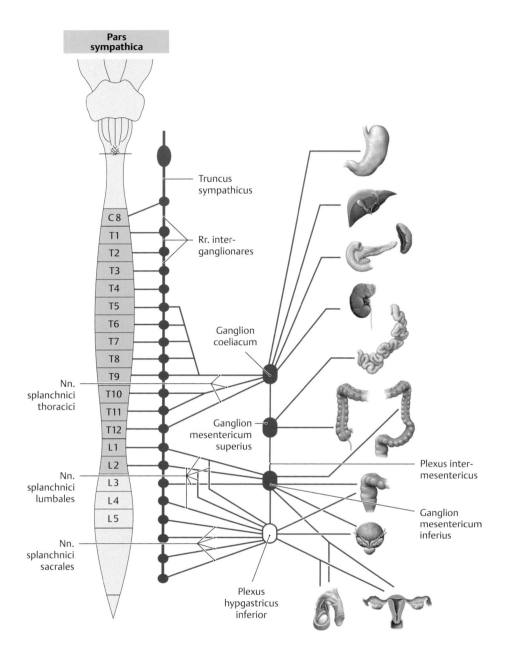

Pars sympathica

Truncus sympathicus

C 8
T1
T2
T3
T4
T5
T6
T7
T8
T9
T10
T11
T12
L1
L2
L3
L4
L5

Rr. inter-ganglionares

Nn. splanchnici thoracici

Nn. splanchnici lumbales

Nn. splanchnici sacrales

Ganglion coeliacum

Ganglion mesentericum superius

Ganglion mesentericum inferius

Plexus inter-mesentericus

Plexus hypgastricus inferior

B Effects of the pars sympathica of the nervous system on organs in the abdomen and pelvis

Organ, organ system	Pars sympathica effects
• Gastrointestinal tract	
– Longitudinal and circular muscle fibers	Decreased motility
– Sphincter muscles	Contraction
– Glands	Decreased secretions
• Capsula splenis	Contraction
• Hepar	Increased glycogenolysis/ gluconeogenesis
• Pancreas	
– Endocrine pancreas	Decreased insulin secretion
– Exocrine pancreas	Decreased secretion
• Vesica urinaria	
– M. detrusor vesicae	Relaxation
– Functional bladder sphincter	Contraction
• Vesicula seminalis	Contraction (ejaculation)
• Ductus deferens	Contraction (ejaculation)
• Uterus	Contraction or relaxation, depending on hormonal status
• Arteries	Vasoconstriction

A Organization of the pars sympathica of the nervous system in the abdomen and pelvis

The first, or presynaptic, neurons of the pars sympathica that supply the **organs of the abdomen** are located in the cornua lateralia of segmenta T5–T12 medullae spinalis. Their presynaptic axons pass *without synapsing* through the ganglia of the truncus sympathicus and form the thoracic splanchnic nerves (nn. splanchnici major and minor, and occasionally a n. splanchnicus imus from T 12). The *synapse with the second, or postsysnaptic, neuron* is located in the ganglion coeliacum, the ganglion mesentericum superius (or inferius), or the ganglion aorticorenale (see p. 287).

The first, or presynaptic, neurons of the pars sympathica that supply the **organs of the pelvis** are located in the cornua lateralia of segmenta L1 and L2 medullae spinalis. Their presynaptic axons pass through the ganglia lumbalia of the truncus sympathicus and form the nn. splanchnici lumbales. The *synapse with the second, or postsynaptic, neuron* may be located in the ganglia lumbalia, ganglion mesentericum inferius, or

plexus hypogastricus inferior. Beyond that point the postsynaptic fibers of the postsynaptic neuron generally pass to the target organ with its artery, usually accompanied by parasympathetic fibers of the autonomic nervous system.

Note: The peripheral ganglia of the pars sympathica of the nervous system are distributed along the sides of the columna vertebralis (paravertebral). Peripheral ganglia in the abdomen and pelvis are also placed anterior to the columna vertebralis (prevertebral) and os sacrum.

The paravertebral ganglia are interconnected by interganglionic connections to form the truncus sympathicus—two long pathways extending along each side of the columna vertebralis. The ganglia are named for the corresponding levels of the spine (ganglia thoracica, ganglia lumbalia, etc.) and are variable in number. The prevertebral ganglia are located at the origins of the major arteries from the aorta abdominalis and are named accordingly (ganglion coeliacum, ganglia mesenterica superius and inferius, etc.).

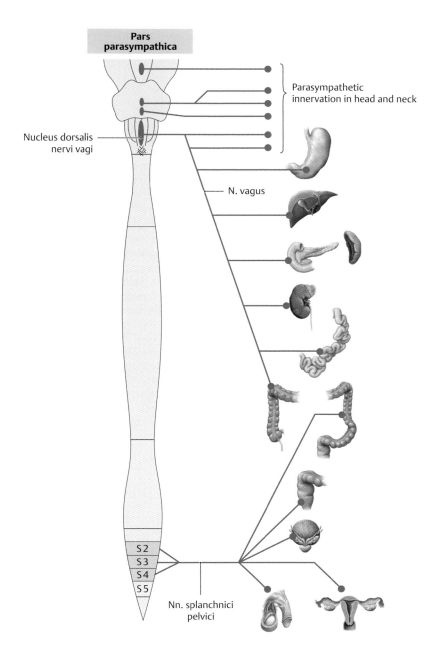

Pars parasympathica

Nucleus dorsalis nervi vagi

Parasympathetic innervation in head and neck

N. vagus

S2
S3
S4
S5

Nn. splanchnici pelvici

D Effects of the pars parasympathica of the nervous system on organs in the abdomen and pelvis

Organ, organ system	Pars parasympathica effects
• Gastrointestinal tract	
– *Longitudinal and circular muscle fibers*	Increased motility
– *Sphincter muscles*	Relaxation
– *Glands*	Increased secretions
• Capsula splenis	–
• Hepar	–
• Pancreas	
– *Endocrine pancreas*	–
– *Exocrine pancreas*	Increased secretion
• Vesica urinaria	
– *M. detrusor vesicae*	Contraction
– *Functional bladder sphincter*	–
• Vesicula seminalis	–
• Ductus deferens	–
• Uterus	–
• Arteries	Vasodilation of the arteries in the penis or clitoris (erection)

Note the special role played by the suprarenal medulla and kidneys: the suprarenal medulla is phylogenetically and functionally analogous to a "sympathetic ganglion." It is thus part of the sympathetic nervous system and is therefore not listed in this table. The renal vessels are not regulated by the sympathetic or parasympathetic nervous systems, but by autoregulation (occurs only for renal blood flow). For functional reasons, the kidneys self-regulate renal blood pressure.

C Organization of the pars parasympathica of the nervous system in the abdomen and pelvis

Contrasting with the thoracolumbar organization of the pars sympathica of the nervous system, the pars parasympathica in the abdomen and pelvis consists of *two topographically distinct systems*: a pars cranialis and a pars pelvica. This system also differs from the pars sympathica in that the synapse of the first, or presynaptic, neuron with the second or postsynaptic neuron is located in the intramural ganglia of the organ walls.

• **Pars cranialis of the pars parasympathica in the abdomen and pelvis:** The presynaptic neuron is located in the nucleus posterior nervi vagi (i.e., the nucleus of n. cranialis X in the medulla oblongata). The axons (presynaptic nerve fibers) course with the n. vagus to visceral or intramural ganglia, where they synapse with the postsynaptic neuron. The *distribution* of the pars cranialis includes the gaster, hepar, vesica biliaris, pancreas, duodenum, ren, gl. suprarenalis, intestinum tenue, and the intestinum crassum from the colon ascendens to near the flexura coli sinistra.

• **Pars pelvica of the pars parasympathica in the abdomen and pelvis:** Its origin is located in the cornua lateralia of segmenta S2–S4 medullae spinalis (sacral nucleus intermediolateralis). The axons (presynaptic nerve fibers) run a very short distance with nn. spinales S2–S4, then separate from them and course as the nn. splanchnici pelvici to ganglion cells in the plexus hypogastricus inferior or organ wall, where they synapse with the postsynaptic neuron. The *distribution* of the pars pelvica of the pars parasympathica of the nervous system in the abdomen and pelvis includes flexura coli sinistra, the colon descendens and sigmoideum, rectum, canalis analis, vesica urinaria, urethra, and the internal and external genitalia.

3.1 Gaster: Location, Shape, Divisions, and Interior View

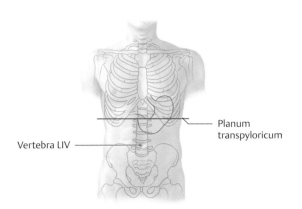

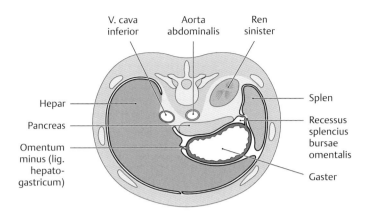

A Projection onto the trunk

Anterior view.

The gaster is intraperitoneal and located in the left upper quadrant (epigastrium).

Note the planum transpyloricum (halfway between the superior border of the symphysis pubica and superior border of the manubrium sterni, see p. 360). It serves as an important anatomical landmark: the pylorus is located at or slightly below the planum transpyloricum. Unlike other parts of the gaster, the pylorus hardly moves at all since it is connected to the duodenum, which is retroperitoneal (and thus relatively immobile).

B Topographical relationships

Transverse section at approximately the T12/L1 level. Viewed from above.

Note the relationship of the gaster to the splen, pancreas, hepar, and bursa omentalis: The curvatura major extends to the splen; the lobus hepatis sinister extends in front of the gaster and into the left upper quadrant. When the abdomen is opened, very little of the gaster is visible as most of it is obscured by the hepar. Posterior to the gaster lies a narrow peritoneal space called the bursa omentalis. Its posterior wall is largely formed by the pancreas. Due to its peritoneal covering, the gaster is very mobile relative to the neighboring organs. This is important for facilitating the gaster's peristaltic movements. Due to its embryonic placement in the mesogastrium ventrale and dorsale (see p. 42), the gaster has direct peritoneal attachments to the splen and hepar.

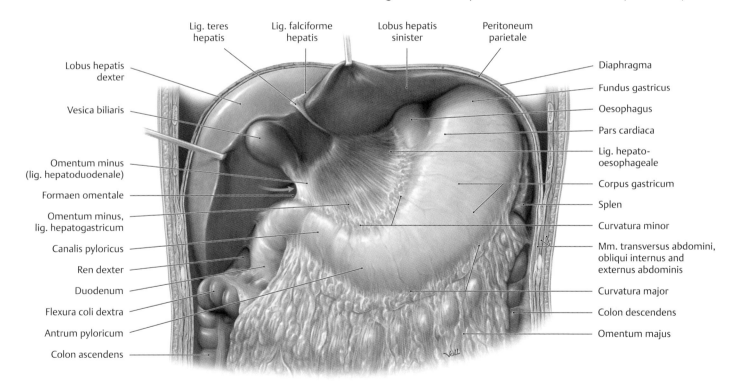

C The gaster in situ

Anterior view of the opened upper abdomen. The hepar has been retracted superolaterally, and the oesophagus has been pulled slightly downward for better exposure. The arrow points to the foramen omentale, the opening in the bursa omentalis behind the omentum minus. Peritoneal adhesions are visible between the hepar and the pars descendens duodeni. The omentum minus is visibly subdivided into a relatively thick lig. hepatoduodenale (transmitting neurovascular structures to the porta hepatis) and a thinner lig. hepatogastricum, which is attached to the curvatura minor of the gaster. A lig. hepatooesophageale can also be identified. The curvatura major of the gaster is closely related to the splen in the left upper quadrant (LUQ). The omentum majus is a duplication of peritoneum that covers the colon transversum and drapes over the loops of intestinum tenue (not visible here).

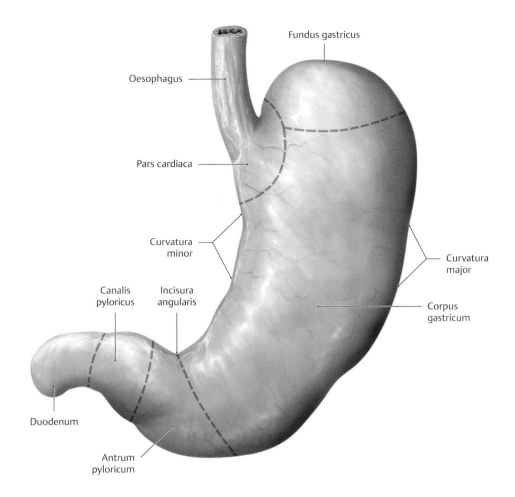

D Shape and anatomical divisions
Anterior view of the paries anterior. The body (corpus) of the gaster is the largest part of the gaster. It terminates blindly at the fundus gastricus, which in the standing patient is the highest part of the gaster and is usually filled with air (visible on radiographs as the "gastric bubble").

Note: The cardia is the area of the gastric inlet where the oesophagus opens into the gaster (at the ostium cardiacum). While the oesophagus is invested by adventitial connective tissue (tunica adventitia), the gaster has a visceral peritoneal covering or tunica serosa. The transition from tunica adventitia to tunica serosa is sharply defined, and occasionally the tunica serosa continues a short distance onto the lower end of the oesophagus.

The part of the gaster that opens into the duodenum, the pars pylorica, consists of a broad antrum pyloricum, a narrow canalis pyloricus, and the pylorus itself (ostium pyloricum). The stratum circulare of the tunica muscularis of the gaster is markedly thickened at the end of the canalis pyloricus to form the m. sphincter pyloricus (not visible here), which produces a visible external constriction of the canalis pyloricus.

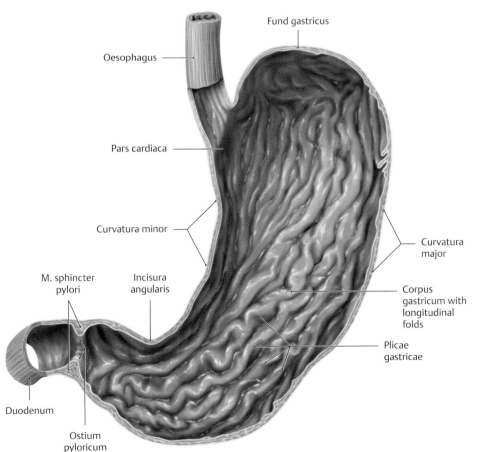

E Interior of the gaster
Anterior view of the gaster with the paries anterior removed. For clarity, small portions of the oesophagus and duodenum are also shown. The gastric tunica mucosa forms prominent folds (plicae gastricae) that serve to increase its surface area. These folds are directed longitudinally toward the pylorus, forming "canales gastrici." The plicae gastricae are most prominent in the corpus gastricum and along the curvatura major and diminish in size toward the pyloric end. The tunica mucosa imparts a glossy sheen to the stomach lining.

Note: The ostium pyloricum is quite large in this dissection. Normally, the orifice usually opens to a luminal diameter of only 2–3 mm.

229

3.2 Gaster: Wall Structure and Histology

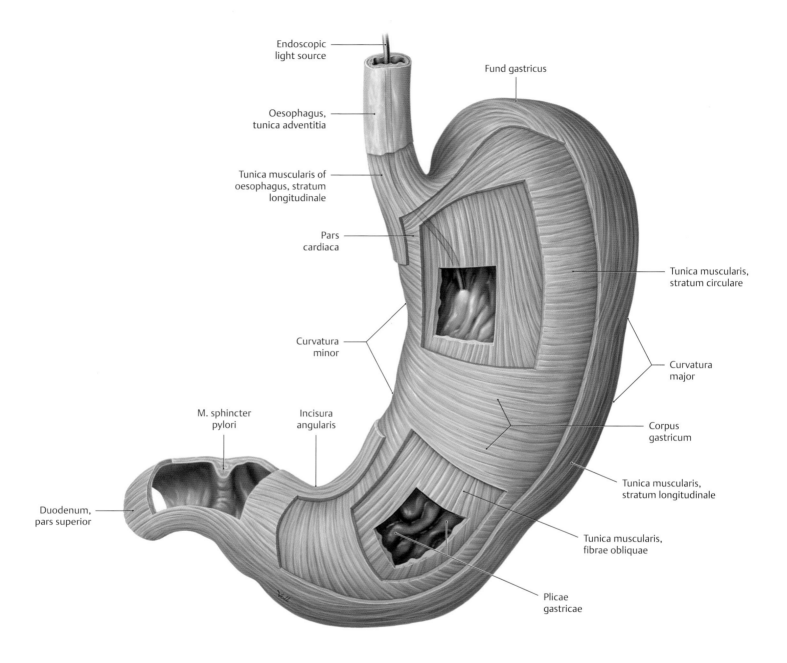

Endoscopic light source

Fund gastricus

Oesophagus, tunica adventitia

Tunica muscularis of oesophagus, stratum longitudinale

Pars cardiaca

Tunica muscularis, stratum circulare

Curvatura minor

Curvatura major

M. sphincter pylori

Incisura angularis

Corpus gastricum

Duodenum, pars superior

Tunica muscularis, stratum longitudinale

Tunica muscularis, fibrae obliquae

Plicae gastricae

A Muscular layers

Anterior view of the paries anterior gastricus with the tunica serosa and tela subserosa removed. The tunica muscularis of the gaster has been windowed at several sites. The *entire stomach wall* ranges from 3 mm to approximately 10 mm in thickness (see **B** for individual layers). Most of its tunica muscularis consists not of two layers (as in other hollow organs of the gastrointestinal tract) but of *three* muscular layers:

- An outer stratum longitudinale, which is most pronounced along the curvatura major (greatest longitudinal expansion)
- A middle stratum circulare, which is well developed in the corpus gastricum and most strongly developed in the canalis pyloricus (anular m. sphincter pyloricus, see p. 229)

- An innermost layer of fibrae obliquae, which is derived from the stratum circulare and is clearly visible in the corpus gastricum.

The three-layered structure of its muscular wall enables the gaster to undergo powerful churning movements. The muscles can forcefully propel solid food components against the gastric wall in the acidic gastric juice, breaking the material up into particles approximately 1 mm in size that can pass easily through the pylorus. The longitudinally oriented plicae gastricae (reserve folds that disappear when the gaster is distended) form channels, called canales gastrici, that rapidly convey liquids from the gastric inlet to the pylorus.

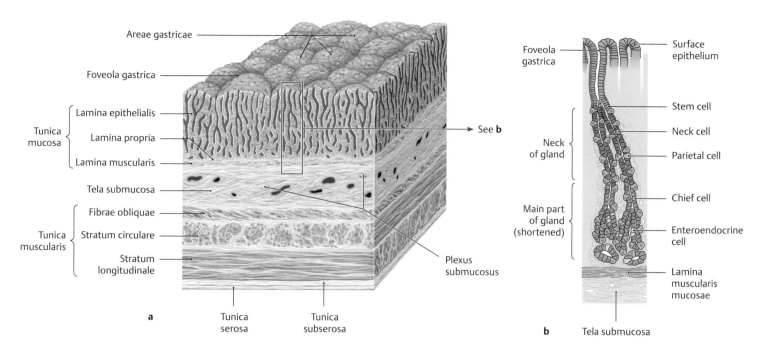

a

Tunica serosa	Tunica subserosa

b   Tela submucosa

B Structure of the gaster wall and gll. gastricae

a The **structure of the gaster wall** illustrates the layered wall structure that is typical of the hollow organs throughout the gastrointestinal tract. The gaster is unique, however, in that its tunica muscularis consists of three rather than two layers (see **A**).

Note: The tunica serosa (visceral layer of the peritoneum) and tela subserosa (connective-tissue layer giving attachment to the tunica serosa and transmitting neurovascular structures for the tunica muscularis) are present only in areas where the organ in question is covered by peritoneum viscerale. In wall areas that lack a peritoneal covering (e.g., large portions of the duodenum and colon), the tunica serosa and tela subserosa are replaced by a fibrous tunica adventitia, which connects the wall of the organ to the connective tissue of surrounding structures.

The *tunica mucosa* contains specialized cells that are aggregated into *glandulae* (visible microscopically). The glandular *orifices* open at the base of the foveolae gastricae (see **b**). In the corpus and pylorus of the gaster these glands extend down to the muscular layer of the mucosa, the lamina muscularis mucosae (deeper glands = more cells = higher secretory output). The *tela submucosa* (layer of connective tissue transmitting neurovascular structures for the tunica muscularis) contains the *plexus submucosus* for visceromotor and

viscerosensory control of the hollow organs in the gastrointestinal tract. This plexus, like the *plexus myentericus* (located in the tunica mucosa for visceromotor control of the visceral muscle, not shown here), is part of the *enteric* nervous system (plexus entericus), which contains, in total, millions of scattered ganglion cells.

b **Structure of the gll. gastricae** (after Lüllmann-Rauch) (simplified schematic of a gland from the corpus gastricum). Several types of cells are distinguished in the fundus and corpus gastricum:

- Surface epithelial cells: cover the surface of the tunica mucosa and secrete a mucous film.
- Neck cells: produce mucin to strengthen the mucous film (make it more anionic).
- Parietal cells: produce HCl and intrinsic factor, which is necessary for vitamin B_{12} absorption in the ileum.
- Chief cells: produce pepsinogen, which is converted to pepsin (for protein breakdown) in the stomach.
- Enteroendocrine cells: different subtypes producing gastrin (G cells), somatostatin (D cells), or other factors controlling motility and secretion
- Stem cells: reservoir for replenishing the surface epithelial cells and gland cells

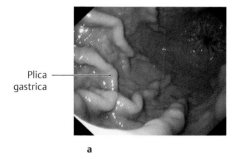

a

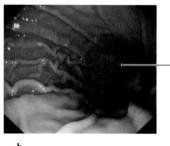

b

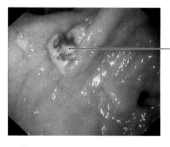

c

C Endoscopic appearance of the gastric tunica mucosa

a, b Healthy gastric tunica mucosa with a glistening surface; **c** Gastric ulcer.

a View into the corpus gastricum, which has been moderately distended by air insufflation. The tunica mucosa is raised into prominent, tortuous plicae gastricae that form the canales gastrici.

b Inspection of the antrum pyloricum shows less prominent folds than in the corpus gastricum.

c Fibrin-covered gastric ulcer with hematin spots. A gastric ulcer is defined as a tissue defect that extends at least into the lamina muscularis mucosae, but many ulcers extend much deeper into the stomach wall. Most gastric ulcers are caused by infection with *Helicobacter pylori*, a bacterium that is resistant to stomach acid (from Block, Schachschal, and Schmidt: *The Gastroscopy Trainer.* Stuttgart: Thieme, 2004).

231

3.3 Intestinum Tenue: Duodenum

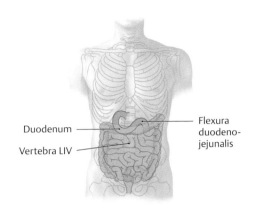

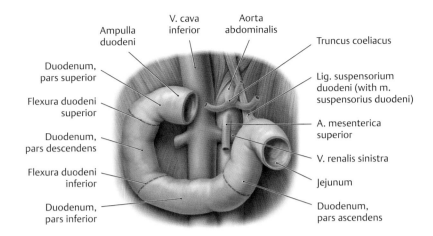

A Projected onto the columna vertebralis

The duodenum is a C-shaped loop of intestinum tenue lying predominantly on the right side of the columna vertebralis in the right upper quadrant (RUQ) and encompassing the L1 through L3 vertebrae and occasionally extending to L4. The concavity of the duodenum normally encloses the caput pancreatis at the L2 level (see **D**).

B Parts of the duodenum

Anterior view. The anatomical parts of the duodenum (partes superior, descendens, horizontalis, and ascendens with intervening flexures) have a total length of approximately 12 fingerwidths (L. *duodeni* = "twelve at a time"). *Note* the lig. suspensorium duodeni (called also the ligament of Treitz), which often

contains smooth-muscle fibers. Mobile loops of intestinum tenue may wrap around this ligament and become entrapped between the ligament and the vessels behind it (most notably the pars abdominalis aortae). This "Treitz hernia" may cause mechanical obstruction of the affected bowel loop and strangulate its blood supply.

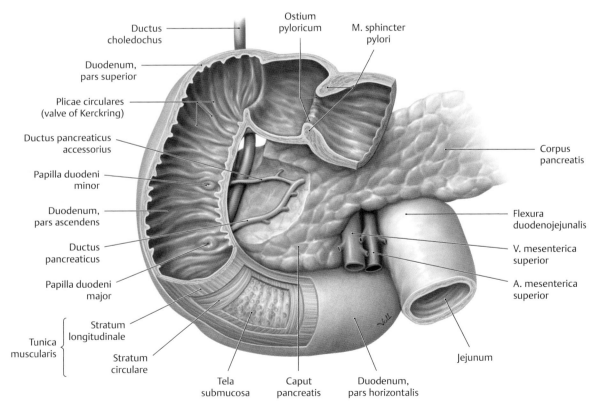

C Wall structure and duct orifices

Anterior view. Most of the duodenum has been opened. The ostium pyloricum (here greatly dilated) opens to a luminal diameter of only about 2–3 mm for the passage of chyme. The duodenum has basically the same wall structure as the other hollow organs of the gastrointestinal tract (see **B**, p. 231). The structure of the tunica mucosa is shown in **F**. The pars descendens of the duodenum has two small elevations

along its inner curve: the papilla duodeni minor, which bears the orifice of the ductus pancreaticus accessorius, and the papilla duodeni major (called also the papilla of Vater), which has a common orifice for the ductus pancreaticus and ductus choledochus. Thus, the release of bile and pancreatic juice to aid digestion takes place in the upper part of the duodenum.

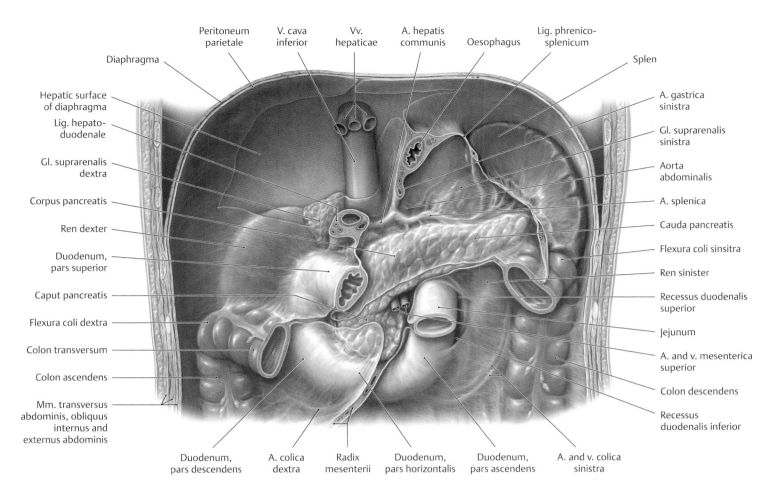

Labels (clockwise from top):
Peritoneum parietale · V. cava inferior · Vv. hepaticae · A. hepatis communis · Oesophagus · Lig. phrenico-splenicum

Diaphragma

Splen

Hepatic surface of diaphragma

A. gastrica sinistra

Lig. hepato-duodenale

Gl. suprarenalis sinistra

Gl. suprarenalis dextra

Aorta abdominalis

Corpus pancreatis

A. splenica

Ren dexter

Cauda pancreatis

Duodenum, pars superior

Flexura coli sinsitra

Caput pancreatis

Ren sinister

Flexura coli dextra

Recessus duodenalis superior

Colon transversum

Jejunum

Colon ascendens

A. and v. mesenterica superior

Mm. transversus abdominis, obliquus internus and externus abdominis

Colon descendens

Recessus duodenalis inferior

Duodenum, pars descendens · A. colica dextra · Radix mesenterii · Duodenum, pars horizontalis · Duodenum, pars ascendens · A. and v. colica sinistra

D The duodenum in situ

Anterior view. The gaster, hepar, intestinum tenue, and large portions of the colon transversum have been removed. The retroperitoneal fat and connective tissue, including the capsula adiposa, have been substantially thinned. The caput pancreatis lies in the concavity of the C-shaped loop of the duodenum. The first 2 cm of the pars superior of the duodenum is still intraperitoneal (attached to the hepar by the lig. hepatoduodenale), but most of the duodenum is retroperitoneal. Owing largely to the proximity of the duodenum and the caput pancreatis, lesions of the pancreas (tumors) or malformations (anular pancreas) may cause duodenal obstruction. The peritoneum at the duodenojejunal junction forms the recessus duodenales superior and inferior. Mobile loops of intestinum tenue may enter these peritoneal recesses and become entrapped there (*internal hernia*), causing a potentially life-threatening bowel obstruction.

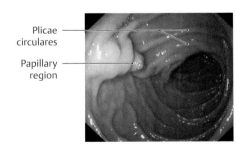

Plicae circulares

Papillary region

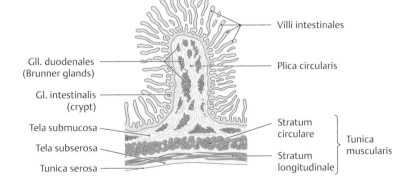

Villi intestinales

Gll. duodenales (Brunner glands)

Plica circularis

Gl. intestinalis (crypt)

Tela submucosa

Stratum circulare ⎫ Tunica muscularis

Tela subserosa

Stratum longitudinale ⎭

Tunica serosa

E Endoscopic view

The endoscope is pointing down into the pars descendens of the duodenum. The papillary region where the ductus biliaris and ductus pancreaticus open into the duodenum is visible on the left side of the image at approximately the 10 o'clock position. The plicae circulares (valves of Kerckring) are typical of those found in the intestinum tenue, diminishing in size in the proximal to distal direction (from Block, Schachschal, and Schmidt: *Endoscopy of the Upper G I Tract.* Stuttgart: Thieme, 2004).

F Histological structure

Longitudinal section through the duodenal wall. The duodenum has basically the same histological structure as the other hollow organs of the gastrointestinal tract (see **B**, p. 231), with some notable differences such as the presence of gll. duodenales (Brunner) (secrete mucins and bicarbonate to neutralize the acidic gastric juice) and valves of Kerckring (specialized plicae circulares). Other features that distinguish the duodenum from the jejunum and ileum are its more prominent mucosal folds, which diminish in size toward the end of the intestinum tenue.

Note: The tunica muscularis externa of *all* portions of the intestinum, unlike that of the gaster, consists of only two layers: an inner stratum circulare and an outer stratum longitudinale.

233

3.4 Intestinum Tenue: Jejunum and Ileum

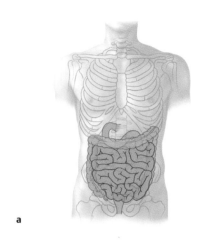

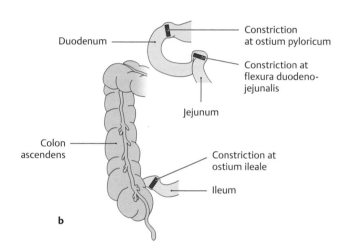

a

b

A Parts of the intestinum tenue: overview (a) and anatomical constrictions (b)
Anterior view. The intestinum crassum surrounds the loops of intestinum tenue like a frame. Because the intestinum tenue loops are intraperitoneal and therefore very mobile, it is not possible to define their location by reference to skeletal landmarks. If the intestinal loop rotates normally during embryonic development (see p. 46), the duodenum lies *behind* the colon transversum. If the intestinal loop rotates in the wrong direction, the duodenum will come to lie *in front* of the colon transversum.
Note the following normal anatomical constrictions:

- Junction of the pylorus and duodenum (luminal diameter of the ostium pyloricum is only about 2–3 mm)
- Flexura duodenojejunalis
- Ostum ileale

Swallowed foreign bodies may become lodged at these sites, obstructing intestinal transit and causing mechanical intestinal paralysis (*mechanical ileus*, a life-threatening condition that is an absolute indication for surgical treatment).

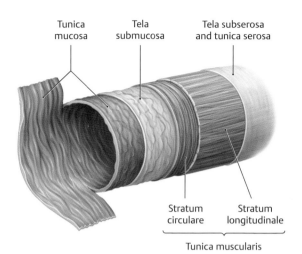

B Wall structure of the jejunum and ileum
The wall layers of the intestinum tenue are displayed in a "telescoped" cross-section. The tunica mucosa has been incised longitudinally and opened. The jejunum and ileum have basically the same wall structure as the other hollow organs of the gastrointestinal tract (see **B**, p. 231), but local differences are observed in the plicae circulares (see **C**) and vascular supply (see p. 268).

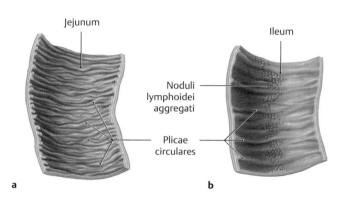

a   **b**

C Differences in the wall structure of the jejunum and ileum
Macroscopic views of the jejunum (**a**) and ileum (**b**), which have been opened longitudinally to display their mucosal surface anatomy.
Note: The transversely oriented plicae circulares in the jejunum are spaced much closer together than in the ileum. Lymphatic follicles are particularly abundant in the wall of the ileum (from the lamina propria to the tela submucosa) for mounting an immune response to antigens in the intestinal contents (noduli lymphoidei aggregati, Peyer's patches).

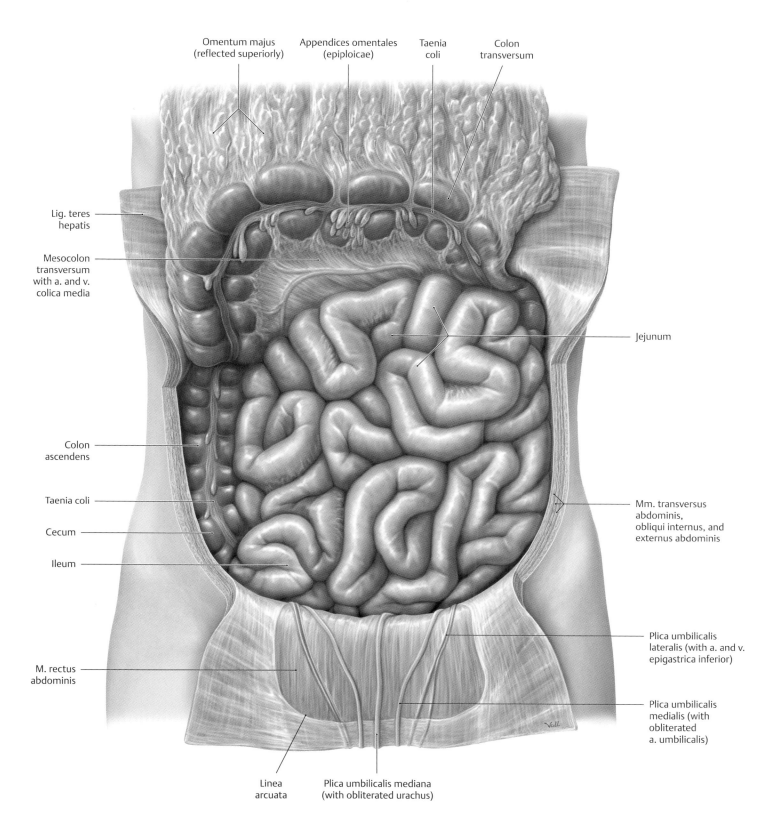

Omentum majus
(reflected superiorly)

Appendices omentales
(epiploicae)

Taenia
coli

Colon
transversum

Lig. teres
hepatis

Mesocolon
transversum
with a. and v.
colica media

Jejunum

Colon
ascendens

Taenia coli

Mm. transversus
abdominis,
obliqui internus, and
externus abdominis

Cecum

Ileum

Plica umbilicalis
lateralis (with a. and v.
epigastrica inferior)

M. rectus
abdominis

Plica umbilicalis
medialis (with
obliterated
a. umbilicalis)

Linea
arcuata

Plica umbilicalis mediana
(with obliterated urachus)

D The jejunum and ileum in situ

Anterior view. The abdominal wall has been opened and the colon transversum has been reflected upward. Coils of jejunum and ileum completely fill the four quadrants of the cavitas peritonealis below the mesocolon transversum and are framed by the colon segments. In this dissection the loops of intestinum tenue have been displaced slightly to the left in front of the colon descendens, hiding it from view. The colon ascendens and caecum are visible along the right flank of the abdomen.

235

3.5 Intestinum Crassum: Colon Segments

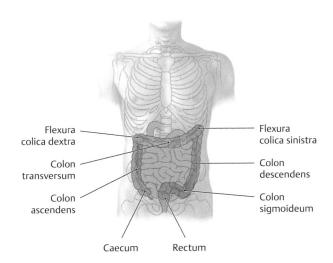

A Projection of the intestinum crassum onto the skeleton
Because of the embryonic rotation of the primary intestinal (midgut) loop, the intestinum crassum typically forms a frame encompassing the intestinum tenue. The position and length of the colon segments may vary, however, depending on the course of intestinal rotation. For example, when the intestinal loop rotates normally, the colon ascendens acquires a "normal" length (as shown here). If intestinal rotation is incomplete, the colon ascendens is shortened. The colon transversum is particularly mobile owing to its mesocolon, while the cola ascendens and descendens are less mobile because they are fixed to the posterior wall of the cavitas peritonealis. The flexura coli sinistra usually occupies a somewhat higher level than the flexura coli dextra due to the space occupied by the large lobus hepatis dexter. Also, the colon descendens is usually more posterior than the colon ascendens.

B Distinctive morphological features of the intestinum crassum
There are four morphological features—three visible externally and one internally—that distinguish the intestinum crassum from the intestinum tenue. It should be noted that these features do not occur equally in all parts of the intestinum crassum and are absent in the caecum, appendix vermiformis, and rectum.

Taeniae coli	In most portions of the intestinum crassum, the longitudinal muscle fibers do not form a continuous layer around the intestinal wall but are concentrated to form three longitudinal bands, the taeniae (see **C**). Taeniae are not present in the rectum or appendix vermiformis. The three taeniae converge to form the muscularis externa of the appendix.
Appendices epiploicae	Fat-filled protrusions of the tunica serosa, scattered over the surface of the intestinum crassum except on the caecum (absent or sparse) and rectum (absent).
Haustra (haustrations)	Saccular wall protrusions between the transverse folds of the intestinum crassum (see p. 238), absent in the rectum.
Plicae semi-lunares coli	Visible only *internally*, in contrast to the external features above. They are functional features caused by contraction of the tunica muscularis. The internal plicae correspond to external constrictions that separate the haustra.

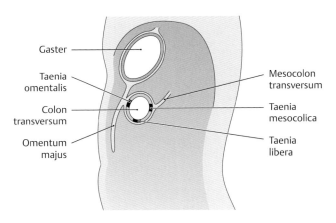

C The three taeniae of the colon
Sagittal section, viewed from the left side. The three taeniae are named for their position on the colon:

- Taenia libera (free taenia)
- Taenia omentalis (the taenia at the attachment of the omentum majus)
- Taenia mesocolica (the taenia at the attachment of the mesocolon)

D Anatomical divisions of the intestinum crassum

The intestinum crassum consists of the following divisions in the proximal-to-distal direction:

- Caecum with the appendix vermiformis
- Colon, consisting of four parts:
  - Colon ascendens
  - Colon transversum
  - Colon descendens
  - Colon sigmoideum
- Rectum

Note: For various reasons, some authors consider the rectum to be a separate section of the intestine, and not a part of the intestinum crassum. However, according to the *Terminologia Anatomica*, which serves as the international standard on human anatomic terminology, the rectum is a segment of the intestinum crassum.

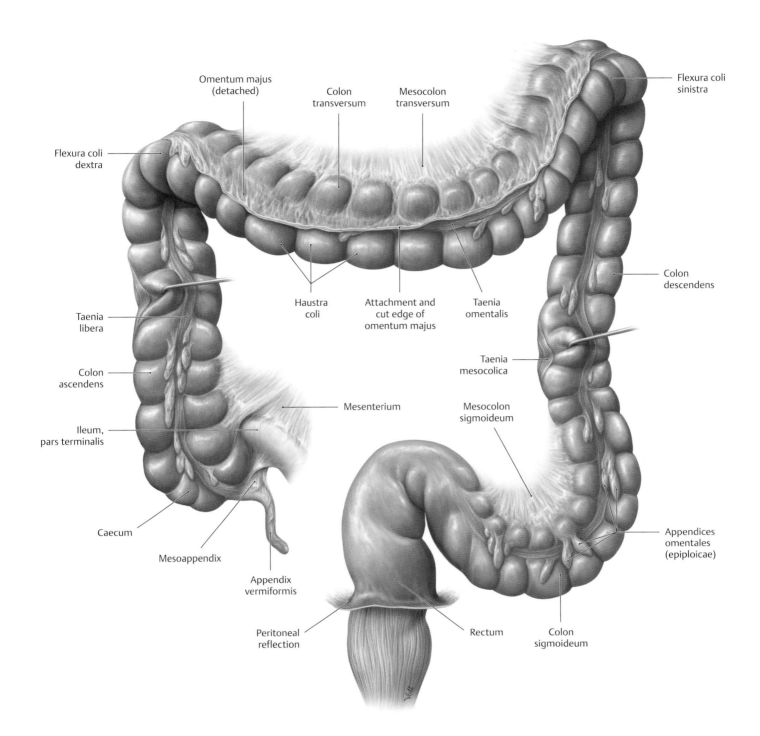

Omentum majus (detached)

Colon transversum

Mesocolon transversum

Flexura coli sinistra

Flexura coli dextra

Haustra coli

Attachment and cut edge of omentum majus

Taenia omentalis

Colon descendens

Taenia libera

Taenia mesocolica

Colon ascendens

Mesenterium

Mesocolon sigmoideum

Ileum, pars terminalis

Caecum

Mesoappendix

Appendix vermiformis

Peritoneal reflection

Rectum

Colon sigmoideum

Appendices omentales (epiploicae)

E Intestinum crassum: Segments, shape, and distinctive features
Anterior view, intestinum crassum. The pars terminalis of the ileum and portions of the mesocola transversum and sigmoideum are shown. The cola ascendens and transversum have been rotated to display their taeniae.

Note: Colorectal cancer, which has become one of the most common cancers in industrialized countries, has a special predilection for the rectosigmoid junction and the rectum itself (i.e., sites distal to the flexura coli sinistra).

The various colon segments possess all the morphological characteristics of the intestinum crassum (haustra, taeniae, appendices epiploicae, see **B**). Typically these features disappear past the rectosigmoid

junction. As the taeniae disappear, they are replaced on the rectum by a continuous stratum longitudinale. Instead of haustra, the rectum has three permanent constrictions that are produced by internal plicae transversae (see p. 248). The peritoneal reflection on the anterior rectal wall represents the site where the peritoneum is reflected onto the posterior wall of the uterus (in the female) or onto the upper surface of the vesica urinaria (in the male).

Note: The cola ascendens and descendens are (secondarily) retroperitoneal and therefore, unlike the cola sigmoideum and transversum, they do *not* have a mesocolon and are covered only anteriorly by peritoneum. The rectum is extraperitoneal in the pelvis minor, lacks a "suspensory ligament," and bears other unique features.

3.6 Intestinum Crassum: Wall Structure, Caecum, and Appendix Vermiformis

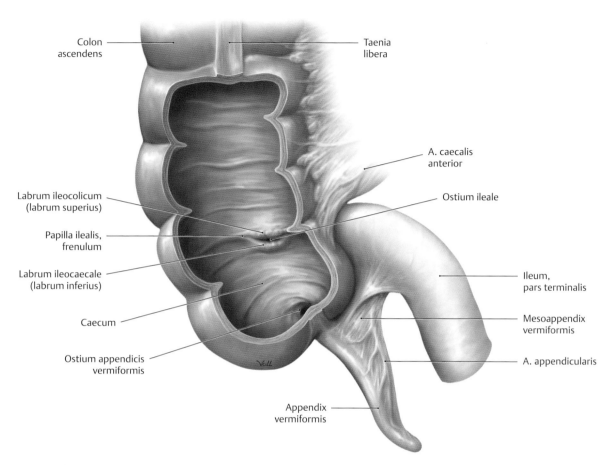

Colon ascendens

Taenia libera

A. caecalis anterior

Labrum ileocolicum (labrum superius)

Ostium ileale

Papilla ilealis, frenulum

Labrum ileocaecale (labrum inferius)

Ileum, pars terminalis

Caecum

Mesoappendix vermiformis

Ostium appendicis vermiformis

A. appendicularis

Appendix vermiformis

A Caecum and pars terminalis ilei

Anterior view. The caecum is unique in its end-to-side connection with the pars terminalis of the intestinum tenue (ileum) and the presence of the appendix vermiformis. As a result, there are two openings in the wall of the caecum: the *ostium ileale* on a small papilla (papilla ilealis) and, below that, the *ostium appendicis vermiformis*. The ostium ileale is approximately round in the living individual but is often slit-like in the postmortem condition. It is bounded by superior and inferior flaps or "lips," the labrum ileocolicum (labrum superius) and the labrum ileocaecale (labrum inferius). Both are continued as a narrow ridge of mucosa, the frenulum ostii ilealis.

Note: Inflammation of the appendix vermiformis (appendicitis) is one of the most common surgically treated diseases of the gastrointestinal tract. If acute appendicitis goes untreated, the inflammation may perforate into the free cavitas peritonealis (a "ruptured appendix" in popular jargon). This creates a route by which bacteria in the bowel lumen can enter the cavitas peritonealis and gain access to the large peritoneal surface, quickly inciting a life-threatening inflammation of the peritoneum (peritonitis).

B Ostium ilealis

Anterior view of a longitudinal coronal section of the cecum and ileum. The ostium ilealis hermetically seals the pars terminalis ilei from the caecum and prevents the reflux of contents from the intestinum crassum (structural constriction, see **A**, p. 234). At the ostium ilealis, the end of the ileum evaginates the stratum circulare of the tunica muscularis of the intestinum crassum into the cecal lumen. All layers of the ileal wall except the stratum longitudinale of the tunica muscularis and peritoneum contribute to the structure of the ileocecal orifice. The strata circulares tunicarum muscularium of the ileum and caecum function as a sphincter, which periodically opens the ostium. This allows the contents of the intestinum tenue to enter the intestinum crassum while effectively preventing reflux. The function of the sphincter is similar to that of the pylorus.

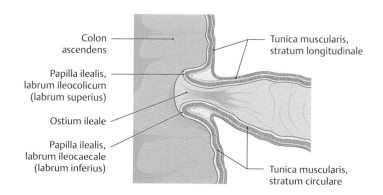

Colon ascendens

Tunica muscularis, stratum longitudinale

Papilla ilealis, labrum ileocolicum (labrum superius)

Ostium ileale

Papilla ilealis, labrum ileocaecale (labrum inferius)

Tunica muscularis, stratum circulare

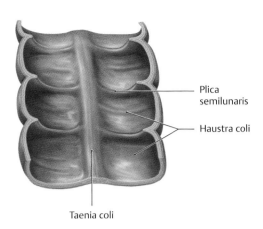

Plica semilunaris

Haustra coli

Taenia coli

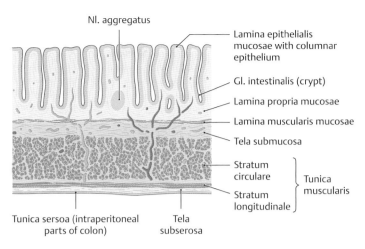

Nl. aggregatus

Lamina epithelialis mucosae with columnar epithelium

Gl. intestinalis (crypt)

Lamina propria mucosae

Lamina muscularis mucosae

Tela submucosa

Stratum circulare

Stratum longitudinale

Tunica muscularis

Tunica sersoa (intraperitoneal parts of colon)

Tela subserosa

C Interior of the colon

The interior of the colon is marked by transversely oriented folds called plicae semilunares. They are formed by the shortness of the muscular taenia of the colon wall and are visible externally as anular constrictions. The sacculations between the folds are the haustra coli. The plicae semilunares are inconstant features that depend on the muscular tension in the taenia. The plicae and haustra move slowly down the colon with waves of peristaltic activity.

D Wall structure of the colon and caecum

Longitudinal section through the bowel wall. All the typical wall layers of the gastrointestinal canal are present: the tunica mucosa, tela submucosa, tunica muscularis externa, and tunica serosa (or adventitia in the retroperitoneal parts of the colon, see **B**, p. 231). There are several features, however, that distinguish the wall structure of the colon and caecum from that of the gaster and intestinum tenue:

- The tunica mucosa is *devoid* of villi (i.e., the total surface area is not enlarged as much as in the intestinum tenue). Instead of villi, there are large numbers of deep *crypts* (Lieberkühn crypts, glandulae intestinales), more numerous than in the intestinum tenue.
- The epithelial layer of the tunica mucosa contains large numbers of goblet cells (for clarity, not shown here).
- The colonic mucosal surface undulates in large-scale, crescent-shaped, plicae semilunares (see **C**).
- The tunica muscularis externa consists of an inner stratum circulare and an outer stratum longitudinale, which is concentrated in three longitudinal bands, the taeniae coli (see p. 236).

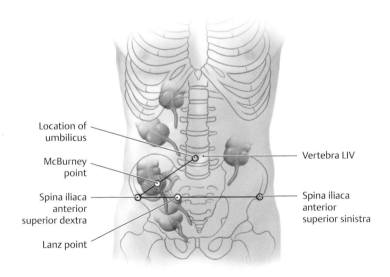

Location of umbilicus

McBurney point

Spina iliaca anterior superior dextra

Lanz point

Vertebra LIV

Spina iliaca anterior superior sinistra

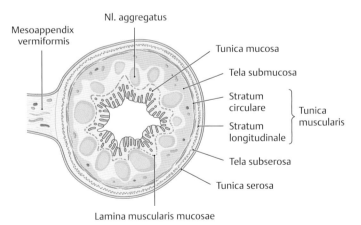

Nl. aggregatus

Mesoappendix vermiformis

Tunica mucosa

Tela submucosa

Stratum circulare

Stratum longitudinale

Tunica muscularis

Tela subserosa

Tunica serosa

Lamina muscularis mucosae

E Variants in the position of the appendix vermiformis

Disturbances in the rotation of the embryonic gut can result in numerous positional variants of the caecum and appendix vermiformis. The appendix may even come to lie in the left side of the abdomen. The inflammation of an appendix in the *typical position* is characterized by tenderness at two points:

- McBurney point: Position on a line connecting the umbilicus and the right spina iliaca anterior superior. The McBurney point is one-third of the distance along this line from the spina iliaca.
- Lanz point: Position on a line connecting the the spinae iliacae anteriores superiores. The Lanz point is one third of the distance along this line from the right spina.

Although very useful, these are not definitive clinical signs. Tenderness may be felt at other abdominal sites, especially if the appendix is in an atypical position.

F Wall structure of the appendix vermiformis

The appendix vermiformis has the typical wall structure of an intraperitoneal intestinal tube. One striking feature is the abundance of lymphatic follicles (noduli lymphoidei aggregati) in the tela submucosa (also present in the colon and caecum, but in much smaller numbers). With its high degree of immunological activity, the appendix has been characterized as the "intestinal tonsil." The mucosa has numerous deep crypts that are in intimate contact with the noduli lymphoidei aggregati in the lamina propria and the tela submucosa (crypts and noduli lymphoidei aggregati are not visible here). Since the appendix vermiformis is intraperitoneal, it possesses a small mesenterium, the mesoappendix, which transmits neurovascular structures.

3.7 Intestinum Crassum: Location, Shape, and Interior View of Rectum

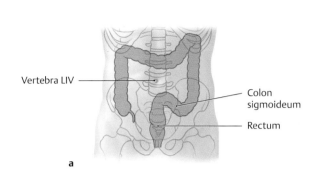

a

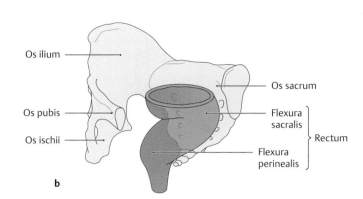

b

A Location and curves of the rectum

Anterior view (**a**) and left anterior view (**b**). The rectum is 15–16 cm long and extends approximately from the superior border of the third sacral vertebra to the perineum. It is "straight" only in the frontal projection (as shown in **a**); it presents two flexures in the sagittal projection (see **b**):

the flexura sacralis (retroperitoneal) and the flexura perinealis (extraperitoneal), which represents the start of the canalis analis and is already extraperitoneal. The flexura sacralis—conforming to the shape of the os sacrum—is concave anteriorly. The flexura perinealis is an important functional component of rectal continence (see p. 242f).

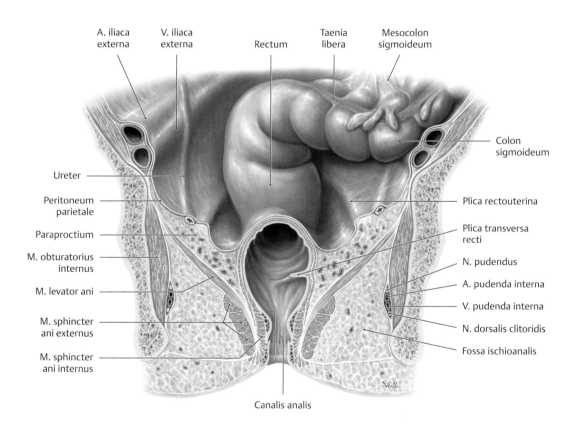

C Distinct morphological features of the rectum

The mucosa and wall structure of the rectum does not differ from the intestinum crassum, including the colon and caecum. Nevertheless, it lacks several colonic characteristics:

- no taeniae, the rectum has a continuous stratum longitudinale tunicae muscularis;
- no appendices epiploicae;
- no haustra;
- no plicae semilunares, the rectum has plicae transversae recti
- the wall of rectum is devoid of ganglion cells;
- embryonic development: the part above the anorectal line, like the colon, is derived from endoderma, the canalis analis is derived from ectoderm (which is why some authors don't consider it part of the rectum).

B The rectum in situ

Coronal section of the female pelvis, anterior view, with the rectum opened from about the level of the plica transversa inferius recti media. The taeniae of the sigmoid colon are not continued onto the rectum. The constrictions in the outer wall of the rectum correspond to the transverse folds on the inner wall. The rectum (which would appear in this form only if the ampulla were full) is shown in a slightly raised position. Below the levator ani muscle is the powerful external anal

sphincter, the muscular component of the rectal continence organ. The pararectal connective tissue below the peritoneal cavity contains numerous vessels that supply the rectum. This drawing was made from the dissection of a female cadaver. Thus, the peritoneum would be reflected from the anterior wall of the rectum onto the posterior wall of the uterus. Although both the anterior rectal wall and uterus are not visible here (anterior to this plane of section), parts of the rectouterine folds are still visible.

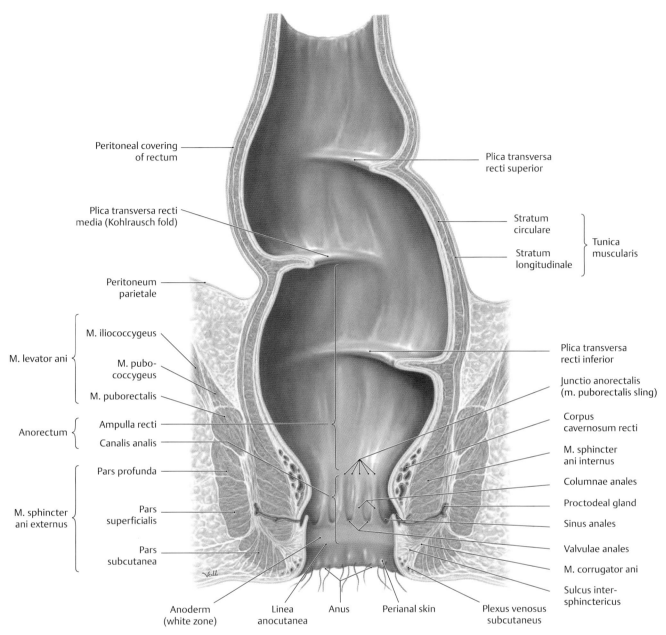

Peritoneal covering of rectum — Plica transversa recti superior — Plica transversa recti media (Kohlrausch fold) — Stratum circulare — Tunica muscularis — Stratum longitudinale — Peritoneum parietale — M. levator ani { M. iliococcygeus, M. pubo-coccygeus, M. puborectalis } — Plica transversa recti inferior — Junctio anorectalis (m. puborectalis sling) — Corpus cavernosum recti — Anorectum { Ampulla recti, Canalis analis } — M. sphincter ani internus — M. sphincter ani externus { Pars profunda, Pars superficialis, Pars subcutanea } — Columnae anales — Proctodeal gland — Sinus anales — Valvulae anales — M. corrugator ani — Sulcus intersphinctericus — Anoderm (white zone) — Linea anocutanea — Anus — Perianal skin — Plexus venosus subcutaneus

D Rectum and canalis analis: Divisions, internal surface and wall structure

Anterior view of the rectum in coronal section with the anterior wall removed. Instead of plicae semilunares, the rectum contains three permanent plicae transversae. The distal portion of the rectum, also known as the *anorectum*, is recognizable by a palpable protrusion (m. puborectalis sling or junctio anorectalis) which is visible on the mucosal surface. The anorectum is divided into two segments, the *ampulla recti* and the *canalis analis*.

- **Ampulla recti:** the lowest portion of the rectum between the middle plica transversa recti (Kohlrausch fold, flexura intermediosinistra lateralis) and the junctio anorectalis. The ampulla recti is the most distensible part of the rectum and, contrary to popular opinion, does not serve as a reservoir for holding stool but is usually empty (see mechanism of defecation, p. 245). The middle plica transversa, which projects into the rectum from its right posterior wall, is approximately 6–7 cm from the anus and can just be reached with the palpating finger. Rectal tumors located below the Kohlrausch fold may therefore be palpable.
- **Canalis analis:** located below the junctio anorectalis at the distal flexura perinealis (see **A**). It is approximately 4 cm long and normally kept closed by the mm. sphincteres ani. The clinically important "*surgical*

anal canal" begins at the level of the junctio anorectalis and extends to the linea anocutanea, which is also palpable. It is a groove located between the margins of the mm. sphincteres ani internus and externus (sulcus intersphinctericus) at the junction of the anoderm (zona alba), a region with very dense somatic innervation, and the pigmented perianal skin (see p. 242 **B**). Above the anoderm are located 8–10 longitudinal mucosal folds (columnae anales), produced by the arterial corpus cavernosum recti (hemorrhoidal plexus), located in the submucosa (see p. 242). The distal ends of the columnae anales are connected by valve-like transverse folds (valvulae anales). All valvulae anales together form the linea pectinata, which is an important landmark because it is visible. Behind the valvulae anales are pocket-like depressions (sinus anales or pouches of Morgagni), into which empty 6–8 outflow ducts of the rudimentary mucus-secreting anal glands (proctodeal glands). The most common site of these glands is the commissura laborium posterior (approximately at 6 o'clock in the lithotomy position), either in the tela submucosa or intersphincteric (between the mm. sphincteres ani interni and externi) space, so that the outflow ducts partially transverse the m. sphincter ani internus.

Note: Bacterial infections of the glands may cause perianal abscesses and anal fistulas, which are difficult to treat (see p. 247).

241

3.8 Continence Organ: Structure and Components

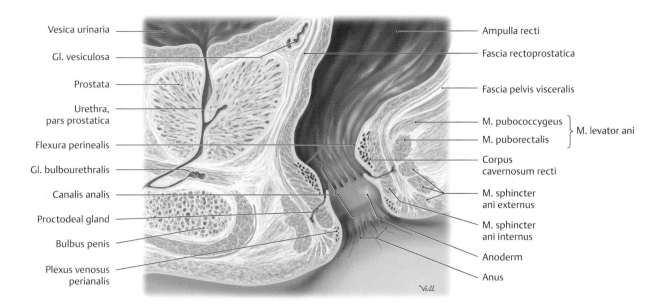

Vesica urinaria

Gl. vesiculosa

Prostata

Urethra, pars prostatica

Flexura perinealis

Gl. bulbourethralis

Canalis analis

Proctodeal gland

Bulbus penis

Plexus venosus perianalis

Ampulla recti

Fascia rectoprostatica

Fascia pelvis visceralis

M. pubococcygeus
M. puborectalis } M. levator ani

Corpus cavernosum recti

M. sphincter ani externus

M. sphincter ani internus

Anoderm

Anus

A Components of the continence apparatus
Midsagittal section at the level of the canalis analis in the male, viewed from the left side.

The continence apparatus, or continence *organ*, controls the closing (continence) and opening (defecation) of the rectum and provides a tight closure before and after evacuation of solid, liquid and gas bowel contents.

It consists of a distensible hollow organ as well as vascular and muscular continence mechanisms, including their neural control. These angiomuscular continence mechanisms are integrated into a structurally narrow segment, which begins at the level of the flexura perinealis and continues along the canalis analis:

- Distensible hollow organ:
  - rectum with stretch receptors, mainly in the ampulla recti (viscerosensory innervation)
  - anus with distensible skin in the canalis analis (somatosensory innervation);

- Muscular continence:
  - m. sphincter ani internus (visceromotor innervation)
  - m. sphincter ani externi (somatomotor innervation)
  - m. levator ani, especially the m. puborectalis (somatomotor innervation);
- Vascular continence:
  - hemorrhoidal plexus (permanently distended cavernous tissue that subsides only during defecation);
- Neural control:
  - visceral and somatic nervous system (mainly from S2–S4) with the nn. splanchnici pelvici, n. pudendus and plexus rectales.

Functionally, both continence and defecation are the result of a fine-tuned feedback loop between receptors and effectors of the continence apparatus with involvement of the central nervous system (see p. 244 f).

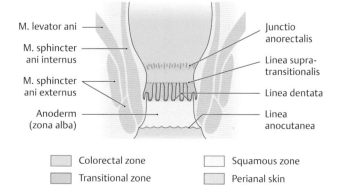

M. levator ani

M. sphincter ani internus

M. sphincter ani externus

Anoderm (zona alba)

Junctio anorectalis

Linea supra-transitionalis

Linea dentata

Linea anocutanea

☐ Colorectal zone   ☐ Squamous zone
☐ Transitional zone   ☐ Perianal skin

B Epithelial regions of the canalis analis (after Lüllmann-Rauch)
In the canalis analis, the unilayered columnar epithelium of the colorectal tunica mucosa at the level of the zona transitionalis analis is continuous with the stratified squamous epithelium of the anoderm and perianal skin. The transition occurs near characteristic landmarks. The canalis analis can be divided into the following epithelial regions:

- **colorectal zone** between junctio anorectalis and supratransitional line; homogeneous colorectal mucosa with crypts;
- **zona transitionalis** at the level of the columnae anales (between supratransitional line and linea pectinata) mosaic patterns of colorectal mucosa, unilayered columnar epithelium and stratified squamous epithelium;
- **squamous zone** between linea pectinata and linea anocutanea: evenly covered by stratified, nonkeratinized squamous epithelium, which is intimately attached to the underlying m. sphincter ani internus, hence its whitish appearance (white zone). Deep sensory innervation with touch, pressure, temperature and mainly pain receptors (clinically: anoderm);
- **perianal skin** below the linea anocutanea: start of the stratified squamous epithelium of the outer layer of the skin (heavy pigmentation, eccrine and apocrine sweat glands and hair follicles).

Note: Knowledge about the epithelial regions of the canalis analis is important mainly for the differentiation between rectal (usually adenocarcinoma) and anal carcinoma (of keratinizing or non-keratinizing squamous epithelium).

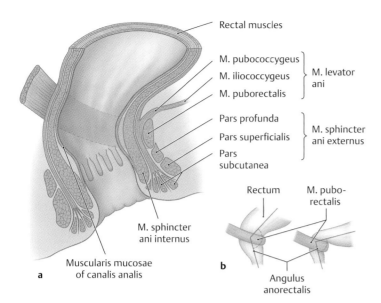

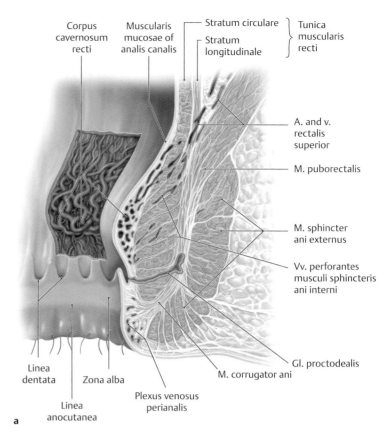

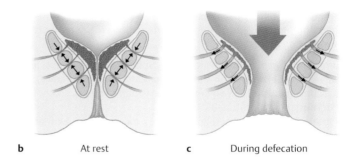

C Structure of the muscular continence mechanism

a Midsagittal section, viewed from the left side; **b** M. puborectalis sling and anorectal angle: relaxed muscle (left) and contracted muscle (right).

The complex system of anal sphincters involves both smooth and striated muscles. Whereas the smooth muscles represent the direct continuation of the muscles of the rectal wall, the striated muscles are formed by specialized areas of the pelvic floor muscles. Thus, these muscular continence mechanisms are maintained under both somatic-voluntary and visceral-involuntary control.

Involuntarily innervated smooth muscles:

- *M. sphincter ani internus:* most significant smooth muscle; as the continuation of the stratum circulare tunicae muscularis of the rectum, it forms a strong circular ring. Sympathetic nerve fibers and a significantly reduced number of enteric ganglion cells (hypoganglionosis) allow it to maintain constant tonic activity to help constrict the canalis analis (the internal sphincter is responsible for 70% of fecal continence);
- *Lamina muscularis mucosae of the canalis analis:* as the continuation of the lamina muscularis mucosae, it extends beyond the hemorrhoidal plexus and ends at the linea pectinata; stabilizes the hemorrhoidal plexus and holds it in place;
- *Corrugator ani:* as the continuation of the stratum longitudinale of the tunica muscularis of the rectum, the muscle fibers extend beyond the canalis analis, permeate through the subcutaneous part of the m. sphincter ani externus and insert into the perianal skin. M. corrugator ani owes its name to the fact that muscle contraction produces radial wrinkles on the perianal skin.

Voluntarily innervated striated muscles:

- *M. sphincter ani externus:* cylindrical muscle that encircles the outside wall of the canalis analis, made up of three recognizable parts: partes profunda, superficialis, and subcutanea. Whereas the partes profunda and subcutanea are arranged in circular layers, the pars superficialis extends between the anteriorly located corpus perineale and the posterior lig. anococcygeum and surrounds the canalis analis and serves as a clamp. It is largely composed of type I fibers, which are slow, durable, and fatigue resistant.
- *M. puborectalis:* as the innermost portion of the m. levator ani, it forms a strong sling of muscle, which loops around the rectum at the level of the junctio anorectalis and is closely aligned to the pars profunda of the m. sphincter ani externus. It arises from the fixed end of the os pubis, so when the m. puborectalis contracts it creates a "kink" between canalis analis and rectum at the anorectal angle.

D Structure of the vascular continence mechanism

a Longitudinal section of the canalis analis with the hemorrhoidal plexus windowed; **b** and **c** Hemorrhoidal plexus at rest and during defecation.

Above the linea pectinata at the level of the columnae anales in the submucosa lies a cavernous body, the hemorrhoidal plexus. Its elasticity largely ensures liquid- and gas-tight closure of the rectum. The circular configuration of the hemorrhoidal plexus is similar in structure to the corpus cavernosum penis but differs in that it is permanently distended. The hemorrhoidal plexus is a network of cavernous tissue and is almost exclusively supplied by three branches of the a. rectalis superior (at 3, 7 and 11 o'clock in the lithotomy position), which further divide near the columnae anales (see p. 273). Blood reaches the venous drainage system via arteriovenous anastomoses through transsphincteric veins—largely along the m. sphincter ani internus—and reaches the drainage area of the v. mesenterica inferior (and is carried to the v. portae hepatis) but also partially through the vv. rectales mediae and inferiores to the perianal veins of the external venous plexus. When the sphincter apparatus relaxes during defecation, it allows blood to drain from the hemorrhoidal plexus.

Note: Abnormal dilation (hyperplasia) of the hemorrhoidal plexus beyond the physiological range leads to hemorrhoidal disease, one of the most common proctological disorders (see p. 246 f).

3.9 Continence Organ: Function

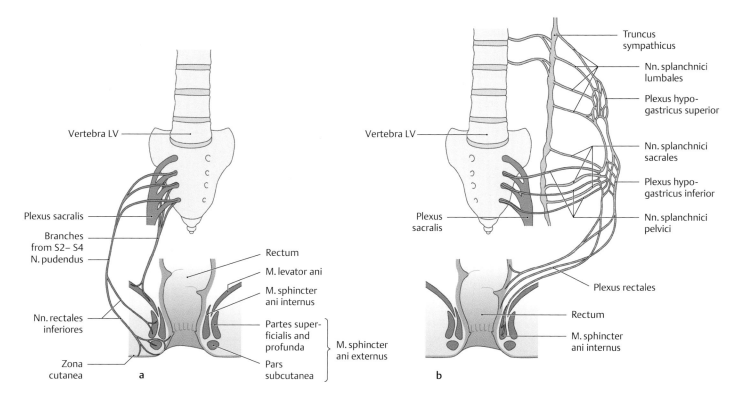

A Innervation (after Stelzner)
a Somatomotor and somatosensory innervation; **b** Visceromotor and viscerosensory innervation.

- Somatomotor: n. pudendus for the m. sphincter ani externus, levator nerves for the m. levator ani (especially the m. puborectalis). They provide active, partially voluntary innervation of the m. sphincter ani externus and m. levator ani.
- Somatosensory: nn. rectales inferiores for the anus and perianal skin. Arising from the n. pudendus, they transmit touch and especially pain sensation. The skin of the anus is extremely sensitive to pain. Even small tears in the anal skin, which often show inflammatory changes, tend to be extremely painful.

- Visceromotor: pelvic splanchnic nerves (S2–S4) for the internal anal sphincter. The resting tone of the internal sphincter (nn. splanchnici lumbales et sacrales) helps to maintain closure of the anal canal and inhibits venous drainage from the hemorrhoidal plexus; the cavernous body remains distended, contributing to fecal continence and flatus control. Topographically, the pelvic splanchnic nerves are closely related to the rectal plexuses.
- Viscerosensory: pelvic splanchnic nerves (S2–S4) supply the wall of the rectum, particularly the stretch receptors in the rectal ampulla. Stretching of the ampulla by the fecal column triggers a subjective awareness of the need to defecate.

B Mechanism of defecation (after Wedel; see right page)
a Filling of the ampulla recti; **b** Relaxation of the voluntarily controlled sphincters and propulsion of fecal column.
Both defecation and continence are under central nervous system control involving different anatomical structures ranging from the cortex cerebri to the perianal skin, with the anorectum being one of multiple effectors. Directly involved are the diaphragma pelvis, muscles used during squatting, the abdominal press as well as autonomic and sensory nerves along with their higher nerve centers.

Filling of the ampulla recti and stimulation of local stretch receptors in the ampullary wall: When the fecal bolus is propelled into the ampulla recti by anterogradely propagating waves, mechanoreceptors detect distension and transmit the information via visceral afferents in the funiculus posterior medullae spinalis to the sensory cortex, which perceives the urge to defecate. Olfactory, visual, or acoustic stimuli can either accelerate or decelerate the perception and subsequent voluntary action, which results in defecation.

Rectoanal inhibitory reflex and relaxation of the voluntarily innervated sphincters: When the ampulla fills with feces, the intrarectal

pressure increases and the m. sphincter ani internus relaxes, followed by voluntary relaxation of the m. puborectalis sling and the m. sphincter ani externus. As a result, the anorectal angle straightens and the canalis analis widens.

Propulsion of fecal column: Rectal evacuation is assisted by a direct involuntary increase in pressure in the rectal area and by simultaneous increase in pressure by the contraction of voluntarily innervated muscles: abdominal (abdominal press), perineal (pelvic floor lift), diaphragmatic (diaphragma contraction) and glottic (glottis closure) muscles. The squatting position further increases abdominal pressure (flexor reflex). With the propulsion of the fecal column, the hemorrhoidal cushions are drained and pushed out.

Completion of defecation: After the sphincter apparatus allows the fecal column to pass through, it comes in contact with the highly sensitive anoderm, which perceives the volume, consistency, and location of the stool. This perception initiates the voluntary process of completing defecation. Defecation is completed once the sphincter apparatus contracts and the hemorrhoidal plexus fills up.

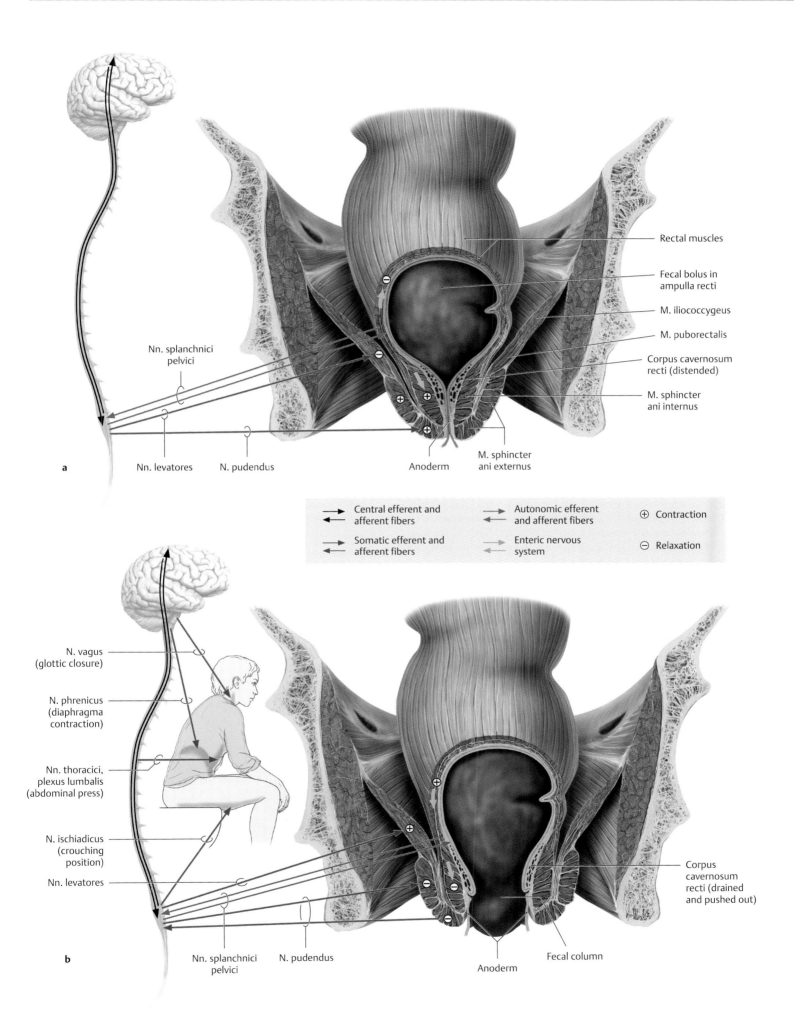

Rectal muscles

Fecal bolus in
ampulla recti

M. iliococcygeus

M. puborectalis

Corpus cavernosum
recti (distended)

M. sphincter
ani internus

Nn. splanchnici
pelvici

Nn. levatores

N. pudendus

Anoderm

M. sphincter
ani externus

a

→ Central efferent and afferent fibers	→ Autonomic efferent and afferent fibers
→ Somatic efferent and afferent fibers	→ Enteric nervous system

⊕ Contraction

⊖ Relaxation

N. vagus
(glottic closure)

N. phrenicus
(diaphragma
contraction)

Nn. thoracici,
plexus lumbalis
(abdominal press)

N. ischiadicus
(crouching
position)

Nn. levatores

Corpus
cavernosum
recti (drained
and pushed out)

Nn. splanchnici
pelvici

N. pudendus

Anoderm

Fecal column

b

3.10 Disorders of the Canalis Analis: Hemorrhoidal Disease, Anal Abscesses, and Anal Fistulas

Grade I
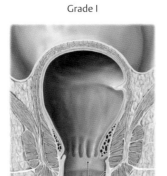

Grade II
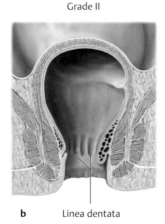

Grade III
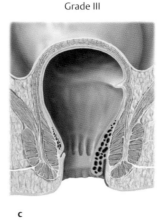

Grade IV
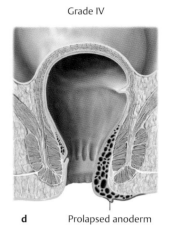

a   Anoderm   **b**   Linea dentata   **c**   **d**   Prolapsed anoderm

A Hemorrhoidal disease

Hemorrhoidal disease is one of the most common proctological disorders. The site of origin is the circular hemorrhoidal plexus of the cavernous body of the rectum located above the linea pectinata. It is largely responsible for the fine adjustment of anal continence. *Hemorrhoid* is a general term used to describe hyperplasia (enlargement) of a corpus cavernosum with arterial blood supply, a condition which initially does not cause any symptoms. Hemorrhoids become pathological once they become symptomatic (bleeding is bright red from arterial blood, mucus discharge, itching, burning, fecal soiling, etc.) and when they require treatment (hemorrhoidal disease). Most commonly, hemorrhoids result from increased pressure on the anus during defecation, often caused by chronic constipation as a result of a lack of fiber and fluids in the diet. Another cause is impaired venous return due to increased m. sphincter ani tone as this may lead to the hemorrhoidal plexus taking on a gnarled appearance. Diagnosis and classification of hemorrhoids are based on examination, palpation, and proctoscopy of the canalis analis. Depending on the severity of the hemorrhoids and their symptoms, they are divided into four grades:

- **Grade I (a):** swollen, elastic cushions of tissue that are visible only on proctoscopy (located above the linea pectinata) and may cause painless bright red bleeding (painless because the swollen cushions are located above the anoderm);

- **Grade II (b):** visibly hyperplastic vascular cushions, which can prolapse inside or outside of the canalis analis during defecation or while pressing but retract immediately after emptying the bowels. Dripping blood and mucus discharge may cause oozing or itching, a condition also known as perianal eczema;
- **Grade III (c):** during defecation or while the intra-abdominal pressure is increased, hemorrhoids prolapse spontaneously and require manual repositioning. Possible thrombosis or incarceration of the prolapsed knot may cause significant pain;
- **Grade IV (d):** at this stage, the nodular enlargements and large parts of the canalis analis, including the highly pain-sensitive anoderm, are permanently prolapsed (irreducible) and attached to the anal margin (also known as an anal prolapse).

Note: Unlike in the German medical terminology, the Anglo-American and Swiss terminology distinguish between *internal* and *external hemorrhoids*. Internal hemorrhoids originate from the internal plexus venosus rectalis, external hemorrhoids are subcutaneous clots at the margin of the anus (e.g., perianal thromboses). In our assessment, however, external hemorrhoids are simply hyperplastic vascular cushions of the plexus venosus rectalis with their arterial blood supply that have prolapsed to the outside.

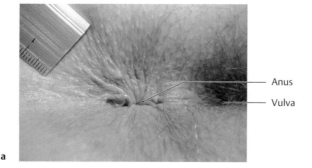

Anus
Vulva

a

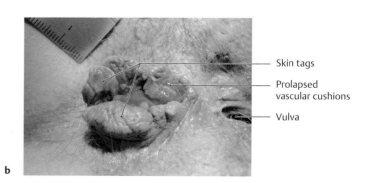

Skin tags
Prolapsed vascular cushions
Vulva

b

B Conditions of the perianal skin with and without hemorrhoidal disease
a Normal anatomy of the perianal area in a 38-year-old female patient;
b Grade IV hemorrhoids in a 54-year-old female patient: mucosal

prolapse at the commissura laborium anterior combined with right- and left-lateral anal skin tags (harmless, generally asymptomatic perianal skin folds) (from Rohde, H.: Lehratlas der Proktologie. Thieme, Stuttgart 2006).

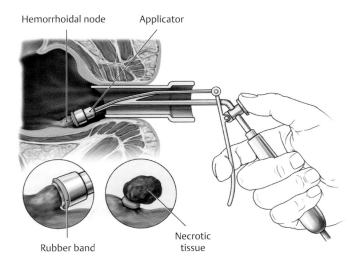

Hemorrhoidal node   Applicator

Rubber band   Necrotic tissue

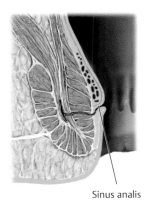
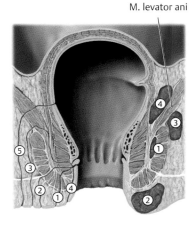

M. levator ani

Sinus analis

a   Proctodeal gland   **b**   Anal fistulas   Anal abscesses

C Therapeutic possibilities in hemorrhoidal disease

Treatment for hemorrhoidal disease is mainly aimed at prevention, removal of hemorrhoids, and restoration of the normal anatomy and physiology of the affected areas. Thus, the therapeutic possibilities can be divided into preventive measures and symptomatic (conservative, semi-invasive, surgical) treatment:

- **Preventive measures:** focus on informing patients about advisable nutritional habits (switching to a fiber-rich, low-fat diet with sufficient fluid intake, avoiding alcohol, tobacco, and hot spices) and improving bowel habits (defecating only when feeling the urge to have a bowel movement, avoid straining, no laxatives, proper but not excessive anal hygiene);
- **Conservative measures:** local treatment using ointments, suppositories, anal tampons, and sitz baths to alleviate symptoms;
- **Semi-invasive measures:** sclerotherapy (e.g., after Blond), rubber band ligation (after Barron), and Doppler ultrasound-guided hemorrhoidal arterial ligation have proven effective as treatments especially for grade I and grade II hemorrhoids. In sclerotherapy, 0.5–1.0 ml polidocanol is injected submucosally above the linea pectinata. Polidocanol is a sclerosing agent that damages the endothelium of the blood vessels, which are then replaced by fibrous tissue. This treatment is aimed at fixing the hemorrhoids. Rubber band ligation is the preferred method to treat grade II hemorrhoids (see fig.). Using a special applicator, excess hemorrhoidal tissue is tied off with a rubber band. The necrotic tissue falls off within one to two weeks. Hemorrhoidal artery ligation (HAL) helps to reduce the blood supply to the enlarged vascular cushions and makes them shrink.
- **Surgical measures:** grade III and grade IV hemorrhoids require surgical intervention. Common surgical procedures include hemorrhoidectomy after Millian-Morgan and a procedure known as stapled hemorrhoidopexy after Longo. Hemorrhoidectomy involves radial-segmental excision and ligation of the enlarged cushions. For stapled hemorrhoidopexy, a special device is inserted with which to reposition the prolapsed hemorrhoids and to resect a ring of mucosa from the proximal canalis analis along with parts of the hemorrhoidal tissue. A circular stapler is used to fix the remaining tissue in place. This procedure offers a significant advantage in that it results in less post-operative pain because the staple line is placed in the area of the rectal mucosa that does not receive sensory innervation.

D Anal fistulas and anal abscesses

The symptoms of both of these conditions are closely related and are almost always caused by the same disorder: an infection of the rudimentary proctodeal glands (see p. 241). Usually, the anal abscess represents the acute and the anal fistula the chronic manifestation of the cryptoglandular infection. Based on the anatomy of the proctodeal glands—which most commonly are located within the intersphincteric space near the commissura laborium posterior and open into the sinus anales (**a**)—anal fistulas and anal abscesses (**b**) are classified according to their course or location relative to the sphincter apparatus:

- **Anal fistulas** (typical fistulas are complete, meaning they have an internal opening into the canalis analis and an external opening in the skin; hence two openings—one in the sinus analis and one in the perianal skin):

  ① Intersphincteric fistula: 50–70% of all anal fistulas, pierces the m. sphincter ani internus;
  ② Transsphincteric fistula: 30–40% of all anal fistulas, pierces both the mm. sphincteres ani internus and externus;
  ③ Suprasphincteric fistula: approximately 5% of all anal fistulas, passes upward between the sphincters and crosses the m. puborectalis sling;
  ④ Subcutaneous or subanodermal fistula: 5–10% of all anal fistulas, does not pierce either sphincter but passes directly below the canalis analis and opens in the perianal skin (synonym: marginal fistula);
  ⑤ Atypical fistula: approximately 5% of all anal fistulas, does not begin at the proctodeal glands but passes from the ampulla recti through the m. levator ani and has an external opening on the skin (also known as extrasphincteric fistula), common symptom of Crohn's disease.

- **Anal abscesses** (result from fistulas that don't have an external opening and thus end blindly):

  ① Intersphincteric abscess: within the proctodeal glands;
  ② Subcutaneous or subanodermal abscess: perianal or around the canalis analis;
  ③ Ischiorectal or infralevator abscess: below m. levator ani in the fossa ischioanalis;
  ④ Pelvirectal or supralevator abscess: between the rectum and m. levator ani funnel in the pararectal fascia.

Note: Anal fistulas and anal abscesses always require adequate surgical therapy. Anal abscesses in particular are accompanied by severe pain, fever, and leukocytosis and are generally an indication for emergency treatment. The aim of surgical treatment of anal fistulas in addition to sealing the fistula channel is to treat the infection of the proctodeal glands to prevent relapse. Exact knowledge of the anatomical relationships is crucial for a successful treatment.

3.11   Rectal Carcinoma

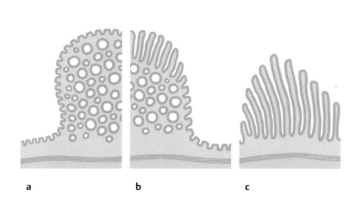

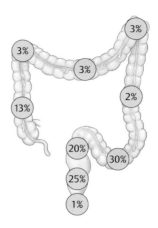

A Adenomatous polyps of the intestinum crassum
a Tubular; **b** Tubulovillous; **c** Villous polyps.

Adenoma is a type of benign epithelial tumor (neoplasia) that originates in glandular tissue. When it originates in the large bowel mucosa, it often extends beyond the mucosa and grows in a polypous fashion (hence the term "large bowel polyps"). According to their morphological appearance, they are divided into

- Tubular adenomas (75% of all large bowel polyps): most commonly pedunculated and smaller than 2cm;
- Tubulovillous adenomas (15% of all large bowel polyps): mixed, significantly higher risk of malignant transformation than tubular adenoma;
- Villous adenomas (10% of all large bowel polyps; high—30%–risk of malignant transformation): hairy-appearing surface and overall flatter than tubular adenomas; because they are broad-based they are more difficult to remove endoscopically, hence there is a high risk of relapse.

Note: All adenomas can develop into cancer. The risk of malignant transformation correlates with the size of the polyp, its histological type, and the degree of dysplasia (e.g., degree of differentiation).

B Frequency and risk factors of colorectal carcinoma
Colorectal carcinoma is the most common cancer of the gastrointestinal tract in the Western world. In Europe and the United States, colorectal carcinoma accounts for 15% of all newly diagnosed cancers with increasing incidence rates. In Germany alone, with 60,000 new cases each year, colorectal adenocarcinoma is the second most common form of cancer regardless of gender (more than half of patients die from it). Almost 45% of these tumors develop in the rectum (see fig.). It is not clear what causes colorectal cancer but the following exogenous and endogenous risk factors appear to play a role:

- **Exogenous risk factors**:
  - high-meat, high-fat, low-fiber diet
  - insufficient intake of vitamins (folic acid, vitamins A, C, E) and trace elements (selenium)
  - alcohol consumption
  - asbestos exposure
  - low socioeconomic status (associated with malnutrition, see above)
  - physical inactivity;
- **Endogenous risk factors**:
  - adenomatous polyps of the intestinum crassum
  - frequent occurrence of colon cancer in families
  - inflammatory bowel diseases (e.g., ulcerative colitis, Crohn's disease).

Note: Colorectal cancer does not include canalis analis tumors (1%).

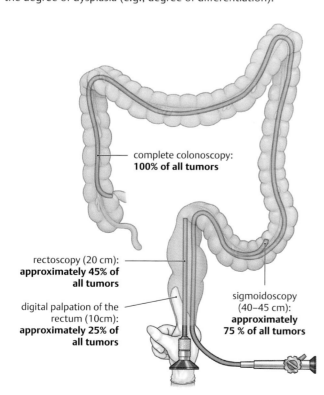

complete colonoscopy:
100% of all tumors

rectoscopy (20 cm):
approximately 45% of all tumors

digital palpation of the rectum (10cm):
approximately 25% of all tumors

sigmoidoscopy (40–45 cm):
approximately 75 % of all tumors

C Cancer screening
Early detection of cancer through screening is particularly helpful in the case of colorectal carcinoma. This is due to the relatively long latency period of several years that it takes for the primarily benign adenoma to transform into cancer. Benign colorectal tumors predominantly begin as polypoid changes in the colorectal mucosa (tubular, villous, and tubulovillous adenomas that may be pedunculated or broad-based and occur as solitary or multiple lesions), with the greatest tendency for malignant change in villous adenomas (30%) (see **A**). Guideline-recommended colorectal cancer screenings include annual fecal occult blood testing (hemoccult testing to begin at age 40), digital rectal examination and a colonoscopy (to begin at age 55) with the option of direct primary intervention to remove Neoplastic cells. CT colonography (virtual colonoscopy) offers an additional, less invasive alternative to the conventional endoscopic examination. An extensive body of research shows that endoscopic diagnosis results in an impressive reduction of the incidence and mortality rate by 60–80%.

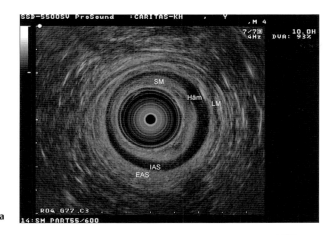

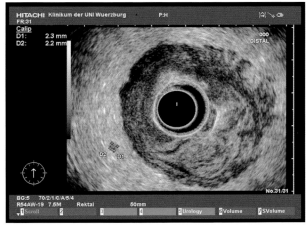

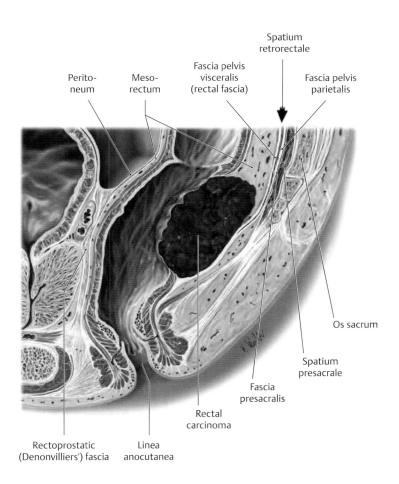

D Rectal and anal endosonography

In rectal and anal endosonography, the layers of the anorectal wall and surrounding structures are clearly displayed with high spatial resolution. Whereas endorectal ultrasound images display primarily the layers of the rectal wall, the endoanal ultrasound allows the evaluation of the mm. sphincteres and the diaphragma pelvis. In order to correctly assess results of endosonographic imaging, thorough knowledge of the anatomy is crucial. The transverse orientation with a 360-degree transducer is the most commonly used imaging plane employed in endosonography; it facilitates precise anatomical localization of the displayed structures.

a Anal endosonography: technique to display the sphincter apparatus in the canalis analis; the circular hypoechoic m. sphincter ani internus (IAS), which is continuous with the hyperechoic tela submucosa (SM) (parts of the hemorrhoidal plexus), serves as landmark. Outside the m. sphincter ani internus lies the m. sphincter ani externus (EAS), which exhibits a mixed echogenic pattern. As a continuation of the stratum longitudinale tunica muscularis (LM), fibers of the m. corrugator ani are visible as a thin hypoechoic layer in the intersphincteric space.

b Rectal endosonography: large circular rectal tumor that infiltrates the perirectal fat tissue. Rectal endosonography is used in the preoperative staging of rectal carcinoma to determine the depth of penetration into the rectal wall and the number of malignant nodi lymphoidei regionales. This information is essential with regards to the surgical approach: complete removal of the rectum (abdominoperineal excision), preserving fecal continence (total mesorectal excision, see **E**), or localized treatment (from: Dietrich, Ch. [Hrsg]: Endosonography, Lehrbuch und Atlas des endoskopischen Ultraschalls. Thieme, Stuttgart 2007).

E Total mesorectal excision (TME)

Sphincter preservation can be achieved in 80% of surgeries for rectal cancer. One precondition for a sphincter sparing procedure is that the distal margin of the tumor is at least 6 cm above the linea anocutanea. Introduction of total mesorectal excision (TME) has significantly improved oncologic outcomes (reduction of local recurrence rates) especially for carcinomas situated in the middle or lower third of the rectum. TME takes into account the pattern of regional metastasis not only by removing the tumor, which may have infiltrated the perirectal fat tissue, but also by completely resecting the regional lymphatic drainage area. Additionally, the surgical treatment is guided by the plexus autonomici of the pelvis (plexus hypogastricus inferior) mainly to prevent voiding and prostata dysfunction. Hence, the procedure is also referred to as nerve-oriented or nerve-guided mesorectal excision (see p. 381).

Operative approach: After preparing the lymphovascular pedicle of the superior rectal vessels, the a. and v. mesentericae inferiores are ligated centrally (vascular ligation). The a. mesenterica inferior is ligated 2 cm distal to its origin so as not to damage the plexus autonomicus around the aorta. In the posterior direction, the actual TME includes the entire retrorectal pad of fat (i.e., the mesorectum is included in the mobilized segment) and occurs along the retrorectal space (black arrow; see also p. 381) between the fasciae pelvis visceralis (rectal fascia) and parietalis. In the anterior direction the mobilization occurs in the prerectal space along the fascia rectoprostatica (Denonvilliers'), and in lateral direction the entire area extending to the pelvic wall (the pararectal fascia) is mobilized while protecting the nn. hypogastricus and splanchnici pelvici. After mobilization of the rectum to the m. levator ani and after the m. puborectalis sling has been identified, the rectum is resected with a safety margin of 2 cm. A stapling device is used to attach the colon to the rectal stump, a procedure known as a coloanal anastomosis.

3.12 Hepar: Position and Relationship to Adjacent Organs

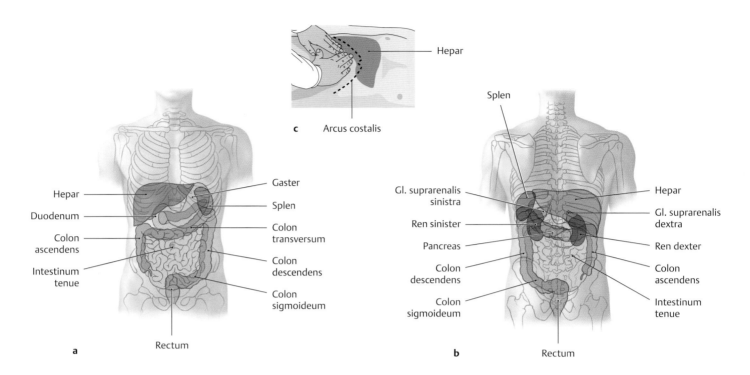

c   Arcus costalis

a

b

A Projection of the hepar onto the trunk and adjacent organs; palpation of the hepar

a Anterior view, **b** posterior view, **c** palpation of the liver.
The hepar is situated mainly in the right upper quadrant but extends across the epigastrium into the left upper quadrant, lying anterior to the gaster. The lobus hepatis dexter is closely related to the right ren and flexura coli dextra. Owing to the dome of the hemidiaphragm, the cavitas pleuralis overlaps the anterior and posterior surfaces of the hepar. Because the hepar is attached to the inferior surface of the diaphragma, its position is significantly affected by respiratory excursions.

It also depends on posture and age: The hepar descends in the standing position, and it is also affected by the gradual settling of organs that occurs with aging. The hepar is palpated (**c**) most easily by having the patient lie supine with the abdominal wall relaxed (legs drawn up) and exhale fully (the hepar rises with the diaphragma), followed by a full inhalation. This causes the hepar to fall, and its sharp margo inferior (see **B**) can be palpated at the margin of the ribs. If the hepar is abnormally enlarged (hepatomegaly), it may occasionally extend to the apertura pelvis superior.

B Liver in situ: Location of the hepar in the cavitas abdominis

Anterior view of the opened abdomen, the cor and pulmones have been removed; the lig. falciforme and lig. teres hepatis have been transected anteriorly.
The hepar occupies the right regio hypochondriaca and extends across the regio epigastrica and into the left upper quadrant. The gaster is visible at the margo inferior of the lobus hepatis sinister, and the vesica biliaris is visible at the margo inferior of the lobus dexter.
Note: Owing to the dome-shaped structure of the diaphragma, the hepar and cavitas thoracica lie on the same horizontal plane and they partially overlap. Thus, perforating injuries of the cavitas thoracis containing the pulmones may also involve the cavitas abdominis containing the hepar. This is known as a multicavity injury.

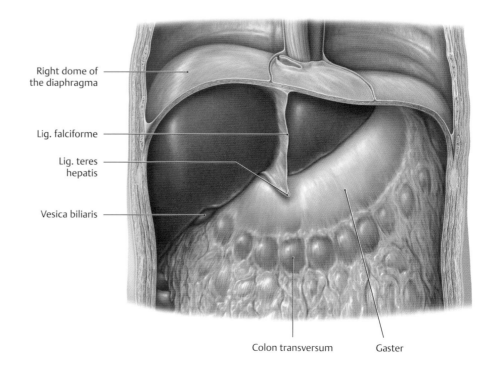

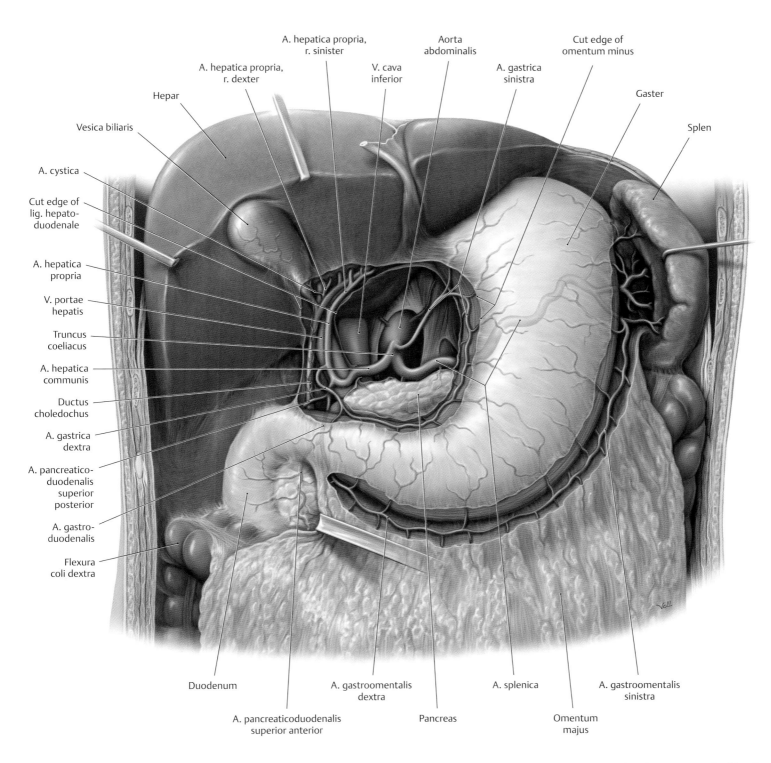

A. hepatica propria, r. sinister
A. hepatica propria, r. dexter
Hepar
Vesica biliaris
A. cystica
Cut edge of lig. hepato-duodenale
A. hepatica propria
V. portae hepatis
Truncus coeliacus
A. hepatica communis
Ductus choledochus
A. gastrica dextra
A. pancreatico-duodenalis superior posterior
A. gastro-duodenalis
Flexura coli dextra

Aorta abdominalis
V. cava inferior
A. gastrica sinistra
Cut edge of omentum minus
Gaster
Splen

Duodenum
A. pancreaticoduodenalis superior anterior
A. gastroomentalis dextra
Pancreas
A. splenica
Omentum majus
A. gastroomentalis sinistra

C The hepar in situ after the omentum minus has been opened

Anterior view of the opened upper abdomen, the hepar and splen have been lifted.

The omentum minus has been opened allowing a direct view into the bursa omentalis. A small section of the cavitas pleuralis is visible immediately to the right and slightly above the lobus hepatis dexter (see p. 253). The anterior border of the hepar, which points downward in situ, has a sharp edge that is clearly palpable when the hepar is enlarged. The inferior surface of the hepatis bears a fossa for the vesica biliaris (see p. 256), whose fundus is directed anteriorly toward the abdominal wall and extends slightly past the margo inferior hepatis. The right portion of the omentum minus, the lig. hepatoduodenale, transmits the blood vessels of the hepar (a. hepatica propria and v. portae hepatis) and the ductus choledochus. The contour of the right ren can be seen on the inferior surface of the lobus hepatis dexter.

Note: The opening of the vv. hepaticae into the v. cava inferior is located just below the diaphragma (see p. 257), just a few centimeters from the atrium dextrum of the cor. Thus, in cases where the right side of the cor has lost pumping power (right-sided heart failure), blood may engorge the liver, causing palpable hepatic enlargement. When palpating the liver, the examiner should take into account the variable position of the organ (see **Ac**).

3.13 Hepar: Peritoneal Relationships and Shape

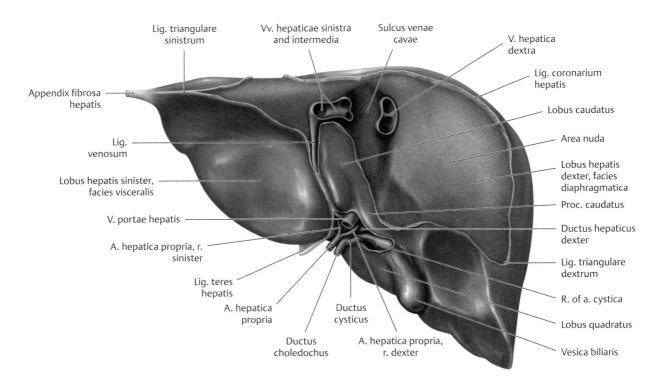

A Peritoneal covering of the hepar

Posterior view of the upper part of the facies diaphragmatica of the hepar. The hepar is surrounded by a capsula fibrosa with extensions that pass into the hepar and transmit neurovascular structures. Most of the *surface* of the hepar is covered by glistening peritoneum viscerale, which is external to the capsula fibrosa. Only the area nuda, which is highly variable in extent, *lacks a peritoneal covering*; it has a rough appearance because the capsula fibrosa forms its surface. The vv. hepaticae (usually three in number) leave the hepar in the area nuda, and thus *outside* the peritoneal covering. This is different from all other intraperitoneal

organs, which have mesenteric structures for transmitting their veins and arteries. In the case of the hepar, only the *afferent* artery, *afferent* v. portae hepatis, and ductus choledochus course in the lig. hepatoduodenale (see **Cb**), while the efferent veins do not. At sites where the peritoneum viscerale is reflected into the peritoneum parietale on the inferior surface of the diaphragma, the delicate peritoneal epithelium is often backed by connective tissue to form a ligamentous band (lig. coronarium hepatis, see **Ca**). This connective tissue is drawn out into a tapered band at the extremity of the lobus hepatis sinister (appendix fibrosa hepatis).

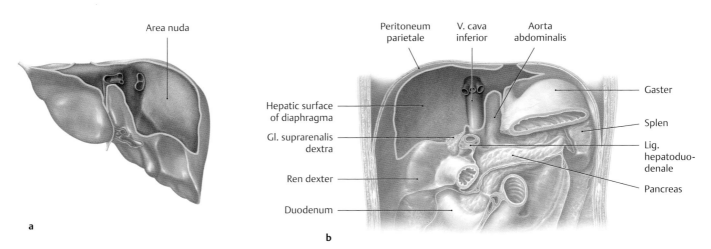

B Area nuda of the hepar and the hepatic surface of the diaphragma

Posterior view of the facies diaphragmatica of the hepar (**a**) and the inferior surface of the diaphragma (**b**). The lines of peritoneal reflection on the hepar and diaphragma demonstrate the mirror-image

correspondence of the area nuda with the hepatic surface of the diaphragma. The area nuda is firmly attached to the inferior surface of the diaphragma by peritoneal reflection (ligg. coronaria), rendering the hepar immobile despite its intraperitoneal location.

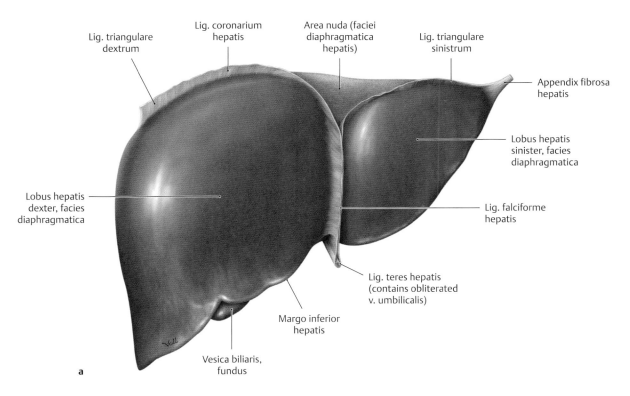

a

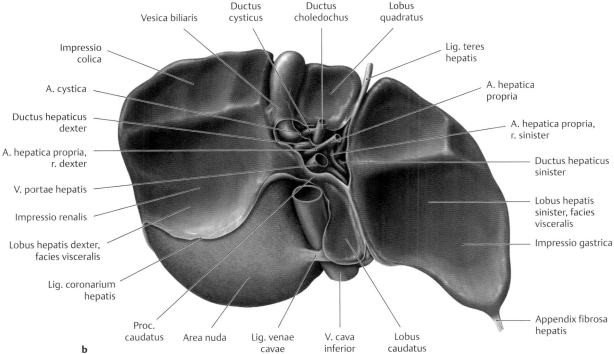

b

C Hepar: Facies diaphragmatica and visceralis

a **Anterior view of the facies diaphragmatica.** Two lobi are visible in this view: the larger lobus dexter and the smaller lobus sinister. Between the two lobi is the lig. falciforme of the hepar, a "ventral mesentery" that extends to the anterior abdominal wall.

b **Inferior view of the facies visceralis.** Two more of the four hepatic lobes are visible in this view: the lobus caudatus and lobus quadratus. The facies visceralis also contains the porta hepatis where neurovascular structures enter and leave the hepar (ductus hepaticus communis, a. hepatica propria, v. portae hepatis). Topographically, the lig.

hepatoduodenale is a component of the omentum minus. The extent of the lig. hepatoduodenale can be appreciated by noting the cut edge of peritoneum viscerale surrounding the trias hepatica. Along with the lig. hepatogastricum, it creates a "dorsal mesentery" for the liver. The numerous impressions from adjacent organs are seen this plainly only in a hepar that has been chemically preserved. The vesicula biliaris is closely applied to the facies visceralis of the hepar. Its fundus extends slightly past the margo inferior hepatis, and its neck is directed toward the porta hepatis, where it comes into contact with the extrahepatic bile ducts.

253

3.14 Hepar: Segmentation and Histology

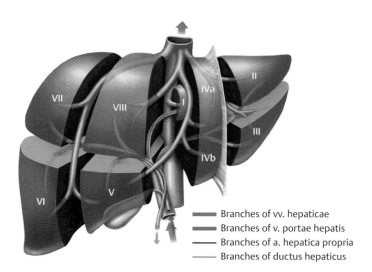

- ▬ Branches of vv. hepaticae
- ▬ Branches of v. portae hepatis
- — Branches of a. hepatica propria
- — Branches of ductus hepaticus

A Segmentation of the hepar

Anterior view. The a. hepatica propria, v. portae hepatis, and ductus hepaticus communis enter/exit the hepar at the porta hepatis as the "trias hepatica." The central branch first divides into two larger branches, functionally subdividing the hepar into partes hepatis sinistra (yellow) and dextra (purple). The boundary between the partes hepatis sinistra and dextra is an imaginary line that roughly connects the fossa vesicae biliaris to the v. cava inferior (caval-gallbladder line, see **Cb**). Thus it is not identical to the externally visible boundary formed by the lig. falciforme (see p. 253). The trias hepatica continues to ramify within the liver, forming a total of eight segmenta that are more or less functionally independent of one another. This allows the surgeon to resect one or more hepatic segmenta without damaging the hepar as a whole. Additionally, the remaining hepatic segmenta have a high regenerative potential. In the diagram above, the hepar has been "exploded" at its virtual segmental boundaries to demonstrate the position and shape of its segmenta (numerical designations are shown in **B** and **C**).

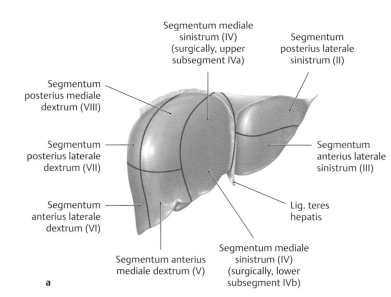

a

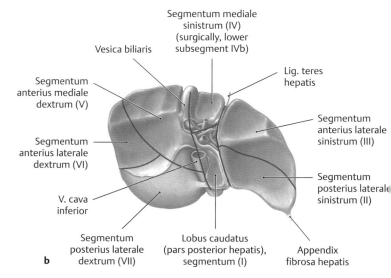

b

C Projection of segmental boundaries onto the surface of the hepar

Views of the facies diaphragmatica (**a**) and facies visceralis of the hepar (**b**).* The segments defined by the divisions of the portal vascular triad (see **A**) are projected onto the surface of the hepar with their virtual boundaries. In this way the pattern of hepatic segmentation, which is based on vascular distribution, can be directly compared with the traditional division of the liver into four lobi based on external morphological criteria. For surgical purposes, it is useful to group the segmenta by partes and divisiones (see **B**) because the portion of the liver selected for surgical resection may encompass not just one segmentum but two neighboring segmenta or the entire pars hepatis dextra or sinistra. Surgeons can positively identify the hepatic segmenta by ligating the feeding vessels until the segmentum or segmenta become discolored due to loss of blood supply.

* Blue line in **b**: caval-gallbladder line

B Hepatic segmenta grouped by parts and divisions

Pars hepatis sinister	• Segmentum posterius lobus caudatus	• Segmentum I
	• Divisio lateralis sinistra	• Segmentum posterius laterale sinistrum (segmentum II) • Segmentum anterius laterale sinistrum (segmentum III)
	• Divisio medialis sinistra	• Segmentum mediale sinistrum (segmentum IV), subdivided into subsegment IVa (above) and IVb (below)
Pars hepatis dextra	• Divisio medialis dextra	• Segmentum anterius mediale dextrum (segmentum V) • Segmentum posterius mediale dextrum (segmentum VIII)
	• Divisio lateralis dextra	• Segmentum anterius laterale dextrum (segmentum VI) • Segmentum posterius laterale dextrum (segmentum VII)

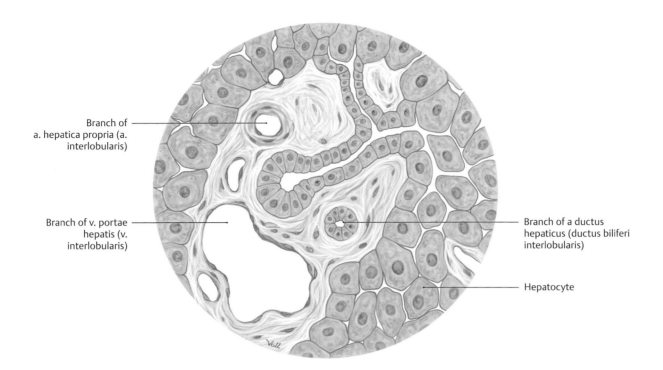

D Histological appearance of a portal area

Hematoxylin and eosin stain, magnification approximately 540x. The trias hepatica of the hepar, while grossly visible at the porta hepatis, ramifies into a network of microscopic branches embedded in connective tissue: the portal area. The trias hepatica at this level consists of the a. hepatica propria, which becomes the a. interlobularis (situated between several lobules), the v. portae hepatis, which becomes the v. interlobularis, and the ductus hepaticus communis, which becomes the ductus bilifer interlobularis. These structures are easily distinguished from one another by differences in their calibers, wall thickness, and wall structure:

- A. interlobularis: thick wall, squamous epithelium, small lumen
- V. interlobularis: thin wall, squamous epithelium, large lumen

- Ductus bilifer interlobularis: cuboidal epithelium and very small lumen

Cirrhosis of the liver is characterized by a proliferation of connective tissue in the liver that is most conspicuous in the portal area and about the vv. centrales. Necrotic hepatocytes are permanently replaced by scar tissue. The sinuses—the capillary bed of the liver—are obliterated in the scarred areas, progressively diminishing the blood flow through the hepar. The afferent blood vessels are still carrying the same amount of blood to the hepar, however. This causes obstruction of portal venous flow and an abnormal pressure increase (portal hypertension). In many cases the blood is returned to the right cor by an alternate route (portosystemic collaterals, see p. 218).

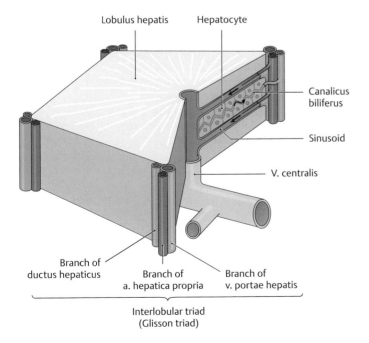

Interlobular triad
(Glisson triad)

E Structure of a central venous lobule (lobulus hepatis)

This is a *three-dimensional structural model* of a lobulus hepatis based on studies of numerous histological sections (see **D**). It shows that each polyhedral lobulus hepatis is composed of hepatocytes that are arrayed around a v. centralis (hence the term "central venous lobule"). Ultimately the vv. centrales return their blood to the vv. hepaticae. The portal area (see **D**) in this model is located *between* adjacent lobuli at the points where the lobuli interconnect (hence the term "interlobularis" for the artery, vein, and bile duct).

While the a. and v. interlobularis convey their blood into sinusoids that have a stable wall (see **D**), the canaliculi biliferi that transfer bile to the ductus bilifer interlobularis do not have their own walls. They also course between the hepatocytes, but on the opposite side from the sinusoids. If biliary stasis develops between adjacent hepatocytes (e.g., due to hepatitis), the hepatocytes may separate and lose their intercellular contacts. Abnormally large interspaces may form, allowing the bile to escape from the canaliculi biliferi and seep to the opposite side of the cells, where it can enter the sinusoids and bloodstream, causing a yellowish discoloration of the skin and mucous membranes (jaundice).

255

3.15 Vesica Biliaris and Ductus Biliares: Location and Relationships to Adjacent Organs

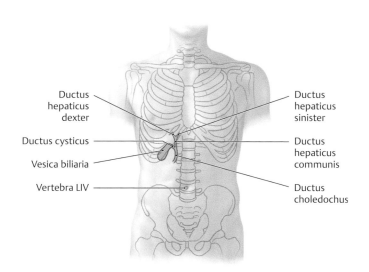

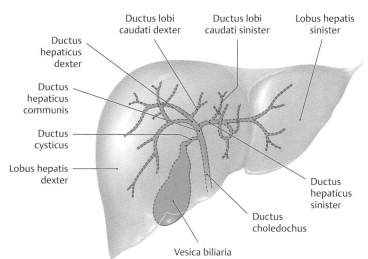

A Projection of the extrahepatic bile ducts onto the skeleton

Viewed from the front, the vesica biliaris is projected at a point where the mid-clavicular line intersects the margo inferior of the ninth rib. The orifice of the ductus choledochus (which generally opens jointly with the ductus pancreaticus on the papilla duodeni major) lies approximately at the level of the corpus vertebrae L2. The vesica biliaris emerges beneath the right arcus costalis at approximately the L1/L2 level. In certain diseases (e.g., cholecystitis), tenderness to pressure may be noted at this location.

B Projection of the intra- and extrahepatic bile ducts onto the surface of the hepar

Anterior view. Bile flows through the canaliculi biliferi (microscopic) into the small ductuli biliferi interlobulares in the portal area (see p. 255). These ducts coalesce to form increasingly larger units that drain a hepatic segmentum. The bile from all the segmenta ultimately drains into two large collecting vessels, the ductus hepatici sinister and dexter, which receive the small ductus lobi caudati sinister and dexter, respectively, while still inside the hepar. The ductus hepatici dexter and sinister unite to form the ductus hepaticus communis. Almost immediately the excretory duct of the vesica biliaris, the ductus cysticus, enters the side of the ductus hepaticus communis, which then becomes the ductus choledochus.

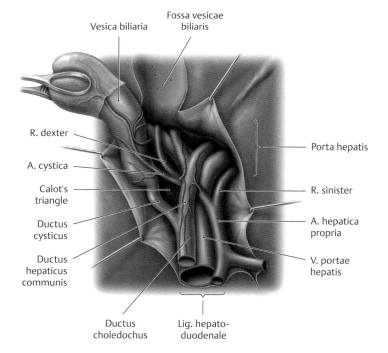

C Topography of Calot's triangle at the fissura portalis

Inferoanterior view. The anterior margin of the lobus dexter has been pushed upward, the vesica biliaris has been lifted from its fossa and retracted to the right. The peritoneum has been opened in the area of the fissura portalis and the lig. hepatoduodenale. For better exposure, nerves, nodi lymphoidei and their pathways have been removed (after von Lanz and Wachsmuth). 95% of injuries to the extrahepatic ductus biliares are sustained intraoperatively, most commonly during cholecystectomies. Particularly with the minimally invasive surgical method to remove the vesica biliaris (laparoscopic cholecystectomy), the precise identification of anatomical structures is an essential aspect of this surgical procedure. Thus, before transecting the a. cystica and the ductus cysticus it is important to identify Calot's triangle (trigonum cystohepaticum), which is bordered by the a. cystica, ductus cysticus and ductus hepaticus communis. The fundus vesicae biliaris is grasped and retracted slightly superiorly to expose and open the trigonum cystohepaticum. The structures that are to be transected are ligated with clips.

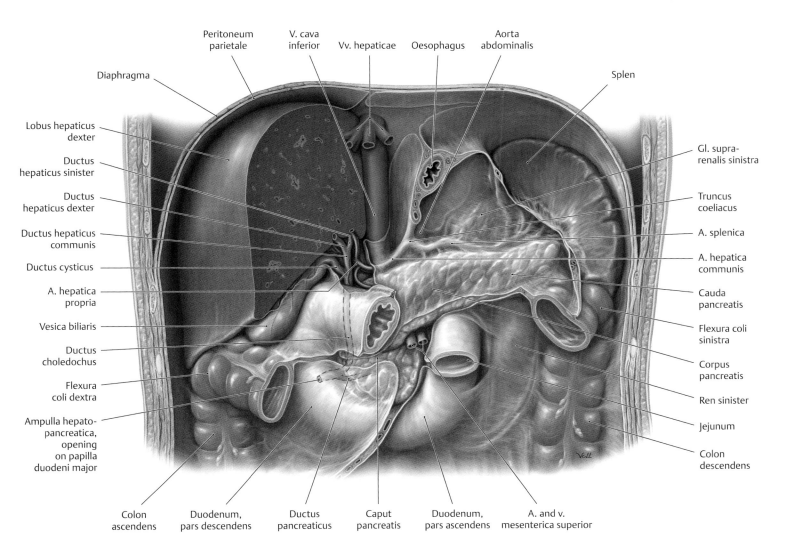

Peritoneum parietale — V. cava inferior — Vv. hepaticae — Oesophagus — Aorta abdominalis — Splen

Diaphragma

Lobus hepaticus dexter

Ductus hepaticus sinister

Ductus hepaticus dexter

Ductus hepaticus communis

Ductus cysticus

A. hepatica propria

Vesica biliaris

Ductus choledochus

Flexura coli dextra

Ampulla hepato-pancreatica, opening on papilla duodeni major

Gl. supra-renalis sinistra

Truncus coeliacus

A. splenica

A. hepatica communis

Cauda pancreatis

Flexura coli sinistra

Corpus pancreatis

Ren sinister

Jejunum

Colon descendens

Colon ascendens — Duodenum, pars descendens — Ductus pancreaticus — Caput pancreatis — Duodenum, pars ascendens — A. and v. mesenterica superior

D Relationship of the biliary tract to adjacent organs
Anterior view of the opened abdomen. The gaster, intestinum tenue, colon transversum, and large portions of the hepar have been removed, and the peritoneum has been divided in the area of the lig. hepatoduo-denale. The vesica biliaris is partially contained in a fossa on the facies visceralis of the hepar. The ductus choledochus passes behind the duo-denum toward the caput pancreatis. After passing through the caput pancreatis, the ductus biliaris frequently unites with the ductus pancre-aticus, as shown here. Both ducts then open together at the papilla duo-deni major in the pars descendens of the duodenum (see p. 258).

E Bile: Secretion, composition and function

Secretion:
Bile is a thin secretion (up to 1200 ml/day) produced by the hepar (hepatic bile). After water and salts have been removed, the bile is stored in the vesica biliaris (gallbladder bile) or runs into the duodenum via bile ducts. The major driving force for the secretion of bile is ATP-powered pumps, which transport mainly bile acids and other substances to the canaliculi biliferi, and into which water follows by osmosis.

Composition:
Water, bile acids or their salts (e.g., cholate, deoxycholate), phospholipids (mainly lecithin), bile pigments (e.g., bilirubin), cholesterol, inorganic salts, etc.

Enterohepatic circulation:
98 % of the bile salts secreted into the vesica biliaris are reabsorbed in the pars terminalis ilei, returned to the hepar via the v. portae hepatis, and secreted again from hepatocytes. In this way, bile salts are recycled up to 10 times per day before they are excreted in the feces.

Function:
Bile has essentially two major functions:
- Absorption of fat in the intestinum tenue: together with phospholip-ids, the bile salts emulsify insoluble lipids (through formation of lipid micelles);
- Route for excretion of cholesterol and other waste products (e.g., bili-rubin, a by-product of hemoglobin breakdown).

Gallstones:
Gallstones are caused by changes in vesica biliaris bile composition (cho-lesterol and pigment stones). The stones themselves usually do not pro-duce any symptoms. Only the obstruction or inflammation of the bile ducts caused by the gallstones leads to symptoms (cholelithiasis, cholecystitis).

3.16 Extrahepatic Ductus Biliares and Ductus Pancreatici

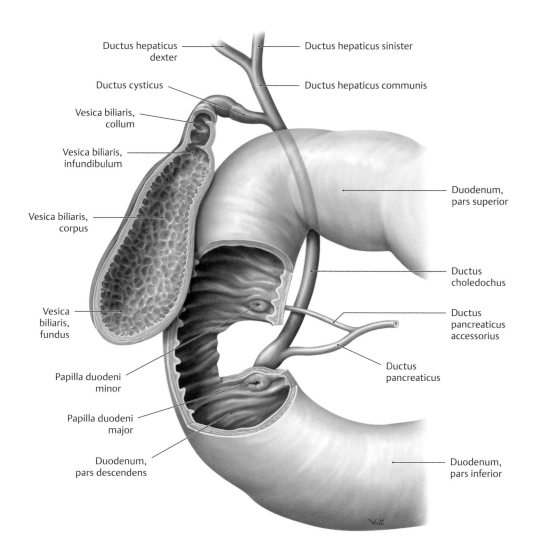

Ductus hepaticus dexter
Ductus hepaticus sinister
Ductus cysticus
Ductus hepaticus communis
Vesica biliaris, collum
Vesica biliaris, infundibulum
Duodenum, pars superior
Vesica biliaris, corpus
Ductus choledochus
Vesica biliaris, fundus
Ductus pancreaticus accessorius
Papilla duodeni minor
Ductus pancreaticus
Papilla duodeni major
Duodenum, pars descendens
Duodenum, pars inferior

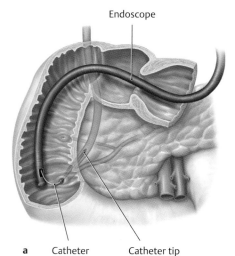

Endoscope

a   Catheter   Catheter tip

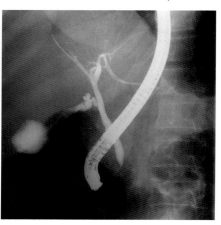

b

A Divisions of the extrahepatic ductus biliares

Anterior view. The vesica biliaris has been opened, and the duodenum has been opened and windowed. The web-like pattern of plicae mucosae in the tunica mucosa vesicae biliaris is plainly seen. The mucosa between the plicae may be deepened to form crypts that can trap bacteria (with risk of cholecystitis). The largest part of the vesica biliaris is the *corpus* vesicae biliaris, which is joined to the collum vesicae biliaris by the funnel-shaped infundibulum vesicae biliaris. The collum leads to the ductus cysticus, which opens end-to-side into the ductus hepaticus communis, formed by the union of the *ductus hepatici dexter* and *sinister*. The large duct formed by the union of the ductus cysticus and ductus hepaticus communis is called the *ductus choledochus*. This duct often receives the ductus pancreaticus, both of which then discharge their secretions into the duodenum at the papilla duodeni major (of Vater). A short distance superior to the papilla duodeni major is the papilla duodeni minor, whose associated duct (ductus pancreaticus accessorius) crosses in front of the ductus choledochus. The diagram illustrates a normal pattern of development in which the ductus hepaticus communis and pancreaticus unite to form an ampulla (variants are shown in **D**).

Note: The combined termination of the ductus choledochus and ductus pancreaticus has two important implications: A tumor in the caput pancreatis may obstruct the ductus choledochus (causing biliary reflux into the hepar with jaundice), and a gallstone that has migrated from the vesica biliaris into the ductus choledochus may obstruct the terminal part of the ductus pancreaticus. The obstruction of pancreatic secretions may incite a life-threatening pancreatitis.

B Endoscopic retrograde cholangiopancreatography (ERCP)

a Anterior view, duodenum opened anteriorly;
b Image of the corresponding region using ERCP (**b** from: Möller, T.B,. E. Reif: Taschenatlas der Röntgenanatomie, 3. Aufl. Thieme, Stuttgart 2006).

ERCP is a technique that uses radiographic contrast (see **b**) to display the ductus biliares, vesica biliaris and ductus pancreaticus. An endoscope is used to locate the papilla duodeni (major or minor) and to inject contrast agent into the papillary orifice. A radiograph of the contrast-filled duct system can then be evaluated. ERCP can also be used to remove gallstones that have become impacted at the papilla (endoscopic papillotomy) with the help of a scissor-cutting device fitted to the tip of the endoscope. Thus, ERCP is used for diagnosis and treatment.

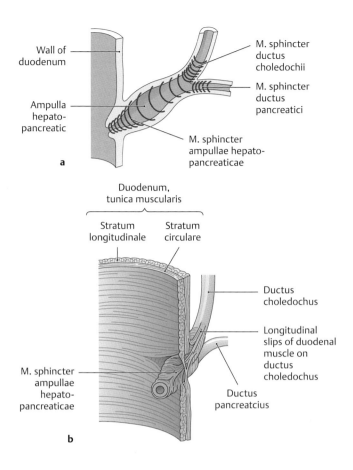

a

Wall of duodenum

Ampulla hepato-pancreatic

M. sphincter ductus choledochii

M. sphincter ductus pancreatici

M. sphincter ampullae hepato-pancreaticae

b

Duodenum, tunica muscularis

Stratum longitudinale

Stratum circulare

Ductus choledochus

Longitudinal slips of duodenal muscle on ductus choledochus

M. sphincter ampullae hepato-pancreaticae

Ductus pancreatcius

C Function and structure of the biliary sphincter system

a Sphincters of the ductus choledochus and ductus pancreaticus. Each duct has its own sphincter system. Typically both of the ducts unite to form a large ampulla, the hepatopancreatic ampulla, which also has its own sphincter. The sphincter mechanism is supported by adjacent venous pads (not shown here) in the walls of the ducts.

b Integration of the sphincter system in the duodenal wall. The muscles of both ducts blend with the sphincter muscle of the hepatopancreatic ampulla, which passes through the duodenal wall.

Note: The ampullary sphincter system works independently of the circular muscle layer of the duodenal wall, allowing the sphincters to function even during fasting when the duodenum is relaxed. In this state the ductal sphincters are contracted and bile is stored. When food is ingested, the sphincter system opens and allows bile to flow into the duodenum. The sphincter system forms a normal anatomical constriction where a gallstone may become lodged, obstructing the outflow of bile and pancreatic juice (pancreatitis, see **A**). The function of the sphincters, the discharge of bile by the vesica biliaris, and the production of bile by the hepar are controlled partially by the autonomic nervous system (especially the parasympathetic system) and partially by gastrointestinal hormones (e.g., cholecystokinin and secretin).

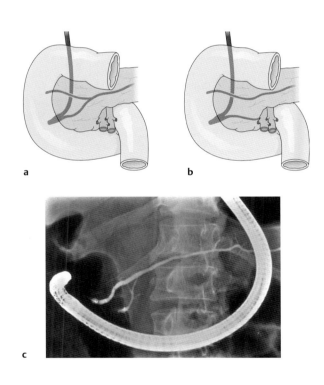

a   **b**

c

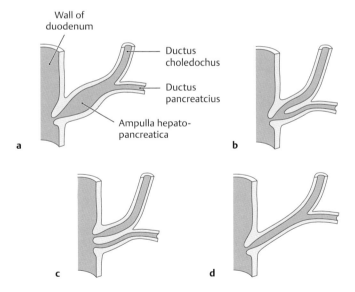

a

Wall of duodenum

Ductus choledochus

Ductus pancreatcius

Ampulla hepato-pancreatica

b

c   **d**

D Extrahepatic bile ducts: Typical anatomy and variants

Variants in the termination of the ductus choledochus and ductus pancreaticus.

a Typical anatomy: Both ducts open at the papilla duodeni major by way of a common ampulla hepatopancreatica (the most common form).

b–d Variants:

b Varying degrees of septation of the common ampulla hepatopancreatica.

c Complete septation of the ampulla hepatopancreatica, with a separate opening for each duct.

d The ducts unite without forming a true ampulla.

E Pancreas: Normal anatomy and variants

a Gemmae pancreaticae have fused; **b** Pancreas divisum (in up to 10% of examined patients); **c** Pancreas divisum at ERCP (**c** from Brambs, H.-J.: Pareto Reihe Radiologie. Gastrointestinal system. Thieme, Stuttgart 2007).

Failure of the gemma pancreatica dorsalis to fuse with the gemma pancreatica ventralis (see p. 43) leads to a divided pancreas (pancreas divisum; no clinical disease, usually presents as an incidental finding). The ducts of both buds remain completely separate. The duct of the gemma pancreatica ventralis opens into the papilla duodeni major and the duct of the gemma pancreatica dorsalis into the papilla duodeni minor. In ERCP (see **c**) both ducts were filled separately via the two papillae.

3.17 Pancreas

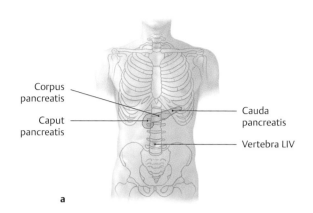

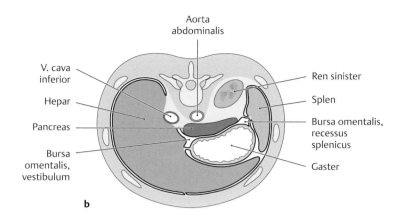

a

b

A Location of the pancreas

a Projection onto the vertebral column; **b** Transverse section through the abdomen at approximately the T 12/L 1 level, viewed from above. *Note:* The head of the pancreas is below the plane of section which is why the pancreas appears shortened at this level.

The pancreas is an elongated organ that is oriented transversely in the right and left upper quadrants, lying mainly in the epigastric region.

Whereas most of the body of the pancreas crosses the midline at the L 1/L 2 level. Caput pancreatis is directed to the right and extends to the L 2/L 3 level. The tail of the pancreas may closely approach the spleen in the LUQ. The pain associated with diseases of the pancreas is often a "girdling pain" that encircles the upper abdomen and even the lower thorax (see p. 284).

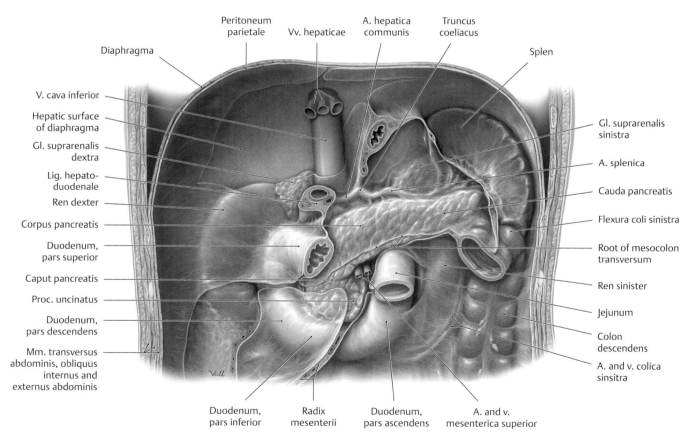

B The pancreas in situ

Anterior view. The hepar, gaster, intestinum tenue, and intestinum crassum have been removed proximal to the flexura coli sinistra. The retroperitoneal fat and connective tissue and the capsula adiposa have been greatly thinned to better demonstrate the structures in the retroperitoneum. The pancreas is a secondarily retroperitoneal organ located on the posterior wall of the bursa omentalis. Its head (caput pancreatis) lies in the C-shaped loop of the duodenum. The mesocolon transversum is attached to the facies anterior of the pancreas. Because of its position posterior to or adjacent to other organs and large vessels, it is difficult to access surgically. At the same time, owing to its proximity, pancreatic tumors may invade and encase the a. and v. mesenterica superior (leading to impaired circulation of the organs they supply, such as the jejunum, ileum, and colon ascendens). Inflammation of or tumors in the caput pancreatis may also lead to obstruction of the ductus choledochus (leading to obstructive jaundice).

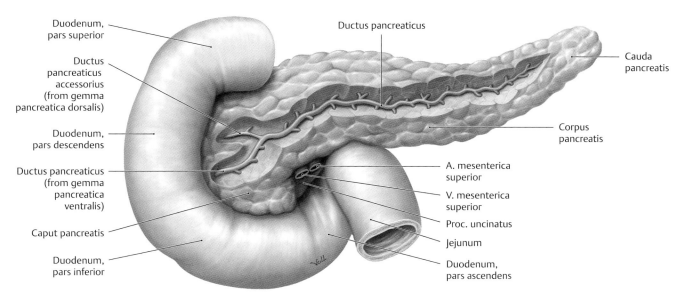

Labels for the upper figure:
- Duodenum, pars superior
- Ductus pancreaticus accessorius (from gemma pancreatica dorsalis)
- Duodenum, pars descendens
- Ductus pancreaticus (from gemma pancreatica ventralis)
- Caput pancreatis
- Duodenum, pars inferior
- Ductus pancreaticus
- Cauda pancreatis
- Corpus pancreatis
- A. mesenterica superior
- V. mesenterica superior
- Proc. uncinatus
- Jejunum
- Duodenum, pars ascendens

C Location and course of the ductus pancreatici

Anterior view. The anterior side has been partially dissected. The ducts of the former gemmae pancreaticae ventralis and dorsalis have united to form a common duct, which is referred to as the main ductus pancreatis (formed from the ductus pancreaticus ventralis in the caput pancreatis and the distal portion of the ductus pancreatis dorsalis (most common case). It traverses the entire length of the pancreas and opens into the pars descendens of the duodenum, usually sharing an orifice with the ductus choledochus, on the papilla duodeni major. The small ductus pancreatis accessorius (the remaining proximal portion of the former ductus pancreaticus dorsalis in the caput pancreatis) opens into the duodenum on the papilla duodeni minor (see p. 259). Several variants of ductal anatomy may exist:

- both ducts remain separate and open on two different papillae (pancreas divisum, see p. 259),
- both ducts unite to form a single duct that opens on one papilla,
- in both cases (though rarely), the ductus choledochus may open into the duodenum by a separate orifice.

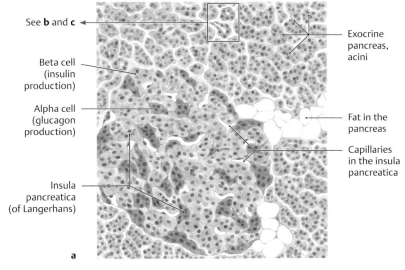

Labels for figure a:
- See **b** and **c**
- Beta cell (insulin production)
- Alpha cell (glucagon production)
- Insula pancreatica (of Langerhans)
- Exocrine pancreas, acini
- Fat in the pancreas
- Capillaries in the insula pancreatica

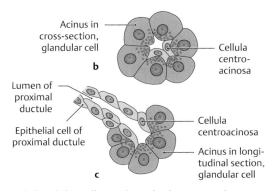

Labels for figures b and c:
- Acinus in cross-section, glandular cell
- **b**
- Cellula centroacinosa
- Lumen of proximal ductule
- Epithelial cell of proximal ductule
- Cellula centroacinosa
- Acinus in longitudinal section, glandular cell
- **c**

levels, and the alpha cells produce the hormone glucagon. Other islet cell types include delta (D) and F cells, which produce somatostatin or pancreatic polypeptide. Special staining methods are used to make these cell types visible. The islet cells release hormones directly into the bloodstream (which is why there are many capillaries present in the insulae pancreaticae).

Note: A decrease in the number of beta-cells and deficient or defective production of insulin leads to the clinical picture of diabetes mellitus.

b The **acinar cells** produce approximately 2 liters of "pancreatic juice," an enzyme-rich secretion (containing numerous proteins) per day, which is passed into the duodenum via the ductus pancreaticus. This secretion is important for digestion. Thus, hypofunction of the exocrine pancreas leads to maldigestion.

Note: Acinar cells usually stain intensely with conventional techniques. Nonetheless, they don't appear equally dark in histological sections. The parts that transport secretions (the ductule cells) stain less intensely than the parts that produce secretions. Because the initial portion of the part that transports secretions is invaginated into the center of the acinus, which stains more intensely, they are conspicuous in histological sections. These cells that lie at the center of the acinus, but belong to the secretion-transporting part, are referred to as cellulae centroacinosae. The pancreas is the only exocrine gland that cellulae centroacinosae.

D Histological structure of the pancreas

a Pancreatic tissue; **b** and **c** Detail from **a**: Higher magnification views of acini shown in transverse and longitudinal sections.

a Histologically, the pancreas consists of two functionally distinct types of glandular tissue:

- The **exocrine pancreas** (98 % of the organ mass, light pink in the upper part of the figure) consists of myriad berry-shaped glands (acini pancreatis, see **b** and **c**), which secrete an enzyme-rich fluid through the ductus pancreaticus into the duodenum. Produced at a rate of approximately 2 liters/day, this fluid contains enzymes that assist numerous digestive processes in the bowel. Insufficiency of the exocrine pancreas leads to impaired digestive function.
- The **endocrine pancreas** (2 % of the organ mass) also known as the islet apparatus: approximately 1 million epithelial cells (islets of Langerhans, insulae pancreaticae), which can be divided into alpha (A) cells (20 % of islet cells) and beta (B) cells (80 % of islet cells). The beta cells produce insulin, which lowers blood glucose

261

3.18   Splen

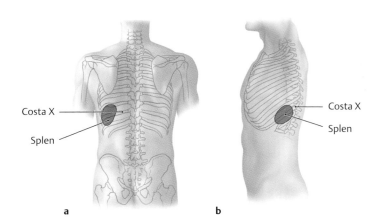

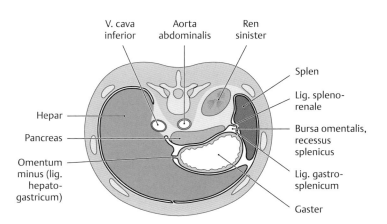

A Projection of the splen onto the skeleton
Posterior view (**a**) and left lateral view (**b**). The splen is located in the left upper quadrant. Its position varies considerably with respiration because it lies just below the diaphragma and is directly affected by its movements, even though (unlike the hepar) it is not attached to the diaphragma. At functional residual capacity (the resting position between inspiration and expiration), the hilum splenicum crosses the tenth rib on the left side. Generally a healthy, unenlarged splen is not palpable on physical examination.

B Location of the splen
Transverse section through the abdomen, viewed from above. This section demonstrates the relationship of the splen to neighboring organs. The intraperitoneal splen lies in its own compartment and is attached by folds of peritoneum to the posterior trunk wall (lig. splenorenale) and to the stomach (lig. gastrosplenicum). A recess of the bursa omentalis (recessus splenicus) extends to the splen.

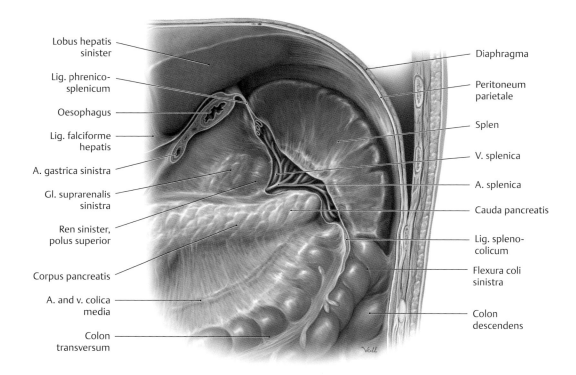

C The splen in situ: Peritoneal relationships
Anterior view into the LUQ with the gaster removed. When the splen is abnormally enlarged, it may press heavily upon the gaster and colon, causing pain. The drawing illustrates the close proximity of the splen to the cauda pancreatis and flexura coli sinistra, which is also called the flexura coli splenica.
Note the peritoneal attachment between the splenica and colon transversum (lig. splenocolicum, part of the omentum majus).

Embryologically, the omentum majus is a mesenterium dorsale in which the splen develops. During rotation of the gaster in the embryo, the splen moves from its original position posterior to the gut into the LUQ. A "side stitch" (piercing sensation felt below the cavea thoracica during exercise) is believed to be caused by stretching of the peritoneal covering and lig. splenocolicum due to swelling of the splen during physical exercise.

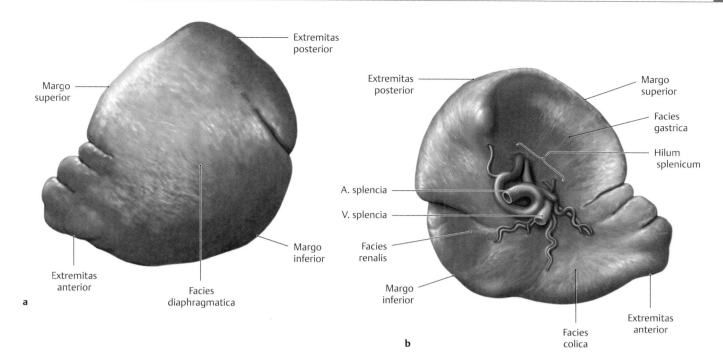

a

- Extremitas posterior
- Margo superior
- Extremitas anterior
- Facies diaphragmatica
- Margo inferior

b

- Extremitas posterior
- Margo superior
- Facies gastrica
- Hilum splenicum
- A. splencia
- V. splencia
- Facies renalis
- Margo inferior
- Facies colica
- Extremitas anterior

D Splen: Shape and surface anatomy

Views of the facies diaphragmatica (**a**) and facies visceralis (**b**) of the organ. The splen is highly variable in its conformation in different people, but because this very soft organ is covered by a firm fibrous capsula, it maintains a relatively constant external shape ("coffee bean"). Since it is very difficult to suture the soft splenic tissue, it is not uncommon to treat splenic injuries by splenectomy, which eliminates a potential source of severe intraperitoneal bleeding. The blood vessels that enter and leave the organ at the hilum splenicum are usually tortuous and form multiple coils.

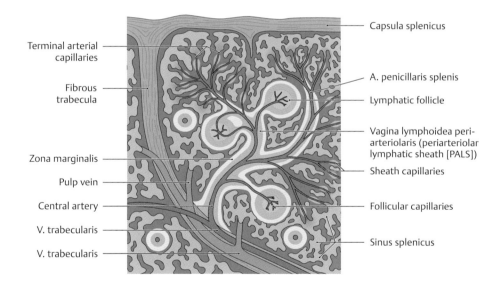

- Terminal arterial capillaries
- Fibrous trabecula
- Zona marginalis
- Pulp vein
- Central artery
- V. trabecularis
- V. trabecularis
- Capsula splenicus
- A. penicillaris splenis
- Lymphatic follicle
- Vagina lymphoidea peri-arteriolaris (periarteriolar lymphatic sheath [PALS])
- Sheath capillaries
- Follicular capillaries
- Sinus splenicus

E Structure of the splen

The splen is the single largest lymphoid organ and the only lymphatic organ that is incorporated directly into the bloodstream (to screen out abnormal cells, see below). Strands of connective tissue called trabeculae splenicae extend from the firm fibrous capsula (tunica fibrosa) toward the hilum splenicum, subdividing the splenic tissue into small chambers. The branches of the fibrous trabeculae splenicae and the vessels they transmit (*trabecular arteries and veins*) determine the architecture of the splen. Between the fibrous trabeculae splenicae is a meshwork of fine reticular connective tissue, the pulpa splenica. On entering the pulpa, the blood vessels become known as the *pulp arteries* (central arteries) and *pulp veins*. The terminal arterial branches have the appearance of the mycelia of bread mold (*penicillium*), and are thus named aa. penicillares splenis. Two types of pulpa splenica are distinguished: pulpa rubra and pulpa alba:

- The pulpa rubra consists of cavities (sinus splenici) that are engorged with blood in the living organism (aggregation of large masses of red blood cells), accounting for its red color and its name (in the section shown here, the pulpa rubra is devoid of blood and is colorless). The function of the pulpa rubra is to screen out aging and defective erythrocytes from the bloodstream. The numerous sinuses within the reticular meshwork give the splen its soft, spongy consistency.
- The pulpa alba consists of noduli lymphoidei splenici (Malpighian bodies)—variable-sized aggregations of lymphocytes (vaginae lymphoideae periarteriolares, lymphatic follicles) that consist of clones of beta cells that are proliferatory in response to antigens.

The lymphatic aggregations of the pulpa alba ensheath the central arteries in varying degrees to ensure close contact between the blood and lymphocytes. The central arteries ramify extensively before delivering their blood to the sinuses of the pulpa rubra. From there the blood is conveyed by pulp veins to the trabecular veins, which in turn empty into the v. splenica.

3.19 Branches of the Truncus Coeliacus: Arteries Supplying the Gaster, Hepar, and Vesica Biliaris

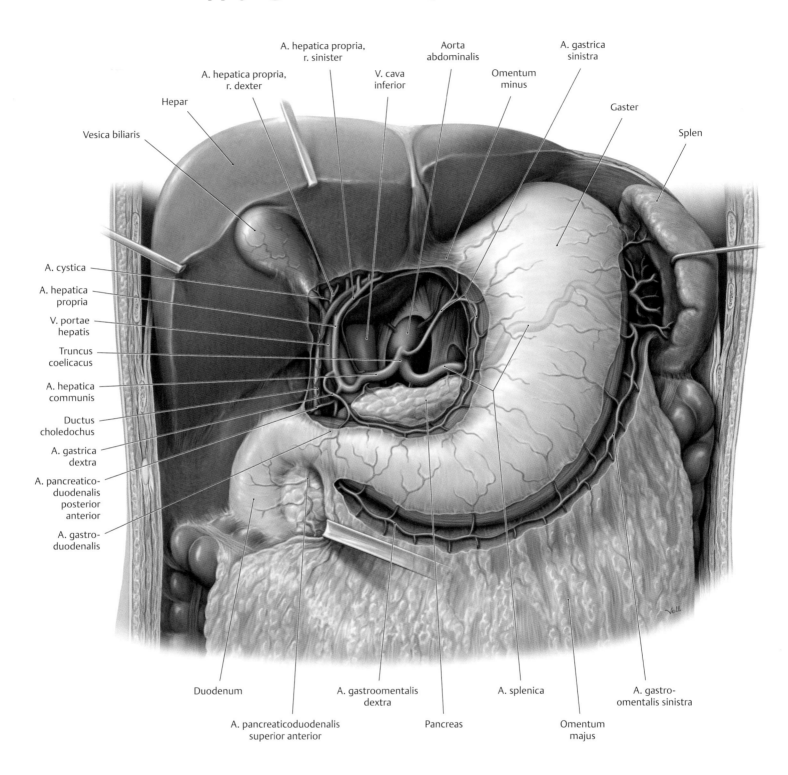

A. hepatica propria, r. sinister

A. hepatica propria, r. dexter

Hepar

Vesica biliaris

Aorta abdominalis

V. cava inferior

Omentum minus

A. gastrica sinistra

Gaster

Splen

A. cystica

A. hepatica propria

V. portae hepatis

Truncus coelicacus

A. hepatica communis

Ductus choledochus

A. gastrica dextra

A. pancreatico- duodenalis posterior anterior

A. gastro- duodenalis

Duodenum

A. pancreaticoduodenalis superior anterior

A. gastroomentalis dextra

Pancreas

A. splenica

Omentum majus

A. gastro- omentalis sinistra

A Truncus coeliacus and arteries to the gaster, hepar, and vesica biliaris

Anterior view. The omentum minus has been opened to display the truncus coeliacus. The omentum majus has been incised to demonstrate the aa. gastroomentales.

The truncus coeliacus is the first anterior visceral branch of the aorta abdominalis (see p. 211). It is only about 1 cm long. In 25% of cases it divides into three arterial branches in a tripod-like configuration, as illustrated here. The principal variants of the truncus coeliacus are shown in **C**.

Note that the a. hepatica propria, v. portae hepatis, and ductus choledochus reach the hepar by passing through the lig. hepatoduodenale, which is part of the omentum minus. These vessels must be protected in surgical operations on the vesica biliaris and ductus choledochus.

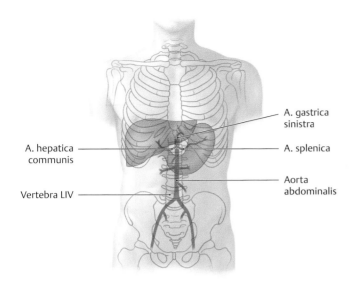

B Projection of the truncus coeliacus onto the columna vertebralis (T 12) and its relationship to the hepar and gaster

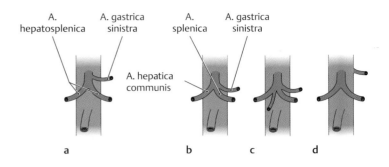

C Variants of the celiac trunk (after Lippert and Pabst)
a The truncus coeliacus divides into the a. gastrica sinistra and a. hepatosplenica (approximately 50 % of cases).
b The a. hepatica communis, a. gastrica sinistra, and a. splenica have a common origin (approximately 25 % of cases).
c The truncus coeliacus gives off a fourth branch to the pancreas (approximately 10 % of cases).
d The a. gastrica sinistra branches directly from the aorta abdominalis (approximately 5 % of cases). All other variants have an incidence less than 5 %.

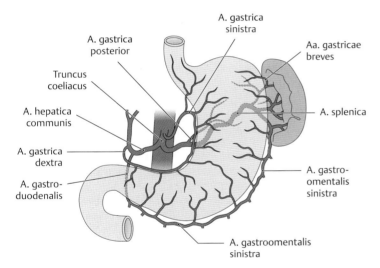

D Arteries of the gaster
Note that the *paries posterior* of the gaster is supplied by the a. gastrica posterior, which arises from the a. splenica in 60 % of cases. Variants of the aa. gastricae do occur, but for simplicity they are not illustrated here.

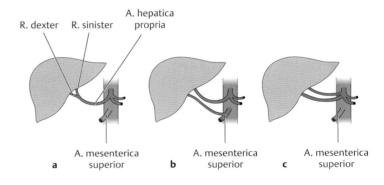

E Variants in the arterial supply to the hepar (after Lippert and Pabst)
a Typical division of the a. hepatica propria into rr. dexter and sinister (approximately 75 % of cases).
b The r. dexter arises from the a. mesenterica superior (approximately 10 %).
c Both branches arise separately from the truncus coeliacus (less than 5 %).

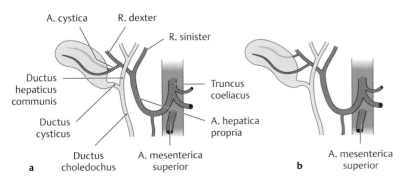

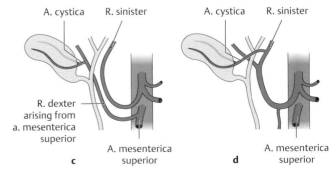

F Common variants of the arteria cystica (after Lippert and Pabst)
a A. cystica divides and passes to the anterior and posterior aspect of the vesica biliaris (46 % of cases).
b Two aa. cysticae supply the vesica biliaris (13 % of cases),

c A. cystica arising from the r. dexter (arteriae hepaticae) arising from the a. mesenterica superior (12 % of cases),
d A. cystica arising from the r. sinister of the a. hepatica propria (5 % of cases).

3.20 Branches of the Truncus Coeliacus: Arteries Supplying the Pancreas, Duodenum, and Splen

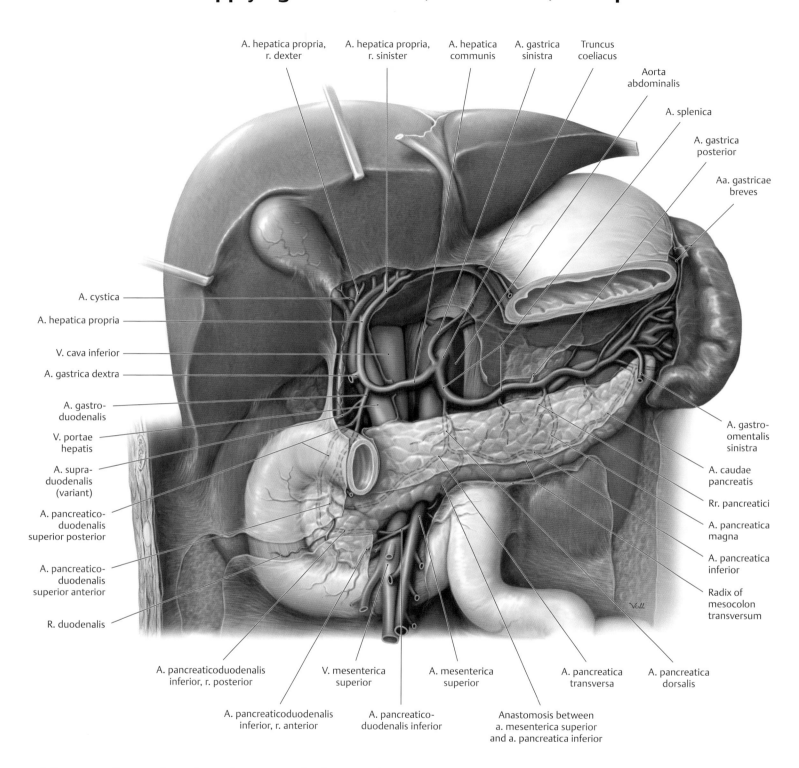

A. hepatica propria, r. dexter

A. hepatica propria, r. sinister

A. hepatica communis

A. gastrica sinistra

Truncus coeliacus

Aorta abdominalis

A. splenica

A. gastrica posterior

Aa. gastricae breves

A. cystica

A. hepatica propria

V. cava inferior

A. gastrica dextra

A. gastro-duodenalis

V. portae hepatis

A. supra-duodenalis (variant)

A. pancreatico-duodenalis superior posterior

A. pancreatico-duodenalis superior anterior

R. duodenalis

A. gastro-omentalis sinistra

A. caudae pancreatis

Rr. pancreatici

A. pancreatica magna

A. pancreatica inferior

Radix of mesocolon transversum

A. pancreaticoduodenalis inferior, r. posterior

V. mesenterica superior

A. mesenterica superior

A. pancreatica transversa

A. pancreatica dorsalis

A. pancreaticoduodenalis inferior, r. anterior

A. pancreatico-duodenalis inferior

Anastomosis between a. mesenterica superior and a. pancreatica inferior

A Truncus coeliacus and arteries to the pancreas, duodenum, and splen

Anterior view with the corpus gastricum, pylorus, omentum minus, and colon removed. For better exposure of the vascular structures, the peritoneum parietale has been partially removed.

The a. gastrica sinistra passes to the left and runs superiorly to the curvatura minor of the gaster. The a. hepatica propria in the lig. hepatoduodenale passes to the right and runs to the hepar. Before reaching the splen, the a. splenica gives off branches to supply blood to the pancreas (close to the splen) and to the gaster via the a. gastromentalis sinistra. The a. (and v.) mesenterica superior runs in an inferior direction and in close proximity to the caput pancreatis (while giving off branches to supply blood to the pancreas, see **C**). Pancreatic tumors may compress the artery and vein and restrict their blood flow. The truncus coeliacus is the uppermost of the three arteries that supply the organs of the digestive system (plus the splen).

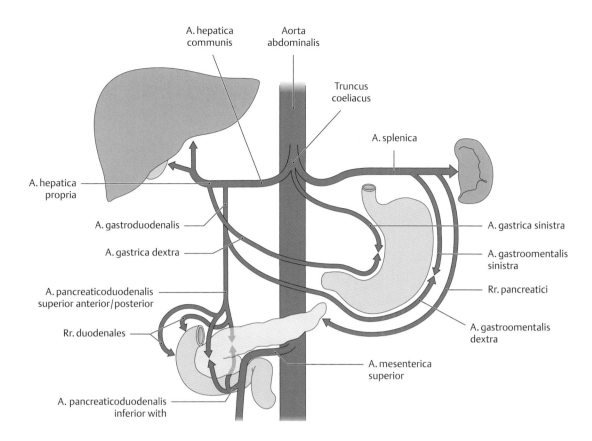

B Schematic overview of the distribution of the truncus coeliacus

Note: The pancreas is additionally supplied by branches from the a. mesenterica superior.

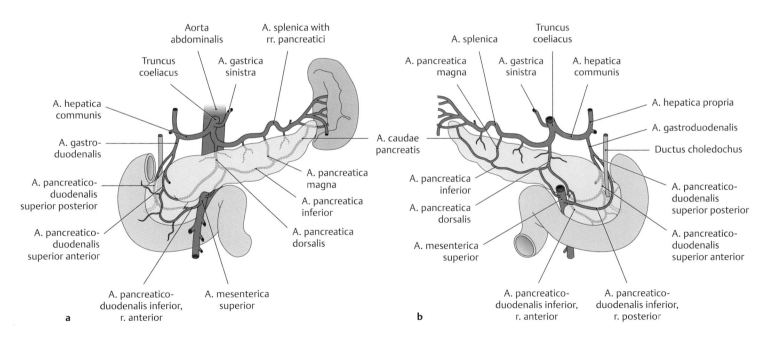

C Arterial supply to the pancreas

a Anterior view; **b** Posterior view. In **b**, the aorta abdominalis has been removed to show the origins of the truncus coeliacus and a. mesenterica superior.

Note that the pancreas is supplied by branches from the truncus coeliacus as well as branches from the a. mesenterica superior. The superior and inferior arteries that supply the pancreas are arranged in an anastomosing system called the "pancreatic arcade." The largest of the anastomoses between the a. splenica and a. pancreatica inferior is called the a. pancreatica magna.

3.21 Branches of the Arteria Mesenterica Superior: Arteries Supplying the Pancreas, Intestinum Tenue, and Intestinum Crassum

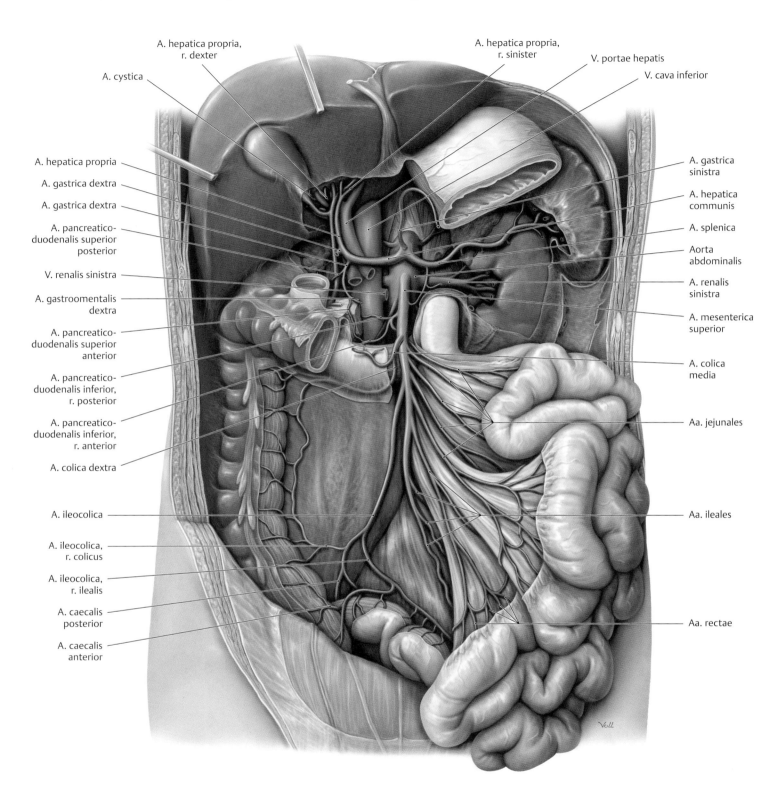

A. hepatica propria, r. dexter

A. cystica

A. hepatica propria, r. sinister

V. portae hepatis

V. cava inferior

A. hepatica propria

A. gastrica dextra

A. gastrica dextra

A. pancreatico-duodenalis superior posterior

V. renalis sinistra

A. gastroomentalis dextra

A. pancreatico-duodenalis superior anterior

A. pancreatico-duodenalis inferior, r. posterior

A. pancreatico-duodenalis inferior, r. anterior

A. colica dextra

A. ileocolica

A. ileocolica, r. colicus

A. ileocolica, r. ilealis

A. caecalis posterior

A. caecalis anterior

A. gastrica sinistra

A. hepatica communis

A. splenica

Aorta abdominalis

A. renalis sinistra

A. mesenterica superior

A. colica media

Aa. jejunales

Aa. ileales

Aa. rectae

A Distribution of the arteria mesenterica superior

Anterior view. For clarity, the gaster and peritoneum have been partially removed or windowed, leaving intact most of the retroperitoneal connective tissue below the colon transversum.

The a. mesenterica superior arises from the front of the aorta abdominalis at the level of the first lumbar (L1) vertebra. It passes anteriorly and inferiorly, distributing most of its numerous branches to the right side. Thus, it is clearly accessible to inspection and dissection only when the loops of intestinum tenue are reflected to the left side, as illustrated here. This view also displays the series of arcades formed by

the intestinal branches of the a. mesenterica superior (only one set of arches is present along the jejunum, but the arches increase distally and form multiple sets along the ileum). Straight arteries (vasa recta) extend from the arcades to the associated bowel segments. The a. mesenterica superior and its numerous branches supply the intestinum tenue, portions of the pancreas (see p. 267), and a considerable part of the intestinum crassum (see **C**), almost as far as the flexura coli sinistra (not visible here). The trunk of the a. mesenterica superior passes over the duodenum and v. renalis sinister (see **D**).

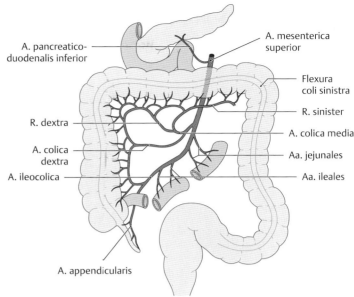

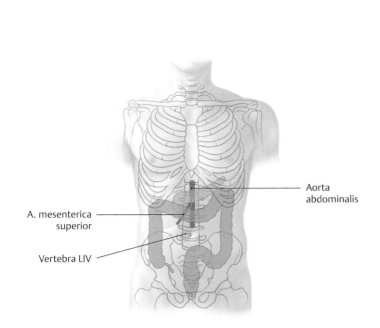

B Projection of the arteria mesenterica superior onto the columna vertebralis and its relationship to the intestinum crassum and pancreas

The a. mesenterica superior arises at the level of the first lumbar vertebra.

C Sequence of branches from the arteria mesenterica superior
(see also **E**)

Relationship of the a. mesenterica superior to specific organs. The territory of the a. mesenterica superior ends just proximal to the flexura coli sinistra, at which point the supply by the a. mesenterica inferior begins (see p. 271). It is common for multiple anastomoses to exist between the two mesenteric systems (see p. 213).

Note: The diagram is highly schematic and does not incorporate the topographical relationships between the distinct structures.

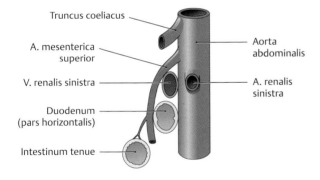

D Relationship of the arteria mesenterica superior to the duodenum and left vena renalis

Left lateral view.

Note: The a. mesenterica superior descends in front of the duodenum and left v. renalis. The left v. renalis lies within the aorticomesenteric angle, where it may become entrapped and compressed.

E Branches of the arteria mesenterica superior, listed in the sequence of the organs they supply

- A. pancreaticoduodenalis inferior
- Aa. jejunales and ileales (approximately 14–20)
- A. ileocolica with aa. caecales anterior and posterior and a. appendicularis
- A. colica dextra
- A. colica media

The arteries to the intestina tenue and crassum form numerous arcades from which small straight arteries (vasa recta) pass through the mesenterium to supply the various parts of the intestinum.

Note: The a. colica dextra varies in its origin. According to Lippert and Pabst (1985), as well as Kuzu et al. (2017), it arises directly from the a. mesenterica superior in only 40% of all cases. In 20% of all cases the a. colica dextra shares a truncus communis with the a. colica media, and in 15% of cases it arises directly from the a. ileocolica. In 25% of cases, the a. colica dextra is actually absent.

269

3.22 Branches of the Arteria Mesenterica Inferior: Arteries Supplying the Intestinum Crassum

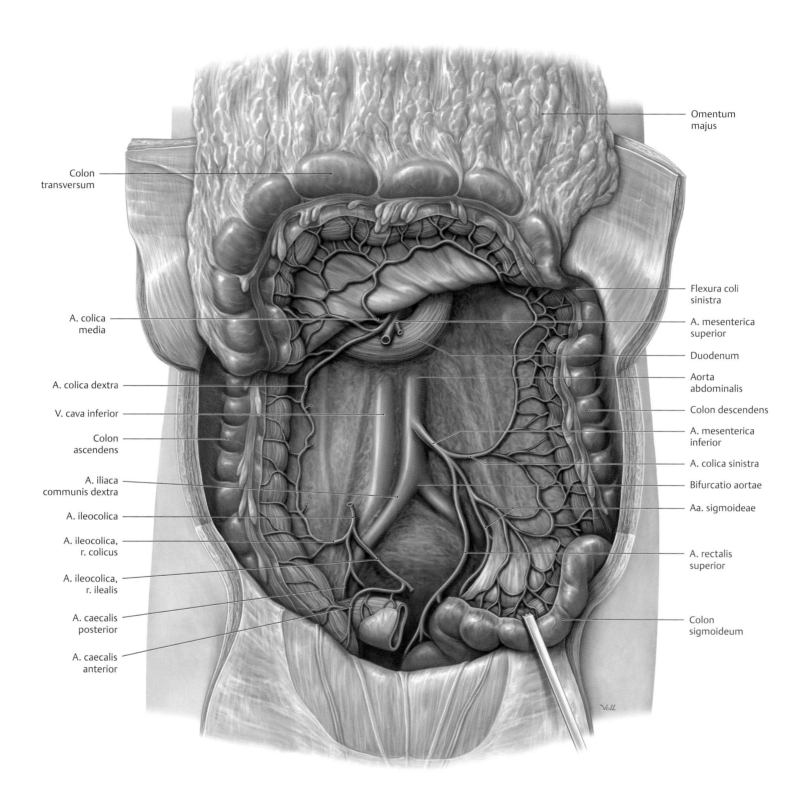

Colon transversum

A. colica media

A. colica dextra

V. cava inferior

Colon ascendens

A. iliaca communis dextra

A. ileocolica

A. ileocolica, r. colicus

A. ileocolica, r. ilealis

A. caecalis posterior

A. caecalis anterior

Omentum majus

Flexura coli sinistra

A. mesenterica superior

Duodenum

Aorta abdominalis

Colon descendens

A. mesenterica inferior

A. colica sinistra

Bifurcatio aortae

Aa. sigmoideae

A. rectalis superior

Colon sigmoideum

A Arterial supply to the intestinum crassum from the arteriae mesentericae superior and inferior

Anterior view. The jejunum and most of the ileum have been removed, and the colon transversum has been reflected superiorly. The peritoneum has been windowed or removed at several sites, leaving part of the retroperitoneal connective tissue in place. The a. mesenterica inferior arises from the aorta abdominalis at the level of the L3 vertebra (see **B**) and descends toward the left side. Thus, it is clearly accessible to inspection and dissection only when the loops of intestinum tenue are reflected to the right side (bowel loops have been removed here). This view also displays the numerous sets of arcades formed by the branches of the a. mesenterica inferior. This artery supplies the distal portions of the intestinum crassum, starting approximately at the flexura coli sinistra.

Note: The rectum is supplied by three arteries (see **D**), only one of which, the a. rectalis superior, is visible in this dissection.

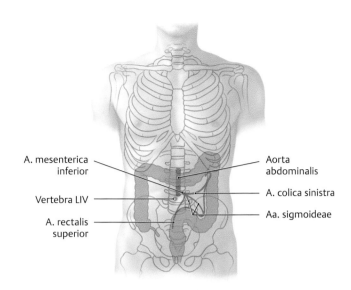

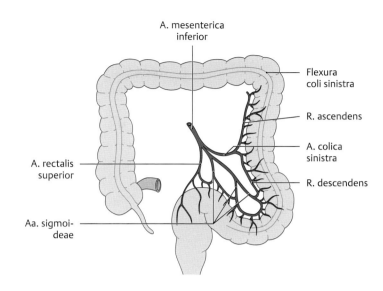

B Projection of the arteria mesenterica inferior onto the columna vertebralis and its relationship to the intestinum crassum

The a. mesenterica inferior branches from the aorta abdominalis at the level of the L3 vertebra.

C Sequence of branches from the arteria mesenterica inferior

(see p. 213)

A. colica sinistra, aa. sigmoideae (two or three), a. rectalis superior. Note that the flexura coli sinistra marks the approximate boundary between the blood supply by the aa. mesentericae superior and inferior.

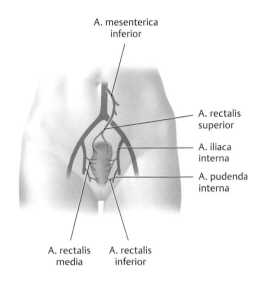

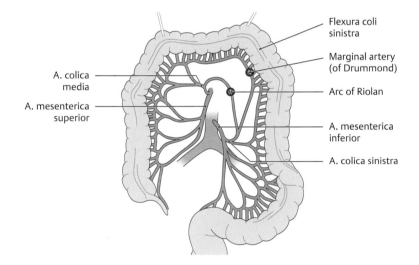

D Contribution of the arteria mesenterica inferior to the rectal blood supply

The rectum is supplied by three different arteries or branches (see p. 273):

- The a. mesenterica inferior (or its branch, the a. rectalis superior)
- The a. rectalis media (directly)
- The a. pudenda interna (or its branch, the a. rectalis inferior)

The a. mesenterica inferior supplies most of the rectum from above, while the other two arteries supply the smaller, lower portions of the rectum.

E Shortcircuits between arteries of the intestinum crassum

Shortcircuits between arteries of the intestinum crassum have two consequences: Abnormally low blood flow in one artery can be compensated for via a shortcircuit with blood from an adjacent artery. The portion of the colon with the initially low flow can still be sufficiently supplied. When performing a resection of a portion of the colon, the supplying vessel is tied off and the shortcircuit disconnected to prevent blood loss via a neighboring vessel. Because of their size, two shortcircuits are described below:

- Riolan's arcade: a direct connection between the a. colica media and the a. colica sinistra (usually close to the trunk where the aa. colicae media and sinistra arise from the superior and inferior, respectively);
- Marginal artery of Drummond (a. marginalis coli): close to the margin of the intesti-

nal tube, connects the arteries of the entire colon.

Such shortcircuits are referred to—often imprecisely—as anastomoses.

Due to the extensive anastomoses described above, occlusive arterial diseases are very rare in the region of the colon. Vascular obstruction leads to symptoms only if two of the three major vessels (truncus coeliacus, a. mesenterica superior or inferior) are severely constricted. In that case, patients complain of upper abdominal pain approximately 15 minutes after eating. The pain is caused by ischemia resulting from vascular occlusion that follows an increase in oxygen demand by the colon after eating large meals. As a consequence, the patient eats only small portions (small meal syndrome) but more often. Because of the smaller portions, blood flow to the colon does not need to increase.

3.23 Branches of the Arteria Mesenterica Inferior: Supply to the Rectum

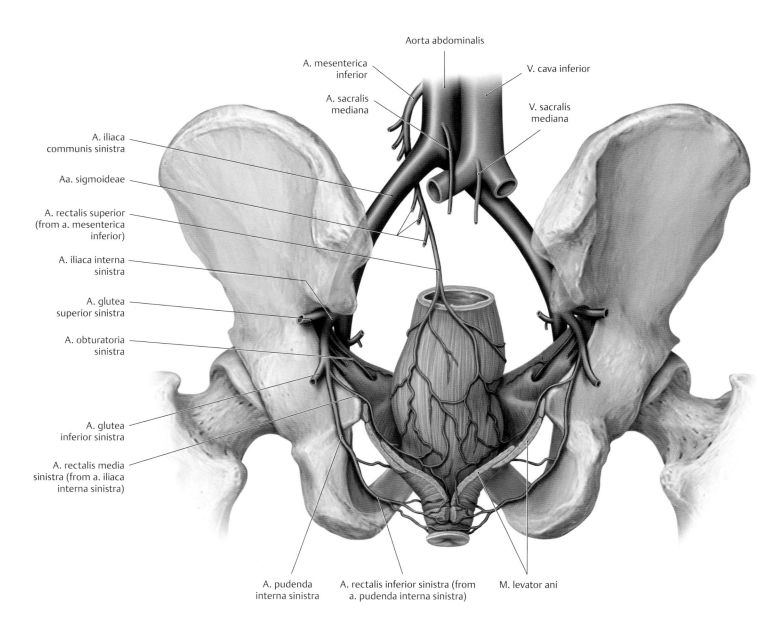

Aorta abdominalis

A. mesenterica inferior

V. cava inferior

A. sacralis mediana

V. sacralis mediana

A. iliaca communis sinistra

Aa. sigmoideae

A. rectalis superior (from a. mesenterica inferior)

A. iliaca interna sinistra

A. glutea superior sinistra

A. obturatoria sinistra

A. glutea inferior sinistra

A. rectalis media sinistra (from a. iliaca interna sinistra)

A. pudenda interna sinistra

A. rectalis inferior sinistra (from a. pudenda interna sinistra)

M. levator ani

A Arterial supply of the rectum

Posterior view. For clarity, portions of the ilium are shown translucent. *Note:* The unpaired a. rectalis *superior* (from the unpaired a. mesenterica inferior) divides into two branches on reaching the rectum. The right, sturdier branch further divides into two equally strong arterial branches. From these two or three major branches originate multiple collaterals that form anastomotic networks. The aa. rectales *mediae* (from the aa. iliacae internae) and the aa. rectales inferiores (from the aa. pudendae internae) are paired owing to their origin from paired parent vessels. In females, it is not unusual for the a. rectalis media to arise from the a. uterina.

The a. rectalis *inferior* leaves the a. pudenda interna in the canalis pudendalis (*Alcock's canal*). The a. rectalis superior approaches the rectum from above and posteriorly, also coming in contact with the peritoneal covering of the rectum (for clarity, not shown here). The course of this artery is also described as "peritoneal." It runs in the mesorectum where it further divides before it descends in the corpus cavernosum recti. The aa. rectales mediae and inferiores approach the rectum from the sides, the m. levator ani forming a well-defined partition between them: The aa. rectales mediae pass to the rectum above that muscle, the aa. rectales inferiores below it. Because the m. levator ani forms an essential part of the diaphragma pelvis (see p. 395), the course of the aa. rectales mediae and inferiores is also described as *supradiaphragmatic* and *infradiaphragmatic*, respectively. The aa. rectales frequently accompany the vv. rectales for a considerable distance.

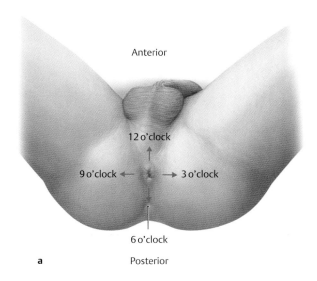

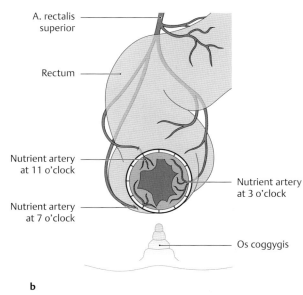

B Arterial supply of the corpus cavernosum recti (hemorrhoidal plexus)

a Caudal view with the patient supine in the lithotomy position and the examiner having a view of the perineum, clock face orientation is used. The hemorrhoidal plexus is a permanently distended corpus cavernosum (see p. 243), which is supplied by three main branches (**b**) at the typical positions (3, 7, and 11 o'clock) where they form three major cushions (**c**) in the area of the columnae anales. The three major vessels divide into four branches and form minor cushions (**d**) at the 1, 5, 6, and 9 o'clock positions. Together, these circular cavernous structures filled with blood serve as a very effective continence mechanism that ensures liquid- and gas-tight closure. The sustained contraction of the muscular sphincter apparatus inhibits venous drainage, and blood is allowed to drain from the corpus cavernosum when the sphincters relax during defecation.

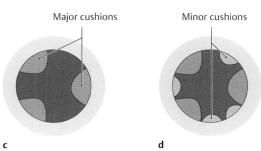

Note: Abnormal dilation (hyperplasia) of the hemorrhoidal plexus beyond the physiological range leads to hemorrhoidal disease, one of the most common proctological disorders (see p. 246 f).

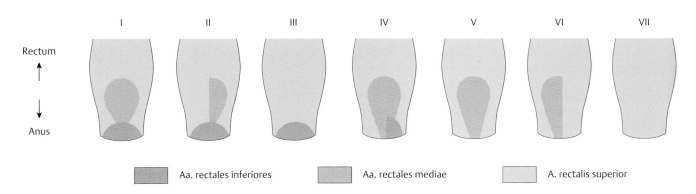

C Areas supplied by the arteriae rectales

Schematic representation of the distinct types of arterial supply in the sagittally cut rectum. Rendered from radiographs obtained after the injection of radiographic contrast agent into the supplying arteries. View of the anterior wall of the splayed out colon (after Stelzner).

There are 7 distinct patterns of arterial supply to the rectum (I–VII). The most common pattern is I (36% of cases). The upper three-quarters are supplied almost exclusively by the unpaired a. rectalis superior, the lower one quarter is supplied by the smaller caliber aa. rectales mediae (from the aa. iliacae internae) and the aa. rectales inferiores (from the aa. pudendae internae). All three arteries form extensive anastomoses.

Note: The common notion that the a. rectalis superior supplies the upper-third of the rectum, the aa. rectales mediae the middle-third, and the aa. rectales inferiores the lower third, is thus incorrect.

3.24 Vena Portae Hepatis: Venous Drainage of the Gaster, Duodenum, Pancreas, and Splen

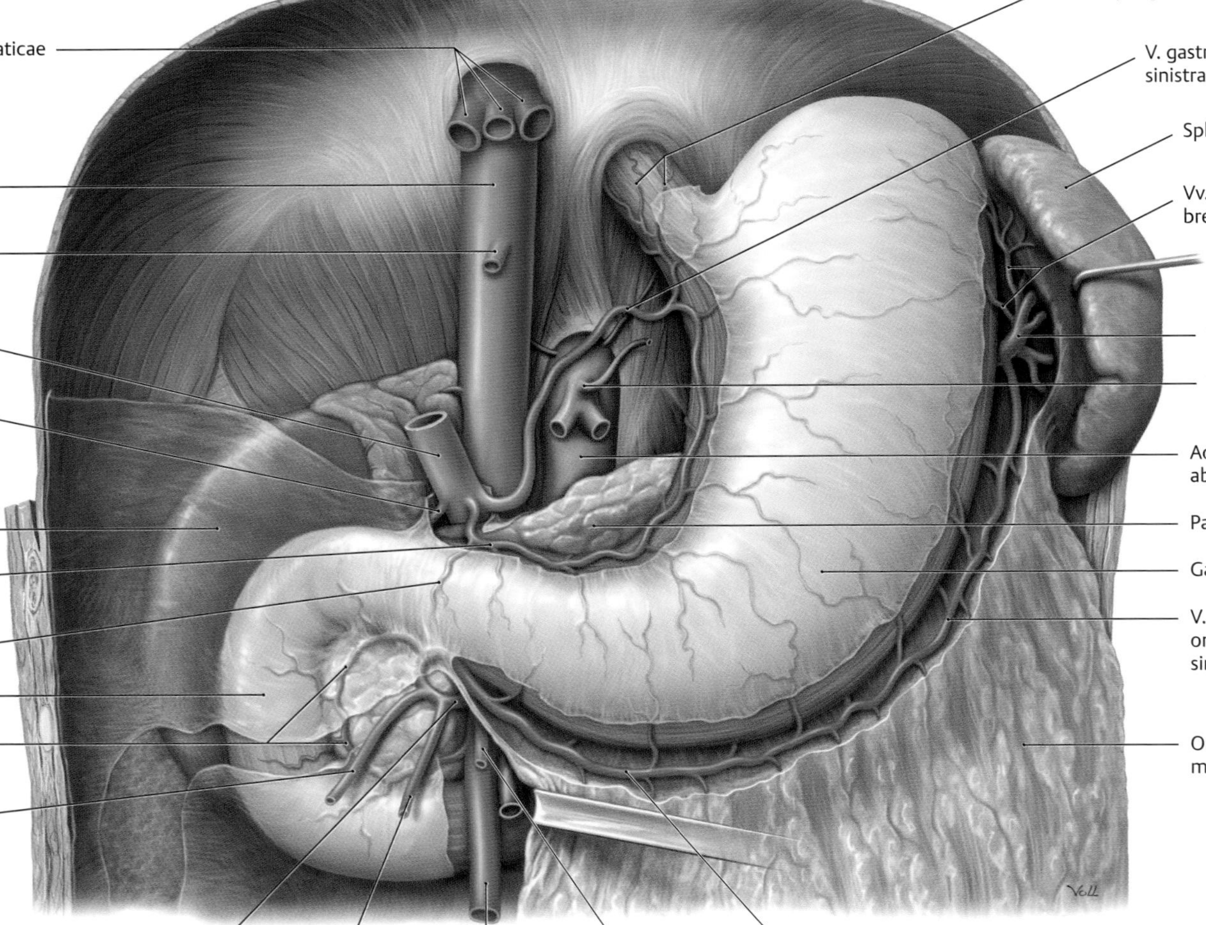
Vv. oesophageales
Vv. hepaticae
V. gastrica sinistra
Splen
V. cava inferior
Vv. gastricae breves
Vein for the lobus caudatus
V. splenica
V. portae hepatis
Truncus coeliacus
V. pancreatico-duodenalis superior posterior
Aorta abdominalis
Ren dexter
Pancreas
V. gastrica dextra
Gaster
V. prepylorica
V. gastro-omentalis sinistra
Duodenum
Vv. pancreatico-duodenales
Omentum majus
V. colica dextra superior
Truncus gastro-pancreaticocolicus
V. colica dextra
V. mesenterica superior
V. colica media
V. gastro-omentalis dextra

A Venous drainage of the gaster and duodenum
Anterior view. The hepar and omentum minus have been removed, and the omentum majus has been opened and retracted to the left. The gaster has been pulled slightly inferiorly, and the peritoneum has been removed or windowed at several sites to display the termination of the vv. hepaticae in the v. cava inferior and the communication of the vv. gastricae with the portal venous system.
Blood from the *curvatura minor gastris* generally flows directly into the v. portae hepatis, while blood from the *curvatura major* reaches the v. portae hepatis by way of the v. splenica and v. mesenterica superior. The lower portions of the duodenum drain chiefly to the v. mesenterica superior, while the upper portions usually drain directly to the v. portae hepatis. Variants are common, however.
Note how the esophageal veins drain into the v. portae hepatis by way of the vv. gastricae sinistrae. This is important in the portacaval collateral circulation (see **B** and p. 218).

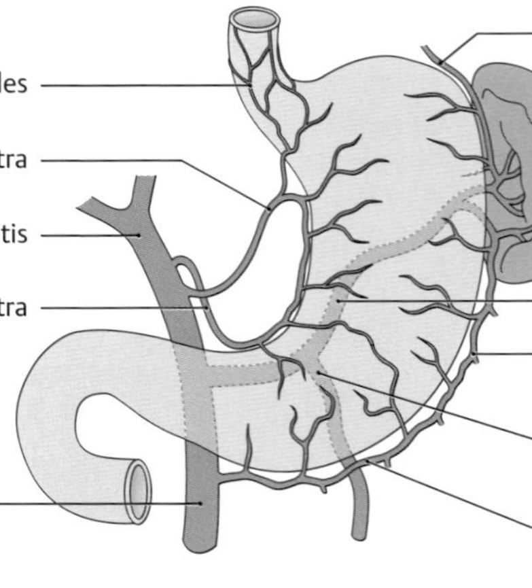
Vv. gastricae breves
Vv. oesophageales
V. gastrica sinistra
V. portae hepatis
V. splenica
V. gastrica dextra
V. gastro-omentalis sinistra
V. mesenterica inferior
V. mesenterica superior
V. gastro-omentalis dextra

B Junction of the vena mesenterica inferior and vena splenica
Anterior view. This view, with the gaster translucent, demonstrates the site where the v. mesenterica inferior typically opens into the v. splenica behind the gaster.

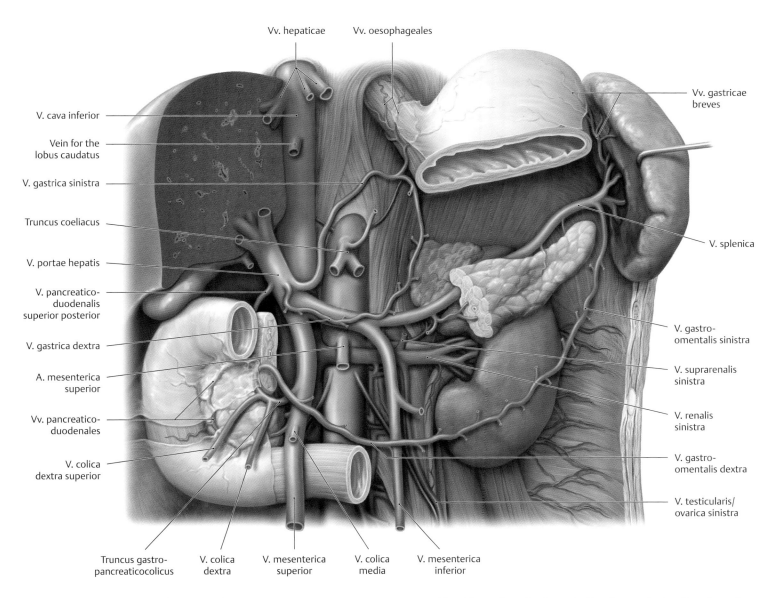

Labels (clockwise from top):
Vv. hepaticae
Vv. oesophageales
Vv. gastricae breves
V. cava inferior
V. splenica
Vein for the lobus caudatus
V. gastrica sinistra
Truncus coeliacus
V. portae hepatis
V. pancreatico-duodenalis superior posterior
V. gastro-omentalis sinistra
V. gastrica dextra
V. suprarenalis sinistra
A. mesenterica superior
V. renalis sinistra
Vv. pancreatico-duodenales
V. gastro-omentalis dextra
V. colica dextra superior
V. testicularis/ovarica sinistra
Truncus gastro-pancreaticocolicus
V. colica dextra
V. mesenterica superior
V. colica media
V. mesenterica inferior

C Venous drainage of the pancreas and splen

Anterior view. The gaster has been partially removed and pulled slightly inferiorly for better exposure, and most of the peritoneum has been removed. This dissection clearly shows how the v. portae hepatis is formed by the junction of the v. mesenterica superior and v. splenica near the hepar. In 70% of cases the v. splenica receives the v. mesenterica inferior, as shown here, before uniting with the v. mesenterica superior (see also **B**).

Venous blood from the splen is carried by the v. splenica directly to the v. portae hepatis, while blood from the pancreas takes various routes: Most of the vv. pancreaticae (mainly from the cauda and corpus pancreatis) open into the v. splenica. A few, along with the veins draining the gaster and colon ascendens, open into the v. mesenterica superior via the truncus gastropancreaticocolicus.

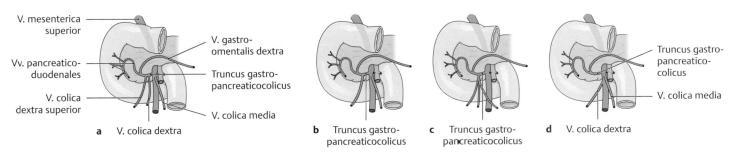

Labels:
V. mesenterica superior
V. gastro-omentalis dextra
Vv. pancreatico-duodenales
Truncus gastro-pancreaticocolicus
V. colica dextra superior
V. colica media
a V. colica dextra
b Truncus gastro-pancreaticocolicus
c Truncus gastro-pancreaticocolicus
d V. colica dextra
Truncus gastro-pancreatico-colicus
V. colica media

D Variants of the truncus gastropancreaticocolicus (Trunk of Henle) (after Jin et al and Ignjatovic et al)

a 45%; **b** 33%; **c** 11%; and **d** 11% of cases.

In 90% of cases, the venous truncus gastropancreaticocolicus provides drainage of the colon ascendens (v. colica dextra) and the flexura coli dextra (v. colica dextra superior) in addition to the gaster (v. gastroomentalis dextra) and caput pancreatis/duodenum (vv. pancreaticoduodenales). In 11% of cases, the truncus gastropancreaticocolicus also receives the v. colica media (**c**). The truncus gastropancreaticocolicus drains into the v. mesenterica superior at the level of the processus uncinatus.

Note: The truncus gastropancreaticocolicus is an important landmark for surgeons, particularly in operations on the caput pancreatis and the flexura coli dextra.

275

3.25 Venae Mesentericae Superior and Inferior: Venous Drainage of the Intestina Tenue and Crassum

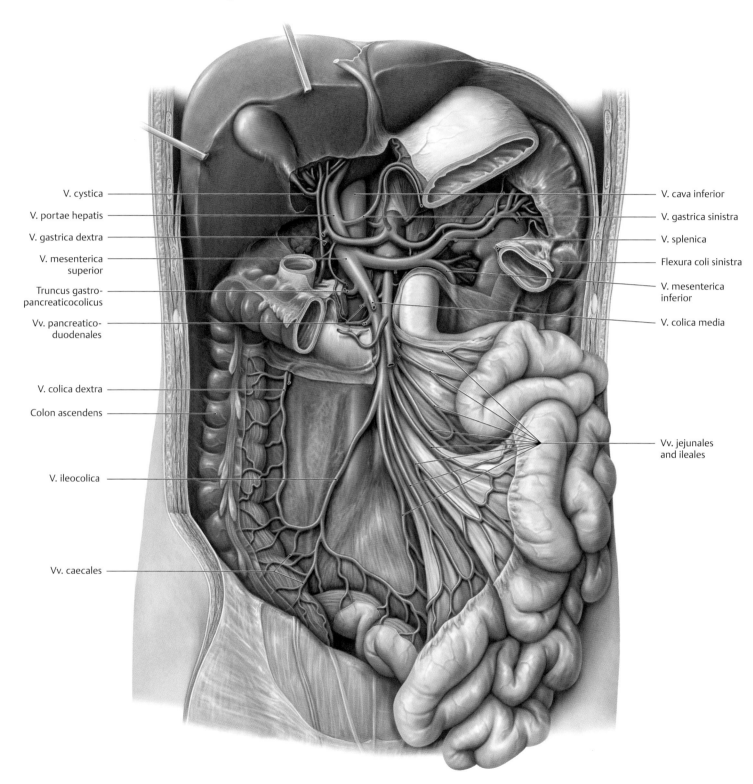

V. cystica

V. portae hepatis

V. gastrica dextra

V. mesenterica superior

Truncus gastro-pancreaticocolicus

Vv. pancreatico-duodenales

V. colica dextra

Colon ascendens

V. ileocolica

Vv. caecales

V. cava inferior

V. gastrica sinistra

V. splenica

Flexura coli sinistra

V. mesenterica inferior

V. colica media

Vv. jejunales and ileales

A Tributaries of the vena mesenterica superior

Anterior view. Most of the gaster has been removed, and the peritoneum has been removed or windowed at multiple sites, leaving some of the retroperitoneal connective tissue in place. The mesenterium and colon transversum have been partially removed, and the loops of intestinum tenue have been displaced to the left. The v. mesenterica superior unites with the v. splenica at the L1 level to form the v. portae hepatis (see **B**, p. 274).

The intestinum tenue drains exclusively into branches of the v. mesenterica superior. The v. mesenterica superior also collects blood from the caecum, appendix vermiformis, colon ascendens, and two-thirds of the colon transversum almost to the flexura coli dextra. From that point the colon is drained by the v. mesenterica inferior. As with the aa. mesentericae, multiple anastomoses are present between these two large veins. The v. mesenterica superior drains a much larger territory than the v. mesenterica inferior. Thus, the venous drainage of the intestina tenue and crassum follows the pattern of their arterial supply.

Note: The colon ascendens, which is secondarily retroperitoneal, may also be drained by veins in the retroperitoneum (vv. lumbales) that empty into the v. cava inferior. This is another example of a portacaval collateral pathway (see p. 218).

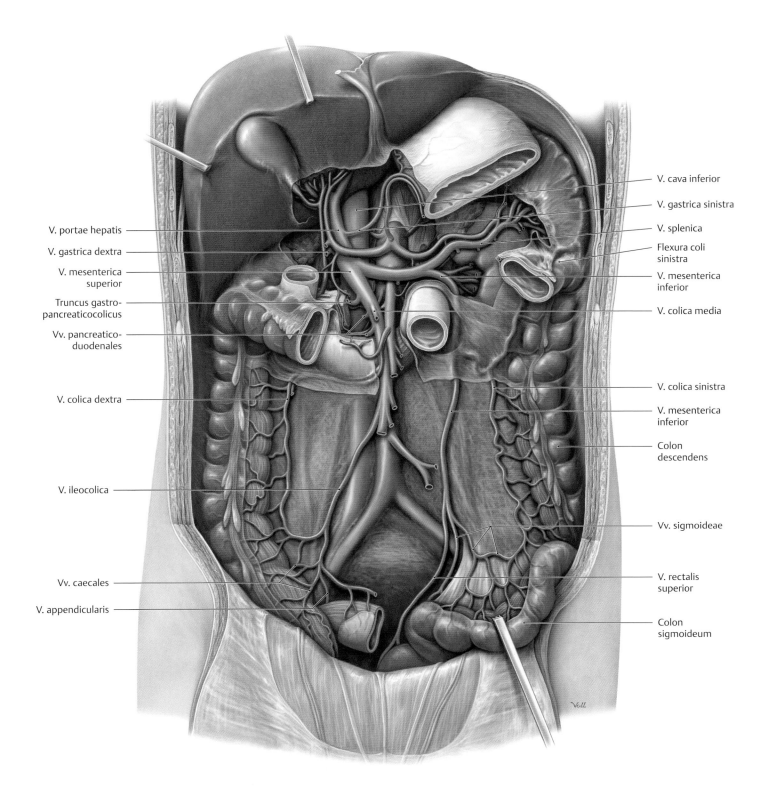

V. cava inferior

V. gastrica sinistra

V. splenica

Flexura coli sinistra

V. mesenterica inferior

V. colica media

V. colica sinistra

V. mesenterica inferior

Colon descendens

Vv. sigmoideae

V. rectalis superior

Colon sigmoideum

V. portae hepatis

V. gastrica dextra

V. mesenterica superior

Truncus gastro-pancreaticocolicus

Vv. pancreatico-duodenales

V. colica dextra

V. ileocolica

Vv. caecales

V. appendicularis

B Tributaries of the vena mesenterica inferior

Anterior view. Most of the gaster, pancreas, and intestinum tenue have been removed. The peritoneum has been removed or windowed at several sites, leaving some of the retroperitoneal connective tissue in place. The v. mesenterica inferior is formed by the union of the v. colica sinistra, vv. sigmoideae, and v. rectalis superior. Unlike the v. mesenterica *superior*, the v. mesenterica *inferior* runs separate from the artery and generally opens into the v. splenica behind the gaster and pancreas (see p. 275). Thus, the v. mesenterica inferior returns blood *only from the intestinum crassum*. The boundary between the territories of the vv. mesentericae superior and inferior is usually located in the colon transversum near the flexura coli sinistra, although multi-

ple anastomoses exist between the two vv. mesentericae. The colon descendens, which is secondarily retroperitoneal, may also be drained by veins in the retroperitoneum (vv. lumbales), again establishing a portacaval collateral pathway.

Note: Blood from the *upper rectum* drains through the v. rectalis *superior* to the v. mesenterica inferior before entering the *v. portae hepatis*. The *lower rectum* (not shown here) is drained by the vv. rectales mediae and inferiores, which drain into the *v. cava inferior* by way of the vv. iliacae (see p. 278). A portacaval anastomosis may also be present in this region. This explains why malignant tumors of the upper rectum metastasize to the hepar, while malignant tumors of the lower rectum tend to metastasize to the pulmo.

3.26 Branches of the Vena Mesenterica Inferior: Venous Drainage of the Rectum

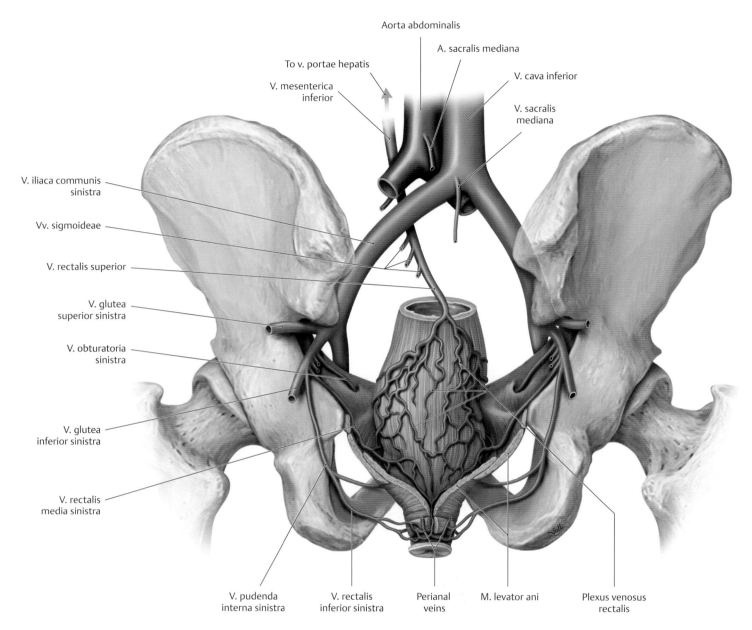

Aorta abdominalis

A. sacralis mediana

To v. portae hepatis

V. cava inferior

V. mesenterica inferior

V. sacralis mediana

V. iliaca communis sinistra

Vv. sigmoideae

V. rectalis superior

V. glutea superior sinistra

V. obturatoria sinistra

V. glutea inferior sinistra

V. rectalis media sinistra

V. pudenda interna sinistra

V. rectalis inferior sinistra

Perianal veins

M. levator ani

Plexus venosus rectalis

A Venous drainage of the rectum
Posterior view. Portions of the ilium are shown translucent for clarity.
Note: The unpaired v. rectalis *superior* (to the unpaired v. mesenterica inferior) divides into two branches on reaching the rectum. By contrast, the vv. rectales *mediae* (to the vv. iliacae internae) and vv. rectales *inferiores* (to the vv. pudendae internae) are paired owing to their termination in paired venous trunks.

Because the vv. rectales accompany the corresponding arteries for some distance, their course is analogous to that previously described for the arteries: The v. rectalis superior follows an abdominal route, while the vv. rectales mediae and inferiores take supra- and infradiaphragmatic routes. The v. rectalis superior drains to the hepatic portal system by way of the v. mesenterica inferior (see **B**).

Note: Tumors in the region drained by the v. rectalis *superior* can metastasize through the portal venous system to the capillary bed of the hepar (hepatic metastases), whereas tumors in the region drained by the vv. rectales *mediae* and *inferiores* metastasize through the v. cava inferior to the capillary bed of the pulmo (pulmonary metastases). Note also the importance of these veins as portacaval collaterals (see **B**).

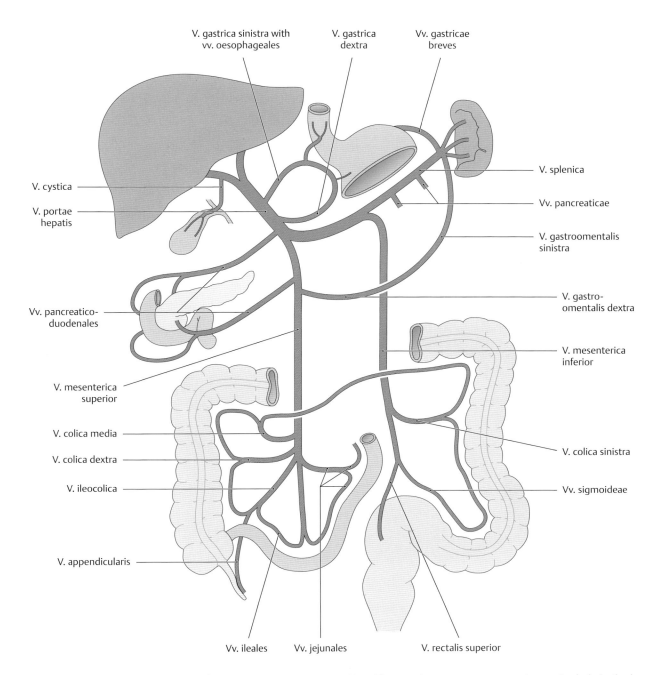

V. gastrica sinistra with vv. oesophageales

V. gastrica dextra

Vv. gastricae breves

V. cystica

V. portae hepatis

Vv. pancreatico- duodenales

V. mesenterica superior

V. colica media

V. colica dextra

V. ileocolica

V. appendicularis

V. splenica

Vv. pancreaticae

V. gastroomentalis sinistra

V. gastro- omentalis dextra

V. mesenterica inferior

V. colica sinistra

Vv. sigmoideae

Vv. ileales

Vv. jejunales

V. rectalis superior

B Draining of the vena rectalis superior into the vena portae hepatis

The rectum sends most of its venous drainage to the v. rectalis superior, which drains into the v. portae hepatis. Particularly the upper two-thirds of the rectum are drained this way. However, venous blood of the lower third of the rectum is carried via the vv. rectales inferiores and mediae to the vv. iliacae internae, which drain into the v. cava inferior. Along the perirectal veins (plexus venosus rectalis), numerous anastomoses exist between the two drainage areas (to the v. portae hepatis and to the v. cava inferior), which under certain circumstances (e.g., portal hypertension resulting from intrahepatic drainage disorders) may form a portacaval anastomosis.

Note: The rectal venous anatomy varies particularly in the lower third of the rectum, similar to the arterial anatomy. Blood from the vv. rectales drains not only into the v. cava inferior but also into the v. portae hepatis and thus reaches the hepar. This plays an important role in the rectal administration of drugs (e.g., in the form of suppositories). The idea is to bypass the hepar and the first-pass-effect (intestinal drug absorption and presystemic elimination in the liver) to ensure systemic distribution of the drug throughout the entire body, which because of the variable venous anatomy of the rectum, is not guaranteed. Thus, there are varying degrees of absorption and systemic distribution of drugs that are administered rectally. Rectal delivery is particularly suited for children as an alternative to the often difficult to perform venipuncture.

3.27 Lymphatic Drainage of the Gaster, Splen, Pancreas, Duodenum, and Hepar

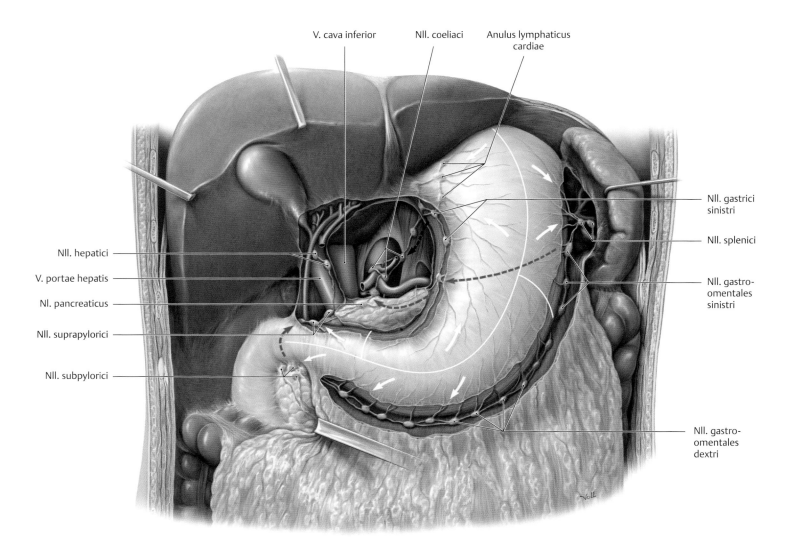

A Lymphatic drainage of the gaster
Anterior view. The omentum minus has been removed, the omentum majus has been partially opened along the curvatura major of the gaster, and the hepar has been retracted slightly superiorly. The following lymphatic pathways are important in this region:

- Drainage toward the **curvatura major and minor of the gaster**. Initial drainage is to the nodi lymphoidei regionales: the nll. gastrici dextri and sinistri (toward the curvatura minor) or the nodi

gastroomentales dextri and sinistri (toward the curvatura major, see white lines and arrows). These nodi lymphoidei regionales convey lymph either directly or indirectly to the nll. coeliaci (indirectly by way of the nll. pylorici and splenici). From there the lymph drains to the truncus intestinalis.
- Drainage from the **fundus and cardia**: initially to the inconstant (not always present) anulus lymphaticus cardiae, then to the truncus intestinalis.

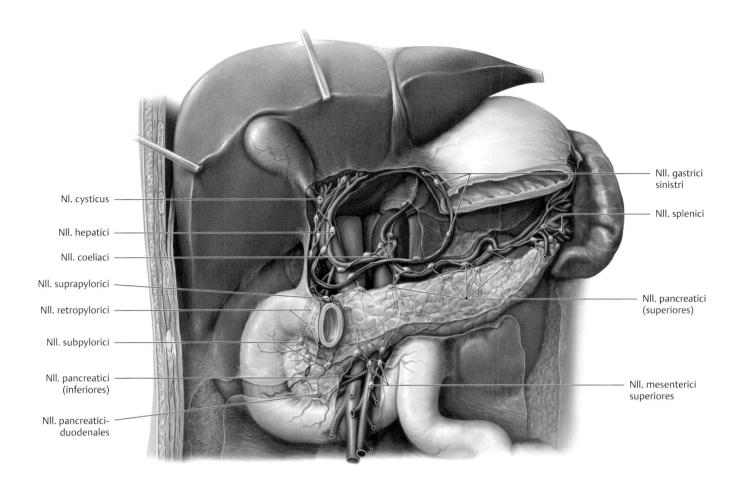

NI. cysticus

NII. hepatici

NII. coeliaci

NII. suprapylorici

NII. retropylorici

NII. subpylorici

NII. pancreatici
(inferiores)

NII. pancreatici-
duodenales

NII. gastrici
sinistri

NII. splenici

NII. pancreatici
(superiores)

NII. mesenterici
superiores

B Lymphatic drainage of the splen, pancreas, and duodenum
Anterior view. Most of the gaster has been removed, the colon has been detached, and the hepar has been retracted upward. The following nodi lymphoidei and groups of nodi are important in this region:

- **Splen:** Drains initially to the *nll. splenici*, then directly or indirectly to the *truncus intestinalis* (the indirect route may be through the superior nll. pancreatici alone or through the superior nll. pancreatici and the nodi coeliaci).
- **Pancreas:** Drains initially to the *superior and inferior nll. pancreatici*, then directly or indirectly (via the nodi coeliaci) to the truncus intestinalis; or drains initially to the *nll. pancreaticoduodenales superiores and*

inferiores (mainly on the posterior side of the pancreas), then directly or indirectly via the nodi mesenterici superiores to the truncus intestinalis.

- **Duodenum:** The *pars superior* of the duodenum drains initially to the *nll. pylorici* (see **C**), then to the nll. pancreaticoduodenales superiores and from there to the nll. hepatici, or directly to the nll. coeliaci in some cases, before entering the truncus intestinalis. The *lower portion* of the duodenum first drains to the *nll. pancreaticoduodenales superiores and inferiores*, then directly to the truncus intestinalis.

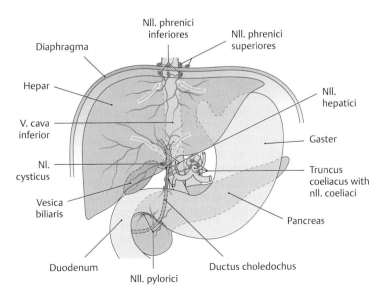

Diaphragma

NII. phrenici
inferiores

NII. phrenici
superiores

Hepar

V. cava
inferior

NI.
cysticus

Vesica
biliaris

Duodenum

NII. pylorici

Ductus choledochus

Pancreas

Truncus
coeliacus with
nll. coeliaci

Gaster

NII.
hepatici

C Lymphatic pathways for the hepar and biliary tract
Anterior view. The following lymphatic pathways are important in this region:
Hepar and intrahepatic ductus biliares (three drainage pathways):

- Most lymph drains inferiorly through the nodi hepatici to the nll. coeliaci and then to the truncus intestinalis and cisterna chyli, or it may drain directly from the nll. hepatici to the truncus intestinalis and cisterna chyli.
- A small amount of lymph drains cranially through the nll. phrenici inferiores to the truncus lumbalis.
- In some cases lymph drains through the diaphragma (partly through the foramen venae cavae and partly through muscular openings in the diaphragma) to the nll. phrenici superiores and then to the truncus bronchomediastinalis.

Vesica biliaris: Lymph from the vesica biliaris drains initially to the nodus cysticus, then follows the pathway described above.
Ductus choledochus: Lymph from the ductus choledochus drains through the nll. pylorici (nll. supra-, sub-, and retropylorici) and the nl. foraminalis to the nll. coeliaci, then to the truncus intestinalis.

3.28 Lymphatic Drainage of the Intestina Tenue and Crassum

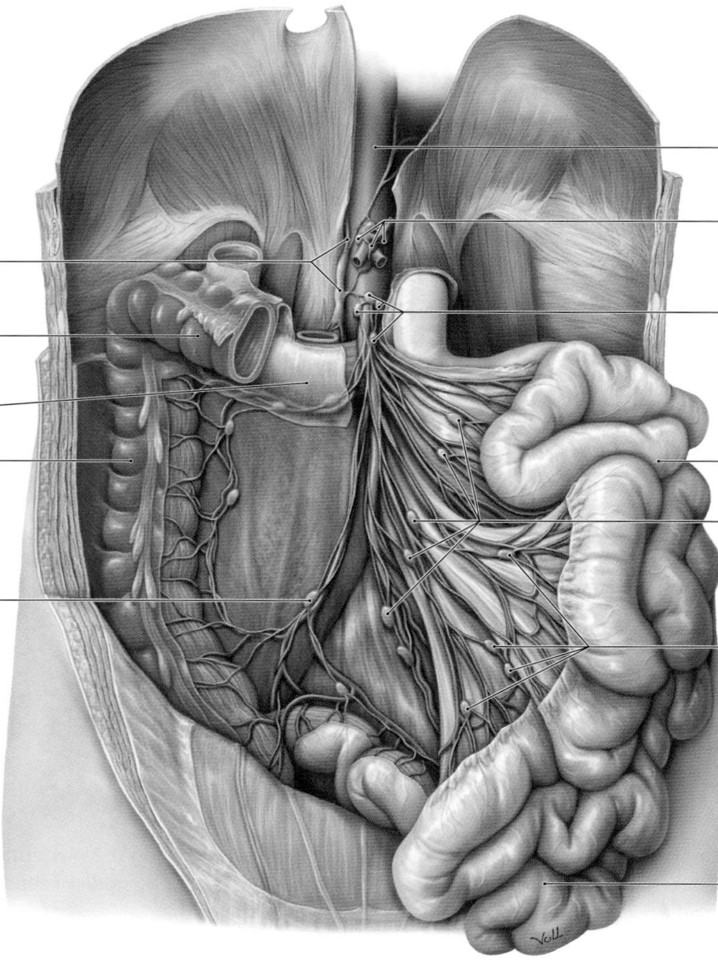

Aorta abdominalis
Nll. coeliaci
Ductus thoracicus with cisterna chyli
Nll. mesenterici superiores
Colon transversum
Duodenum
Colon ascendens
Jejunum
Nll. mesenterici intermedii
Nl. ileocolicus
Nll. juxta-intestinales
Ileum

A Nodi lymphoidei and lymphatic drainage of the jejunum and ileum

Anterior view. The gaster, hepar, pancreas, and most of the colon have been removed. The nodi lymphoidei of the intestinum tenue are the largest group of nodi lymphoidei in the human body, numbering approximately 100 to 150 nodes of greatly varying size. For clarity, the above drawing shows only a few nodi lymphoidei that are representative of larger groups. Lymph from both the jejunum and ileum drains initially to nodi lymphoidei regionales (nodi juxtaintestinales), then to the nodi mesentericae superiores, and finally to the truncus intestinalis. The nll. lymphoidei and vasa lymphatica in the *mesenterium* basically follow the distribution of the arteries and veins.They are called "intermediate" because they are situated *between* visceral and collecting nodi lymphoidei (the nodi mesenterici superiores and inferiores). In patients with a malignant tumor, it is desirable to remove as many nodi lymphoidei as possible along a drainage pathway to ensure the removal of any micrometastases (metastases not grossly visible) that may be present in the nodes. In the case of the duodenum, this means that the resection should include not only the affected part of the duodenum but also the attached portion of the mesenterium and the (intermediate) nodi lymphoidei that it contains. Occasionally even the nodi mesenterici superiores and inferiores are also removed.

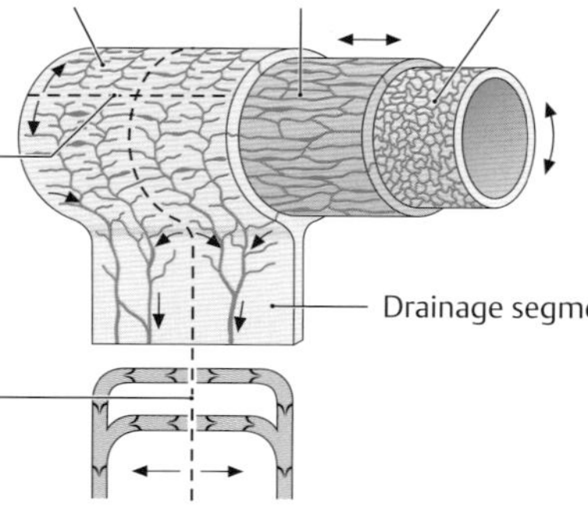

Subserosal collectors
Plexus muscularis
Plexus serosus
Drainage boundary along the intestine
Drainage segment
Drainage boundary across the intestine

B Lymphatic drainage of the intestinum by segments (after Földi and Kubik)

Lymph is collected in several plexuses (networks of vasa lymphatica and lymph collectors) in the intestinal wall. The lymphatics accompany the aa. and vv. mesentericae through the mesenterium, and in principle they drain the intestinal segment that is supplied by those vessels. Valves in the subserous collectors determine the direction of flow and define the boundaries of the individual drainage segments in the intestinal wall. Because of these segmental boundaries, it is rare for a tumor to spread extensively along the intestinum by the lymphatic route. Arrows: principal direction of lymphatic drainage.

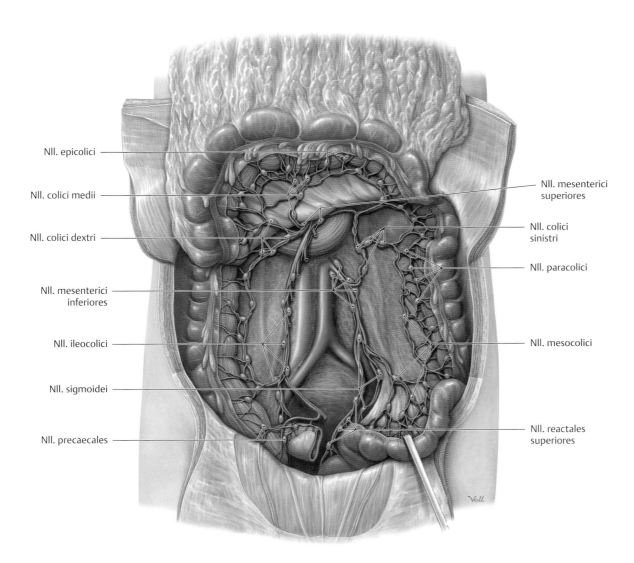

NII. epicolici

NII. colici medii

NII. colici dextri

NII. mesenterici inferiores

NII. ileocolici

NII. sigmoidei

NII. precaecales

NII. mesenterici superiores

NII. colici sinistri

NII. paracolici

NII. mesocolici

NII. reactales superiores

C Lymphatic drainage of the intestinum crassum
(modified from Földi and Kubik)
Anterior view. The colon transversum and omentum majus have been reflected superiorly. The following lymphatic pathways are important in this region:

- **Colon ascendens, caecum, and colon transversum:** Lymph from these structures drains initially to the *nll. colici dextri and medii*, then to the *nll. mesenterici superiores*, and finally to the *truncus intestinalis*.
- **Descending colon:** Lymph from the descending colon drains initially to regional lymph nodes, the *left colic lymph nodes*, then to the *inferior mesenteric lymph nodes*, and then drains into the truncus intestinalis via the *left lumbar lymph nodes* (not visible here) into the *left lumbar trunk* (not visible here).
- **Colon sigmoideum:** Lymph from the colon sigmoideum drains initially to the nll. sigmoidei, then follows the pathway described for the colon descendens (above).

- **Upper rectum** (see also **D**): Lymph from the upper rectum drains initially to the *nll. rectales superiores*, then follows the pathway described for the colon sigmoideum (above).

Thus, a malignant tumor undergoing lymphogenous spread must negotiate several nodus lymphoideus groups (all of which should be removed in tumor resections) before the malignant cells can reach the truncus intestinalis and ductus thoracicus and finally enter the bloodstream. This long route of lymphogenous spread improves the prospects for a cure. The nodi lymphoidei of the intestinum crassum can be classified *clinically* and *functionally* into more groups than by anatomical criteria alone: nodi lymphoidei of the intestinal wall (nodi epicolici), nodi lymphoidei near the intestinum (nodi paracolici), nodi lymphoidei at the origins of the three large intestinal arteries (central group), and nodi lymphoidei at the origins of the aa. mesentericae (collecting lymph nodes). In standard anatomical nomenclature, the epicolic nodes are not distinguished as a seperate group, and the nll. paracolici and central groups are considered collectively as nll. mesocolici.

D Lymphatic drainage of the rectum
Anterior view. The rectum has three levels and three principal directions of lymphatic drainage (direct or indirect via the pararectal nodi lymphoidei on the rectal wall):

- Upper level: through nll. rectales superiores (not shown here) to nll. mesenteric inferiores (→ truncus intestinalis and left truncus lumbalis).
- Middle level: nl. iliaci interni (→ right and left trunci lumbales).
- Lower level:
  - Columnar zone: to nll. iliaci interni.
  - Cutaneous zone: through nll. inguinales superficiales to nodi iliaci externi (→ trunci lumbales).

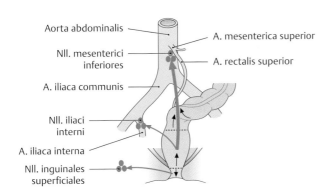

Aorta abdominalis

NII. mesenterici inferiores

A. iliaca communis

NII. iliaci interni

A. iliaca interna

NII. inguinales superficiales

A. mesenterica superior

A. rectalis superior

283

3.29 Autonomic Innervation of the Hepar, Vesica Biliaris, Gaster, Duodenum, Pancreas, and Splen

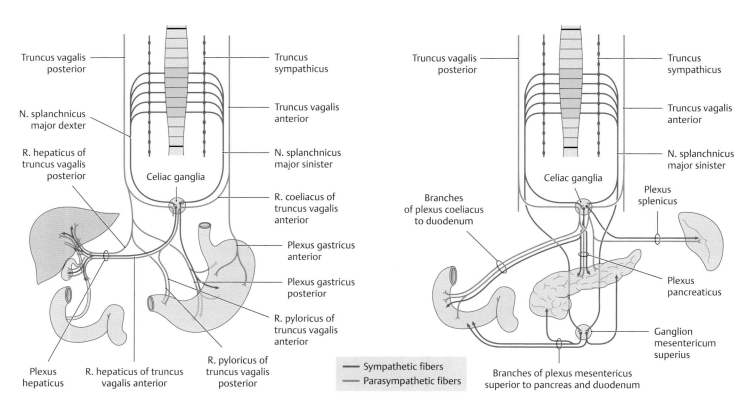

Left diagram labels:

Truncus vagalis posterior
Truncus sympathicus
N. splanchnicus major dexter
Truncus vagalis anterior
R. hepaticus of truncus vagalis posterior
N. splanchnicus major sinister
Celiac ganglia
R. coeliacus of truncus vagalis anterior
Plexus gastricus anterior
Plexus gastricus posterior
R. pyloricus of truncus vagalis anterior
Plexus hepaticus
R. hepaticus of truncus vagalis anterior
R. pyloricus of truncus vagalis posterior

Right diagram labels:

Truncus vagalis posterior
Truncus sympathicus
Truncus vagalis anterior
N. splanchnicus major sinister
Branches of plexus coeliacus to duodenum
Celiac ganglia
Plexus splenicus
Plexus pancreaticus
Ganglion mesentericum superius
Branches of plexus mesentericus superior to pancreas and duodenum

—— Sympathetic fibers
—— Parasympathetic fibers

A Autonomic innervation of the hepar, vesica biliaris, and gaster
These organs receive their **sympathetic supply** from the ganglia coeliaca. The *postsynaptic* fibers course with the branches of the truncus coeliacus, while the *presynaptic* fibers form the nn. splanchnici (mainly the n. splanchnicus major) and synapse with the postsynaptic neuron in the ganglion. They receive their **parasympathetic supply** from the vagal trunks (presynaptic fibers). The truncus vagalis *anterior* (preponderance of left n. vagus fibers) terminates at the gaster, while the truncus vagalis *posterior* goes on to supply large portions of the intestinum. The anterior and posterior plexus gastrici are distributed to the parietes anterior and posterior of the gaster. The synapse with the postsynaptic parasympathetic neuron occurs in small ganglia located directly on the stomach wall.
Sympathetic and parasympathetic fibers pass along the a. hepatica propria to the porta hepatis as the plexus hepaticus. After dividing at the hepar, this plexus also distributes fibers to the vesica biliaris and the intra- and extrahepatic bile ducts.

B Autonomic innervation of the pancreas, duodenum, and splen
These organs receive their **sympathetic supply** from the ganglia coeliaca and ganglion mesentericum superius. The *postsynaptic* fibers pass along the branches of the truncus coeliacus and a. mesenterica superior. The *presynaptic* fibers form the nn. splanchnici major and minor. They receive their **parasympathetic supply** from the trunci vagales (mainly the truncus vagalis posterior).
Sympathetic and parasympathetic fibers course with the a. splenica to the splen as the *plexus splenicus*, and they course with branches of the a. splenica and a. mesenterica superior to the pancreas as the *plexus pancreaticus*. The fibers to the duodenum reach that organ via the a. gastroduodenalis, a. pancreaticoduodenalis, and rr. duodenales as part of the *plexus mesentericus superior*. The synapse with the second parasympathetic neuron occurs in small ganglia located near the organs.

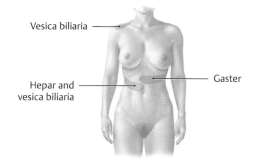

Vesica biliaria
Hepar and vesica biliaria
Gaster

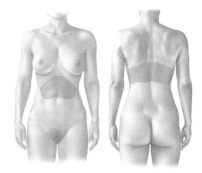

C Referred pain from the hepar, vesica biliaris, and gaster
The Head zones (see p. 73) of the hepar, vesica biliaris, and gaster extend from the right and left regiones hypochondriacae to the regio epigastrica. Vesica biliaris pain may also radiate to the right shoulder (C 4, n. phrenicus). (There are no Head zones associated with the duodenum and splen.)

D Referred pain from of the pancreas
The Head zone of the pancreas girdles the abdomen. Pain due to pancreatic disease may be perceived not just in the upper abdomen but also in the back. The anterior Head zone overlaps with the zones of the hepar and gaster.

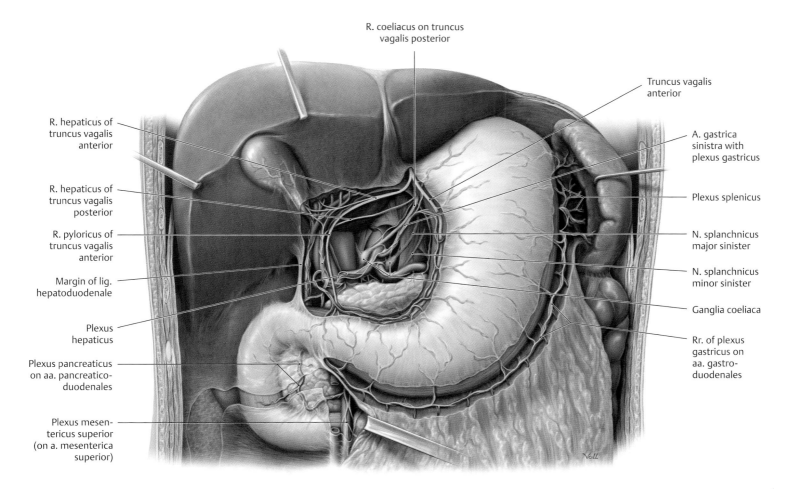

R. coeliacus on truncus
vagalis posterior

R. hepaticus of
truncus vagalis
anterior

R. hepaticus of
truncus vagalis
posterior

R. pyloricus of
truncus vagalis
anterior

Margin of lig.
hepatoduodenale

Plexus
hepaticus

Plexus pancreaticus
on aa. pancreatico-
duodenales

Plexus mesen-
tericus superior
(on a. mesenterica
superior)

Truncus vagalis
anterior

A. gastrica
sinistra with
plexus gastricus

Plexus splenicus

N. splanchnicus
major sinister

N. splanchnicus
minor sinister

Ganglia coeliaca

Rr. of plexus
gastricus on
aa. gastro-
duodenales

E Innervation of the hepar, vesica biliaris, gaster, duodenum, pancreas, and splen

Anterior view. The omentum minus has been broadly removed, and the omentum majus has been opened. The colon ascendens and part of the colon transversum have been removed. The retroperitoneal fat and connective tissue has been partially removed to improve the exposure. The plexus viscerales arising from the ganglion coeliacum mainly accompany the arteries as they pass to their target organs.

Note: The pylorus is generally supplied by separate rr. pylorici that arise from the trunci vagales (parasympathetic supply) and often run initially with the rr. hepatici. Because of this arrangement, the function of the pylorus is not impaired when the trunci vagales are divided distal to the origin of the rr. pylorici, as it is by a *selective proximal vagotomy* (see **F**).

Thus it is possible to reduce acid production by the parietal cells in the corpus and fundus of the gaster without affecting necessary gastrin production in the antrum pyloricum and pylorus or compromising the motor function of the pylorus.

The **ductus hepaticus and bile ducts** receive their autonomic supply from *parasympathetic* rr. hepatici that join the *sympathetic* fibers in the plexus hepaticus. The *plexus hepaticus* accompanies the a. hepatica propria to the hepar and gives off branches that supply the vesica biliaris and biliary tract. The **splen and pancreas** receive autonomic fibers from the plexus splenicus and pancreaticus. The **duodenum** derives part of its supply from the ganglion mesentericum superius and plexus mesentericus superior.

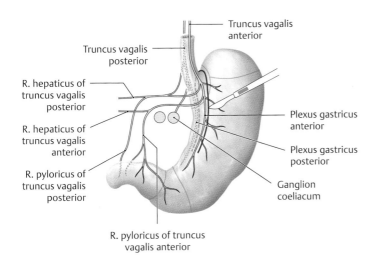

Truncus vagalis
anterior

Truncus vagalis
posterior

R. hepaticus of
truncus vagalis
posterior

R. hepaticus of
truncus vagalis
anterior

R. pyloricus of
truncus vagalis
posterior

Plexus gastricus
anterior

Plexus gastricus
posterior

Ganglion
coeliacum

R. pyloricus of truncus
vagalis anterior

F Selective proximal vagotomy

Impulses from the n. vagus stimulate the production of HCl (hydrochloric adic). Thus, a selective syroximal vagotomy may be considered for the treatment of gastric hyperacidity that is *refractory to medical treatment*. This is an operation in which the vagus fibers that stimulate the acid-producing parietal cells (mainly in the corpus gastricum and fundus gastricus) are transected on the stomach wall, at a site which is past the origin of the rr. pylorici from the trunci vagales. The rr. pylorici are left intact, ensuring the maintenance of normal pyloric function.

285

3.30 Autonomic Innervation of the Intestinum: Distribution of the Plexus Mesentericus Superior

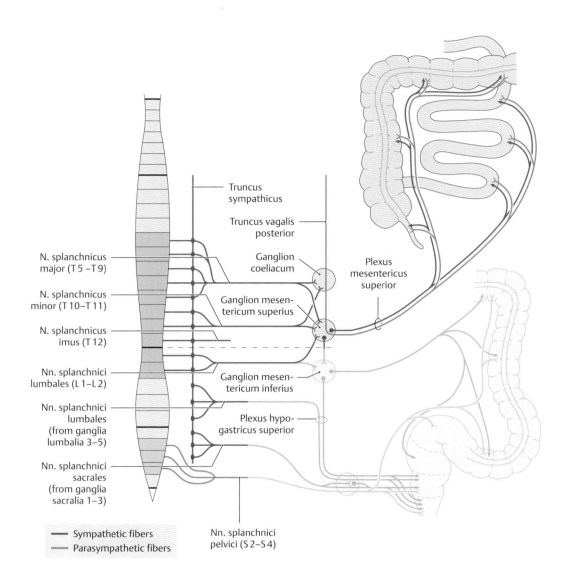

- Truncus sympathicus
- Truncus vagalis posterior
- N. splanchnicus major (T 5 –T 9)
- N. splanchnicus minor (T 10–T 11)
- Ganglion coeliacum
- Plexus mesentericus superior
- Ganglion mesentericum superius
- N. splanchnicus imus (T 12)
- Nn. splanchnici lumbales (L 1–L 2)
- Ganglion mesentericum inferius
- Nn. splanchnici lumbales (from ganglia lumbalia 3–5)
- Plexus hypogastricus superior
- Nn. splanchnici sacrales (from ganglia sacralia 1–3)
- Nn. splanchnici pelvici (S 2–S 4)

—— Sympathetic fibers
—— Parasympathetic fibers

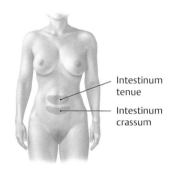

- Intestinum tenue
- Intestinum crassum

B Referred pain from the intestina tenue and crassum
In many cases the pain associated with intestinal diseases is not localized precisely to the bowel. Frequently the pain is projected to the color-shaded areas on the abdominal wall.

A Autonomic distribution of the plexus mesentericus superior
While a clear distinction is drawn between the intestina tenue and crassum topographically and histologically, autonomic innervation is based on the supply of a particular intestinal segment by a particular plexus, regardless of whether that segment is part of the intestinum tenue or intestinum crassum. The main distinction to be made is whether the intestinal segment is supplied by the plexus mesentericus *superior* or *inferior*. This principle is illustrated in the above diagram:

Sympathetic innervation:
- The *jejunum, ileum, caecum, colon ascendens*, and the *proximal two-thirds of the colon transversum* are supplied by postsynaptic branches of the ganglion mesentericum superius via the plexus mesentericus superior, which is distributed to the various intestinal segments along the branches of the a. mesenterica superior.
- Similarly, the *distal third of the colon transversum*, the *colon descendens, colon sigmoideum*, and *upper rectum* are innervated by postsynaptic branches of the ganglion mesentericum inferius and the associated plexus, which is distributed along the branches of the a. mesenterica inferior.
- The *middle and lower rectum* are supplied by the nn. splanchnici lumbales and sacrales via the plexus hypogastricus inferior (the supply to the three levels of the rectum is shown on p. 288).

The ganglion mesentericum superius, then, provides sympathetic innervation to the entire intestinum tenue and part of the intestinum crassum, supplying by far the greater portion of the entire bowel.

The **parasympathetic innervation** of the intestina tenue and crassum is analogous to their sympathetic innervation.
- The *intestinum tenue, caecum, colon ascendens*, and *proximal two-thirds of the colon transversum* are supplied by the *truncus vagalis* and its branches.
- The remaining *colon* and *rectum* are innervated by the *nn. splanchnici pelvici* from segments S2–S4 (see p. 288). Some of these nerves have their synapses in ganglion cells within the plexus hypogastricus inferior and some in ganglion cells on the organ wall.

Thus, the truncus vagalis (i.e., elements of the pars cranialis of the pars parasympathica of the nervous system) provides **parasympathetic** innervation to the entire intestinum tenue and part of the intestinum crassum, supplying the greater portion of the entire bowel. A site on the colon transversum called the *Cannon-Böhm point* marks the boundary between the proximal and distal territories of the autonomic nervous system.

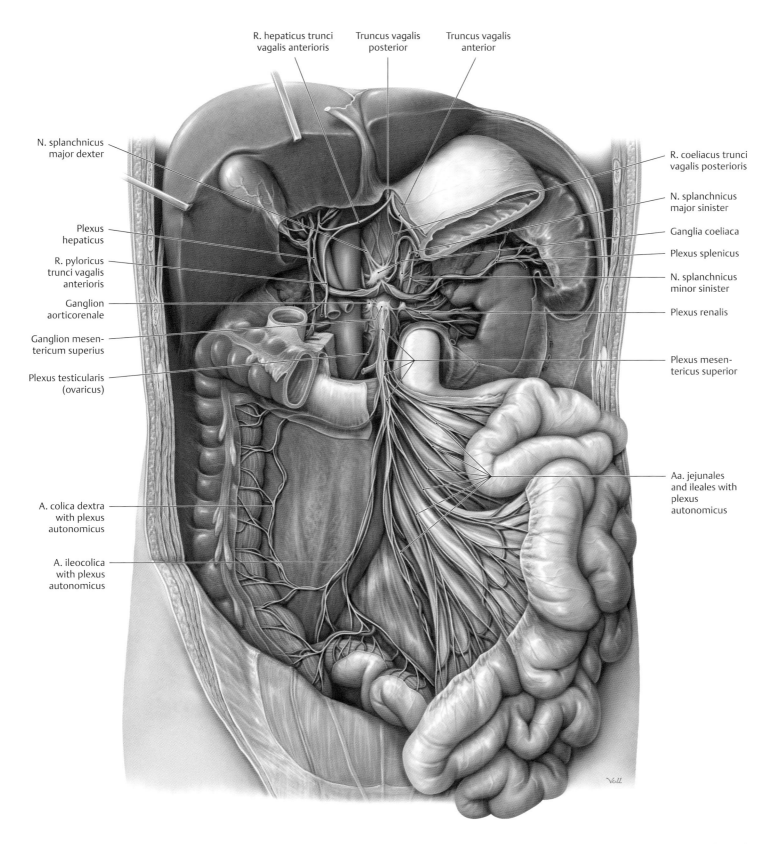

R. hepaticus trunci vagalis anterioris

Truncus vagalis posterior

Truncus vagalis anterior

N. splanchnicus major dexter

Plexus hepaticus

R. pyloricus trunci vagalis anterioris

Ganglion aorticorenale

Ganglion mesentericum superius

Plexus testicularis (ovaricus)

A. colica dextra with plexus autonomicus

A. ileocolica with plexus autonomicus

R. coeliacus trunci vagalis posterioris

N. splanchnicus major sinister

Ganglia coeliaca

Plexus splenicus

N. splanchnicus minor sinister

Plexus renalis

Plexus mesentericus superior

Aa. jejunales and ileales with plexus autonomicus

C Autonomic distribution of the plexus mesentericus superior to the intestinum

Anterior view. The hepar has been retracted superiorly, and the gaster and pancreas have been partially removed. Most of the distal part of the colon transversum has been removed, and all loops of intestinum tenue have been reflected toward the left side.

The postsynaptic branches of the ganglion mesentericum superius (**sympathetic supply**) pass along the branches of the a. mesenterica superior in the mesenterium as the plexus mesentericus superior, being distributed to the jejunum, ileum, caecum (and appendix vermiformis), and the colon as far as the junction of the middle and distal thirds of the colon transversum. Past that point the bowel receives its sympathetic innervation from the ganglion mesentericum inferius (not visible here). **Parasympathetic innervation** from the jejunum to the distal third of the colon transversum is supplied by the truncus vagalis and its branches. The innervation of the remaining colon and rectum is described on p. 288.

3.31 Autonomic Innervation of the Intestinum: Distribution of the Plexus Mesentericus Inferior and Plexus Hypogastricus Inferior

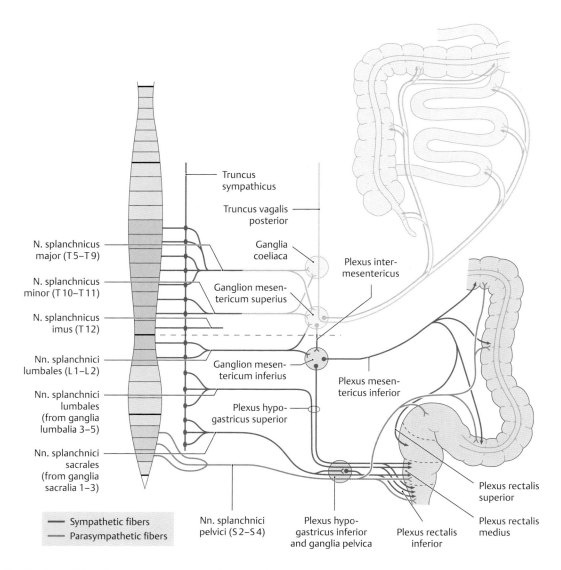

Truncus sympathicus

Truncus vagalis posterior

N. splanchnicus major (T 5–T 9)

N. splanchnicus minor (T 10–T 11)

N. splanchnicus imus (T 12)

Nn. splanchnici lumbales (L 1–L 2)

Nn. splanchnici lumbales (from ganglia lumbalia 3–5)

Nn. splanchnici sacrales (from ganglia sacralia 1–3)

Ganglia coeliaca

Plexus inter-mesentericus

Ganglion mesen-tericum superius

Ganglion mesen-tericum inferius

Plexus mesen-tericus inferior

Plexus hypo-gastricus superior

Plexus rectalis superior

—— Sympathetic fibers
—— Parasympathetic fibers

Nn. splanchnici pelvici (S 2–S 4)

Plexus hypo-gastricus inferior and ganglia pelvica

Plexus rectalis inferior

Plexus rectalis medius

A Autonomic distribution of the plexus mesentericus inferior and plexus hypogastricus inferior

Note: The autonomic innervation of the bowel is not divided anatomically between the intestina tenue and crassum. It is best understood in terms of the particular bowel segment that is supplied by a particular plexus (plexus mesentericus superior or inferior, plexus hypogastricus

inferior). Because this unit is concerned mainly with the distribution of the plexus mesentericus inferior and plexus hypogastricus inferior (see also **C**), the regions supplied by these plexuses are highlighted in the above diagram. Further details on the innervation pattern are given on p. 225.

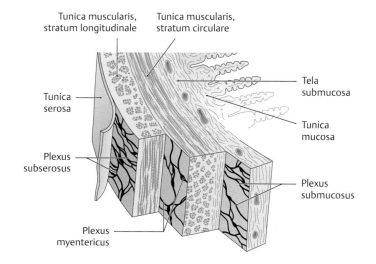

Tunica muscularis, stratum longitudinale

Tunica muscularis, stratum circulare

Tunica serosa

Plexus subserosus

Plexus myentericus

Tela submucosa

Tunica mucosa

Plexus submucosus

B Organization of the plexus entericus

The plexus entericus is the portion of the autonomic nervous system that specifically serves *all the organs of the gastrointestinal tract.* Located within the wall of the digestive tube (intramural nervous system), it is subject to both sympathetic and parasympathetic influences. Congenital absence of the plexus entericus leads to severe disturbances of gastrointestinal transit (e.g., Hirschsprung disease). The plexus entericus has basically the same organization throughout the gastrointestinal tract, although there is an area in the wall of the lower rectum that is devoid of ganglion cells (see p. 243). Three subsystems are distinguished in the plexus entericus:

• Plexus submucosus (Meissner's plexus)
• Plexus myentericus (Auerbach's plexus)
• Plexus subserosus

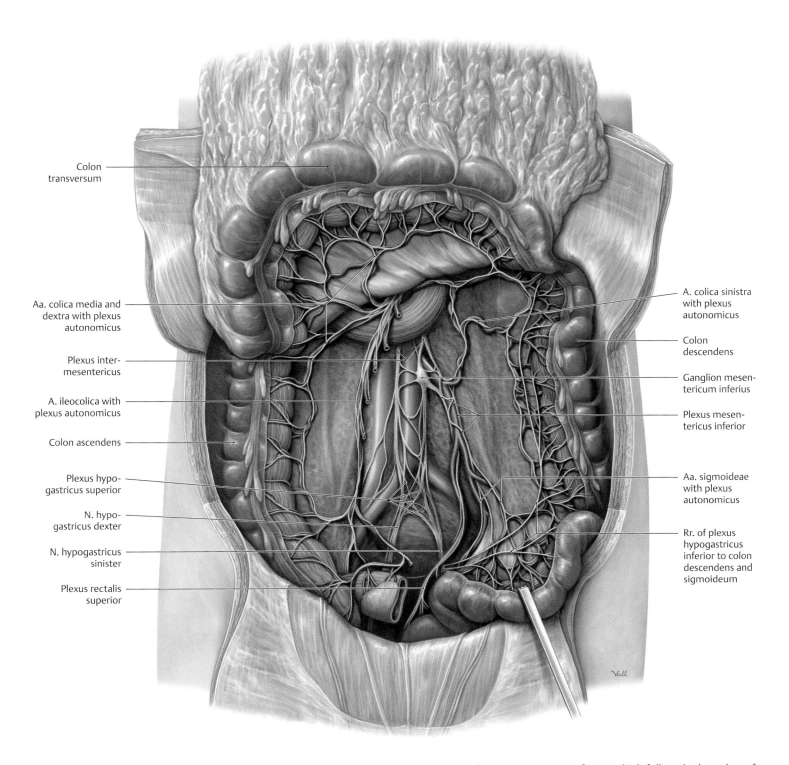

Colon transversum

Aa. colica media and dextra with plexus autonomicus

Plexus inter-mesentericus

A. ileocolica with plexus autonomicus

Colon ascendens

Plexus hypo-gastricus superior

N. hypo-gastricus dexter

N. hypogastricus sinister

Plexus rectalis superior

A. colica sinistra with plexus autonomicus

Colon descendens

Ganglion mesen-tericum inferius

Plexus mesen-tericus inferior

Aa. sigmoideae with plexus autonomicus

Rr. of plexus hypogastricus inferior to colon descendens and sigmoideum

C Autonomic distribution of the plexus mesentericus inferior and plexus hypogastricus inferior to the bowel

Anterior view. The jejunum and ileum have been removed, leaving a short ileal stump on the caecum. The colon transversum has been reflected superiorly, and the colon sigmoideum has been retracted inferiorly.

Sympathetic innervation:

- The *caecum, appendix vermiformis, colon ascendens*, and *proximal two-thirds of the colon transversum* (plus all of the intestinum tenue, not visible here) are supplied by postsynaptic branches of the ganglion mesentericum superius.
- The *distal third of the colon transversum, colon descendens, colon sigmoideum*, and *upper rectum* are supplied by postsynaptic branches

of the ganglion mesentericum inferius, which follow the branches of the a. mesenterica inferior as the plexus mesentericus inferior.

- The *middle and lower rectum* are supplied by the nn. splanchnici lumbales and sacrales via the plexus hypogastricus inferior (which follows the visceral branches of the a. iliaca interna).

Parasympathetic innervation is also divided at the junction of the middle and distal thirds of the colon transversum:

- The *proximal* portion is innervated by the truncus vagalis and its branches (i.e., the pars *cranialis* of the pars parasympathica of the nervous system).
- The *distal* portion is innervated by the nn. splanchnici pelvici of segments S2–S4 and parts of the plexus hypogastricus inferior (i.e., the pars *sacralis* of the pars parasympathica of the nervous system; see also p. 227).

289

4.1 Overview of the Urinary Organs; the Renes in situ

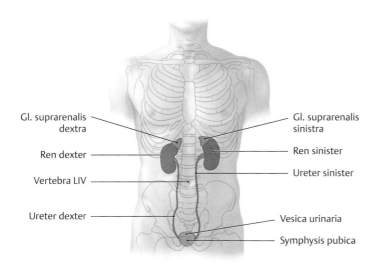

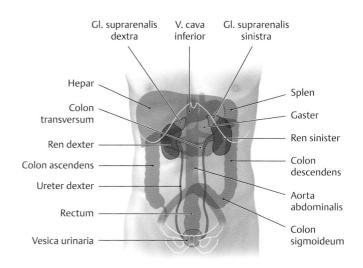

A Projection of the renes and other urinary organs onto the skeleton

Anterior view. The gll. suprarenales are also shown to aid orientation. The renes are located next to the columna vertebralis and are high enough that they overlap the eleventh and twelfth ribs. The hilum renale is situated at the L 1/L 2 level. Usually the right ren is somewhat lower than the left ren due to the space occupied by the hepar (see p. 382). The vesica urinaria is shown fully distended in the diagram. When empty, it is considerably smaller and is hidden behind the symphysis pubica. The ureteres descend in the retroperitoneum and open into the vesica urinaria from the posterior side.

B Projection of the urinary organs onto the organs of the abdomen and pelvis

Anterior view. Owing to its large size, the hepar displaces the right ren slightly inferiorly. The vesica urinaria is shown in a fully distended state. It is anterior to the rectum in the male and anterior to the uterus (not shown here) in the female. Because of this relationship, marked distention of the ampulla recti or enlargement of the uterus due to pregnancy exerts greater pressure on the vesica urinaria, creating an urge to urinate even when the vesica urinaria is not full. Urinary incontinence may develop due to pathological processes of longer duration, such as muscular tumors of the uterus (fibroids), or due to weakening of the vesica closure mechanism as a result of previous vaginal deliveries (descent of the muscular diaphragma pelvis).

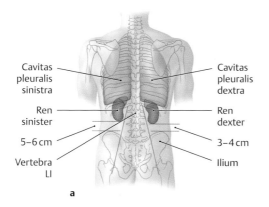

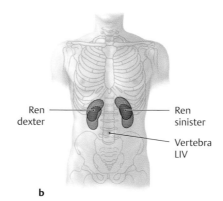

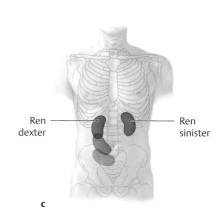

C Location of the renes, normal vs. pathological mobility

a Posterior view. The cavitates pleurales overlap the renes posteriorly owing to the convexity of the diaphragma.

Note that the right ren is lower than the left ren and is closer to the palpable crista iliaca.

b, c Anterior view. The renes are located in the retroperitoneum just below the diaphragma. Hence they move passively with the diaphragma during respiratory excursions, moving inferiorly and slightly laterally during inspiration because of their oblique position (their poli inferiores point away from the spine, see oblique red lines in **a**).

These passive movements may cause respiration-dependent pain in patients with renal disease. A *pathological* increase in renal mobility ("floating kidney," see **c**) results from atrophy of the capsula adiposa that normally surrounds the renes and keeps them in a stable position. A wasting illness (e.g., metastatic tumors of varying origin) may cause such severe fatty atrophy that the renes descend to a lower level in the abdomen. As they are still tethered by the ureter and vascular stalk, this descent may kink the renal vessels or ureter and interfere with renal blood flow or urinary outflow.

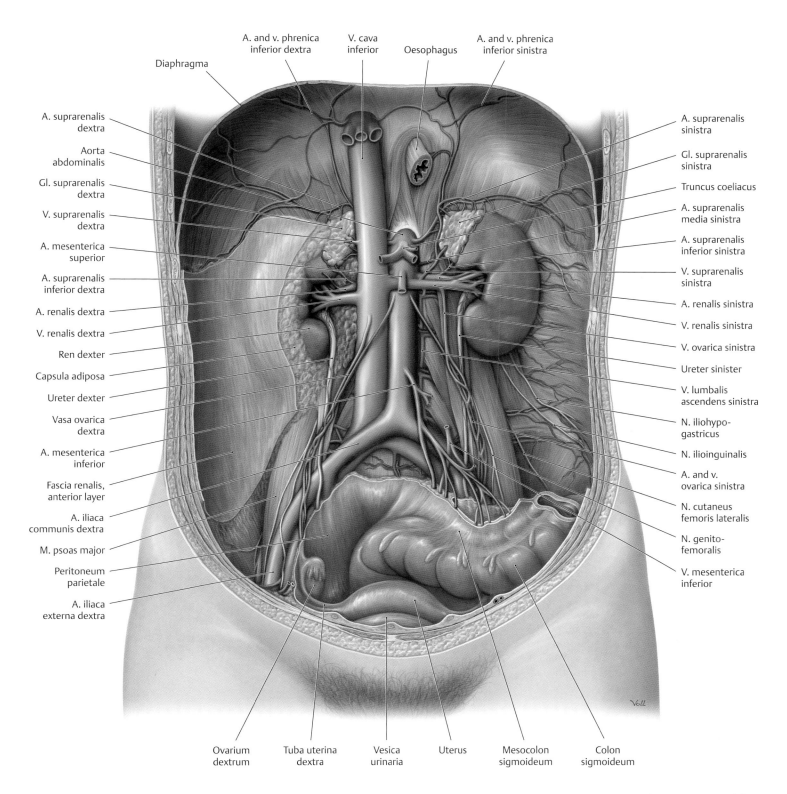

A. and v. phrenica inferior dextra

V. cava inferior

Oesophagus

A. and v. phrenica inferior sinistra

Diaphragma

A. suprarenalis dextra

Aorta abdominalis

Gl. suprarenalis dextra

V. suprarenalis dextra

A. mesenterica superior

A. suprarenalis inferior dextra

A. renalis dextra

V. renalis dextra

Ren dexter

Capsula adiposa

Ureter dexter

Vasa ovarica dextra

A. mesenterica inferior

Fascia renalis, anterior layer

A. iliaca communis dextra

M. psoas major

Peritoneum parietale

A. iliaca externa dextra

A. suprarenalis sinistra

Gl. suprarenalis sinistra

Truncus coeliacus

A. suprarenalis media sinistra

A. suprarenalis inferior sinistra

V. suprarenalis sinistra

A. renalis sinistra

V. renalis sinistra

V. ovarica sinistra

Ureter sinister

V. lumbalis ascendens sinistra

N. iliohypo-gastricus

N. ilioinguinalis

A. and v. ovarica sinistra

N. cutaneus femoris lateralis

N. genito-femoralis

V. mesenterica inferior

Ovarium dextrum

Tuba uterina dextra

Vesica urinaria

Uterus

Mesocolon sigmoideum

Colon sigmoideum

D The urinary organs in situ

Anterior view of an opened female abdomen. The splen and gastrointestinal organs have been removed to the colon sigmoideum, and the oesophagus has been pulled slightly inferiorly. The capsula adiposa remains partially intact on the right side, removed on the left side. The renes and gll. suprarenales are incorporated into the retroperitoneum by the structural fat of this capsule. The moderately distended vesica biliaris is just visible above the symphysis pubica in front of the uterus. The peritoneum parietale has been removed to provide a clear view into the retroperitoneum.

Note: The ureteres pass behind the ovarian vessels and in front of the iliac vessels as they descend in the retroperitoneum. These sites represent clinically important constrictions of the ureter where a stone from the pelvis renalis may become lodged (see **B**, p. 301).

In most cases the renes are not oriented parallel to the coronal plane. The hilum renale, where the blood vessels and ureter enter and leave the renes, is directed anteromedially (see **Ab**, p. 292). Also, the renal poli superiores are closer together than the poli inferiores, so that the renes appear slightly "tilted" toward the midline. Thus the hilum renale also points slightly downward.

4.2 Renes: Location, Shape, and Structure

A Position of the renes in the renal bed
Right renal bed. **a** Sagittal section at approximately the level of the hilum renale, viewed from the right side. **b** Transverse section through the abdomen at approximately the L 1/L 2 level, viewed from above.
The renal bed is located on each side of the spine in the retroperitoneum. It contains the renes, which are invested by a thin **organ capsule** (renal capsula fibrosa), and the gll. suprarenales, which are surrounded by the **perirenal capsula adiposa** that also encloses the kidneys. The capsula adiposa is thicker posteriorly than anteriorly.
Note: Swelling of the ren (usually due to inflammation) may cause severe pain due to stretching of the capsula fibrosa.
The capsula adiposa is surrounded by the **fascia renalis**, which separates it from its surroundings by two layers:

- The anterior layer behind the peritoneum parietale (to which it is fused at some sites)
- The posterior layer, which is partially attached to the fascia transversalis and muscular fasciae on the posterior trunk wall

The fascia renalis, and thus the renal bed, is open inferiorly and medially to allow passage of the ureter and renal vessels. It is closed laterally and superiorly by fusion of the fascial layers. Because of this arrangement, inflammatory processes that are adjacent to the ren but within the fascia renalis tend to spread to the contralateral side or inferiorly and may spread into the pelvis.
Note: The entire renal bed moves downward during inspiratory depression of the diaphragm, *indirectly* causing the ren and gl. suprarenalis to move as well. This differs from the hepar, which is attached to the diaphragma (area nuda) and is *directly* moved by diaphragma excursions.

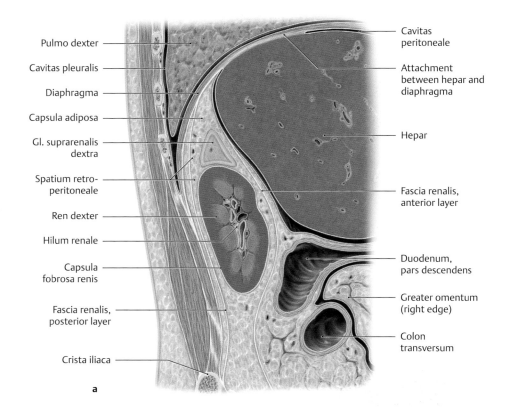

Pulmo dexter
Cavitas pleuralis
Diaphragma
Capsula adiposa
Gl. suprarenalis dextra
Spatium retro-peritoneale
Ren dexter
Hilum renale
Capsula fobrosa renis
Fascia renalis, posterior layer
Crista iliaca

Cavitas peritoneale
Attachment between hepar and diaphragma
Hepar
Fascia renalis, anterior layer
Duodenum, pars descendens
Greater omentum (right edge)
Colon transversum

a

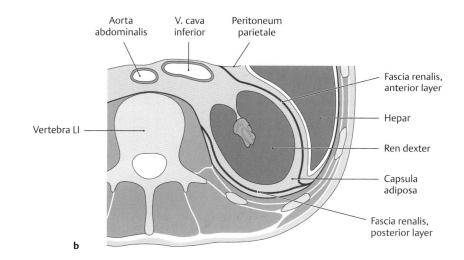

Aorta abdominalis
V. cava inferior
Peritoneum parietale
Vertebra LI

Fascia renalis, anterior layer
Hepar
Ren dexter
Capsula adiposa
Fascia renalis, posterior layer

b

B Renal bed: Fasciae and capsulae of the renes

Capsula fibrosa	Thin, firm connective-tissue capsule that closely invests each ren
Perirenal capsula adiposa	Mass of fat that surrounds the renes and gll. suprarenales and completely occupies the renal bed; it is thickest lateral and posterior to the renes
Fascia renalis	Connective-tissue fascial sac that encloses the perirenal capsula adiposa, portions of the pars abdominalis aortae and v. cava inferior close to the ren (see **Ab**), and the proximal ureter; subdivided into a thin anterior layer and a thick posterior layer (see **Aa**)

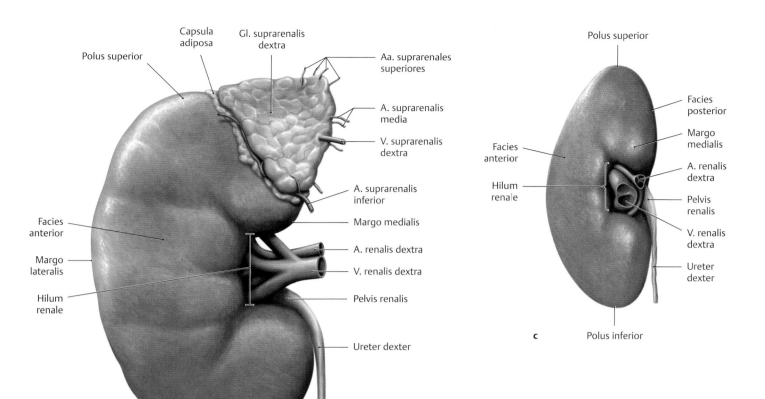

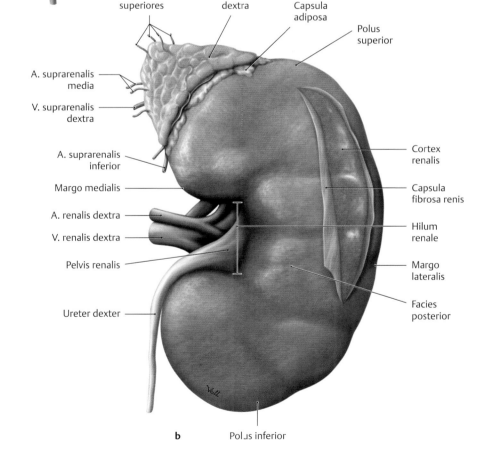

C Structure and shape of the ren

Anterior view (**a**), posterior view (**b**), and medial view (**c**) of the right ren. The gl. suprarenalis is left intact in **a** and **b**, and the ureter has been cut at the level of the polus inferior. The capsula fibrosa that directly invests the ren is intact in **a** and **c** and has been partially opened in **b** to display the underlying renal parenchyma. The sinus renalis (the deep space into which the hilum renalis opens) generally contains a certain amount of structural fat, and so the vascular structures and pelvis renalis are not exposed to view intraoperatively as they are in these drawings. The normal ren measures an average of 12 x 6 x 3 cm (L x W x T) and weighs 150–180 g. It has

- two poles (polus superior and inferior),
- two surfaces (facies anterior and posterior), and
- two borders (margo lateralis and medialis).

The margo medialis bears the hilum renale, where vascular structures and the ureter enter and leave the ren. The shallow surface grooves result from the embryonic lobulation of the ren. The hilar structures are usually arranged as follows from anterior to posterior (as shown in **c**): right v. renalis, right a. renalis, and right ureter.

Note: The a. renalis is usually posterior to the v. renalis because the right a. renalis passes to the right ren *behind* the v. cava inferior (where the vv. renales terminate), while the left v. renalis passes to the left ren *in front of* the pars abdominis aortae (which gives origin to the aa. renales). The left a. renalis may also loop around the left v. renalis from above to occupy an anterior position. The ureter leaves the pelvis renalis (see p. 294) below the vessels and is usually somewhat posterior in relation to the blood vessels.

4.3 Renes: Architecture and Microstructure

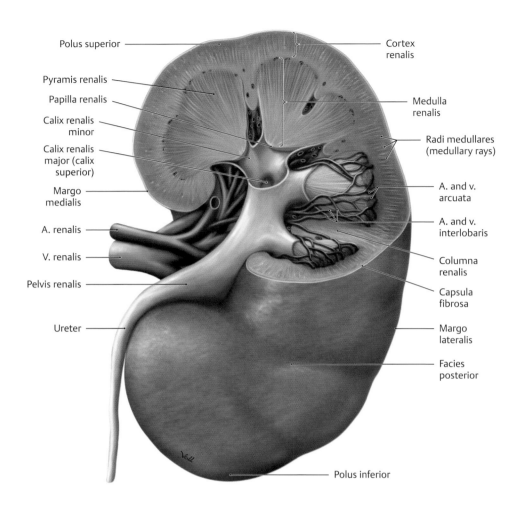

Polus superior

Pyramis renalis

Papilla renalis

Calix renalis minor

Calix renalis major (calix superior)

Margo medialis

A. renalis

V. renalis

Pelvis renalis

Ureter

Cortex renalis

Medulla renalis

Radi medullares (medullary rays)

A. and v. arcuata

A. and v. interlobaris

Columna renalis

Capsula fibrosa

Margo lateralis

Facies posterior

Polus inferior

A Macroscopic structure of the ren
Posterior view of a right ren with the upper half of the ren partially removed. The **renal parenchyma** consists of an outer cortex renalis and inner medulla renalis:

- The *cortex renalis* is a relatively thin layer that lies beneath the capsula fibrosa and forms columns (columnae renales) that extend between the pyramides renales of the medulla. The cortex and columnae contain approximately 2.4 million corpuscula renalia (which contain the glomeruli, see **B**) as well as the proximal and distal renal tubuli (see **C**).
- The *medulla renalis* consists of approximately 10–12 pyramides renales. The bases of the pyramides are directed toward the cortex and capsula, while their apices converge toward the pelvis renalis. The medulla renalis mainly contains the ascending and descending limbs of the renal tubuli.

The **pelvis renalis** is described on p. 296.

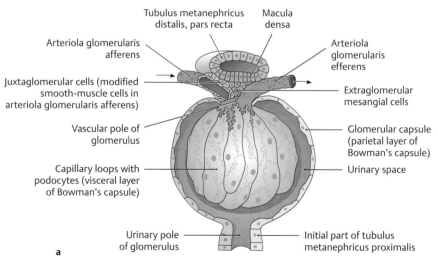

Tubulus metanephricus distalis, pars recta

Macula densa

Arteriola glomerularis afferens

Arteriola glomerularis efferens

Juxtaglomerular cells (modified smooth-muscle cells in arteriola glomerularis afferens)

Extraglomerular mesangial cells

Vascular pole of glomerulus

Glomerular capsule (parietal layer of Bowman's capsule)

Capillary loops with podocytes (visceral layer of Bowman's capsule)

Urinary space

Urinary pole of glomerulus

Initial part of tubulus metanephricus proximalis

a

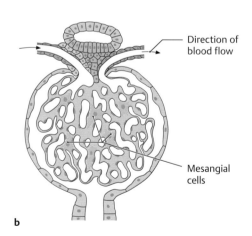

Direction of blood flow

Mesangial cells

b

B Corpusculum renale
a With the capsula glomerularis opened; **b** In section.
The corpusculum renale is the interface between the blood vessels and the excretory portion of the urinary tract (see **C**). It consists of a central convoluted vascular loop, the glomerulus, and a bulbous envelope lined by squamous epithelial cells, the *capsula glomerularis* (Bowman's capsule). Blood enters the *glomerulus* at the vascular pole of the corpusculum renale by flowing through the arteriola glomerularis *afferens*,

and it leaves the glomerulus through the arteriola glomerularis *efferens*. The primary urine is formed within the corpusculum renale and drains through a tubular system at the urinary pole of the glomerulus. The initial portion of this tubular system that is connected to the capsula glomerularis is the tubulus metanephricus proximalis (see **C**).
Note: Specialized cells at the vascular pole of the corpusculum renale regulate the blood pressure that is necessary for ultrafiltration.

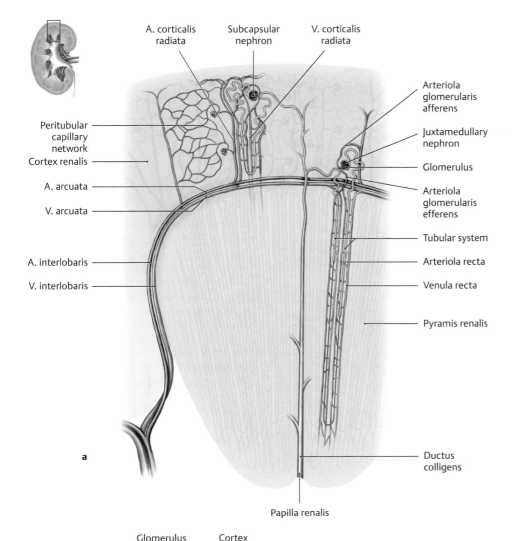

A. corticalis radiata

Subcapsular nephron

V. corticalis radiata

Arteriola glomerularis afferens

Peritubular capillary network

Cortex renalis

A. arcuata

V. arcuata

A. interlobaris

V. interlobaris

Juxtamedullary nephron

Glomerulus

Arteriola glomerularis efferens

Tubular system

Arteriola recta

Venula recta

Pyramis renalis

Ductus colligens

a

Papilla renalis

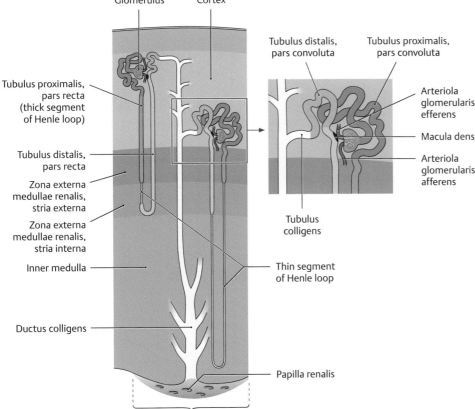

Glomerulus   Cortex

Tubulus proximalis, pars recta (thick segment of Henle loop)

Tubulus distalis, pars recta

Zona externa medullae renalis, stria externa

Zona externa medullae renalis, stria interna

Inner medulla

Ductus colligens

Tubulus distalis, pars convoluta

Tubulus proximalis, pars convoluta

Arteriola glomerularis efferens

Macula dens

Arteriola glomerularis afferens

Tubulus colligens

Thin segment of Henle loop

Papilla renalis

b   Area cribrosa

C Architecture of the renal vessels and intrarenal collecting system

a Renal vessels: Sectional view of a pyramis renalis with adjacent cortical areas. The intrarenal vascular and collecting systems are closely interrelated spatially and functionally. An ultrafiltrate from the blood (primary urine) drains into a microscopically small system of renal tubules. *Blood flow to the ren* (**a**) is supplied by aa. interlobares that pass along the sides of the pyramides renales from the hilum renale. Each a. interlobaris supplies two adjacent pyramides renales and the associated cortical zones (these branches are not shown). At the base of the pyramid, the a. interlobaris gives rise to the a. arcuata, from which the aa. interlobulares are distributed into the cortex renalis as far as the capsula fibrosa. The arteriolae glomerulares *afferentes* that arise from an a. interlobularis each supply one glomerulus. The arteriolae glomerulares *efferentes* that emerge from the glomerulus are still carrying blood at a high oxygen tension; they supply the cortex or medulla renalis.

b Intrarenal collecting system: The smallest functional unit of the kidney is the nephronum, which consists of the corpusculum renale et tubuli metanephrici. Each nephronum drains via a short tubulus metanephricus distalis into a ductus metanephricus colligens duct which collects the urine from about 10–12 nephrona. There are approximately 1 million nephrons, which process approximately 1700 liters of blood daily to form approximately 170 liters of *primary urine*. This primary filtrate enters the tubular system at the urinary pole of the renal corpuscle and reaches the renal papilla as the *final urine*, which drains into the calyceal system (approximately 1.7 liters/day). The *tubular system* consists of the proximal and distal tubules (each with a convoluted and straight portion) and an intermediate tubule (with descending and ascending limbs). The intermediate tubule and the adjacent straight portions of the proximal and distal tubules comprise the *loop of Henle*. While passing through the tubular system, substances contained in the filtrate (mainly water) are reabsorbed while other substances (e.g., ions) are secreted into the filtrate. This process yields the final urine, which passes through a collecting tubule into a collecting duct and drains through the renal papilla into the *caliceal system*. It is conveyed from the calyces and renal pelvis to the ureter by peristalsis.

4.4   Pelvis Renalis and Urinary Transport

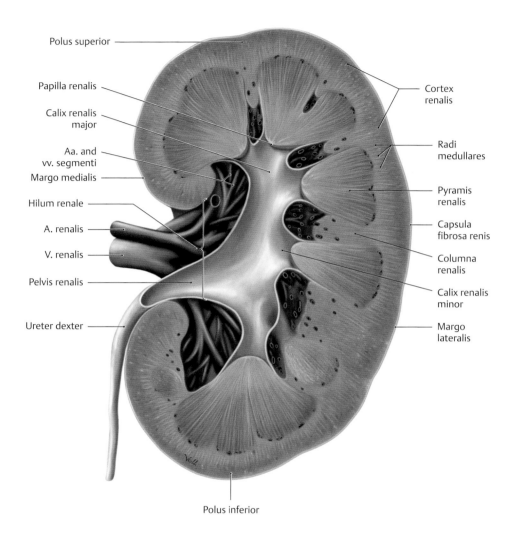

Polus superior

Papilla renalis

Calix renalis major

Aa. and vv. segmenti

Margo medialis

Hilum renale

A. renalis

V. renalis

Pelvis renalis

Ureter dexter

Cortex renalis

Radi medullares

Pyramis renalis

Capsula fibrosa renis

Columna renalis

Calix renalis minor

Margo lateralis

Polus inferior

A Structure and shape of the pelvis renalis
Mid-longitudinal section through a right kidney, posterior view. The pelvis renalis lies posterior to the renal vessels and is continuous inferiorly with the ureter. It may vary in shape (see **B**). It is usually divided into two or three indistinctly separable calices renales majores, which further divide into calices renales minores. They encompass the tips of the papillae renales in such a way that urine drains from the papillae into the calix without entering the renal parenchyma. Smooth-muscle fibers in the calices, pelvis renalis, and ureter (for details about wall structure, see **D**), enable these structures to undergo peristaltic contractions (see **C**).
Note: Stones (see **C**, p. 301) that form in the calices or pelvis renalis may become so large that they more or less fill the cavity and assume its shape (caliceal stone, staghorn calculus).

B Variations in the shape of the pelvis renalis

Anterior view of the left pelvis renalis. The pelvis renalis and ureter develop from an outgrowth of the ductus mesonephricus. This gemma ureterica grows from the bony pelvis toward the renal primordium and unites with it. Branching extensions of the pelvis renalis form the calices renales majores and minores. The calices renales majores in particular vary in number and shape: neighboring calices renales majores may fuse and "become incorporated" into the pelvis renalis. The pelvis renalis is found in basic forms along with transitional forms:

- Typus dendriticus (with extensive branching, also called linear) (**a**): very fine calices majores, narrow pelvis renalis;
- Transitional form (**b**);
- Typus ampullaris (**c**): indistinct calices majores with wide pelvis renalis; calices minores arise "directly" from the pelvis renalis.

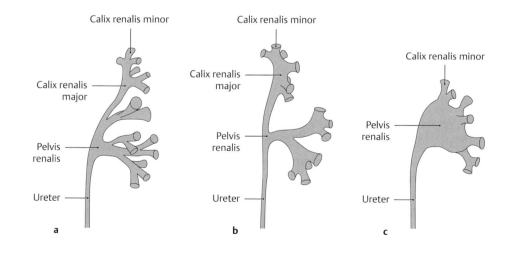

Calix renalis minor

Calix renalis major

Pelvis renalis

Ureter

a

Calix renalis minor

Calix renalis major

Pelvis renalis

Ureter

b

Calix renalis minor

Pelvis renalis

Ureter

c

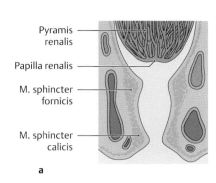

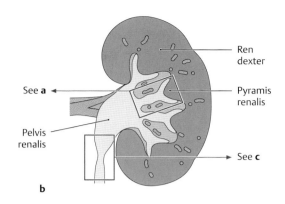

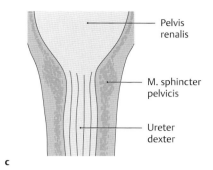

a

b

c

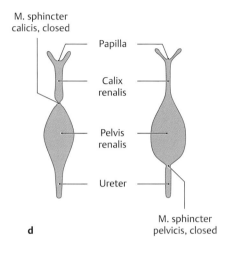

d

C Closure mechanisms of the calices renales and pelvis renalis; urinary transport

(after Rauber and Kopsch)

Schematic representation of a ren (**b**) with magnified sections of a calix renalis (**a**) and pelvis renalis (**c**) and a dynamic functional diagram of the calix and pelvis renalis during urinary transport (**d**). Urine is transported by an active mechanism. The smooth muscula-ture of the mm. sphincteres fornicis and cali-ces (**a**) and the m. sphincter pelvicis (**c**) (the functional sphincter system) enables the wall of the calices and pelvis renales to contract in segments. These contractions are continuous with the peristaltic waves of the ureter, with the result that the urinary tract is never pat-ent over its entire length but is patent in some portions and closed in others (**d**). This main-tains a distal flow of urine from the tip of the papilla renalis into the calix renalis, through the pelvis renalis, into the ureter, and on toward the vesica urinaria while preventing the reflux of urine into the renes.

Note: If this active transport process is impaired (e.g., by renal stones or drugs that inhibit the ureteral muscles), urine may reflux into the ren and incite an inflammatory process in the pelvis renalis. The papillae, calices, and pelvis renales are often affected jointly by disease (e.g., inflammation) because of their close proximity to one another. One of the most common diseases is suppurative bacterial pyelonephritis (*pyelo-*, referring to the pelvis renalis, from Gr. *pyelos*—trough, tub, or vat).

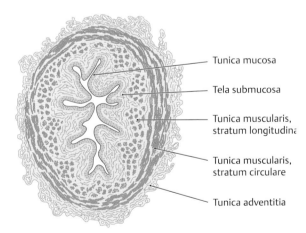

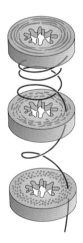

D Wall structure of the ureter

Transverse section through a ureter. A characteristic feature is the stel-late lumen that appears in cross-section due to the longitudinal mucosal folds. As in the urethra and vesica urinaria, the ureteral tunica mucosa consists of a transitional epithelium of varying height (see p. 305). The smooth muscle (tunica muscularis) consists basically of a longitudinal and a circular layer. It is powerfully developed and shows a function-ally spiral architecture (see **E**). When a renal stone enters the ureter, the smooth muscle in the ureteral wall undergoes powerful contractions in an effort to expel the stone, causing very severe pain (renal or ureteral colic). The colic may be relieved by drugs that suppress the activity of the parasympathetic nervous system, though this will also inhibit nor-mal urinary transport to the vesica urinaria. The pelvis renalis is struc-turally analogous to the ureter, including the stellate shape of its lumen.

E Arrangement of the ureteral musculature (after Graumann, von Keyserlingk, and Sasse)

Schematic cross-sections at various levels of the ureter. The longitudi-nal and circular muscle layers of the ureter wall have a slightly oblique arrangement, forming a kind of spiral that propels urine toward the ve-sica urinaria by peristaltic contractions. Although the ureteres are richly innervated, the peristaltic contractions are instigated by spontaneously depolarizing smooth-muscle cells in the walls of the pelvis renalis. Peri-staltic waves of contraction (with a speed of 2–3 cm/s) are propagated through direct electrical connections (gap junctions) between adja-cent smooth-muscle cells. Autonomic motor innervation and local sen-sory reflexes serve to modulate this intrinsic activity. This mechanism may thus have some superficial similarities to the system that controls heartbeat.

297

4.5 Glandulae Suprarenales

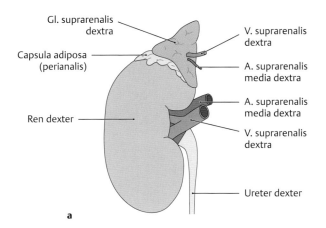

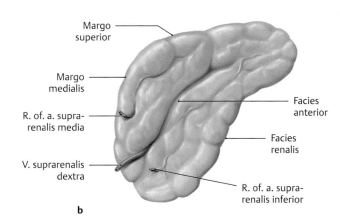

A Location and shape
a Location of the gl. suprarenalis on the right ren. **b** Isolated left gl. suprarenalis, anterior view.
The facies renalis of each v lies upon the polus superior of the associated ren. A thin layer of fat separates the gl. suprarenalis from the *renal capsula fibrosa* (making it easy to dissect the gland from the ren). The *perirenal* capsula adiposa, however, encompasses both the ren and the gl. suprarenalis.
Note: The entire gl. suprarenalis cannot be seen while in situ, and its true size is not appreciated until it has been detached from the ren. Portions descend on the posterior surface of the ren and are not visible in situ.

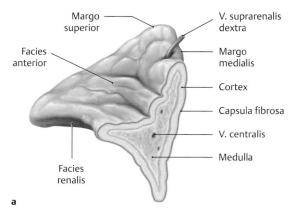

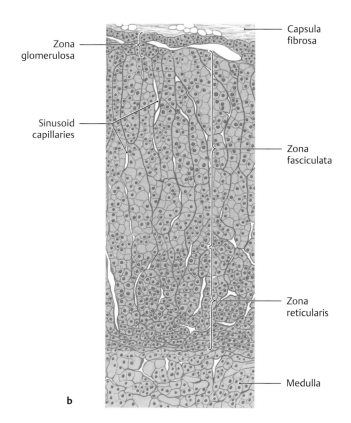

B Structure of the glandula suprarenalis
a Right gl. suprarenalis, cut open. **b** Histological section from a gl. suprarenalis.
The gl. suprarenalis consists of an outer cortex and an inner medulla (see **a**). The **cortex glandulae suprarenalis** is covered by a thin fibrous capsule and consists of three morphologically distinct zones (see **b**) in which adrenocortical hormones are produced and secreted into the bloodstream. These zones are, from outside to inside:

- Zona glomerulosa: mainly secretes mineralocorticoids (aldosterone)
- Zona fasciculata: mainly secretes glucocorticoids (hydrocortisone)
- Zona reticularis: sex hormones (estrogens and androgens)

Note: Loss or deficiency of both cortices glandularum suprarenalium leads to Addison disease, while hyperfunction of the cortex glandulae suprarenalis (or adrenocortical tumors) leads to Cushing syndrome.
The **medulla glandulae suprarenalis** is essentially a completely different endocrine gland, of different origin, that happens to be anatomically (but also functionally) associated with the cortex glandulae suprarenalis. The cortex is derived embryonically from mesoderm lining the posterior abdominal wall. The medulla glandulae suprarenalis is, by contrast, a crista neuralis derivative, and thus has an ectodermal origin. The catecholamines epinephrine and norepinephrine are produced in the medulla glandulae suprarenalis and are released into the bloodstream. From a (neuro)functional standpoint, the medulla glandulae suprarenalis is less a gland than a *ganglion sympathicum:* presynaptic sympathetic neurons pass from the nn. splanchnici major and minor into the medulla glandulae suprarenalis. Because the gll. suprarenales are endocrine glands and ganglia sympathica in one, they can secrete both epinephrine and glucocorticoids (cortisone) in response to stress.

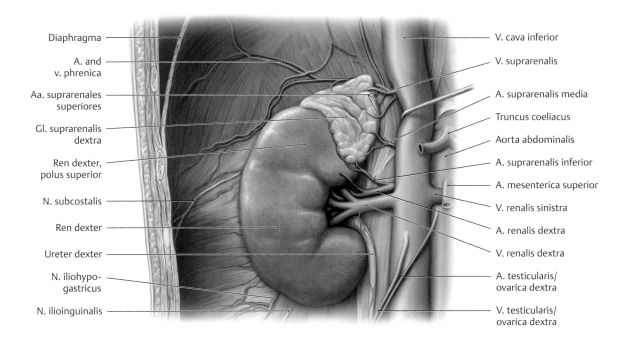

Diaphragma

A. and v. phrenica

Aa. suprarenales superiores

Gl. suprarenalis dextra

Ren dexter, polus superior

N. subcostalis

Ren dexter

Ureter dexter

N. iliohypo-gastricus

N. ilioinguinalis

V. cava inferior

V. suprarenalis

A. suprarenalis media

Truncus coeliacus

Aorta abdominalis

A. suprarenalis inferior

A. mesenterica superior

V. renalis sinistra

A. renalis dextra

V. renalis dextra

A. testicularis/ovarica dextra

V. testicularis/ovarica dextra

a

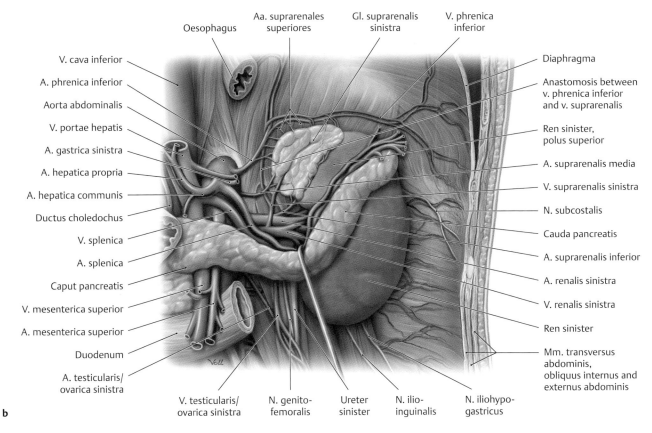

Oesophagus

Aa. suprarenales superiores

Gl. suprarenalis sinistra

V. phrenica inferior

V. cava inferior

A. phrenica inferior

Aorta abdominalis

V. portae hepatis

A. gastrica sinistra

A. hepatica propria

A. hepatica communis

Ductus choledochus

V. splenica

A. splenica

Caput pancreatis

V. mesenterica superior

A. mesenterica superior

Duodenum

A. testicularis/ovarica sinistra

Diaphragma

Anastomosis between v. phrenica inferior and v. suprarenalis

Ren sinister, polus superior

A. suprarenalis media

V. suprarenalis sinistra

N. subcostalis

Cauda pancreatis

A. suprarenalis inferior

A. renalis sinistra

V. renalis sinistra

Ren sinister

Mm. transversus abdominis, obliquus internus and externus abdominis

V. testicularis/ovarica sinistra

N. genito-femoralis

Ureter sinister

N. ilio-inguinalis

N. iliohypo-gastricus

b

C Right and left glandulae suprarenales in situ

Anterior view of the right (**a**) and left (**b**) ren and gl. suprarenalis with the perirenal capsula adiposa removed. To demonstrate the vessels behind the gl. suprarenalis, the v. cava has been retracted medially in **a** and the pancreas has been retracted inferiorly in **b**. The principal differences between the two gll. suprarenales are as follows:

- The right gl. suprarenalis is often somewhat smaller than the left gl. suprarenalis, which frequently extends inferiorly to the hilum renale.

- The right gl. suprarenalis is pyramid-shaped while the large left gl. suprarenalis is more oblong. The right gl. suprarenalis is normally in contact with the v. cava inferior (retracted medially here), but the left gl. suprarenalis is *not* in contact with the aorta abdominalis.

- The v. suprarenalis dexter usually opens *directly* into the v. cava inferior, unlike the v. suprarenalis sinistra, which opens into the left v. renalis.

Note: The gll. suprarenales are richly vascularized because, as endocrine organs, they release their hormones directly into the bloodstream.

4.6 Ureteres in situ

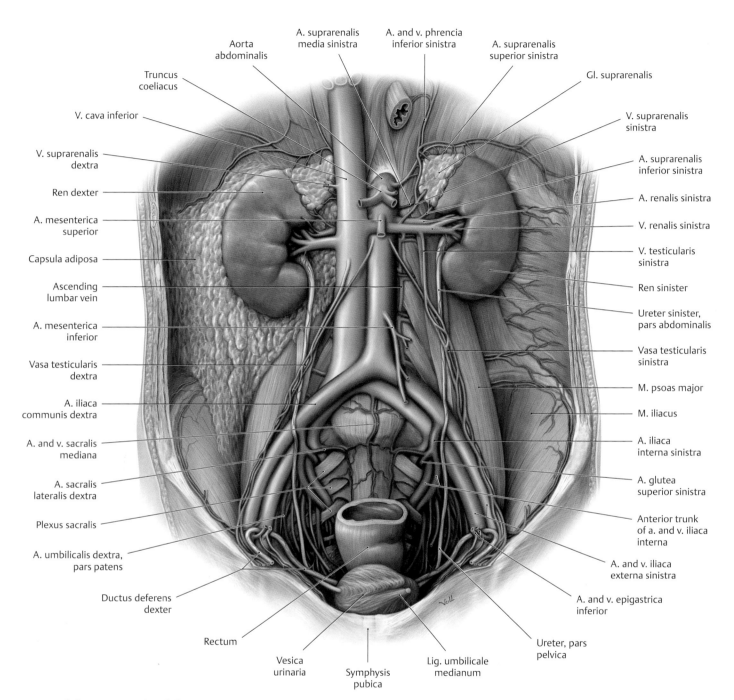

A Course of the ureter in the abdomen and pelvis
Anterior view, male abdomen. All organs have been removed except the urinary organs, gll. suprarenales, and a rectal stump. The oesophagus has been pulled slightly downward, and the capsula adiposa of the right ren has been partially preserved. A prolongation of the pelvis renalis, the ureter passes inferiorly and slightly anterior in the retroperitoneum for a length of approximately 26–29 cm. It opens into the posterior aspect of the vesica urinaria. *Anatomically,* the ureter consists of three parts:

- Pars abdominalis (from the pelvis renalis to the linea terminalis of the bony pelvis)
- Pars pelvica (from the linea terminalis to the bladder wall)
- Pars intramuralis (passes through the bladder wall)

The ureter is also divided into three *clinical* segments, based more on the presence of a free segment and two organ-bound segments than on the anatomical boundary between the partes abdominalis and pelvica:

- Renal segment (connected to the ren)
- Lumbar segment (between the ren and vesica urinaria)
- Vesical segment (in the bladder wall, corresponds anatomically to the pars intramuralis).

The most common *congenital anomalies* of the ureter are duplication anomalies and clefts. They may allow urine to back up to the ren (e.g., a cleft may allow reflux due to deficient vesicoureteral closure), producing an infection that ascends from the vesica urinaria to the pelvis renalis (bacterial pyelonephritis).

B Anatomical constrictions of the ureter

There are three normal *anatomical constrictions* where a stone from the pelvis renalis is apt to become lodged:

- Origin of the ureter from the pelvis renalis (ureteropelvic junction)
- Site where the ureter crosses over the aa. and vv. iliacae externae or communes
- Passage of the ureter through the vesica wall (ureterovesical junction)

Occasionally a *fourth constriction* can be identified where the a. and v. testicularis or ovarica pass in front of the ureter.

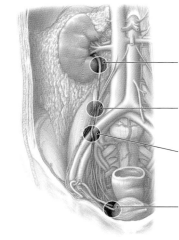

First constriction:
ureter passes over polus
inferior (pars abdominalis)

Possible constriction where
ureter passes behind vasa
testicularia/ovarica

Second constriction:
ureter crosses over vasa
iliaca (pars pelvica)

Third constriction:
ureter traverses the wall of
vesica urinaria
(pars intramuralis)

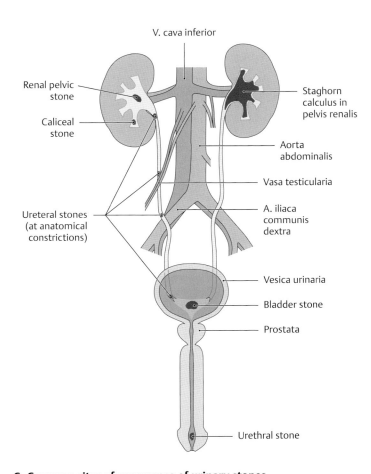

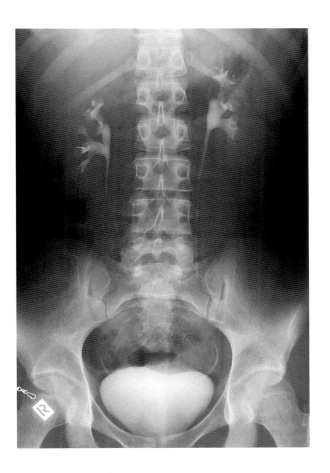

C Common sites of occurrence of urinary stones

When the solubility limit of certain compounds in the urine (e.g., uric acid) is exceeded, the compounds do not remain in solution but are precipitated to form crystallization nuclei. These calculi ("stones") may develop anywhere in the upper urinary tract and may migrate to various sites in any of the urinary organs (renal and renal pelvic stones, ureteral stones, bladder stones, urethral stones). Larger stones are particularly apt to become lodged in the ureter, often stimulating powerful waves of muscular contractions to expel the stone and causing excruciating pain (renal colic, ureteral colic).

D Intravenous urography

With intravenous urography, which is a radiographic examination, iodinated contrast agent is injected and excreted by the rene. The test provides information about renal function, and pathological findings such as anomalies, cysts, urinary obstruction, urinary stones, tumors, etc. (from: Möller, T.B., E. Reif: Taschenatlas der Roentgenanatomie, 3. Aufl. Thieme, Stuttgart 2006).

4.7   Vesica Urinaria in situ

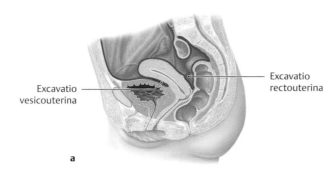

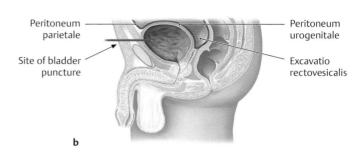

a

b

A Location and peritoneal covering of the female (a) and male (b) vesica urinaria

Midsagittal section, viewed from the left side. The vesica urinaria is shown slightly distended, raising the uterus to a slightly higher position. The peritoneum extends from the posterior surface of the anterior abdominal wall to the superior surface of the vesica urinaria and is reflected onto the organ posterior to the vesica, forming a peritoneal pouch. In the female, it forms the excavatio vesicouterina; in the male, it forms the excavatio rectovesicalis. Most of the vesica urinaria is loosely embedded in pelvic connective tissue.

Note: When the vesica urinaria is distended and thus enlarged, the upper part of the vesica, which is covered by peritoneum urogenitale, is pushed so far cranially that the anterior wall of the vesica, which is embedded in the surrounding connective tissue and not covered with peritoneum, appears superior to the upper margin of the symphysis pubica (like a "sun rising on the horizon"). This provides an access route for percutaneous puncture of the distended vesica urinaria above the symphysis without having to enter the cavitas peritonealis with the needle.

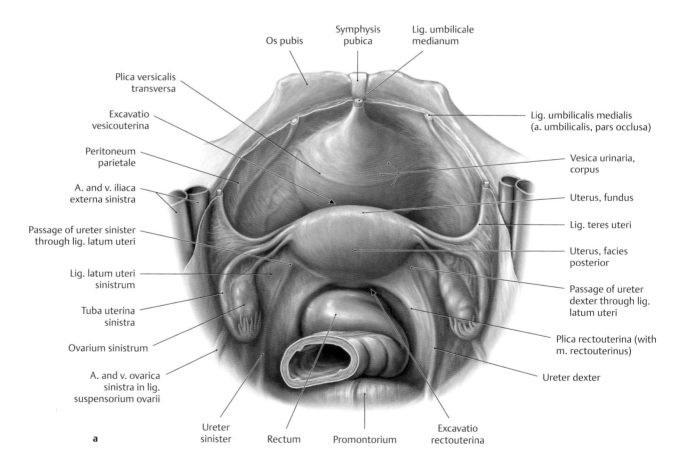

a

B Location of the vesica urinaria in the pelvis and on the diaphragma pelvis

Superior view. The uterus is shown upright for clarity. Most of the intestinum crassum has been removed, leaving the peritoneum urogenitale intact. The plica vesicalis transversa, a peritoneal fold on the surface of the vesica urinaria, is effaced when the vesica is full (as shown here).

In the female, the vesica urinaria lies inferior to the uterus and elevates it when distended. When the structures of the diaphragma pelvis (m. levator ani and its fasciae) are weakened due to injuries sustained in a vaginal delivery, for example, they may allow the vesica urinaria to descend, resulting in incontinence.

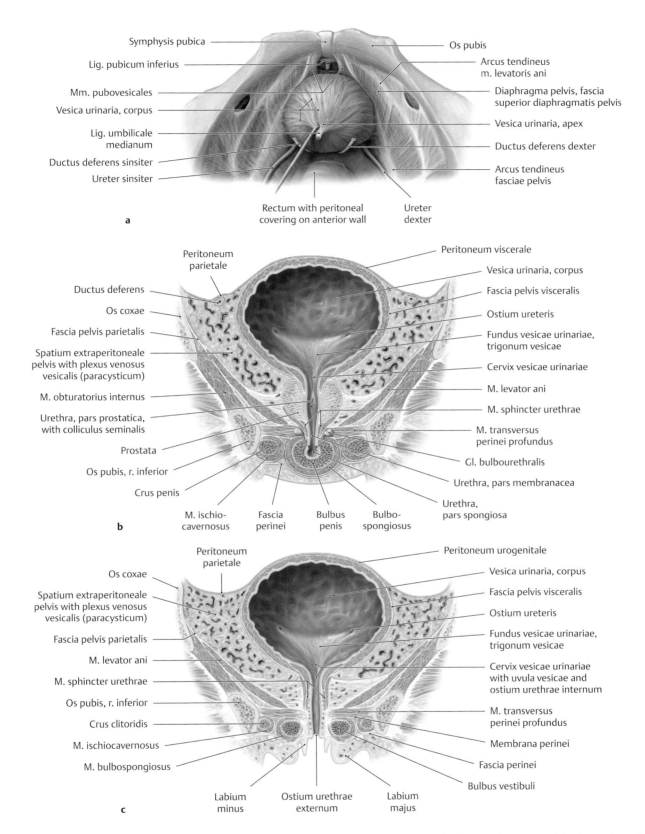

a

Symphysis pubica
Lig. pubicum inferius
Mm. pubovesicales
Vesica urinaria, corpus
Lig. umbilicale medianum
Ductus deferens sinsiter
Ureter sinsiter

Os pubis
Arcus tendineus m. levatoris ani
Diaphragma pelvis, fascia superior diaphragmatis pelvis
Vesica urinaria, apex
Ductus deferens dexter
Arcus tendineus fasciae pelvis

Rectum with peritoneal covering on anterior wall
Ureter dexter

b

Peritoneum parietale
Ductus deferens
Os coxae
Fascia pelvis parietalis
Spatium extraperitoneale pelvis with plexus venosus vesicalis (paracysticum)
M. obturatorius internus
Urethra, pars prostatica, with colliculus seminalis
Prostata
Os pubis, r. inferior
Crus penis

Peritoneum viscerale
Vesica urinaria, corpus
Fascia pelvis visceralis
Ostium ureteris
Fundus vesicae urinariae, trigonum vesicae
Cervix vesicae urinariae
M. levator ani
M. sphincter urethrae
M. transversus perinei profundus
Gl. bulbourethralis
Urethra, pars membranacea
Urethra, pars spongiosa

M. ischio-cavernosus
Fascia perinei
Bulbus penis
Bulbo-spongiosus

c

Peritoneum parietale
Os coxae
Spatium extraperitoneale pelvis with plexus venosus vesicalis (paracysticum)
Fascia pelvis parietalis
M. levator ani
M. sphincter urethrae
Os pubis, r. inferior
Crus clitoridis
M. ischiocavernosus
M. bulbospongiosus

Peritoneum urogenitale
Vesica urinaria, corpus
Fascia pelvis visceralis
Ostium ureteris
Fundus vesicae urinariae, trigonum vesicae
Cervix vesicae urinariae with uvula vesicae and ostium urethrae internum
M. transversus perinei profundus
Membrana perinei
Fascia perinei
Bulbus vestibuli

Labium minus
Ostium urethrae externum
Labium majus

C Comparison of the location of the vesica urinaria in the male (a and b) and female (c)

a Superior view with the vesica urinaria pulled slightly posteriorly. Unlike in **B**, the peritoneum urogenitale has been removed; the vesica urinaria has an almost spherical shape given that it is well distended. The vesica urinaria is located on the muscular sheet of the diaphragma pelvis (lying principally upon the m. levator ani and its fascia = fascia superior diaphragmatis pelvis). This area of contact is smaller in the male than in the female because the pelvis minor also contains the prostata.

b and c slightly angled coronal section with the vesica urinaria and urethra opened. The portions of the vesica urinaria not covered by peritoneum are integrated into the pelvis by a connective tissue space, which has a well-developed venous plexus. This plexus and the mobile peritoneum viscerale allow for considerable changes in vesica size. Like the vesica urinaria itself, the initial portion of the urethra is surrounded by connective tissue, and in the male also by the prostata, which lies upon the m. transversus perinei profundus and the m. levator ani of the diaphragma pelvis.

303

4.8 Vesica Urinaria, Cervix Vesicae, and Urethra: Wall Structure and Function

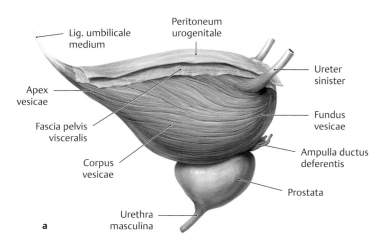

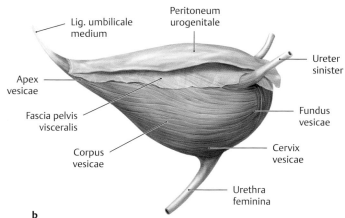

a

b

A External morphology of the vesica urinaria and urethra

Vesica urinaria in a male (**a**) and a female (**b**), viewed from the left side. The vesica urinaria is a hollow muscular organ that collects urine produced by the renes and passes it to the urethra at the right time. The maximum vesica urinaria capacity is between 500 and 700 ml (females > males). The desire to urinate is already experienced when the vesica urinaria contains about 150–200 ml, and even less in pregnant women as the growing uterus ostium urethrae internum pressure on the vesica.

A normal vesica empties fully without retaining residual urine. The vesica urinaria is subdivided into the corpus vesicae, the posterior fundus vesicae, and the anterior apex vesicae, which is continuous with the lig. umbilicale medianum (obliterated urachus) at the inner surface of the anterior trunk wall. The two ureteres, which enter the vesica urinaria dorsolaterally, open into the fundus vesicae. The urethra begins at the ventrocaudal cervix vesicae.

B Muscles of vesica urinaria and urethra

Vesica urinaria in the male, viewed from the left side. The main muscles of the vesica are

- M. detrusor vesicae (bladder emptying) and
- M. sphincter urethrae internalis (bladder closure).

The main muscles of the urethra are

- M. dilator urethrae (urethral dilation) and
- M. sphincter urethrae externus (urethral closure).

According to Dorscher et al (2001), the mm. detrusor vesicae and sphincter urethrae internus are two morphologically separate muscles (see p. 306). The m. detrusor vesicae consists of three layers and is responsible for firmly affixing the vesica urinaria to the pelvis in the anterior-posterior direction. Fibers of its stratum externum longitudinale extend posteriorly to the m. vesicoprostaticus (or m. vesicovaginalis in the female) and in the area of the vesicle node anteriorly to the m. pubovesicalis, which forms an important part of the ventral suspension apparatus (see p. 307). The middle (stratum circulare) and internal (stratum internum longitudinale) layers end posteriorly above the plica intereruterica (see **C**). The m. sphincter urethrae internus is elliptical in shape in the male and circular in the female. Its only function is to close the vesica urinaria. Around its posterior circumference, the internal sphincter forms the morphological basis of the trigonum vesicae (see **C**).

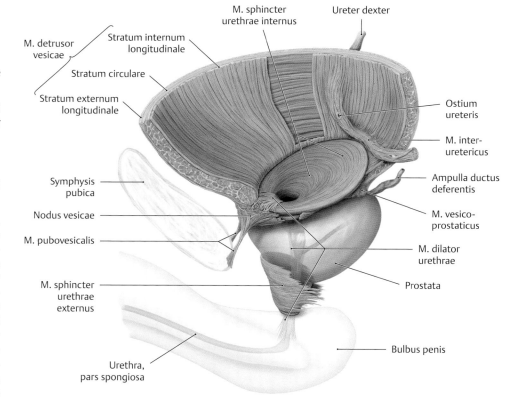

The dilator (see p. 306) is a fan-shaped muscle that arises from the symphysis pubica and the arcus tendineus fasciae pelvis (see p. 307). It extends posteriorly across the ostium urethrae internum and inferiorly at the anterior surface of the urethra, where it inserts on the bulbus penis or the bulbi vestibuli. The m. sphincter urethrae externus consists of an inner layer of smooth muscle fibers and an external layer of striated muscle fibers (for more details see **D**, p. 307).

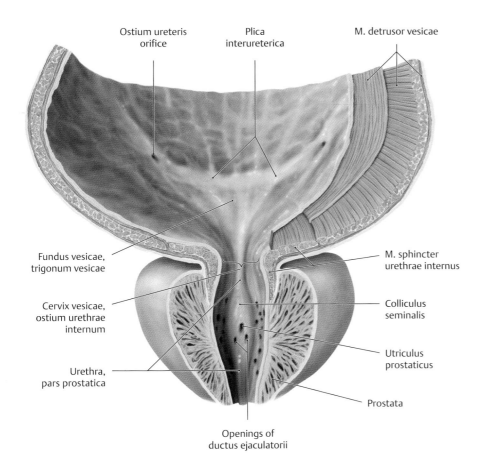

Ostium ureteris orifice

Plica interureterica

M. detrusor vesicae

Fundus vesicae, trigonum vesicae

Cervix vesicae, ostium urethrae internum

Urethra, pars prostatica

M. sphincter urethrae internus

Colliculus seminalis

Utriculus prostaticus

Prostata

Openings of ductus ejaculatorii

C Cervix vesicae, trigonum vesicae, and ostium urethrae internum

Coronal section at the level of the ostium urethrae internum in the male, anterior view.

The interior of the vesica urinaria is lined with a relatively thick tunica mucosa (urothelium and associated underlying connective tissue, see **D**). Except for at the trigonum vesicae, it is easily movable and is thrown into folds when the vesica is not distended. The trigonum vesicae is an area of smooth mucosa at the base of the vesica or at the cervix vesicae between the ostium urethrae internum and the two ureteres, which enter the vesica on its dorsolateral aspect. In the upper border of the trigonum is the plica interureterica, a ridge, produced by the interureteric muscle that extends between the ostia of the two ureteres. Inferiorly, the m. sphincter urethrae internus, shaped like an elliptical cylinder in the male and a circular cylinder in the female, surrounds the ostium urethrae internum.

Note the slit-like ostium ureteris and the oblique transit of the ureter through the vesica wall. This obliquity creates a normal constriction in the pars intramuralis of the ureter (see p. 301). The oblique course, the ureteral muscle, and the bladder-wall muscle provide for functional closure of the ostium ureteris and guard against reflux.

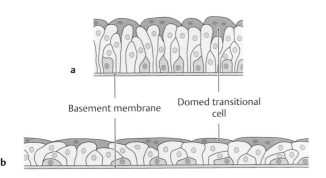

a

Basement membrane

Domed transitional cell

b

D Epithelium of the tunica mucosa

a Vesica urinaria empty: tall epithelium. **b** Vesica urinaria full: flattened epithelium.

Like almost all portions of the urinary tract (except the distal urethra), the vesica urinaria s lined by transitional epithelium (urothelium) whose height and stratification depend on the degree of distention of the urinary tract segment. The transitional epithelium basically consists of multiple cell layers. The conspicuous cells in the surface layer are called "transitional cells" because they change shape.

Note: The total thickness of the vesica wall (tunica muscularis plus tunica mucosa) ranges from 2 to 5 mm in the full vesica and from 8 to 15 mm in the empty vesica.

Emptying and closing the vesica urinaria: Micturition and continence

Micturition is the process of emptying the vesica urinaria. The ability to hold urine with a full vesica is called continence. Coordinated interaction of muscular mechanisms for opening and closing the vesica is crucial for optimal vesica function. Involuntary (autonomic) and voluntary (n. pudendus) control of the muscular apparatus of the vesica urinaria and the urethra play an important role in (cf. p. 316)

- Emptying the vesica urinaria completely during micturition,
- Protecting the ostium ureteris from reflux, and
- Maintaining urinary continence with a full vesica urinaria.

Emptying the vesica urinaria (micturition): activation of the sacral micturition center by a center in the brainstem (pontine micturition center); contraction of the m. detrusor vesicae thereby raising the pressure within the vesica urinaria (supported by an increase in intraabdominal pressure, abdominal press); relaxation of the m. sphincter urethrae internus and contraction of the urethral dilator and m. pubovesicalis, dilating the urethra

(ostium urethrae internum); simultaneous closure of the two ostia ureterum by the ostia ureterum; relaxation of the m. sphincter urethrae externus including both the smooth and striated muscle portions and detumescence of the submucosal venous plexus; voiding of the vesica occurs.

Closing the vesica urinaria (continence): structures responsible for maintaining continence primarily include the muscular mechanisms for closing the bladder and urethra (mm. sphincteres urethrae internus and externus), the ventral suspension apparatus (see p. 307) and parts of the diaphragma pelvis and corpus perineale. Optimal interaction of these distinct structures ensures continence.

Note: At rest, the urethra forms an angle between its posterior margin and the fundus vesicae of 110–120 degrees (posterior vesicourethral angle) in both the male and female. An increased angle due to diaphragma pelvis descent results in incontinence.

4.9 Functional Anatomy of Urinary Continence

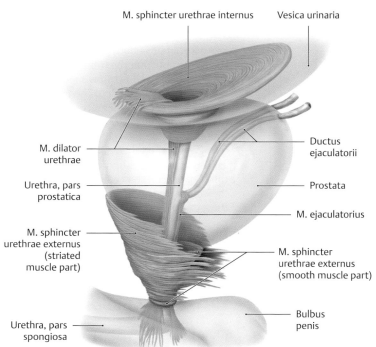

M. sphincter urethrae internus — Vesica urinaria

M. dilator urethrae

Urethra, pars prostatica

M. sphincter urethrae externus (striated muscle part)

Urethra, pars spongiosa

Ductus ejaculatorii

Prostata

M. ejaculatorius

M. sphincter urethrae externus (smooth muscle part)

Bulbus penis

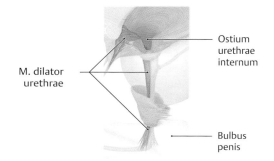

M. dilator urethrae

Ostium urethrae internum

Bulbus penis

A Muscles of the cervix vesicae and proximal urethra in the male

According to Dorschner et al (2001) and Schwalenberg et al (2010), maintaining continence occurs by the interaction of distinct functional units including the anatomically correct positions of the sphincter muscles, tone of the urethral smooth and striated musculature, and a ventral suspensory mechanism at the level of the cervix vesicae. Dysfunction of one of these components may cause urethral hypermobility and result in incontinence. Two muscular systems are differentiated:

- **A system of sphincter muscles:**
  - m. sphincter urethrae internus,
  - m. sphincter urethrae externus with smooth and striated muscle portions,
  - stratum longitudinale tunicae muscularis urethrae with smooth ventral urethral musculature and dorsal longitudinal ejaculatory musculature;
- **A musculofibrous anchoring system in the diaphragma pelvis:**
  - ventral vesicourethral suspension apparatus made up of m. pubovesicalis, lig. pubourethrale and ligg. puboprostatica and the arcus tendineus fasciae pelvis from which the cervix vesicae is suspended;
  - cervix vesicae (corpus perineale) which counters and anchors the m. sphincter urethrae externus.

Note: Except for the dorsal longitudinal ejaculatory muscle, all structures are found in both males and females.

B M. dilator urethrae

This is the ventral stratum longitudinale tunicae muscularis urethrae. It is a fan-shaped muscle that arises from the symphysis pubica and along the arcus tendineus fasciae pelvis (see **E**). It runs over the top of the ventral circumference of the m. sphincter urethrae internus and through the ostium urethrae internum. It extends inferiorly along the anterior surface of the urethra, where it inserts on the bulbus penis. The urethra is shortened and the ostium urethrae internum is widened by the contraction of the longitudinal musculature. This allows initiation of micturition.

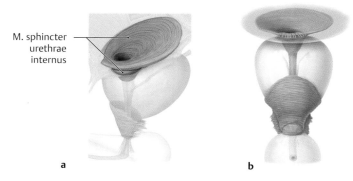

M. sphincter urethrae internus

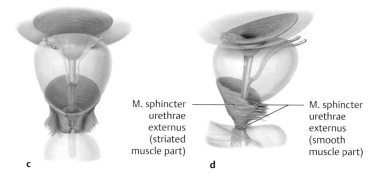

M. sphincter urethrae externus (striated muscle part)

M. sphincter urethrae externus (smooth muscle part)

a   b   c   d

C Mm. sphincteres urethrae internus and externus

a M. sphincter urethrae internus; **b–d** M. sphincter urethrae externus, anterior, posterior, and lateral views.

According to Dorschner et al. (2001), the m. sphincter urethrae internus is a distinct, independent functional sphincter. Its smooth musculature is not related to the m. detrusor vesicae or urethral musculature. Thus, it does not arise from the trigonum vesicaee or m. detrusor vesicae musculature. Generally, the m. sphincter urethrae internus is more distinct in the male than the female, in particular the urethral portion, which extends to the proximal urethra. One reason may be that in the male the m. sphincter urethrae internus ensures not only continence

but also the effective closure of the cervix vesicae to prevent retrograde ejaculation (dual function). According to Dorschner et al (see above), the m. sphincter urethrae externus consists of

- an inner circular layer of smooth muscle, and
- an outer striated layer, which has an omega or horseshoe shape and a depression in its posterior surface.

Note: Numerous studies have shown that the striated m. sphincter urethrae externus (like the m. sphincter urethrae internus) is an independent muscle and is not split off from the m. levator ani or the mm. transversi perinei profundi.

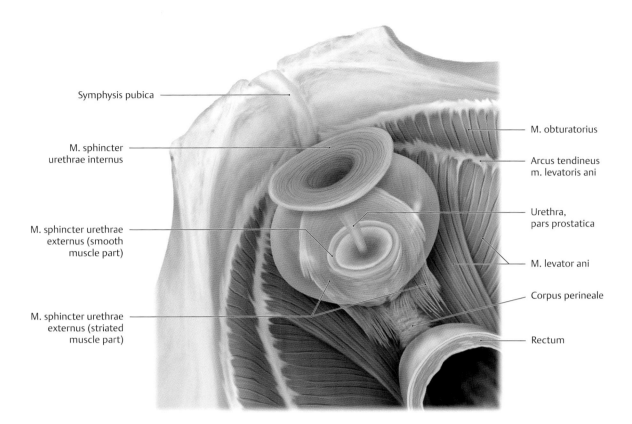

Symphysis pubica

M. sphincter urethrae internus

M. sphincter urethrae externus (smooth muscle part)

M. sphincter urethrae externus (striated muscle part)

M. obturatorius

Arcus tendineus m. levatoris ani

Urethra, pars prostatica

M. levator ani

Corpus perineale

Rectum

D Integration of the m. sphincter urethrae externus into its surroundings

Anteriorly and laterally, the outer portion of the m. sphincter urethrae externus borders the distinct venous plexus (see **E**) and is partially interspersed with veins. According to Wallner et al (2009) and Schwalenberg et al (2010) the lateral fibers of the m. sphincter urethrae externus extends into the fascia of the m. levator ani. Additionally, it has been discussed whether its muscle fibers are anchored to the corpus perineale.

As a result, when the m. sphincter urethrae externus contracts, its fibers stretch to both sides of the m. levator ani, where it is dynamically anchored. Whereas the circular muscle fibers of the smooth m. sphincter urethrae internus exert light but permanent pressure on the membranous urethra, the striated m. sphincter urethrae externus, which receives somatic innervation, together with the corpus perineale and the m. levator ani are able to increase the urethral closure pressure (= improved continence) during diaphragma pelvis contraction.

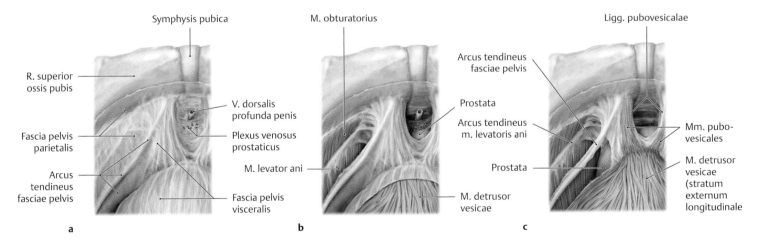

Symphysis pubica

M. obturatorius

Ligg. pubovesicalae

R. superior ossis pubis

V. dorsalis profunda penis

Plexus venosus prostaticus

M. levator ani

Fascia pelvis parietalis

Arcus tendineus fasciae pelvis

Fascia pelvis visceralis

Arcus tendineus fasciae pelvis

Prostata

Arcus tendineus m. levatoris ani

Prostata

M. detrusor vesicae

Mm. pubovesicales

M. detrusor vesicae (stratum externum longitudinale)

a   b   c

E Ventral vesicourethral suspension apparatus

Aside from the anterolateral stabilization of the vesicourethral junction, the most important function of the ventral suspension apparatus in the spatium retropubicum is suspension of the cervix vesicae, which ensures continence (Schwalenberg et al. 2010). Essential components of the ventral suspension apparatus include the mm. pubovesicales and the arcus tendineus fasciae pelvis, which is a thickened band of the fascia pelvis that extends from the symphysis pubica over the diaphragma pelvis to the spina ischiadica. There the visceral and the parietal layers (fascia superior diaphragmatis pelvis) merge. The arcus tendineus fasciae pelvis, partially due to its anterior extensions, serves

as an additional aponeurotic insertion of the mm. pubovesicales that extend as the continuation of the ventral stratum externum longitudinale of the m. detrusor vesicae on both sides of the symphysis pubica to the os pubis. The lig. pubourethrale and lig. puboprostaticum listed in the Nomina Anatomica are not ligaments in the proper sense. They are strong sheets of connective tissue of the fasciae pelvis visceralis and parietalis and extend from the symphysis pubica to the cervix vesicae or prostata.

Note: Protection and restoration of the structures of the ventral suspension apparatus as described above have led to a significant decrease in postoperative incontinence after surgery to remove the prostata.

4.10 Urethra

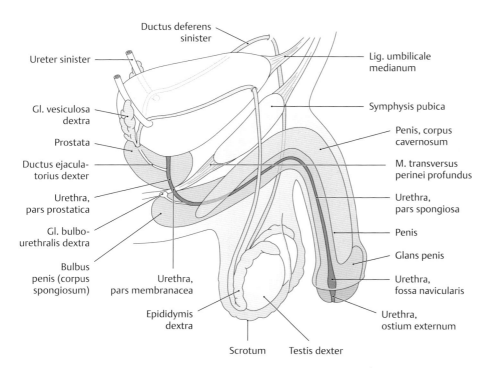

B Wall segments, constrictions, and expansions of the urethra masculina (see also **D**)

Wall segments	Constrictions and expansions
Ostium urethrae internum	
Pars intramuralis	First constriction: m. sphincter urethrae internus
Pars prostatica	First expansion
Pars membranacea	Second constriction: m. sphincter urethrae externus
Pars spongiosa	Second expansion: ampulla Third expansion: fossa navicularis urethrae
Ostium urethrae externum	Third constriction

A Parts of the urethra masculina

Male urogenital system in the pelvis, viewed from the right side. Unlike the urethra feminina, the urethra masculina functions as a common urinary *and* genital passage. It has an average length of 20 cm and consists of four parts with three constrictions and three expansions (see **B**). The pars intramuralis of the urethra in the vesica wall is not shown here. While the urethra feminina is essentially straight (see **E**), the urethra masculina presents two curves: an *infrapubic curve* and a *prepubic curve*. These curves are important in transurethral bladder catheterization (see **F**).

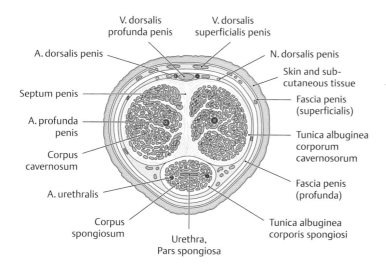

C Location of the urethra masculina in the penis

Transverse section through the penile shaft. The pars spongiosa of the urethra is contained in the corpus spongiosum of the penis. The corpus spongiosum does not become completely hard even at maximum erection, ensuring that the urethra remains patent during ejaculation. The urethral lumen often presents a flattened rather than circular shape in cross-section, with the upper and lower walls touching.

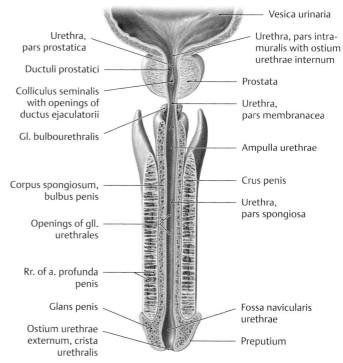

D Urethra masculina in longitudinal section

The whole length of the urethra has been cut open and displayed without curves, and all of the diaphragma pelvis muscles have been removed. The four parts of the urethra masculina can be identified. The urethra masculina extends distally in the corpus spongiosum to its ostium urethrae externa on the glans penis. The pars *prostatica* of the urethra may be greatly narrowed in patients with benign prostatic enlargement (*prostatic hyperplasia*, see p. 338). This condition is often marked by incomplete voiding and the dribbling of urine after micturition. The residual urine left in the vesica urinaria may incite an (often bacterial in nature) inflammation of the vesica (cystitis).

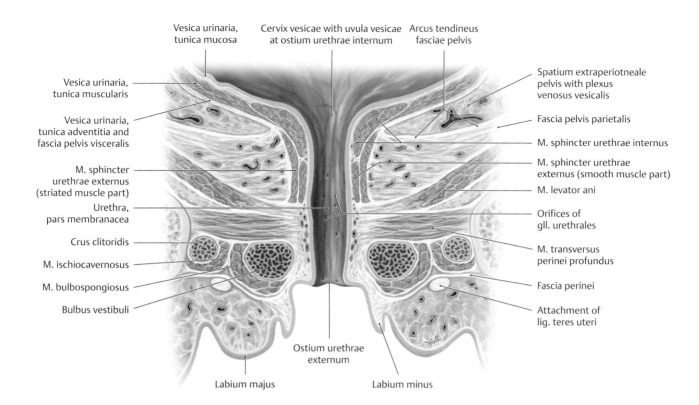

Vesica urinaria, tunica mucosa

Cervix vesicae with uvula vesicae at ostium urethrae internum

Arcus tendineus fasciae pelvis

Vesica urinaria, tunica muscularis

Vesica urinaria, tunica adventitia and fascia pelvis visceralis

M. sphincter urethrae externus (striated muscle part)

Urethra, pars membranacea

Crus clitoridis

M. ischiocavernosus

M. bulbospongiosus

Bulbus vestibuli

Spatium extraperiotneale pelvis with plexus venosus vesicalis

Fascia pelvis parietalis

M. sphincter urethrae internus

M. sphincter urethrae externus (smooth muscle part)

M. levator ani

Orifices of gll. urethrales

M. transversus perinei profundus

Fascia perinei

Attachment of lig. teres uteri

Ostium urethrae externum

Labium majus

Labium minus

E Urethra feminina in longitudinal section

Coronal section tilted slightly posterior, anterior view. Unlike the urethra masculina, the urethra feminina is straight and only about 3–5 cm long. Thus it is much easier to catheterize than in the masculina. At the same time, the short length of the urethra feminina increases susceptibility to urinary tract infections.

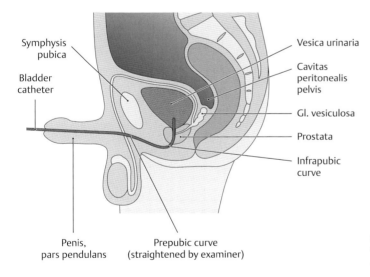

Symphysis pubica

Bladder catheter

Penis, pars pendulans

Prepubic curve (straightened by examiner)

Vesica urinaria

Cavitas peritonealis pelvis

Gl. vesiculosa

Prostata

Infrapubic curve

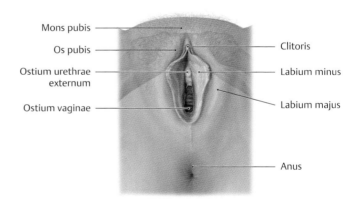

Mons pubis

Os pubis

Ostium urethrae externum

Ostium vaginae

Clitoris

Labium minus

Labium majus

Anus

G Ostium externum of the urethra feminina

Viewed from below. The os pubis is shown in shadow to aid orientation. The ostium urethrae externum is located between the labia minora, anterior to the vagina. Despite its proximity to the female external genitalia, the urethra feminina functions exclusively as a urinary passage. The close topographical relationship of the urethra and external genitalia is important during embryonic development, however: both the urethra and the vagina initially have a common opening at the sinus urogenitalis and become separated only after further development. Failure of this separation results in an abnormal fistulous connection between the vagina and surethra, a *urethrovaginal fistula*. Even with normal embryonic development, the proximity of the urethra (which is physiologically germ-free) to the vagina (which is not a sterile zone) predisposes to bacterial inflammation of the urethra (urethritis). Given the short length of the urethra feminina, the infection can easily ascend to the vesica urinaria (cystitis).

F Transurethral bladder catheterization in the male

The two curves of the urethra masculina (infrapubic and prepubic) and its three constrictions may pose an obstacle to transurethral catheterization. The prepubic curve can be straightened out somewhat by straightening the penile shaft.

4.11 Arteries and Veins of the Renes and Glandulae Suprarenales: Overview

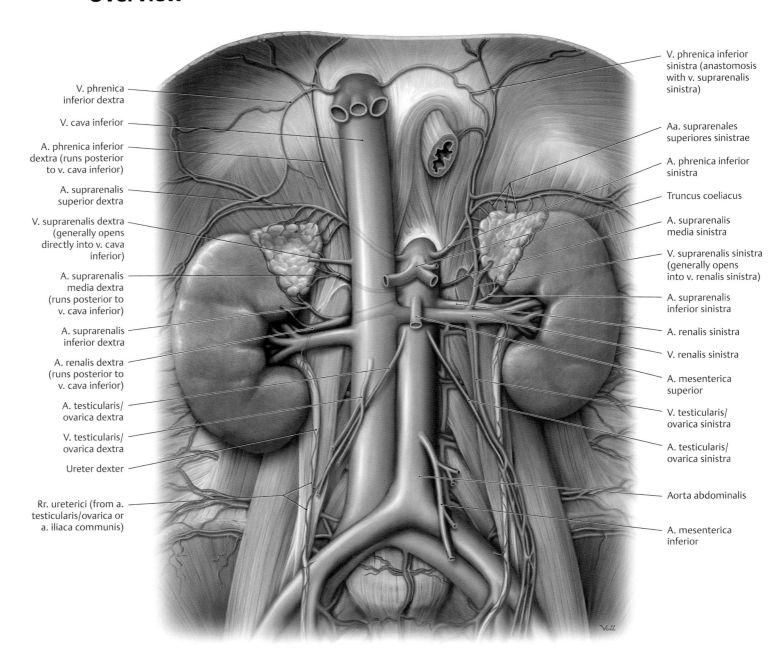

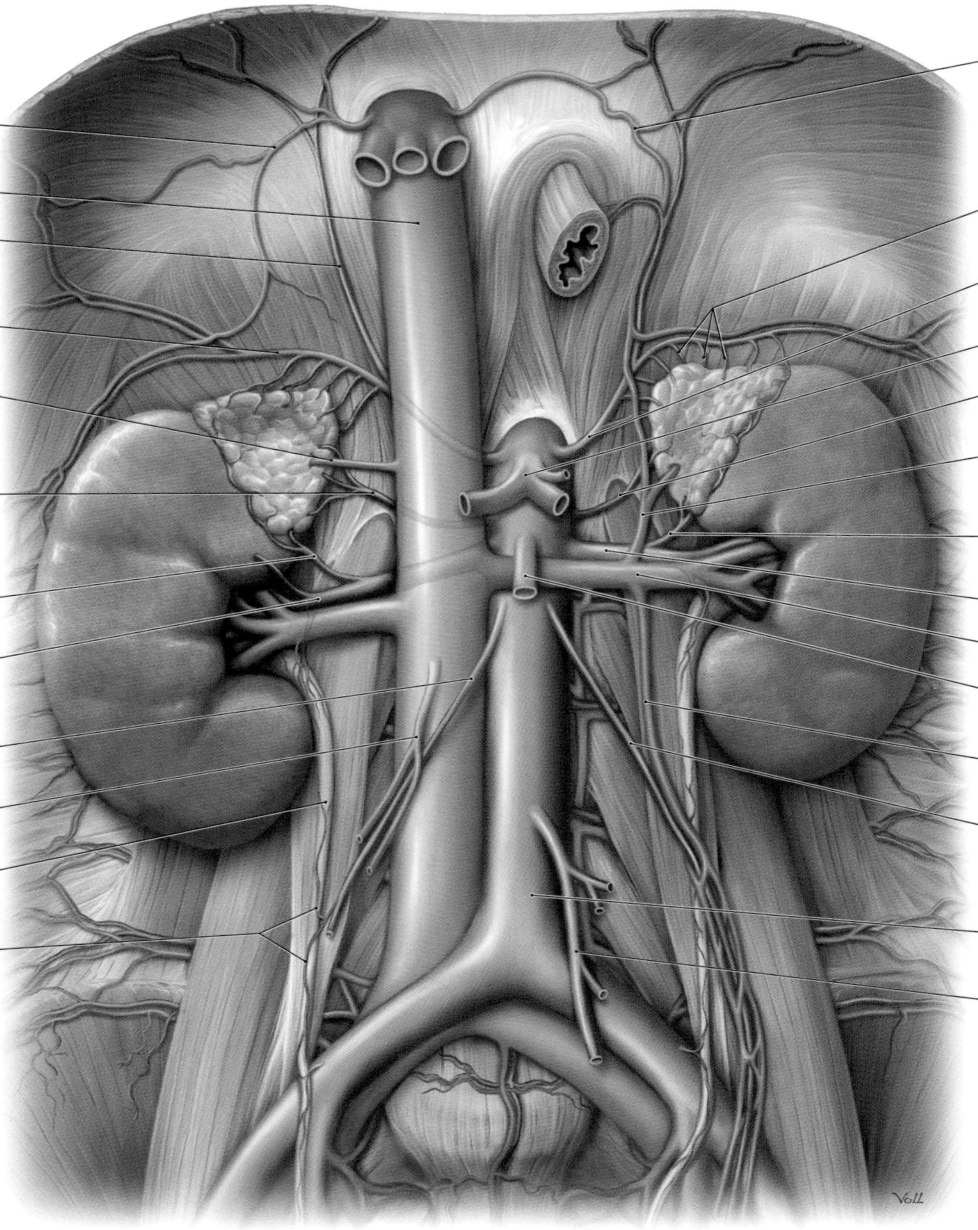
V. phrenica inferior dextra
V. cava inferior
A. phrenica inferior dextra (runs posterior to v. cava inferior)
A. suprarenalis superior dextra
V. suprarenalis dextra (generally opens directly into v. cava inferior)
A. suprarenalis media dextra (runs posterior to v. cava inferior)
A. suprarenalis inferior dextra
A. renalis dextra (runs posterior to v. cava inferior)
A. testicularis/ ovarica dextra
V. testicularis/ ovarica dextra
Ureter dexter
Rr. ureterici (from a. testicularis/ovarica or a. iliaca communis)
V. phrenica inferior sinistra (anastomosis with v. suprarenalis sinistra)
Aa. suprarenales superiores sinistrae
A. phrenica inferior sinistra
Truncus coeliacus
A. suprarenalis media sinistra
V. suprarenalis sinistra (generally opens into v. renalis sinistra)
A. suprarenalis inferior sinistra
A. renalis sinistra
V. renalis sinistra
A. mesenterica superior
V. testicularis/ ovarica sinistra
A. testicularis/ ovarica sinistra
Aorta abdominalis
A. mesenterica inferior
Voll

A Overview of the arteries and veins of the renes and glandulae suprarenales

Anterior view. The oesophagus has been pulled slightly inferiorly, and the right ren and gl. suprarenalis have been pulled away from the v. cava inferior to show the vascular anatomy of the gl. suprarenalis. The other abdominal organs have been removed.

Arteria renalis: The aa. renales branch from the sides of the aorta abdominalis at the level of the L 1/L 2 vertebrae (see **C**). The *right* a. renalis runs *posterior* to the v. cava inferior (shown transparent in the drawing), and the *left* a. renalis runs *posterior* to the left v. renalis. Each a. renalis divides into a r. anterior and r. posterior. The aa. renales give off aa. suprarenales inferiores to the gl. suprarenalis, rr. capsulares to tissue surrounding the ren and to the renal capsule (capsula fibrosa and perirenal capsula adiposa, removed here for clarity), and rr. ureterici to the upper portion of the ureter and the distal pelvis renalis. Possible variants are illustrated in **E**, p. 313.

Arteriae suprarenales: Aa. suprarenales superiores, mediae, and inferiores (from the a. phrenica inferior, aorta abdominalis, and a. renalis, see above).

Vena renalis: The v. renalis on each side is generally formed by the union of two or three venous branches (variants are shown in **F**, p. 313). While the left v. renalis receives the v. suprarenalis sinistra and v. testicularis or ovarica sinistra, the right v. renalis opens directly into the v. cava inferior without receiving these tributaries (see also **D**). The v. renalis also receives vv. capsulares from the capsula fibrosa in addition to small branches from the pelvis renalis and proximal ureter (not shown here).

Venae suprarenales:

Note: The three main arteries of the gll. suprarenales (see above) are generally accompanied *by only one vein* (rarely two), the *v. suprarenalis*. While the v. suprarenalis *sinistra* opens into the left v. renalis, frequently anastomosing with the left v. phrenica inferior (as shown here), the v. suprarenalis *dextra* empties directly into the v. cava inferior (see also **D**).

* The blood vessels supplying the vesica urinaria are discussed together with the neurovascular structures of the internal genital organs that are also located in the pelvis (see p. 346).

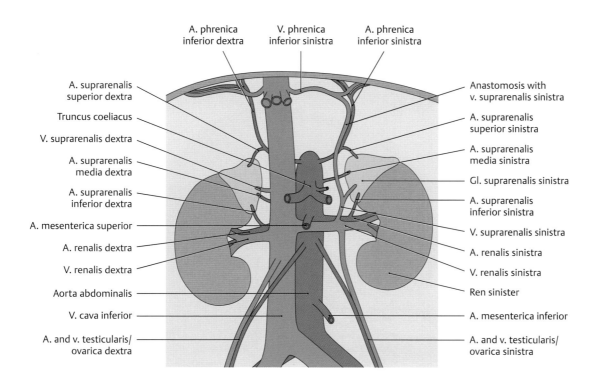

B Arteries and veins of the renes and glandulae suprarenales
Anterior view. The right ren and gl. suprarenalis have been slightly retracted from the v. cava inferior to display their blood vessels more clearly. It is evident in this diagram and in **A** that the gll. suprarenales have a more complex vascular anatomy than the renes: More than 50 small branches may pass from the arterial trunks of the gll. suprarenales (aa. suprarenales superiores, mediae, and inferiores) into the glands.

Note that the three main arteries of the gll. suprarenales are generally accompanied by only one vein, the v. suprarenalis. This vessel opens *directly* into the v. cava inferior on the *right* side and into the renal vein on the *left* side (see **D**).

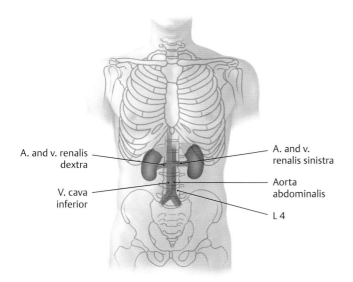

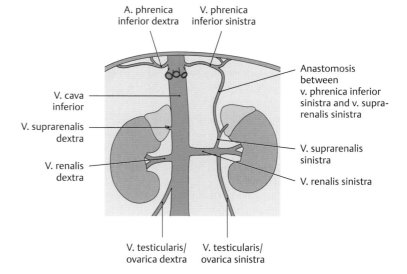

C Projection of the arteriae and venae renales onto the columna vertebralis
The a. renalis arises from the aorta abdominalis at the L 1/L 2 level.
Note: The vv. renales lie anterior to the arteries.

D Tributaries of the left vena renalis
The v. renalis has more tributaries on the left side than on the right. The v. renalis *sinistra* receives the v. suprarenalis sinistra (often anastomosing with the left v. phrenica inferior, see **A**) and the v. testicularis/ovarica sinistra, whereas the corresponding veins on the *right* side open *directly* into the v. cava inferior. Because of this arrangement, varicose dilations of the veins in the funiculus spermaticus (varicoceles) are more common on the left side than on the right.

311

4.12 Arteries and Veins of the Renes and Glandulae Suprarenales: Variants

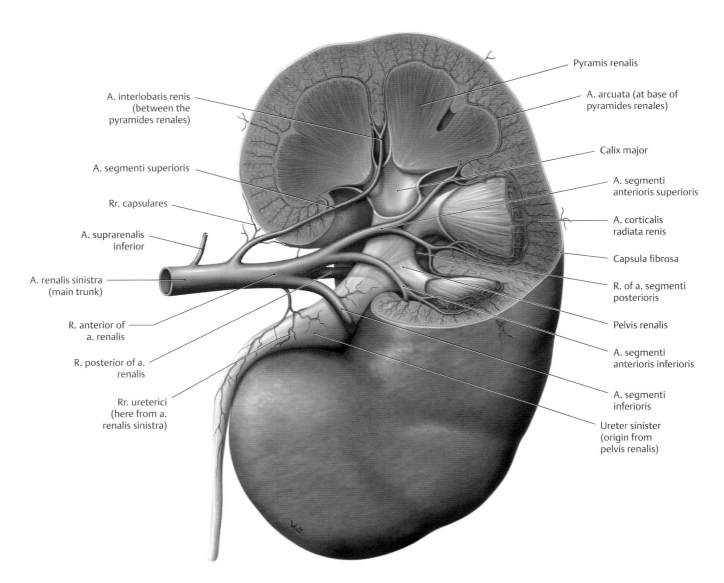

A. interlobaris renis (between the pyramides renales)

A. segmenti superioris

Rr. capsulares

A. suprarenalis inferior

A. renalis sinistra (main trunk)

R. anterior of a. renalis

R. posterior of a. renalis

Rr. ureterici (here from a. renalis sinistra)

Pyramis renalis

A. arcuata (at base of pyramides renales)

Calix major

A. segmenti anterioris superioris

A. corticalis radiata renis

Capsula fibrosa

R. of a. segmenti posterioris

Pelvis renalis

A. segmenti anterioris inferioris

A. segmenti inferioris

Ureter sinister (origin from pelvis renalis)

A Division of the arteria renalis into segmental arteries
Anterior view of the left ren.
The main trunk of the a. renalis divides into a r. anterior and r. posterior.
The r. anterior divides further into four segmental arteries:

- A. segmenti superioris
- A. segmenti anterioris superioris
- A. segmenti anterioris inferioris
- A. segmenti inferioris

The r. posterior gives rise to only one segmental vessel, the a. segmenti posterioris.

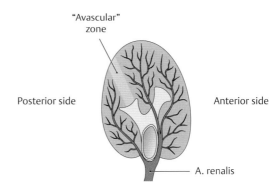

"Avascular" zone

Posterior side

Anterior side

A. renalis

B "Avascular" zone in the ren
Inferior view of the right ren.
Between the segmentum posterius and segmenta anteriora is a relatively avascular zone of the kidney, which otherwise is *very heavily vascularized*. This zone provides an important line of access for intrarenal surgery.

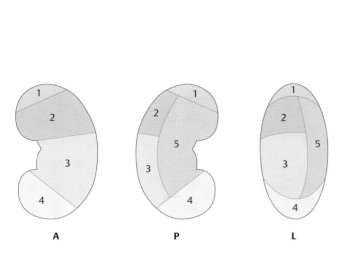

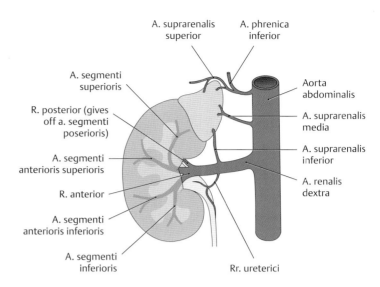

C Vascular segmentation of the ren

Left ren viewed from the anterior (A), posterior (P), and lateral (L) sides. The a. renalis and its branches divide the kidney into five segments:

1 Segmentum superius
2 Segmentum anterius superius
3 Segmentum anterius inferius
4 Segmentum inferius
5 Segmentum posterius

D Relationship of the renal arterial branches to the segmenta renalis

Anterior view of the right ren, demonstrating the origins of the a. renalis, a. suprarenalis media, and a. phrenica inferior from the aorta abdominalis.

Note the division of the a. renalis into a r. anterior (segmenta anteriora, segmenta superiora and inferiora) and a r. posterior (for the segmentum posterius, see also **A**). The upper part of the ureter is supplied by rr. ureterici from the a. renalis.

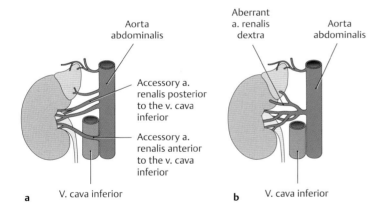

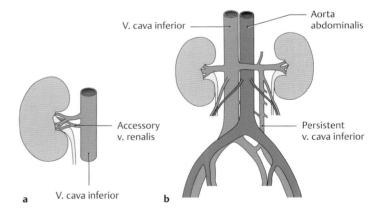

E Variants of the aa. renales

Anterior view of the right ren.

a Two accessory aa. renales (one crossing in front of the v. cava inferior): Accessory aa. renales are extra arteries that pass from the aorta abdominalis to the hilum renale. As a common variant with accessory aa. renales, the a. suprarenalis inferior does not arise from the a. renalis.

b An *aberrant* a. renalis is one that does not enter the ren at the hilum renale.

F Variants of the vv. renales

Anterior view.

a Accessory (supernumerary) vv. renales
b A left v. cava (persistent lower part of the vv. supracardinales) ascends to the level of the left v. renalis and opens into it.

4.13 Lymphatic Drainage of the Renes, Glandulae Suprarenales, Ureter, and Vesica Urinaria

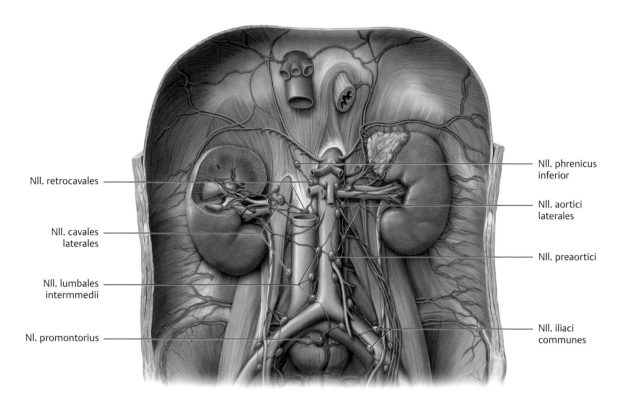

NII. retrocavales

NII. cavales laterales

NII. lumbales intermmedii

NI. promontorius

NII. phrenicus inferior

NII. aortici laterales

NII. preaortici

NII. iliaci communes

A Lymphatic drainage of the ren, glandula suprarenalis, and ureter
(pars abdominalis; the pars pelvica is shown in **C**)
Anterior view. The following lymphatic pathways are important in this region (see also p. 221):

- **Right ren and glandula suprarenalis:** drain to the *nll. lumbales dextri* (nll. cavales laterales, precavales, and retrocavales, see **B**), then to the *right truncus lumbalis*.

- **Left ren and glandula suprarenalis:** drain to the *nll. lumbales sinistri* (nll. aortici laterales, preaortici, and retroaortici, see **B**), then to the *left truncus lumbalis*.
- **Ureter (pars abdominalis):** follows the pathway for the right and left renes and gll. suprarenales (see also **C**).

The nll. lumbales additionally function as collecting lymph nodes for the nll. iliaci communes.

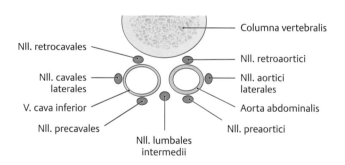

NII. retrocavales

NII. cavales laterales

V. cava inferior

NII. precavales

NII. lumbales intermedii

Columna vertebralis

NII. retroaortici

NII. aortici laterales

Aorta abdominalis

NII. preaortici

B Classification of the nodi lymphoidei lumbales
Transverse section, viewed from above. The nll. lumbales are distributed around the aorta abdominalis and v. cava inferior. They are divided into three groups based on their relationship to these vessels:

- Nll. lumbales sinistri (around the aorta)
- Nll. lumbales intermedii (between the aorta and v. cava inferior)
- Nll. lumbales dextri (around the v. cava inferior)

These groups are further divided into subgroups (see legend of **A**).

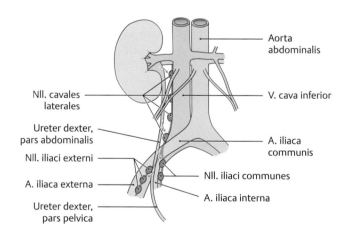

Aorta abdominalis

NII. cavales laterales

Ureter dexter, pars abdominalis

NII. iliaci externi

A. iliaca externa

Ureter dexter, pars pelvica

V. cava inferior

A. iliaca communis

NII. iliaci communes

A. iliaca interna

C Nodi lymphoidei of the ureter
Anterior view of the right ureter.
The lymphatic drainage of the ureter is roughly divided into two levels:

- Pars abdominalis of the ureter: nll. lumbales
  - Right: nll. cavales laterales (nll. lumbales dextri)
  - Left: nll. aortici laterales (nll. lumbales sinistri)
- Pars pelvica of the ureter: nll. iliaci externi and interni.

Both pathways empty into the trunci lumbales.

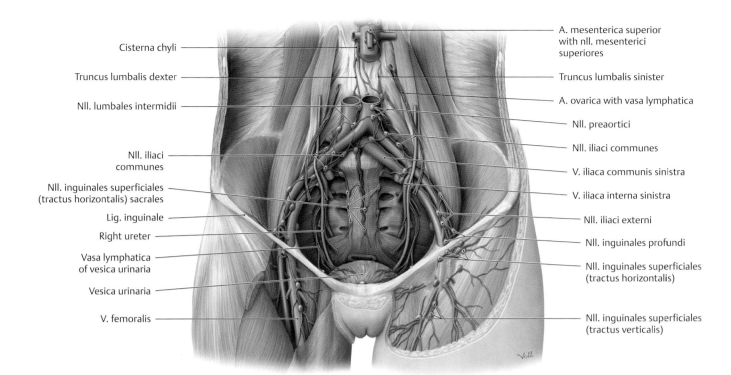

Cisterna chyli

Truncus lumbalis dexter

Nll. lumbales intermidii

Nll. iliaci communes

Nll. inguinales superficiales (tractus horizontalis) sacrales

Lig. inguinale

Right ureter

Vasa lymphatica of vesica urinaria

Vesica urinaria

V. femoralis

A. mesenterica superior with nll. mesenterici superiores

Truncus lumbalis sinister

A. ovarica with vasa lymphatica

Nll. preaortici

Nll. iliaci communes

V. iliaca communis sinistra

V. iliaca interna sinistra

Nll. iliaci externi

Nll. inguinales profundi

Nll. inguinales superficiales (tractus horizontalis)

Nll. inguinales superficiales (tractus verticalis)

D Overview of the nodi lymphoidei pelvis and the lymphatic drainage of the vesica urinaria

Anterior view of an opened female abdomen and pelvis. All organs have been removed except for the vesica urinaria and a small rectal stump, and the peritoneum has been removed. The vesica is distended, making it visible above the symphysis pubica. This drawing clearly shows the numerous nll. parietales that are distributed around the iliac vessels in the pelvis (see **E**). Lymph from the vesica urinaria usually drains first to groups of nodi lymphoidei viscerales: the nll. vesicales laterales and the nll. pre- and retrovesicales (known collectively as the nodi paravesicales). These nodes are embedded in the pelvic connective tissue surrounding the vesica urinaria and lie so deep within the pelvis that they are not visible here. Lymph from these nll. viscerales drains directly or indirectly along two major pathways, reaching nodi lymphoidei lateral to the aorta abdominalis and v. cava inferior (nodi lumbales) and finally entering the trunci lumbales. These pathways are illustrated in **F**.

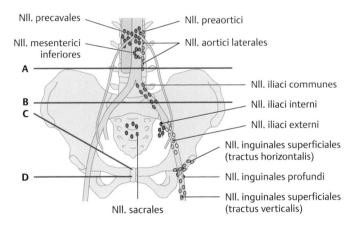

Nll. precavales

Nll. mesenterici inferiores

Nll. preaortici

Nll. aortici laterales

A

Nll. iliaci communes

B

Nll. iliaci interni

C

Nll. iliaci externi

Nll. inguinales superficiales (tractus horizontalis)

D

Nll. inguinales profundi

Nll. sacrales

Nll. inguinales superficiales (tractus verticalis)

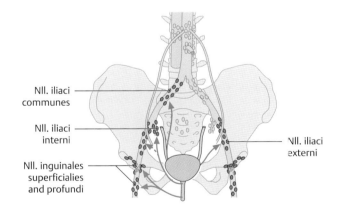

Nll. iliaci communes

Nll. iliaci interni

Nll. inguinales superficialies and profundi

Nll. iliaci externi

E Overview of the nodi lymphoidei pelvis

The nodi lymphoidei pelvis are distributed along major blood vessels and in front of the sacrum. The blood vessels are not visualized by lymphography (contrast radiography of the nodi lymphoidei), however, and so the location of the nodi lymphoidei pelvis must be determined by other means. One method is to use four reference lines based on skeletal landmarks:

A Iliolumbar line: horizontal line tangent to the superior borders of the cristae iliacae

B Iliosacral line: horizontal line through the center of the art. sacroiliaca

C Inguinal line: line along the lig. inguinale

D Obturator line: horizontal line through the center of the foramen obturatum

F Lymphatic drainage of the vesica urinaria and urethra

The **vesica urinaria** is drained by two principal pathways:

- Cranially along the visceral iliac vessels (see **D**)
- To the nll. iliaci interni and externi (mainly at the fundus vesicae)

Portions of the vesica urinaria near the ostium urethrae internum are drained by the nll. inguinales superficiales and profundi. The **urethra** drains chiefly to the nll. inguinales profundi and superficiales (the latter mainly draining areas near the ostium urethrae externum). The proximal portions of the urethra are drained by the nll. iliaci, particularly the nll. iliaci interni.

Note: The penis, like the urethra, is drained by the nll. inguinales superficiales and profundi.

4.14 Autonomic Innervation of the Urinary Organs and Glandulae Suprarenales

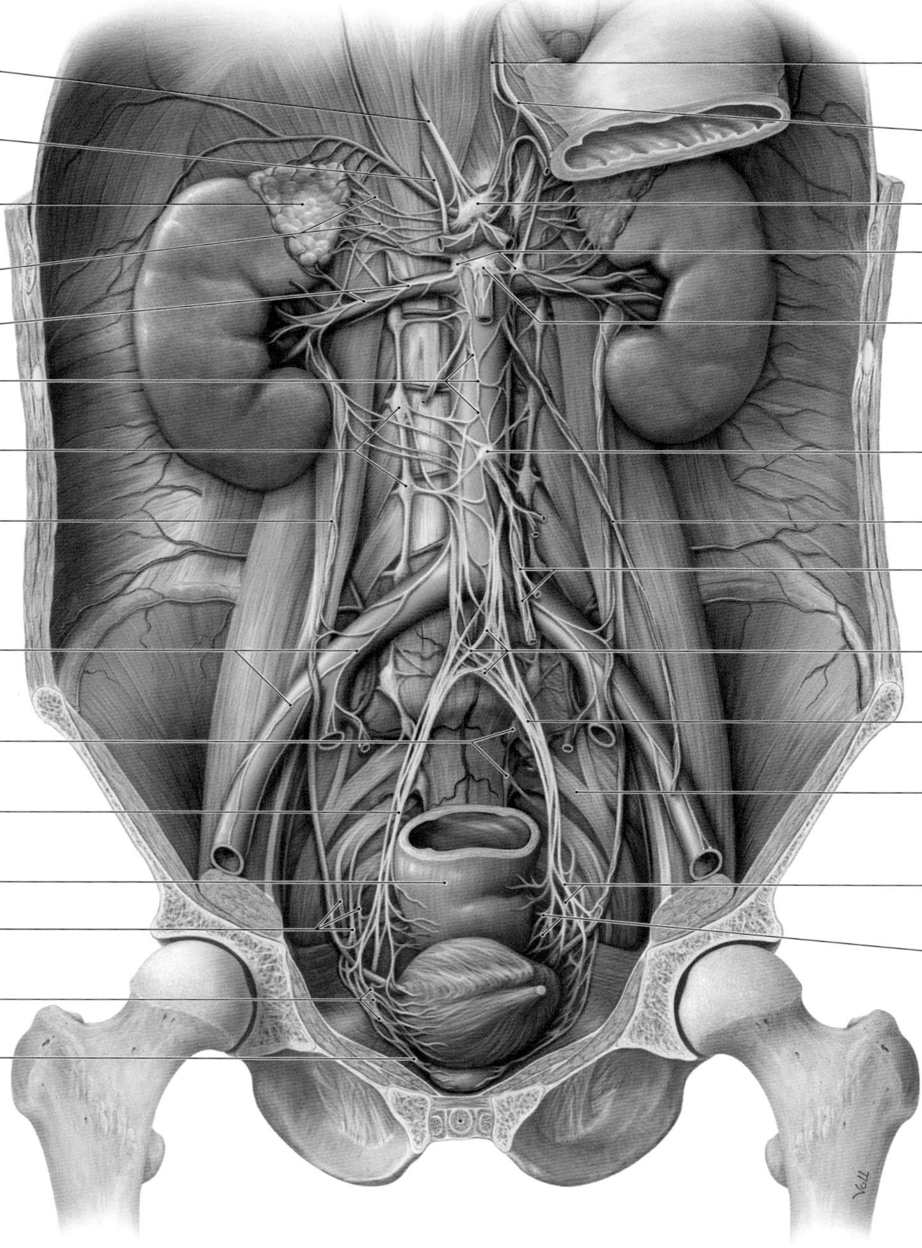
N. splanchnius major dexter
N. splanchnius minor dexter
Gl. suprarenalis dextra
Plexus suprarenalis
Plexus renalis
Plexus inter-mesentericus
Truncus sympathicus, ganglia lumbalia
Plexus uretericus
Plexus iliacus
Truncus sympathicus, ganglia sacralia
N. hypogastricus dexter
Rectum
Nn. splanchnici pelvici
Plexus vesicalis
Plexus prostaticus
Truncus vagalis posterior
Truncus vagalis anterior
Ganglion coeliacum
Ganglia aorticorenalia
Ganglia mesen-tericum superius
Ganglia mesen-tericum inferius
Plexus testicularis
Plexus mesen-tericus inferior
Plexus hypogastricus superior
N. hypogastricus sinister
N. sacralis I, r. anterior
Plexus hypo-gastricus inferior
Plexus rectalis medius (from plexus hypogastricus inferior)

A Overview of the autonomic innervation of the urinary organs and glandulae suprarenales

Anterior view into an opened male abdomen and pelvis. The gaster has been largely removed and pulled slightly inferior with the oesophagus for better exposure. The right ren has been displaced slightly laterally, and the vesica urinaria has been straightened and retracted to the left. The pelvis has been sectioned in a coronal plane passing approximately through the center of the acetabula. The autonomic innervation of the urinary organs and gll. suprarenales varies according to the location of the specific organ:

- The **renes in the retroperitoneum** and portions of the upper urinary tract **(proximal ureteres)** receive *sympathetic* fibers initially from the n. splanchnici minores, imus, and lumbales (see **B**), which synapse with the postsynaptic neuron in the ganglia aorticorenalia or renalia. The *parasympathetic* fibers originate from the truncus vagalis posterior and partly from the nn. splanchnici pelvici (the plexuses are described in **B**).
- The **cortex and medulla glandulae suprarenalis in the retroperitoneum** receive *sympathetic* fibers from the nn. splanchnici major and minor. They receive *parasympathetic* fibers from the truncus vagalis posterior, which pass with the plexus coeliacus to the gll. suprarenales as the plexus suprarenalis. The *sympathetic* autonomic innervation of the suprarenal medulla is exceptional in that the suprarenal medulla is supplied only by presynaptic sympathetic fibers from the plexus suprarenalis. These axons directly innervate the suprarenal medullary cells. At present, there is no convincing evidence that the suprarenal medulla receives *parasympathetic* innervation.
- The **vesica urinaria, most of the partes abdominalis and pelvica of the ureter** (and the **urethra**, not shown here) **in the pelvis** (see **D**) receive *sympathetic* fibers from the nn. splanchnici lumbales and sacrales, and they receive *parasympathetic* fibers from the nn. splanchnici pelvici (S2–S4). The plexuses are shown in **D**.

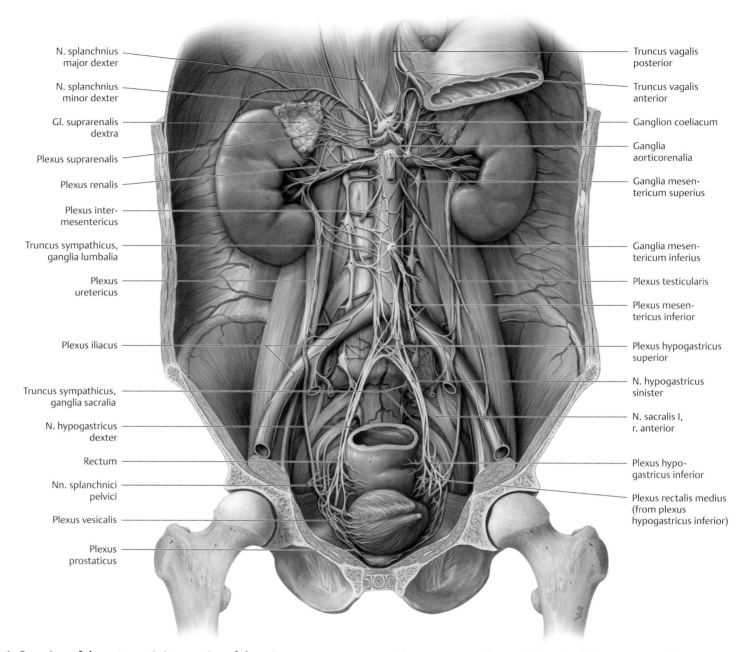

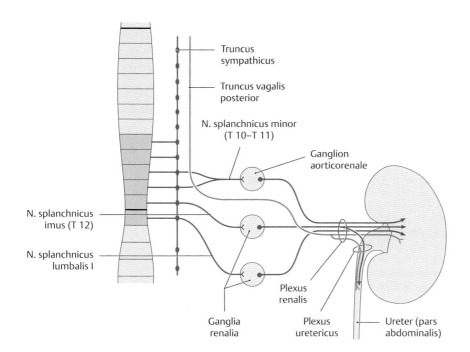

B Autonomic innervation of the ren and upper ureter

The sympathetic fibers from the ganglia aorticorenalia and renalia combine with the parasympathetic fibers from the truncus vagalis posterior to form the *plexus renalis*, which passes to the ren. Branches from that plexus form the *plexus uretericus*, which supplies the pars abdominalis (upper) of the ureter. The presynaptic sympathetic fibers come primarily from the nn. splanchnici thoracici.

Note: Due to their topographic proximity, the ganglia aorticorenalia often merge with the ganglia coeliaca. Illustrations providing an overview, such as on page 70, often show the renes as receiving their innervation from the ganglia coeliaca. Functionally, however, the ganglia aorticorenalia are separate and are thus separately mentioned in the schematic diagram.

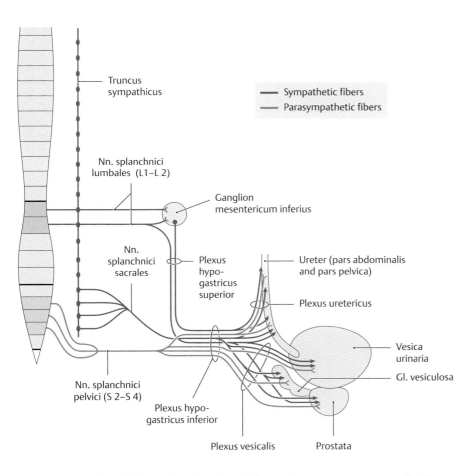

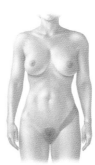

C Referred pain from ren sinister and vesica urinaria

Pain associated with diseases of the ren and vesica urinaria (inflammation, calculi) may be perceived in these skin areas. Occasionally the pain radiates into the groin ("loin to groin pain").

D Autonomic innervation of the vesica urinaria and the partes abdominalis and pelvica of the ureter

Sympathetic fibers from the nn. splanchnici lumbales and sacrales pass with the parasympathetic fibers from the nn. splanchnici pelvici to the plexus hypogastricus inferior. Branches from that plexus are distributed to form additional plexuses, including the plexus vesicalis and uretericus that supply the vesica urinaria and ureter (its partes abdominalis and pelvica). For the *parasympathetic* fibers, the synapse with the postsynaptic neuron is located entirely in the plexus hypogastricus inferior (or organ wall). The *sympathetic* fibers synapse partly in the ganglion mesentericum inferius and partly in the plexus hypogastricus inferior (see the fibers that continue from the plexus hypogastricus superior to the plexus hypogastricus inferior).

Note: With a complete transection of the medulla spinalis, the effect of higher CNS centers on the central parasympathetic neurons of S2–S4 (nn. splanchnici pelvici) is abolished. Because the nn. splanchnici pelvici initiate and control micturition, a complete cord lesion also causes problems of vesica control.

5.1   Overview of the Genital Tract

Classification of the genital organs

The genital organs of the male and female can be classified in various ways:

- Topographically (**A**) as
  - internal genital organs (internal genitalia) or
  - external genital organs (external genitalia)
- Functionally (**B, C**) as
  - organs for germ-cell and hormone production (gonadae) or
  - organs of transport, incubation and copulation, plus accessory sex glands
- Ontogenically (see p. 56) as
  - the undifferentiated gonad primordium (develops into the gonadae)
  - two undifferentiated duct systems (develop into the male and female transport organs, the female uterus, a portion of the female copulatory organ, and one of the accessory sex glands in the male)
  - the sinus urogenitalis and its derivatives (giving rise to the external genitalia of both sexes, the accessory sex glands, and portions of the copulatory organs)

A Male and female internal and external genitalia *

	Male	Female
Internal genitalia	Testis Epididymis Ductus deferens Prostata Gl. vesiculosa Gl. bulbourethralis	Ovarium Uterus Tuba uterina Vagina (upper portion)
External genitalia	Penis and urethra Scrotum and coverings of the testis	Vagina (vestibulum vaginae only) Labia majora and minora Mons pubis Gll. vestibulares major and minor Clitoris

* The *female* external genitalia (pudenda) are known clinically as the *vulva*.

B Functions of the male genital organs

Organ	Function
Testis	Germ-cell production Hormone production
Epididymis	Reservoir for sperm (sperm maturation)
Ductus deferens	Transport organ for sperm
Urethra	Transport organ for sperm and urinary organ
Accessory sex glands (prostata, gll. vesiculosae, and gll. bulbourethrales)	Production of secretions (semen)
Penis	Copulatory and urinary organ

C Functions of the female genital organs

Organ	Function
Ovarium	Germ-cell production Hormone production
Tuba uterina	Site of conception and transport organ for zygote
Uterus	Organ of incubation and parturition
Vagina	Organ of copulation and parturition
Labia majora and minora	Copulatory organ
Gll. vestibulares major and minor	Production of secretions

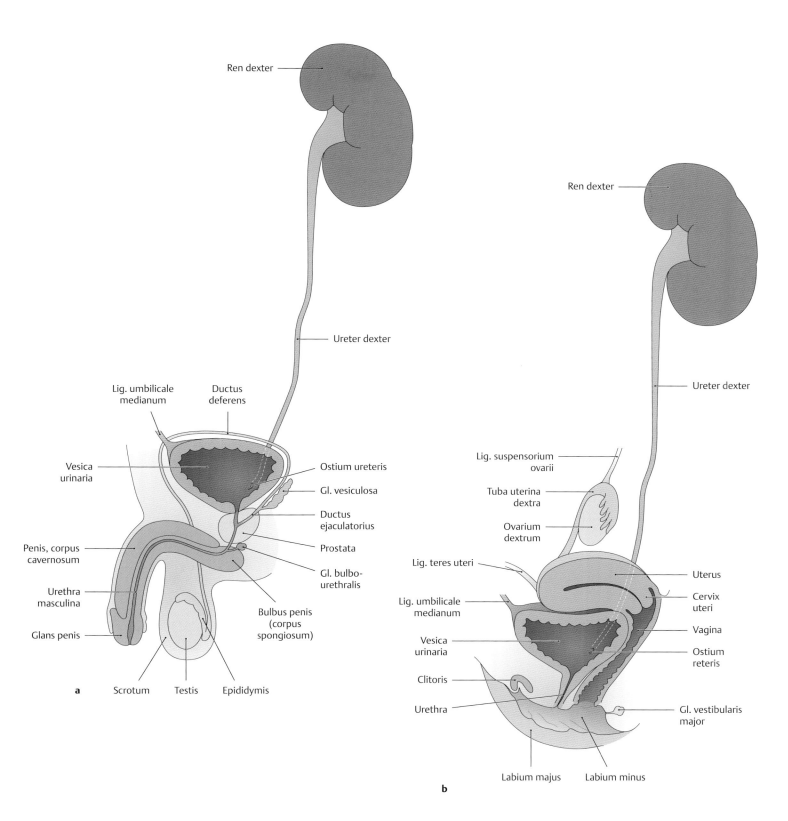

Ren dexter

Ren dexter

Ureter dexter

Ureter dexter

Lig. umbilicale medianum

Ductus deferens

Lig. suspensorium ovarii

Vesica urinaria

Ostium ureteris

Tuba uterina dextra

Gl. vesiculosa

Ovarium dextrum

Ductus ejaculatorius

Lig. teres uteri

Penis, corpus cavernosum

Prostata

Uterus

Gl. bulbo-urethralis

Lig. umbilicale medianum

Cervix uteri

Urethra masculina

Vagina

Bulbus penis (corpus spongiosum)

Vesica urinaria

Glans penis

Ostium reteris

Clitoris

a Scrotum Testis Epididymis

Urethra

Gl. vestibularis major

Labium majus Labium minus

b

D Overview of the urogenital system

Schematic representation of the urogenital apparatus in the male and female, viewed from the left side. Unpaired pelvic organs and the external genitalia are shown in midsagittal section.

a In the **male**, the urinary and genital organs are closely interrelated functionally and topographically. The urethra passes through the prostata, which is derived embryologically from the urethral epithelium. All of the accessory sex glands (prostata, gll. vesiculosae, and gll. bulbourethrales) ultimately discharge their secretions into the urethra.

b In the **female**, the urinary and genital tracts are *functionally* separate from each other. *Topographically*, however, the anterior wall of the uterus is closely related to the vesicula urinaria. In the external genital region as well, the urethra is embedded in the paries anterior of the vagina.

For these reasons, the collective term *urogenital* system is generally used.

319

5.2 Female Internal Genitalia: Overview

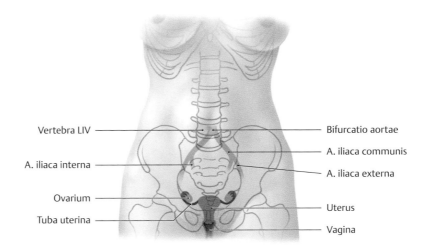

A Projection of the female internal genitalia onto the pelvis
Anterior view. The bifurcatio aortae into the aa. iliacae communes is also shown to aid orientation. The uterus, like the vagina, is located in the pelvic midline while the ovaria are superior, lateral, and posterior to the uterus in the RLQ and LLQ. Each ovarium occupies a fossa located just inferior to the division of the a. iliaca communis. The tubae uterinae do not pass to the ovaria by the shortest route but circle around them from the lateral side, because both of the ductus paramesonephrici (which develop into the tubae uterinae) run lateral to the crista gonadalis in which the ovaria develop.

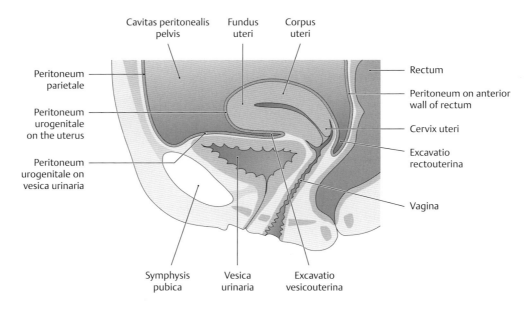

B Uterus and vagina: Relationship to the pelvic organs
Midsagittal section through a female pelvis, viewed from the left side. The peritoneum has been outlined in color. The uterus directly overlies the vesica uterina, and the rectum is posterior to the uterus. The fundus and corpus (body) of the uterus are covered by peritoneum viscerale, which is reflected onto the vesica urinaria and rectum to form the excavatio vesicouterina and excavatio rectouterina. The peritoneum extends farther down the posterior wall of the uterus than its anterior wall, with the result that the *posterior* part of the cervix uteri and upper vagina is covered by peritoneum while the anterior part is not. The vagina is surrounded on all sides by pelvic connective tissue. This tissue is thickened anteriorly and posteriorly to form the septa vesicovaginale and rectovaginale.

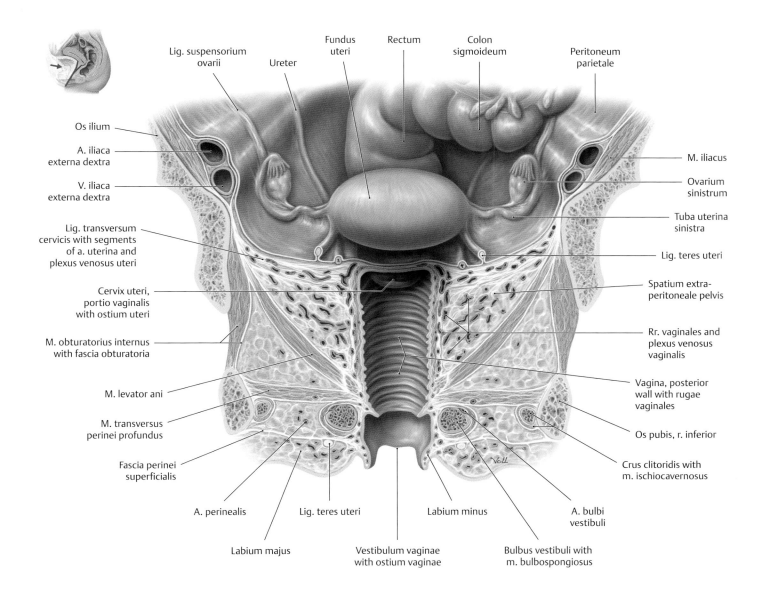

C The female genital organs in situ

Slightly angled coronal section, anterior view. The vesica urinaria, which lies anterior to the vagina and inferior to the fundus uteri (see **B**), is not shown. This illustration represents a compilation of multiple sections to provide a single integrated view. The fundus uteri, which is directed anteriorly owing to its anteverted and anteflexed position (see p. 326),

projects out of the deeper plane of section toward the observer. Around the vagina is a connective-tissue space containing an elaborate venous plexus. This loose connective tissue allows for considerable expansion of the vagina during childbirth. The sections of arterial vessels are arterial rr. vaginales as well as sections of the aa. vesicales inferiores.

5.3 Female Internal Genitalia: Topographical Anatomy and Peritoneal Relationships; Shape and Structure

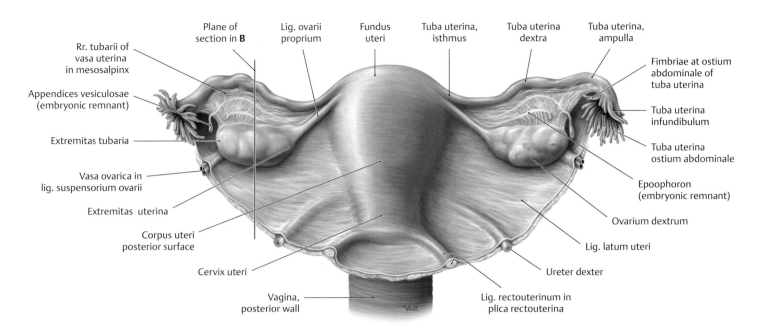

Plane of section in **B** — Lig. ovarii proprium — Fundus uteri — Tuba uterina, isthmus — Tuba uterina dextra — Tuba uterina, ampulla

Rr. tubarii of vasa uterina in mesosalpinx

Appendices vesiculosae (embryonic remnant)

Extremitas tubaria

Vasa ovarica in lig. suspensorium ovarii

Extremitas uterina

Corpus uteri posterior surface

Cervix uteri

Vagina, posterior wall

Fimbriae at ostium abdominale of tuba uterina

Tuba uterina infundibulum

Tuba uterina ostium abdominale

Epoophoron (embryonic remnant)

Ovarium dextrum

Lig. latum uteri

Ureter dexter

Lig. rectouterinum in plica rectouterina

A Uterus and adnexa: Topography and peritoneal relationships
Posterosuperior view of the uterus, adnexa, and the posterior surface of the lig. latum uteri. The uterine adnexa (ovarium and tuba uterina) are attached to the superior border and posterior surface of the lig. latum uteri by folds of peritoneum (mesovarium and mesosalpinx, see **B**). The mesometrium, which follows the anteflexed position of the uterus, attaches the uterus to the pelvic sidewall and transmits the uterine vascular structures.

The ovarium receives its vascular supply through the lig. suspensorium ovarii (these and other ligaments are reviewed in **C**).
Note: The ureteres descend in the retroperitoneum to the base of the lig. latum uteri and run forward between its layers to the vesica urinaria, passing inferior to the a. uterina (not visible here, see p. 351). This relationship must be duly noted in operations on the uterus and lig. latum uteri (risk of ureteral injury).

C Ligaments and peritoneal structures of the female genital organs

Ligamentum latum uteri	Broad fold of peritoneum extending from the lateral pelvic wall to the uterus (transmits vascular structures to the internal genital organs). The ligament has three main parts that extend to specific organs: • Mesometrium = to the uterus • Mesosalpinx = to the tuba uterina • Mesovarium = to the ovarium The connective-tissue space between the two peritoneal layers of the lig. latum uteri is known clinically as the parametrium
Ligamentum transversum cervicis (ligamentum cardinale)	Transverse bands of connective tissue between the cervix uterina and pelvic wall (paracervix)
Ligamentum teres uteri	Distal remnant of the gubernaculum (embryonic cord in both sexes, guides the descent of the testis or ovarium). Extends from the lateral angle of the uterus through the canalis inguinalis into the subcutaneous connective tissue of the labium majus
Plica rectouterina	Peritoneum-covered fold of connective tissue between the uterus and rectum; often contains smooth muscle (m. rectouterinus)
Ligamentum ovarii proprium	Proximal remnant of gubernaculum passing from the extremitas uterina of the ovarium to the angle of the uterus with the tuba uterina
Ligamentum suspensorium ovarii	Fold of peritoneum stretching from the pelvic wall to the ovarium; transmits the ovarian vessels

Peritoneal covering of tuba uterina — Tuba uterina

Mesosalpinx

Mesovarium

Ovarium

Mesometrium with peritoneal covering — Germinal epithelium covering of ovarium

Anterior — **Posterior**

B Folds of peritoneum on the female genital organs
(after Graumann, von Keyserlingk, and Sasse)
Sagittal section through the lig. latum uteri. The ovarium, tuba uterina, and much of the uterus (see **A**) are covered by peritoneum. The tuba uterina is attached to the superior margin of the lig. latum uteri by the mesosalpinx. The ovarium is attached to the posterosuperior surface of the lig. latum uteri by its own peritoneal structure, the mesovarium. These peritoneum-covered bands of connective tissue perform the same functions for the genital organs as the mesenteria do for the bowel and are named accordingly (see **C**): the mesovarium for the ovarium, the mesosalpinx for the tuba uterina (salpinx), and the mesometrium for the uterus. Collectively they form the lig. latum uteri.

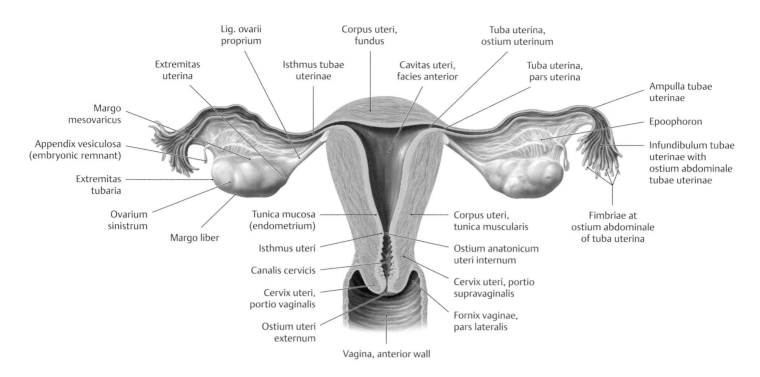

Lig. ovarii proprium

Extremitas uterina

Margo mesovaricus

Appendix vesiculosa (embryonic remnant)

Extremitas tubaria

Ovarium sinistrum

Margo liber

Isthmus tubae uterinae

Corpus uteri, fundus

Cavitas uteri, facies anterior

Tuba uterina, ostium uterinum

Tuba uterina, pars uterina

Ampulla tubae uterinae

Epoophoron

Infundibulum tubae uterinae with ostium abdominale tubae uterinae

Tunica mucosa (endometrium)

Isthmus uteri

Canalis cervicis

Cervix uteri, portio vaginalis

Ostium uteri externum

Corpus uteri, tunica muscularis

Ostium anatonicum uteri internum

Cervix uteri, portio supravaginalis

Fornix vaginae, pars lateralis

Fimbriae at ostium abdominale of tuba uterina

Vagina, anterior wall

D Uterus and tubae uterinae: Shape and structure

Posterior view of a coronal section with the uterus straightened and the mesometrium removed. The uterus consists basically of the corpus (with the fundus) and cervix, the corpus being joined to the cervix by a narrow isthmus approximately 1 cm long. Macroscopically, the isthmus uteri is classified as part of the cervix but histologically it is lined by endometrium. The junction of the corpus and cervix uteri is located at the ostium anatomicum uteri *internum* of the uterus. The lumen of the uterus, called the cavitas uteri, communicates with the vaginal lumen through the isthmus uteri and canalis cervicis uteri. It has a total length ("probe length") of 7–8 cm. The *cavitas uteri* presents a triangular shape

in coronal section. The *cervix uteri* is subdivided into a portio supravaginalis cervicis and portio vaginalis cervicis. The *ostium* uteri is the opening in the portio vaginalis cervicis that is directed toward the vagina. The portio vaginalis cervicis projects into the vagina, forming recesses called the fornices vaginae.

The *tuba uterina* (total length approximately 10–18 cm) is subdivided from lateral to medial into the infundibulum, ampulla, and isthmus tubae uterinae, and pars uterina tubae uterinae. The ostium abdominale tubae uterinae at the infundibulum is surrounded by fimbriae (the "fimbriated end") and opens into the cavitas peritonealis. The ostium uterinum tubae uterinae opens into the cavitas uteri.

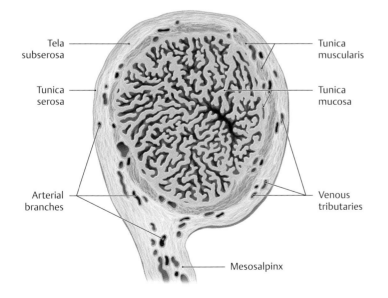

Tela subserosa

Tunica serosa

Arterial branches

Tunica muscularis

Tunica mucosa

Venous tributaries

Mesosalpinx

E Tuba uterina in cross-section: Wall structure

Cross-sectional view of the ampulla of a right tuba uterina. The mesosalpinx extends inferiorly. The three wall layers are clearly distinguishable (wall thickness = 0.4–1.5 cm):

- The **tunica mucosa** is raised into a great many folds that occupy most of the tubal lumen. These folds are of key importance in transporting the zygote to the uterus. Postinflammatory adhesions between the mucosal folds may hamper or even prevent transport of the fertilized ovum (see p. 334).

- The **tunica muscularis** consists of several thin layers of smooth muscle that provide the tuba uterina with its motility (see **B,** p. 332) and propel the zygote toward the uterus by a ciliated epithelium.

- The **tunica serosa** (peritoneal covering) of the tuba uterina is continuous with the mesosalpinx.

5.4 Female Internal Genitalia: Wall Structure and Function of the Uterus

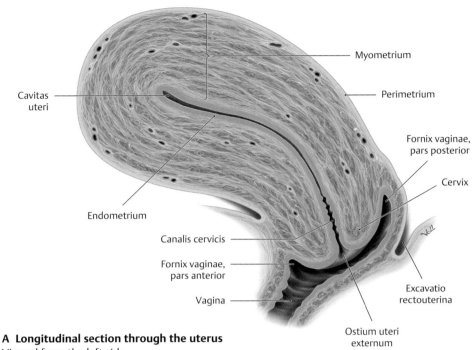

A Longitudinal section through the uterus
Viewed from the left side.

B Wall structure of the uterus

The uterine wall also consists of three layers from inside to outside:

- **Tunica mucosa** or **endometrium** (see **D**): Single layer of columnar epithelium (epithelial layer) on a connective-tissue base (lamina propria)

- **Tunica muscularis** or **myometrium** (see **C**):
Several smooth-muscle layers with a total thickness of approximately 1.5 cm

- **Tunica serosa** or **perimetrium**:
Tunica serosa covering the anterior and posterior sides of the corpus uteri and the posterior wall of the cervix uteri. The tela subserosa adjacent to the myometrium becomes adventitia in areas where the uterus lacks a peritoneal covering (e.g., at the attachment of the lig. latum uteri).

C Layers of the myometrium
(after Rauber and Kopsch)
The myometrium (tunica muscularis) of the uterus consists of three layers from outside to inside:

- **Stratum supravasculare:** thin outermost layer with criss-crossing lamellae; stabilizes the uterine wall
- **Stratum vasculare:** thick intermediate layer with a reticular pattern of muscle fibers; very vascular; the principal source for uterine contractions during labor
- **Stratum subvasculare:** thin innermost layer just below the endometrium; provides for functional closure of the ostium uterinum tubae uterinae. Its contraction promotes separation of the uterine tunica mucosa (shedding of the functional layer) during menses and separation of the placenta after childbirth.

The myometrium performs two seemingly contradictory functions: It must keep the uterus *closed* during pregnancy, but it must *open* the cervix during childbirth. To fulfill these functions, the individual muscle layers (see above) are equipped with longitudinal, oblique, and transverse or circular fibers. The circular muscle fibers are most abundant in the cervical region and serve to maintain closure of the cervix during pregnancy. The longitudinal and oblique muscle fibers are most abundant in the corpus and fundus uteri; they shorten the uterus and lower the fundus during childbirth. The myometrium blends with the circular fibers of the uterine tube muscles at the fundus uteri near the ostium uterinum tubae uterinae. Myometrial contractions are stimulated most effectively by the pituitary hormone oxytocin. These contractions occur not only during labor and delivery but also during menstruation, when they aid in expulsion of the uterine mucosa. Benign tumors of the myometrium (fibroids, myomas) may cause abnormalities of menstrual bleeding.

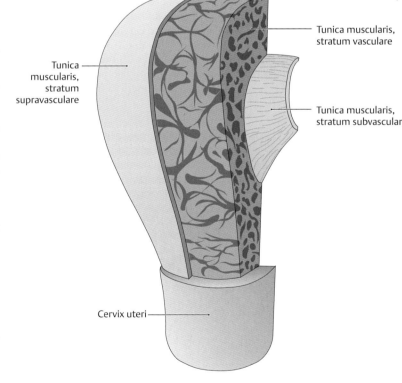

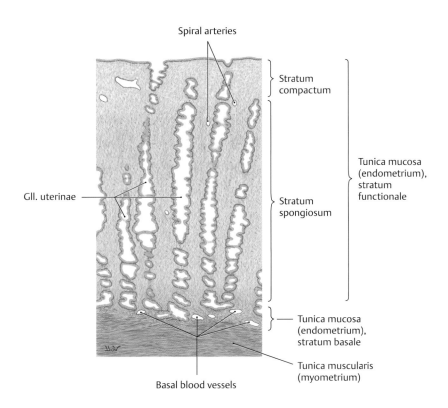

Spiral arteries

Stratum compactum

Gll. uterinae

Tunica mucosa (endometrium), stratum functionale

Stratum spongiosum

Tunica mucosa (endometrium), stratum basale

Tunica muscularis (myometrium)

Basal blood vessels

D Structure of the uterine mucosa (endometrium)

Structurally, the endometrium consists of a simple columnar epithelial cell layer and a lamina propria. The epithelial layer lines the uterine surface and encloses the tubular, coiled endometrial *gll. uterinae*. The lamina propria, which surrounds and supports the gll. uterinae, is made up of connective tissue (stroma) and the vessels embedded in it. The endometrium is *functionally* subdivided into a basal layer (stratum basale) and a functional layer (stratum functionale). The *stratum basale* is approximately 1 mm thick, is largely exempt from the cyclical changes in the endometrium, and is not shed during menstruation. The *stratum functionale* varies in thickness at different phases of the ovarian cycle in women of reproductive age. It is shed at intervals of approximately 28 days during menstruation. It is thickest during the secretory phase of the ovarian cycle, at which time it consists of a superficial stratum compactum and a deeper stratum spongiosum. It receives its blood supply from tortuous vessels called spiral arteries. While in this secretory state, the endometrium is most receptive to the implantation of a zygote. The tunica mucosa of the cervix uteri does not participate in these cyclical changes.

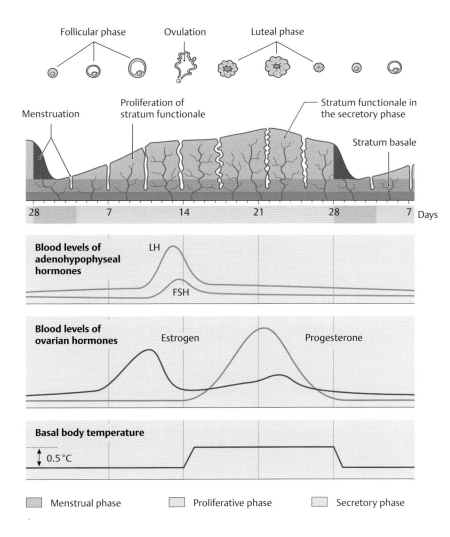

Follicular phase

Ovulation

Luteal phase

Menstruation

Proliferation of stratum functionale

Stratum functionale in the secretory phase

Stratum basale

28   7   14   21   28   7 Days

Blood levels of adenohypophyseal hormones

LH

FSH

Blood levels of ovarian hormones

Estrogen

Progesterone

Basal body temperature

↕ 0.5°C

▨ Menstrual phase   ▨ Proliferative phase   ▨ Secretory phase

E Cyclical changes in the endometrium

The ovarium secretes estrogens (e.g., estradiol) and progestins (e.g., progesterone) on a cyclical basis. Estrogens stimulate proliferation of the endometrium, while progestins induce its secretory transformation. The release of both hormones is controlled chiefly by the hormones FSH (follicle stimulating hormone) and LH (luteinizing hormone), which are secreted cyclically by the hypophysis. While estrogens are produced by the folliculus ovaricus, progestins are produced in significant amounts only by the corpus luteum. If conception does not take place, the corpus luteum regresses and stops producing hormones. As a result of this, the stratum functionale of the endometrium breaks down and is expelled during menstruation. Estrogen production by a new, hypophysis-stimulated folliculus ovaricus initiates a new cycle, which lasts an average of 28 days (1 lunar month). Ovulation usually occurs on day 14 of the cycle.

Note: For practical reasons, the first day of the menstrual period (which lasts about 4 days) is considered day 1 of the cycle, despite the fact that the cycle ends with menstruation. This is because the sudden onset of menstrual bleeding is easier to detect than its more gradual cessation. From the standpoint of the endometrium, however, the last day of the menstrual period (difficult to detect) marks the end of the cycle.

5.5 Female Internal Genitalia: Positions of the Uterus and Vagina

A Curvature and position of the uterus

Midsagittal section of the uterus and upper vagina, viewed from the left side.

Note the two angles that determine the normal anteversion and anteflexion of the uterus (see **D**). Posterior angulation and curvature of the uterus (retroflexion, retroversion) are considered abnormal. A retroverted uterus is more susceptible to descent because it is more closely aligned with the longitudinal axis of the vagina. Moreover, a retroverted uterus that enlarges during pregnancy may become immobile below the promontorium ossis sacri (L5/S1 junction) and jeopardize the further course of the pregnancy by constraining uterine expansion.

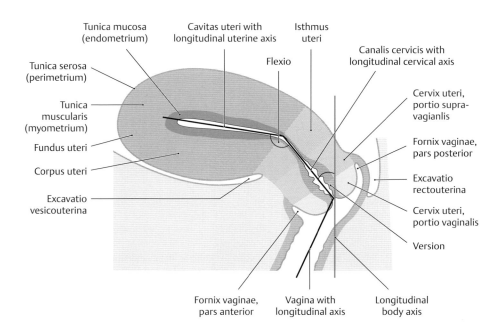

Tunica mucosa (endometrium) — Cavitas uteri with longitudinal uterine axis — Isthmus uteri — Flexio — Canalis cervicis with longitudinal cervical axis — Tunica serosa (perimetrium) — Tunica muscularis (myometrium) — Fundus uteri — Corpus uteri — Excavatio vesicouterina — Cervix uteri, portio supravagianlis — Fornix vaginae, pars posterior — Excavatio rectouterina — Cervix uteri, portio vaginalis — Version — Fornix vaginae, pars anterior — Vagina with longitudinal axis — Longitudinal body axis

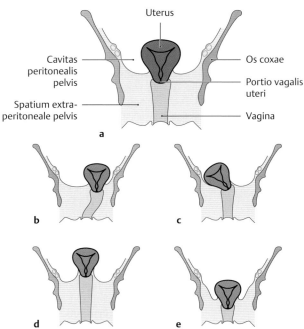

Uterus — Cavitas peritonealis pelvis — Os coxae — Portio vagalis uteri — Spatium extra-peritoneale pelvis — Vagina

a

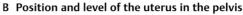

b   c

d   e

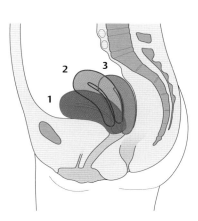

2   3   1

C Physiological changes in uterine position

Midsagittal section of the pelvis, viewed from the left side. Uterine position is directly affected by the varying degrees of vesica urinaria and rectal distention. **1** Vesica and rectum empty; **2** vesica and rectum full; **3** vesica full, rectum empty.

B Position and level of the uterus in the pelvis

Coronal section of the pelvis, anterior view. The uterus has been slightly straightened for clarity. Normally the uterus is located approximately in the median plane (**a**) with its portio vaginalis level with a line connecting the two spinae ischiadicae. The uterus may be displaced from this position to the left or right (sinistroposition or dextroposition, **b** and **c**) or may lie above or below the plane of the spinae ischiadicae (elevation or descent, see **d** and **e**). Anterior and posterior displacement (anteposition, retroposition) may also occur but are not illustrated here. Descent of the uterus usually results from a structural weakness of the diaphragma pelvis (chiefly the m. levator ani, often after numerous vaginal deliveries). Displacement of the uterus may cause complaints and functional disturbances due to pressure on adjacent organs (vesica urinaria, rectum). Descent of the uterus may even cause the portio vaginalis of the uterus to protrude from the vagina (cervical prolapse).

D Describing the position of the uterus in the pelvis

The position of the uterus in the pelvis can be described in terms of version, flexion, and position (angles are shown in **A**).

Version	Inclination of the cervix in the cavitas pelvis; defined by the angle between the cervical axis and the longitudinal axis of the body; the normal condition is *anteversion*
Flexion	Inclination of the corpus uteri relative to the cervix; defined by the angle between the longitudinal axes of the cervix and corpus uteri; the normal condition is *anteflexion*
Position	Position of the portio vaginalis of the uterus in the cavitas pelvis; physiologically, the portio vaginalis of the uterus is at the level of the interspinous line at the center of the pelvis

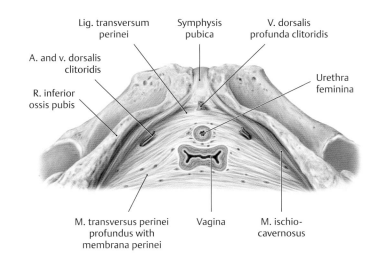

Labium posterior
ostii uteri

Labium anterior
ostii uteri

Columna
rugarum anterior

Vagina,
anterior wall

Ostium urethrae
externum

Clitoris

Cervix uteri, portio
supravaginalis

Ostium uteri

Rugae vaginales

Carina urethralis
vaginae

Vestibulum vaginae
with labium minus

Lig. transversum
perinei

A. and v. dorsalis
clitoridis

R. inferior
ossis pubis

Symphysis
pubica

V. dorsalis
profunda clitoridis

Urethra
feminina

M. transversus perinei
profundus with
membrana perinei

Vagina

M. ischio-
cavernosus

E Vagina
Posterior view. The vagina has been cut open along a coronal plane angled slightly posteriorly to display its paries anterior. The vaginal lumen presents an H-shaped cross section (see **F**), but the lumen in this dissection has been stretched open to a more circular shape (in situ the parietes posterior and anterior are closely apposed). The vaginal tunica mucosa has numerous transverse folds (rugae vaginales) as well as columnae rugarum anterior and posterior formed by the extensive venous plexus in the vaginal wall. The closely adjacent urethra raises the lower paries anterior of the vagina into a prominent longitudinal ridge (carina urethralis vaginae).

F Location of the vagina in the pelvic floor
This drawing illustrates the close proximity of the vagina and urethra. Muscular fibers from the m. transversus perinei profundus encircle the vagina.

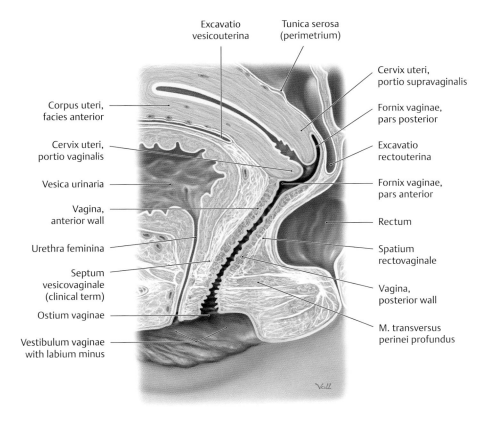

Excavatio
vesicouterina

Tunica serosa
(perimetrium)

Corpus uteri,
facies anterior

Cervix uteri,
portio vaginalis

Vesica urinaria

Vagina,
anterior wall

Urethra feminina

Septum
vesicovaginale
(clinical term)

Ostium vaginae

Vestibulum vaginae
with labium minus

Cervix uteri,
portio supravaginalis

Fornix vaginae,
pars posterior

Excavatio
rectouterina

Fornix vaginae,
pars anterior

Rectum

Spatium
rectovaginale

Vagina,
posterior wall

M. transversus
perinei profundus

G Location of the vagina in the pelvis
Midsagittal section through a female pelvis, viewed from the left side. The longitudinal axis of the vagina is directed posterosuperiorly. The vagina is attached to the pelvic connective tissue anteriorly (vesicovaginal septum), posteriorly (rectovaginal septum), and laterally (not shown here). The vaginal fornix surrounds the vaginal part of the cervix, which itself is directed superiorly and anteriorly. The pars posterior fornicis vaginae is significantly longer than the pars anterior fornicis vaginae and projects further superiorly in the pelvis. The visceral peritoneum extends far down the posterior uterine wall, bringing the posterior part of the vaginal fornix into close proximity to the rectouterine pouch (cul-de-sac, the lowest part of the female peritoneal cavity).

327

5.6 Female Internal Genitalia: Epithelial Regions of the Uterus

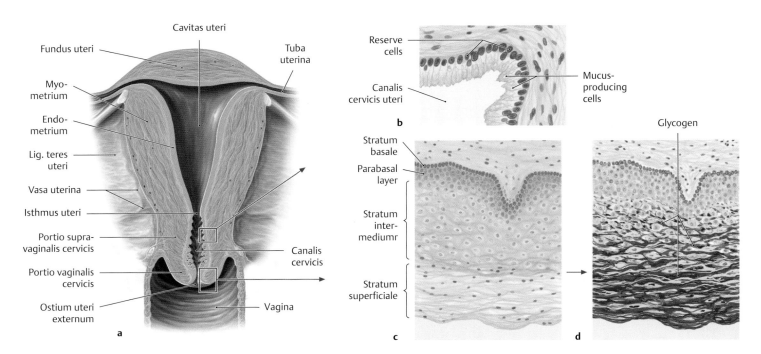

A Epithelial regions of the uterus

a Coronal section through uterus, anterior view; b–d Higher magnification of a: b Mucus-secreting columnar epithelium of the canalis cervicis uteri; c Squamous epithelium of the portio vaginalis cervicis; d Periodic acid–Schiff (PAS) method used to display glycogen (after Luellmann).

The cervix is the lower part uteri. It commences distal to the isthmus of the uterus as the portio supravaginalis cervicis, which is the upper part of the cervix surrounded by connective tissue of the parametrium, and ends at its lower portion that extends into the vagina (portio vaginalis cervicis). At the level of the portio supravaginalis cervicis the uterus is held in place by ligaments (mainly the lig. cardinalis, cf. p. 396). The tubular lumen of the cervix is called the canalis cervicis uteri. It is lined with tunica mucosa and begins at the ostium uteri internum and ends with the ostium uteri at the portio vaginalis of the cervix. The mucosal epithelium of the canalis cervicis uteri is composed of a single layer of mucus-secreting columnar epithelium. A parallel arrangement of folds (plicae palmatae), which form crypts, gives the epithelium a rough appearance on the surface. The function of the reserve cells located at the base of the epithelium is to replenish the cervical epithelium. Unlike the one-layered cervical epithelium, the vagina is lined with stratified,

nonkeratinized squamous epithelium, which depending on the hormonal situation in women may continue to the surface of the portio vaginalis of the cervix. The boundaries of the two epithelial layers can be either endo- or ectocervical (see **C**).

The stratified, nonkeratinized squamous epithelium lining the vagina (and portio vaginalis cervicis) is composed of up to 20 layers of cells and is made up of four tiers: strata basale, parabasale, intermedium, and superficiale. Typically, cells of the two superficial-most layers contain abundant glycogen as a result of differentiation. The epithelium exhibits cyclical changes: whereas at the preovulatory stage, all layers are well developed, at the postovulatory stage cells of the strata superficiale and intermedium desquamate and disintegrate. Glycogen that is released as a result nourishes lactic acid bacteria (lactobacillus acidophilus, Döderlein's bacillus), which inhabit the vagina. The transformation of glycogen into lactic acid leads to the acidic vaginal milieu (pH 4–5), which mainly in the second half of the menstrual cycle protects against pathogens (see **B**). The slightly alkaline cervical mucus has a similar effect as a physiologic barrier against infection. For much of the menstrual cycle, it has a stretchy texture and seals the canalis cervicis uteri with a protective plug (barrier against ascending germs). The mucus is thin only at the time of ovulation and thus becomes penetrable by sperm.

B Defense mechanisms of the vagina and potential dysfunctions

The cavitas peritonealis has an anatomical communication with the exterior of the body (via vagina–canalis cervicis uteri–cavitas uteri–tuba uterina). This exposes the female to ascending infections, and this is why physiologic barriers against infection exist in the form of vaginal defense mechanisms. Dysfunction of these mechanisms may lead to gynecological inflammation and an increased risk of miscarriage.

Protection mechanism	Dysfunction due to
• Physiological acidic vaginal milieu with a pH 4–5 • Effect of estrogens: stimulates vaginal epithelium proliferation and differentiation (glycogen storage) • Effect of progestins: leads to desquamation of superficial and intermediate vaginal cells • Conversion of glycogen into lactic acid through lactobacillus acidophilus (Döderlein's bacillus)	• Elevated pH level: alkalizing effect of menstrual blood/cervical mucus • Lack of glycogen: lack of endogenous estrogen/progestins (childhood/old age/diseases) • Drugs: antibiotics disrupt vagina's normal flora • Exogenous effects: sex life, tampons, improper anal hygiene, using alkaline soaps • Infections: colpitis especially caused by chlamydia, trichomonads and fungi (candida albicans)

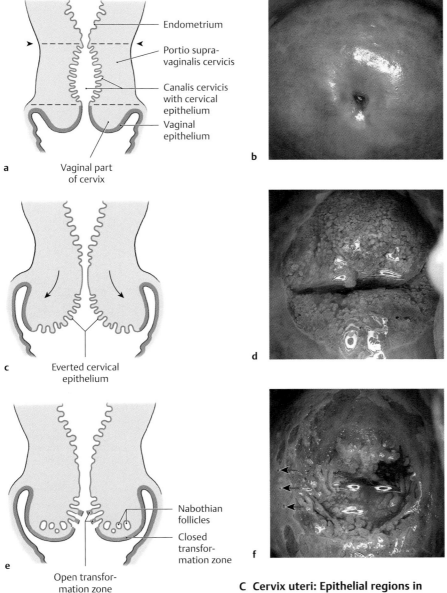

a Vaginal part of cervix

Endometrium

Portio supra-vaginalis cervicis

Canalis cervicis with cervical epithelium

Vaginal epithelium

b

c Everted cervical epithelium

d

e Open transformation zone

Nabothian follicles

Closed transformation zone

f

g

Endocervix

C Cervix uteri: Epithelial regions in pre-reproductive and post-reproductive stages

a, c, e, and g: Highly schematic coronal sections of the uterus and vagina, anterior view; colposcopic images of the portio vaginalis of the cervix before the onset of puberty (**b** nullipara) and during the reproductive phase (**d** and **f** multipara); **b, d,** and **f** from Nauth, H.F.: Gynäkologische Zytodiagnostik. Thieme, Stuttgart 2002).

The arrowheads mark the location of the ostium uteri internus; the dashed lines mark the boundaries of the canalis cervicis uteri (**a**). The boundary between the unilayered mucus-secreting columnar epithelium (cervical epithelium) of the canalis cervicis uteri and the stratified nonkeratinized squamous epithelium of the portio vaginalis cervicis and the vagina varies according to the woman's hormonal status (see below). The visible portion of the uterus is called the ectocervix and the non-visible portion is called the endocervix.

Before the onset of puberty (a and b): Before the onset of the reproductive phase, the portio vaginalis cervicis is covered with squamous epithelium, the ecto-endocervical boundary is located within the canalis cervicis uteri (above the ostium uteri), thus it is not visible from the vagina.

During the reproductive phase (c–f): In response to hormonal stimuli (estrogen) the cervical tunica mucosa is everted and moves inside the vagina. It appears as a glandular field with a very rough surface on the ectocervix (**d**). The sharp boundary with the smooth pink-colored squamous epithelium of the portio vaginalis cervicis is thus located outside of the ostium uteri and is clearly visible from the vagina. The eversion of the cervical glandular field is believed to be related to higher fertility (easier for spermatozoa to enter the cervix). The columnar endocervical epithelium, which has everted onto the ectocervix adjusts to the altered vaginal milieu (acidic milieu in contrast to alkaline milieu of the canalis cervicis uteri) by converting to stratified nonkeratinized squamous epithelium (metaplasia). In this way, it is similar in structure and cyclic behavior to the regular squamous epithelium of the portio vaginalis cervicis. As the mucus-secreting cervical epithelium transforms into squamous epithelium the columnar glands become sealed over (closed transformation zone in contrast to open transformation zone where the glands are not overgrown and occluded, arrows in **f** point to the "open" orifices) leading to the formation of macroscopically visible mucus-filled retention cysts (Nabothian cysts), which are not considered problematic. Squamous epithelium in the transformation zone may become malignant and contribute in prestages (precancerous) to squamous cell carcinoma formation (see p. 330 f).

During postmenopause (g): Lower estrogen levels toward the end of the reproductive phase cause the relocation of cervical epithelium and the boundary of the endo- and ectocervix moves back into the canalis cervicis uteri (similar clinical presentation to **b** although the cervix changes shape after vaginal delivery).

5.7 Female Internal Genitalia: Cytologic Smear, Conization; Cervical Carcinoma

Ectocervical smear

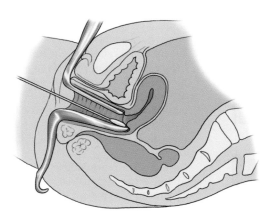

a

Endocervical smear

b

A Cytologic smear: Cell morphology of vaginal and vaginal part of cervical epithelium; early detection of cervical cancer

a and **b** Cytologic smears taken from the portio vaginalis cervicis and the canalis cervicis uteri, **c** transfer of smear material onto glass slide; **d** histological structure and cell morphology of the vaginal and cervical epithelium in the cytologic smear; **e** Pap staining of superficial and intermediate cells (**e** from Nauth H.F.: Gynäkologische Zytodiagnostik. Thieme, Stuttgart 2002).

Especially in the transformation zone of the cervix uteri, where with the onset of puberty the unilayered columnar epithelium of the cervix changes into stratified squamous epithelium (see p. 329), the squamous epithelium may undergo malignant transformation and turn into invasive squamous cell carcinoma. Because cervical cancer usually develops slowly over time, it is possible to detect it in its early stages with the help of cytologic smears. Thus, cytodiagnosis is one of the most important tools in early detection of cervical cancer (see **D**). Cytology testing is an obligatory part of the initial gynecologic examination and cancer screening (in Germany starting at the age of 20) and is also performed to evaluate suspicious changes in cervical tissue. The cytologic smear should always include cells from the uppermost epithelial layer, which if they are normal show signs of differentiation (see p. 328).

Two smears are taken routinely: the first one (**a**) must be taken at the surface of the portio vaginalis cervicis (ectocervix), and the second one (**b**) from the canalis cervicis (endocervix). The smear material is taken with a cotton swab and transferred to a slide and fixed (**c**). After that, the Papanicolaou method (known as Pap stain) is used to stain the cervical smear and evaluate it for characteristics of cell differentiation (cell shape, nuclear shape, nucleus-plasma ratio, see **D**). Because structure, height and the degree of maturation vary with the hormonal status (menstrual cycle) of a woman, it is crucial to confirm at which point during the cycle the smear is taken. If it is taken during the follicular phase (effect of estrogen), it is dominated by eosinophilic superficial cells, which are stained red, and flat, basophilic intermediate cells with pyknotic nuclei, which are stained greenish-blue (**e**). This proliferative phase, during which the uppermost cell layer is constantly regenerated by cells from the basal layer, normally lasts about a week. The postovulatory phase is dominated by cell differentiation and desquamation. Hence, the epithelium is thinner in the second part of the menstrual cycle.

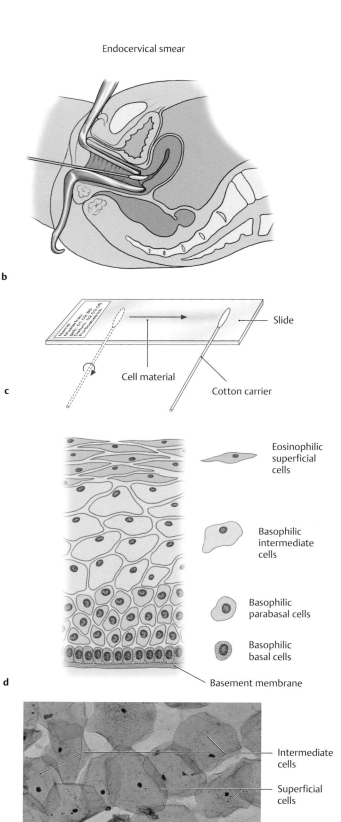

Slide

Cell material

Cotton carrier

c

Eosinophilic superficial cells

Basophilic intermediate cells

Basophilic parabasal cells

Basophilic basal cells

Basement membrane

d

Intermediate cells

Superficial cells

e

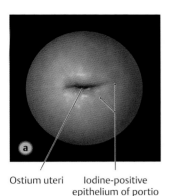

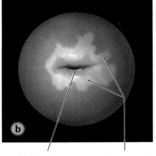

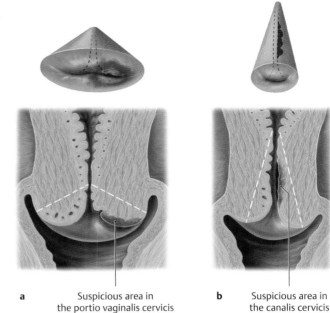

| Ostium uteri | Iodine-positive epithelium of portio vaginalis cervicis | Epithelium lining canalis cervicis | Iodine-negative epithelium of portio vaginalis cervicis |

a   Suspicious area in the portio vaginalis cervicis   b   Suspicious area in the canalis cervicis

B Schiller's iodine test for localization of abnormal epithelial regions

a Normal vaginal cervical epithelium stained by iodine produces a dark brown color; **b** Iodine negative, insufficiently differentiated cervical epithelium.

After inserting a speculum into the vagina, the portio vaginalis cervicis is initially examined macroscopically, if necessary with the help of a colposcope allowing a 6–40 fold magnification of the cervix. For the localization of abnormal areas, Schiller's iodine test utilizes the glycogen content of the surrounding normal squamous epithelium. To that end, iodine solution (Schiller's iodine test) is applied to the surface of the cervix. Normal squamous epithelium, regardless of whether is autochthonous or metaplastic, takes on a dark brown color. However, insufficiently differentiated squamous epithelium with a high or low glycogen content turns only light brown or is iodine negative. Thus, the iodine-unstained areas correspond to the location of undifferentiated epithelium. Iodine-negative areas are not specific but combined with suspicious cytology results (see above cytologic smear) of the same area, point to epithelial abnormalities. Hence, Schiller's iodine test provides a method with which to assess the localization and expansion of cervical changes. Conization (see **C**) is used to remove affected areas.

C Conization

For a histological examination of suspicious findings (iodine-negative areas, dysplastic cells in the smear), a cone-shaped wedge of uterine cervix tissue (conization) is removed while the patient is under anesthesia. In a sexually mature woman, abnormal epithelium is most likely found on the surface of the portio vaginalis cervicis in the transformation zone. When removing a flat and broad wedge of tissue (**a**), this area is included. In postmenopausal women, atypical epithelial cells are usually found in the canalis cervicis uteri. This area is included when removing a sharp cone of tissue (**b**).

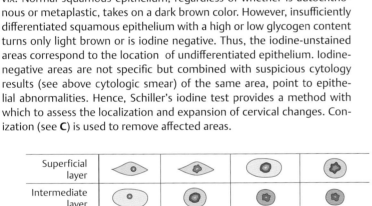

Superficial layer				
Intermediate layer				
Parabasal layer				
Basal layer				
Histology	Normal	Mild dysplasia	Moderate dysplasia	Severe dysplasia

a

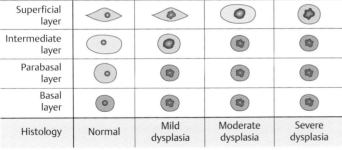

b

D Cervical carcinoma and its pre-stages

a Normal and dysplastic cells in the cytologic smear; **b** Parabasal squamous epithelial cells with atypical and polymorphous nuclei ("immature dyskaryotic cells") (from Nauth, H.F.: Gynäkologische Zytodiagnostik. Thieme, Stuttgart 2002).

Pre-stages of cervical carcinoma are initially confined to the epithelium, and the deeper layers have not yet been infiltrated (see below). Cellular changes that begin at the basal layer and progress to the superficial layer (cell shape, nuclear shape, nucleus-plasma ratio) are signs of increasing differentiation. They are not present when the cells only divide but don't mature (dysplasia = abnormal cells). Dysplastic cells often have enlarged hyperchromatic nuclei, so that the nucleus-plasma ratio shifts in favor of the nucleus. The cytologic smear helps to determine the different degrees of dysplasia, and thus the pre-stages of the cervical carcinoma (**a**). Based on the international classification, they are divided into stages of CIN (CIN = "cervical intraepithelial neoplasia"): mild dysplasia (CIN I); moderate dysplasia (CIN II) severe dysplasia/carcinoma in situ (CIN III). The more severe the dysplasia, the more likely the transformation into

invasive carcinoma. In 50% of cases, mild dysplasia will spontaneously regress. In severe dysplasia (**b**), the atypical changes involve the full thickness of the epithelium and the regular stratification has been lost. However, the carcinoma has not yet perforated the basement membrane (carcinoma in situ). Invasion of the basement membrane is characteristic of an infiltrating growth pattern with subsequent metastasis. Approximately 20% of intraepithelial changes have infiltrative growth patterns, with a latency period between formation of dysplasia and infiltration of more than 10 years.

Cervical carcinoma is the second leading cause of cancer-related deaths in women worldwide. Approximately 500,000 cases are diagnosed each year, and 350,000 die from it despite early detection and treatment. Infection (most commonly sexually transmitted) with certain types of the papilloma virus (HPV-16 and HPV-18) has been identified as one major pathogenetic factor. These viruses inactivate proteins that monitor cell growth (e.g., p53 and Rb). Recently, a vaccination against tumor-producing viruses has become available.

5.8 Female Internal Genitalia: Ovary and Follicular Maturation

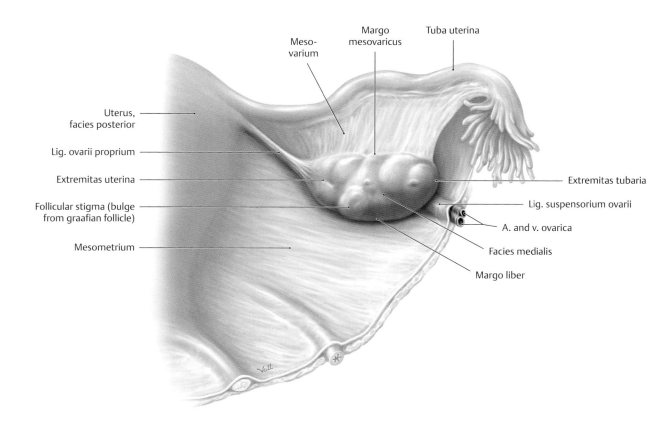

A Ovarium
Posterior view of a right ovarium, showing the peritoneal ligaments that transmit vessels to the ovarium (lig. suspensorium ovarii with the a. and v. ovarica, lig. ovarii proprium with the r. ovaricus of the a. uterina, and portions of the plexus venosus uterinus) along with part of the uterus, tuba uterina, and lig. latum uteri. The ovarium is positioned such that it lies in the fossa iliaca of the pelvis minor.
Note: Given the dual vascular supply to the ovarium from the upper abdomen (the vessels accompany the ovarium during its developmental descent) and the blood supply to the uterus (close to the ovarium), both vascular systems should be ligated during a hysterectomy.
In a woman of reproductive age, the ovarium is 3–5 cm long and has the size and shape of a plum. It consists of a cortex ovarii and medulla ovarii (see **C**) and is surrounded by a tough collagenous capsule (tunica albuginea). The cortex ovarii contains folliculi ovarici at varying stages of development. The folliculi contain an oocyte surrounded by follicular epithelium and a connective-tissue mantle. Female hormones are not produced by the oocyte itself but by the cells that surround it. Although an intraperitoneal organ, the ovarium is covered externally by germinal epithelium (on its tunica albuginea) and has a shiny surface.
Note: The visceral peritoneal covering of the ovarium, a single-layered cuboidal epithelium that surrounds the tunica albuginea, has been referred to traditionally as "germinal epithelium," but it does not participate at all in the principal, reproductive function of the ovarium—egg production—nor is it involved in replenishment of cells in the ovarium itself. However, it is "germinal" in another, unfortunate way—90 % of all malignant ovarian tumors are thought to originate in this cell layer.

B Ovum collection mechanism
Posterior view of a right ovarium and tuba uterina. Both the tuba uterina and the ovarium are motile. The tuba uterina derives its motility from its muscular wall and pulsations of adjacent vessels. Rotational and longitudinal movements of the tuba uterina make it easier for the fimbriated end of the tuba uterina to contact the entire ovarium. The movements stop when the ostium abdominale tubae uterinae has cupped the mound formed by a graafian folliculus ovaricus.

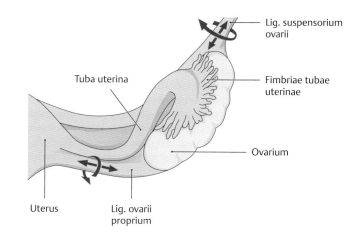

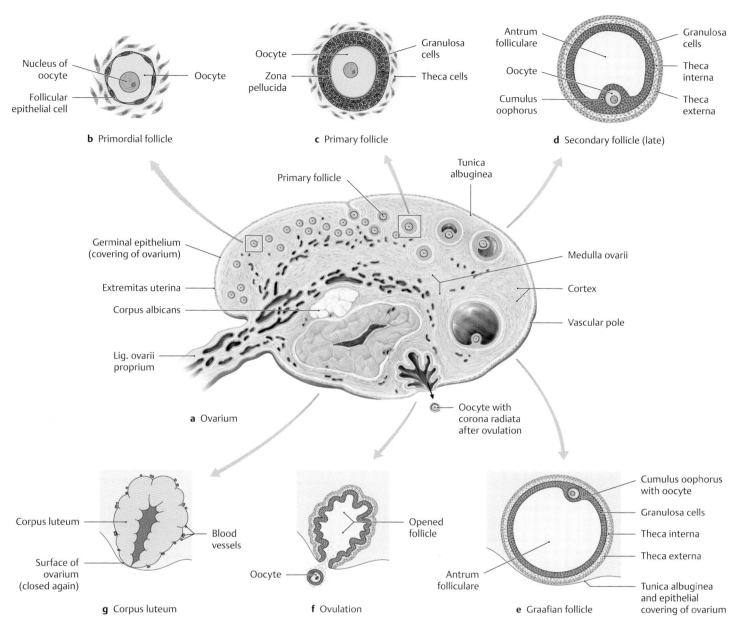

b Primordial follicle

c Primary follicle

d Secondary follicle (late)

a Ovarium

g Corpus luteum

f Ovulation

e Graafian follicle

C Follicular maturation in the ovarium

The sequence of follicular maturation is illustrated in a clockwise direction around the ovarium. The follicular stages are not drawn to scale.

a Ovarium: Section through the ovarium of an adult woman, demonstrating its structure and follicular stages. The central medulla ovarii is surrounded by a cortex ovarii containing folliculi at various stages of development. At the lower edge of the ovarium, an oocyte is being released from a ruptured folliculus (ovulation). After ovulation has taken place, the graafian folliculus initially develops into a hormonally active corpus luteum and later regresses to form a white fibrous scar (corpus albicans).

b Primordial follicle: Oocyte surrounded by a single layer of flat epithelial cells.

c Primary follicle: When the single layer of epithelium around the oocyte becomes multilaminar but without an atrium, the follicle is called a primary follicle.

d Secondary follicle: The epithelium (composed of granulosa cells) becomes stratified with an antrum present, and the epithelium and oocyte are separated from each other by a conspicuous zona pellucida. The fluid-filled spaces between the epithelial cells coalesce to form a single cavity (follicular cavity or antrum) containing follicular fluid. The connective tissue surrounding the follicular epithelium is organized into

a theca externa and theca interna (hormone production), which are separated from the epithelium by a basement membrane.

e Graafian follicle: Preovulatory follicle with a large follicular cavity. The oocyte is located on an eccentric hillock, the cumulus oophorus, together with a large aggregation of epithelial cells, the corona radiata.

Note: The graafian follicle is approximately 2 cm in diameter—large enough to create a distinct bulge on the ovarian surface.

f Ovulation: The follicle ruptures, and the oocyte is expelled with the cumulus oophorus cells into the cavitas peritonealis. Generally the oocyte is caught by the fimbriated end of the tuba uterina. Some spontaneous bleeding occurs into the follicular cavity.

g Corpus luteum: This is a yellowish structure of very high hormonal activity formed by transformation of the graafian follicle. If the ovum is not fertilized, the corpus luteum involutes and degenerates during the menstrual cycle (becoming the corpus luteum of menstruation). If fertilization takes place, the corpus luteum persists (as the corpus luteum of pregnancy) during the first trimester in response to hormonal stimulation from the zygote, lasting until its hormonal function has been replaced by the placenta.

Note: A new follicle matures every 28 days. However, maturation of each individual follicle takes much longer.

5.9 Pregnancy and Childbirth

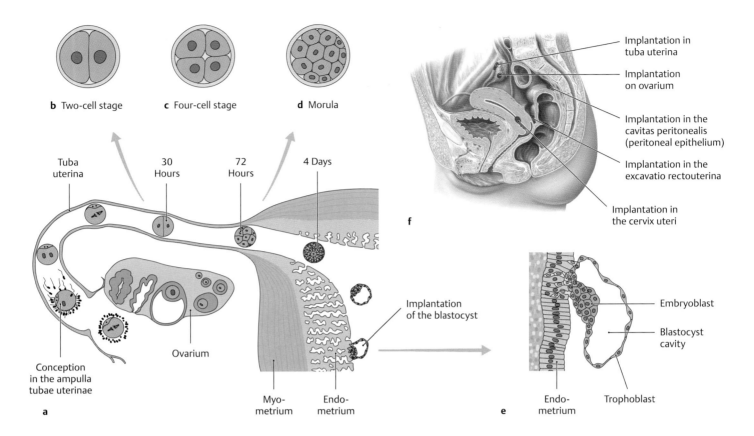

b Two-cell stage   **c** Four-cell stage   **d** Morula

Tuba uterina   30 Hours   72 Hours   4 Days

Implantation in tuba uterina

Implantation on ovarium

Implantation in the cavitas peritonealis (peritoneal epithelium)

Implantation in the excavatio rectouterina

Implantation in the cervix uteri

f

Conception in the ampulla tubae uterinae

Ovarium

Myo-metrium   Endo-metrium

a

Implantation of the blastocyst

Embryoblast

Blastocyst cavity

Endo-metrium   Trophoblast

e

A Phases in the migration of the fertilized ovum and sites of ectopic pregnancy

a Phases in the migration of the fertilized ovum: Normally the zygote migrates to the uterus. The ovum is fertilized in the tuba uterina, usually in the ampulla tubae uterinae. Spermatozoa reach that site by a flagellating tail action that enables them to swim "upstream" against the flow of the ciliated epithelium (positive rheotaxis)—the same current that propels the zygote toward the cavitas uteri. As it migrates through the tuba uterina, the zygote undergoes various stages of development. On approximately the sixth day after ovulation, the blastocyst implants in the endometrium, which has been prepared by secretory transformation (see close-up in **e**).

b–e Show the two- and four-cell stages of development (30 hours), a morula with 16 cells (3 days), and the zygote after implantation (**e**).

f Sites of ectopic pregnancy. Under abnormal conditions, a fertilized ovum may become implanted at various sites outside the cavitas uteri:

- at sites close to the uterus (tubal pregnancy) or
- within the cavitas peritonealis (abdominal pregnancy).

In a tubal pregnancy (e.g., caused by postinflammatory adhesions of the tubal tunica mucosa that hamper zygote migration), there is a risk of tubal wall rupture due to the close confines of the tubal lumen, possibly causing a life-threatening hemorrhage into the cavitas peritonealis.

B Levels of the uterus during pregnancy

a Anterior view; **b** Left lateral view.

The fundus uteri is palpable at different levels during the various lunar months of pregnancy (lunar month = a 28-day period).

Note: At the start of the 10th lunar month, the fundus uteri turns anteriorly and drops to a level that is slightly lower than in the 9th lunar month.

As term approaches, the greatly enlarged uterus presses against almost all the organs in the abdomen and pelvis. In the supine position the uterus may even compress the v. cava inferior, compromising venous return to the heart. In emergency situations, therefore, a pregnant patient should always be placed in the *left lateral decubitus* position to avoid vascular compression.

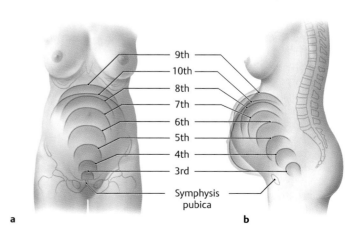

9th
10th
8th
7th
6th
5th
4th
3rd
Symphysis pubica

a   **b**

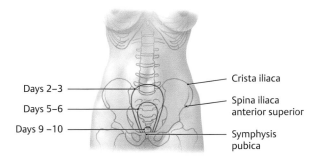

Days 2–3 — Crista iliaca
Days 5–6 — Spina iliaca anterior superior
Days 9–10 — Symphysis pubica

C Postpartum involution of the uterus

Anterior view. With normal postpartum involution of the uterus, the uterine fundus can be palpated and physically examined at various levels. Three palpable bony landmarks (the iliac crest, anterior superior iliac spine, and pubic symphysis) can be helpful in evaluating the level of the uterine fundus.

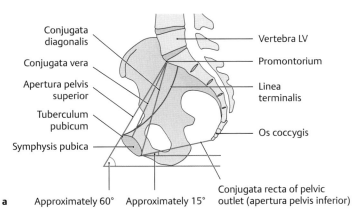

Conjugata diagonalis
Conjugata vera
Apertura pelvis superior
Tuberculum pubicum
Symphysis pubica

Vertebra LV
Promontorium
Linea terminalis
Os coccygis

Conjugata recta of pelvic outlet (apertura pelvis inferior)

a Approximately 60° Approximately 15°

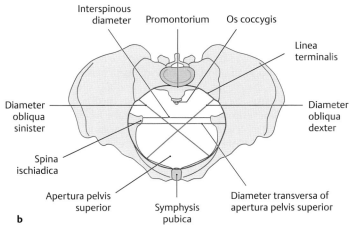

Interspinous diameter Promontorium Os coccygis
Linea terminalis
Diameter obliqua sinister
Diameter obliqua dexter
Spina ischiadica
Apertura pelvis superior
Symphysis pubica
Diameter transversa of apertura pelvis superior

b

D Important obstetric pelvic dimensions: Pelvic planes

a Midsagittal section of the female pelvis, viewed from the left side
b Superior view of a female pelvis.

During parturition, the fetus passes through various planes of the maternal pelvis. The pelvic dimensions of greatest clinical importance are sagittal (smallest anteroposterior diameter). The pelvis has its smallest sagittal diameter at the "true conjugate" (conjugata vera obstetrica),

which is the shortest distance from the posterior surface of the symphysis pubica to the promontorium ossis sacri. That distance should be at least 11 cm; if not, a normal vaginal delivery may be difficult or impossible. The most important fetal dimensions are cranial, particularly the greatest sagittal head diameter. The principal pelvic dimensions are reviewed in **E**.

E Internal dimensions of the female pelvis

Designation	Definition	Length
Conjugata vera obstetrica diameter (true conjugate)	Distance between the promontorium ossis sacri and the posterior border of the symphysis pubica	11 cm
Conjugata diagonalis	Distance between the promontorium ossis sacri and the inferior border of the symphysis pubica	12.5–13 cm
AP diameter of apertura pelvis inferior	Distance between the inferior border of the symphysis pubica and the tip of the os coccygis	9 (+2) cm
Transverse diameter of pelvic inlet plane	Longest distance between the lineae terminales	13 cm
Interspinous diameter	Distance between the spinae ischiadicae	11 cm
Right (I) and left (II) diameter obliqua	Distance between the articulatio sacroiliaca at the level of the linea terminalis and the eminentia iliopubica on the opposite side	12 cm

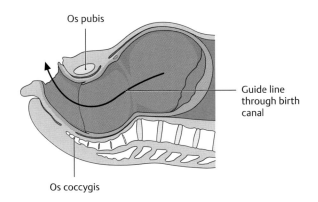

Os pubis
Guide line through birth canal
Os coccygis

F Birth canal in the expulsion phase of labor

(after Rauber and Kopsch)

The cervix uteri, vagina, and diaphragma pelvis have been stretched open to form a "soft-tissue tube." The fetal head, which always rotates its greatest (sagittal) diameter to match the greatest diameter of the current pelvic plane, follows the line indicated. Most babies are delivered in the "occiput anterior" position, with the occiput pointing toward the symphysis pubica.

5.10 Male Genitalia: Accessory Sex Glands

A Accessory sex glands (prostata, glandulae vesiculosae, and glandulae bulbourethrales)

Posterior view of the vesica urinaria, prostata, gll. vesiculosae, and gll. bulbourethrales. The peritoneum and fascia pelvis visceralis have been completely removed; stumps of both ureteres and ductus deferentes have been left in place to aid orientation. Each of the **gll. vesiculosae** consists of a tube approximately 15 cm long that is coiled upon itself to a length of about 5 cm. The secretion from the gll. vesiculosae makes up approximately 70% of the volume of the ejaculate, is slightly alkaline (pH 7.4), and is very high in fructose (energy source for the spermatozoa). The term "seminal vesicle" is misleading in that the gland does not contain spermatocytes. The ductus excretorius of the gl. vesiculosa unites with the ductus deferens to form the ductus ejaculatorius, which passes through the prostata. The gll. vesiculosae develop from the epithelium of the ductus mesonephrici and are situated lateral to the ductus deferentes, which also develop from the ductus mesonephrici. The **gll. bulbourethrales** are embedded in the m. transversus perinei profundus, and their approximately 2- to 4-cm-long ducts open into the posterior aspect of the urethra. They secrete a clear, watery fluid that prepares the urethra for the passage of the sperm. The prostata is described in **B**.

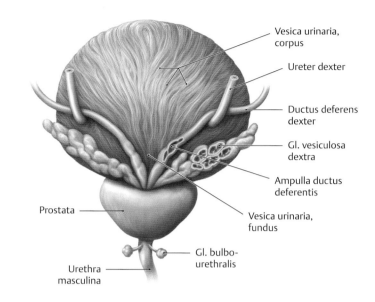

Vesica urinaria, corpus
Ureter dexter
Ductus deferens dexter
Gl. vesiculosa dextra
Ampulla ductus deferentis
Vesica urinaria, fundus
Prostata
Gl. bulbo-urethralis
Urethra masculina

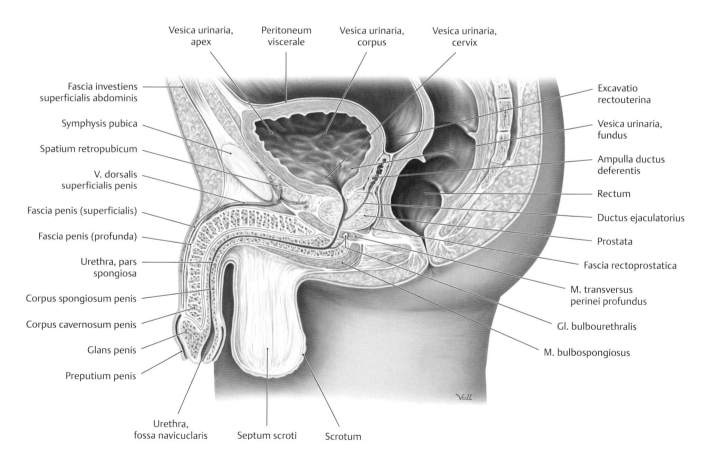

Vesica urinaria, apex
Peritoneum viscerale
Vesica urinaria, corpus
Vesica urinaria, cervix
Fascia investiens superficialis abdominis
Symphysis pubica
Spatium retropubicum
V. dorsalis superficialis penis
Fascia penis (superficialis)
Fascia penis (profunda)
Urethra, pars spongiosa
Corpus spongiosum penis
Corpus cavernosum penis
Glans penis
Preputium penis
Excavatio rectouterina
Vesica urinaria, fundus
Ampulla ductus deferentis
Rectum
Ductus ejaculatorius
Prostata
Fascia rectoprostatica
M. transversus perinei profundus
Gl. bulbourethralis
M. bulbospongiosus
Urethra, fossa navicularis
Septum scroti
Scrotum

B The prostata in situ

Sagittal section through a male pelvis, viewed from the left side, with the vesica urinaria and rectum opened. This drawing is a composite from many planes to demonstrate the peritoneal relationships and the attachment of the gl. vesiculosa to the prostata and urethra. The paramedian ampulla ductus deferentis has been straightened somewhat and projected into the sectional plane with the ductus ejaculatorius and left gl. bulbourethralis. The prostata is located at the ostium urethrae internum and encircles the urethra (see **C**). It borders posteriorly on the anterior wall of the rectum, separated from it by connective-tissue fascia. The prostata has no contact with the peritoneum and lies entirely in the spatium extraperitoneale pelvis. By contrast, the tips of the gll. vesiculosae are frequently covered by peritoneum viscerale.

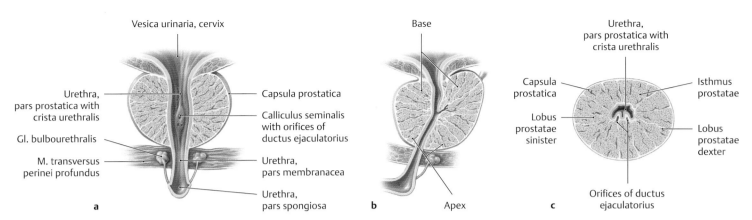

Vesica urinaria, cervix | **Urethra, pars prostatica with crista urethralis**

Urethra, pars prostatica with crista urethralis — Capsula prostatica — Calliculus seminalis with orifices of ductus ejaculatorius — Gl. bulbourethralis — M. transversus perinei profundus — Urethra, pars membranacea — Urethra, pars spongiosa

a **b** Base / Apex **c** Capsula prostatica — Isthmus prostatae — Lobus prostatae sinister — Lobus prostatae dexter — Orifices of ductus ejaculatorius

C Relationship of the prostata to the urethra

a Coronal section (anterior view), **b** sagittal section (left lateral view), and **c** transverse section (superior view) through the prostata and urethra.

The prostata is a chestnut-sized gland consisting of two lateral lobi (dexter and sinister) that are joined posteriorly by the lobus medius and anteriorly by the isthmus prostatae. The entire gland is surrounded by a firm connective-tissue capsule (capsula prostatica). The prostata is a derivative of the urethral epithelium, appearing initially as a posterior epithelial bud that later grows to encircle the pars prostatica urethrae. Histologically, the prostata is composed of 30–50 tubuloalveolar glands that open into the pars prostatica urethrae via approximately 20 excretory ducts. The prostatic secretion makes up approximately 30 % of the volume of the ejaculate. It contains compounds that are important for active sperm motility. The secretion is colorless, watery, and slightly acidic (pH 6.4). It also contains a protein (prostate-specific antigen, PSA) whose serum levels are frequently elevated in patients with a prostatic malignancy.

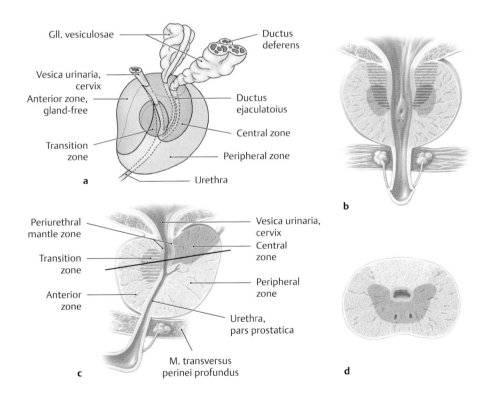

a Gll. vesiculosae — Ductus deferens — Vesica urinaria, cervix — Anterior zone, gland-free — Ductus ejaculatoius — Transition zone — Central zone — Peripheral zone — Urethra

b

c Periurethral mantle zone — Transition zone — Anterior zone — Vesica urinaria, cervix — Central zone — Peripheral zone — Urethra, pars prostatica — M. transversus perinei profundus

d

D Normal values for the male accessory sex glands

Prostata	
Sagittal diameter	ca. 2–3 cm
Width	ca. 4 cm
Thickness	ca. 1–2 cm
Glands	ca. 40 lobules
Duct system	ca. 20 ducts
Secretion	pH 6.4; enzyme-rich
Weight	ca. 20 g

Glandula vesiculosa	
Length – Coiled	ca. 3–5 cm
– Uncoiled	ca. 15 cm
Secretion	pH 7.4; fructose-rich

Glandula bulbourethralis	
Size	Pea-sized
Duct length	ca. 4 cm

E Clinical and histological division of the prostata into zones
(after McNeal)

Schematic representation of the prostata (**a**) viewed in three sections: **b** frontal section, **c** sagittal section; **d** horizontal section.

The most commonly used system for anatomic division of the prostata is based on studies by McNeal. The pars prostatica urethrae serves as a landmark and at the level of the colliculus seminalis angles anteriorly (35 degrees) and divides into a pars proximalis and a pars distalis (**c** and **Cb**). At the level of the colliculus seminalis lies the opening of the utriculus prostaticus (remnant of the ductus paramesonephrici), on each side of which lie the openings of the ductus ejaculatorii. The pars proximalis partis prostaticae urethrae is surrounded like a cuff by the periurethral zone, which is flanked on each side by the transition zone that consists of two lobi that account for not more than 5 % of the glandular tissue of the prostata. Behind it lies the wedge-shaped central zone that accounts for approximately 25% of the prostatic tissue. It is traversed by the ductus ejaculatorii and the utriculus prostaticus. The peripheral zone extends posterolaterally and accounts for 70% of prostatic weight. Anterior prostate tissue consists of a fibromuscular stroma that lacks glands.

Note: Approximately 70 % of prostatic carcinomas occur in the peripheral zone near the capsula prostatica. The most common site of benign prostatic hyperplasia is the transition zone, the volume of which increases significantly as a result (see p. 338).

5.11 Prostate Tumors: Prostatic Carcinoma, Prostatic Hyperplasia; Cancer Screening

Vesica   Subcapsular
urinaria   prostatic carcinoma

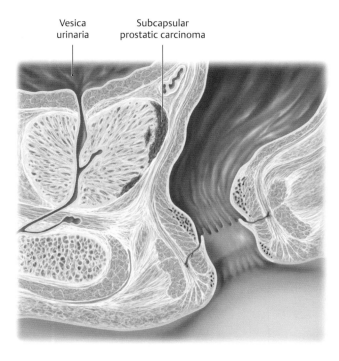

Prostatic   Compressed
hyperplasia   urethra   Rectum

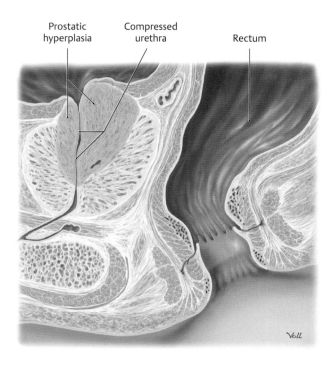

A Prostatic carcinoma

Prostatic carcinoma is the most common urological tumor in males, with 95% of prostatic carcinomas occurring in males between the ages of 45 and 89. The average age at diagnosis is 70. In Germany, 50,000 males are diagnosed each year. It is the third most common cause of cancer related deaths (accounting for 10% of deaths due to cancer). Prostatic carcinomas most often (85%) grow in the peripheral zone of the prostata (see p. 337). Because of its predominantly peripheral location, typical symptoms appear only when the tumor has spread locally. Symptoms indicate bone metastases: back pain, n. ischiadicus pain, and pulling pain in the pelvic region. In almost 50% of patients who are diagnosed with a malignant prostate tumor, the cancer will metastasize which then signifies the incurable stage of the disease. Hence, screening for prostate cancer is crucial to improve the chances of survival. Currently, three tests are routinely performed as part of the screening (see **C**, **D**, and **E**):

- Measurement of prostate-specific antigen (PSA)
- Digital rectal examination (DRE)
- Transrectal ultrasound (TRUS)

Therapeutic concepts: Generally, treatment options are based on the stage of cancer at the time of diagnosis. Usually, a locally confined prostatic carcinoma is treated with surgery (radical prostatectomy) or radiation (e.g., brachytherapy). Because prostate cancers are testosterone-dependent, progressive tumors are often treated with anti-androgens. Testosterone secretion is reduced by suppressing GnRH secretion (GnRH = gonadotropin-releasing-hormone) with the help of synthetic GnRH analogs, which permanently occupy pituitary GnRH receptors (functional castration).

B Benign prostatic hyperplasia (BPH)

Benign prostatic hyperplasia is the most common type of prostatic tumor in older men. BPH is characterized by structural changes accompanied by the formation of nodules particularly in the transition zone (see p. 337), but also often in the peripheral zone, caused by cell proliferation (hyperplasia). Both glandular and stromal proliferation contribute to the hyperplasia (fibromuscular/glandular hyperplasia) and result in an enlarged transition zone and thus the entire prostata. The affected areas are mainly those immediately surrounding the urethra. Compression of the urethra leads to voiding dysfunction including reduction in micturition interval, weak urinary stream and resulting strained efforts to push urine out of the vesica urinaria, and pollakiuria (frequent passing of small volumes of urine). At advanced stages, increasing obstruction of the ostium urethrae internum leads to vesica urinaria wall hypertrophy (trabeculated bladder), residual urine retention and backlog of urine accompanied by the bilateral dilation of the ureteres and the calyceal system of the pelvis renalis.

Diagnostic process: In addition to the patient's history (typical symptoms?) and rectal palpation (enlarged prostata, clearly defined prostata), transvesical and transrectal sonography is used to assess size and structural changes of the prostata and to measure the volume of residual urine. Uroflowmetry measures urine flow (normal values range from 15 to 40 ml/s). Prostate-specific antigen (PSA, see **D**) can be elevated just like with the presence of prostata cancer.

Treatment options: In addition to a "wait and watch" approach (hyperplasia sometimes comes to a standstill), more conservative methods are used to significantly alleviate symptoms (phytotherapy, antiadrenergic therapy, and anti-androgens hormonal treatment–testosterone-dependent hyperplasia). The most common surgical treatment is transurethral resection of the prostata. An electric loop is used to break off small pieces of tissue, which are flushed through the urethra.

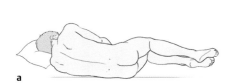

a

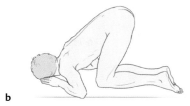

b

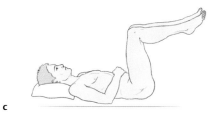

c

C Palpation of the prostata

a Left lateral postion; **b** Knee-elbow position; **c** Lithotomy position; **d** Digital rectal palpation.

The digital rectal examination (DRE) of the prostata is an important screening test and should be performed yearly beginning at age 40. It can be done with the patient in the knee-elbow, lithotomy, or lateral position and starts with the inspection of the rectum. The prostata can be located at the anterior wall of the rectum 7–8 cm from the anus (**d**). Size, surface, and consistency of both lobes, the medial

sulcus, the movability of the rectal mucosa, and the delineation from neighboring tissue are evaluated. The prostata is normally the size of a chestnut and its consistency is like the contracted thenar muscles of the thumb. With benign prostatic hyperplasia (see **B**) the prostata surface is smooth, despite being grossly enlarged, and the rectal tunica mucosa is movable. Prostate cancer (see **A**), however, makes the gland hard and bumpy and reduces the mobility of the rectal tunica mucosa. A soft, tender, ill-defined prostata is a sign of prostate infection.

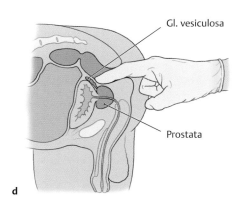

d

D Measurement of prostate-specific antigen (PSA)

Prostate-specific antigen (PSA) is a serine protease that is predominantly produced by the prostata epithelial cells, which are secretorially active. It contributes to the liquefaction of the viscous secretion of the gll. vesiculosae. Thus, PSA is a normal enzyme present in healthy men. Some of it enters the bloodstream and circulates freely (f-PSA) or in a complex formation (c-PSA). Normally, the serum level of total PSA is 4ng/ml, but it can vary for a specific individual. Because PSA formation rate in prostatic carcinoma cells can be up to 10 times higher than in normal

cells, PSA values can be used as a tumor marker (although with some limitations). With slightly elevated levels (4–10 ng/ml), a prostatic carcinoma is detected in 25 % of cases, and in 50 % of cases with a greatly elevated level (greater than 10 ng/ml). Since other benign diseases (benign prostatic hyperplasia, chronic prostatitis), sporting activities (horse riding, bike riding) and simply straining on the toilet due to constipation can lead to elevated PSA levels, the value of PSA-based early detection of prostatic carcinoma is controversial.

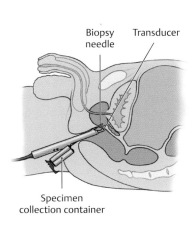

F Prostate biopsy guided by transrectal ultrasound (TRUS)

Ultrasound-guided transrectal trephine biopsy is performed to provide histological proof of prostatic carcinoma. The transrectal ultrasound is used to guide the biopsy needle either to systematically chosen areas of the prostata or to palpable lumps in suspicious areas. The needle, which is passed through the needle guide attached to the probe, is constantly visible on the ultrasound image. In this way, suspicious areas can be precisely located. In trephine biopsy usually 8-18 thin tissue cylinders are obtained, which will then be histologically assessed. The fact that a biopsy only evaluates parts of the prostata limits the conclusiveness of the results.

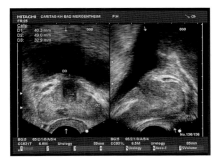

a   b

E Transrectal ultrasound (TRUS)

a Insertion of the ultrasound probe into the rectum; **b** Images of the prostata in transverse and sagittal section for the assessment of prostatic volume (from: Dietrich, CH.: Endosonographie, Lehrbuch und Atlas des endoskopischen Ultraschalls. Thieme, Stuttgart 2008).

Transrectal ultrasound or transrectal prostata sonography is a simple, quick and inexpensive procedure and thus the primary diagnostic imaging technique for evaluating the prostata. A gel-filled condom is placed over a probe,

which is inserted into the rectum. This method allows for optimal coupling to the anterior wall of the rectum to minimize interference with air or feces. With a frequency of 7.5 MHz, high quality images can be taken at a depth of 1–5 cm from the surface of the prostata. To aid orientation, it is first displayed in transverse section. By turning the probe, the prostata can be evaluated in a sagittal section. Displaying the prostata in both sections helps to determine the exact size and thus volume of the prostata.

5.12 Male Genitalia: Scrotum, Testis, and Epididymis

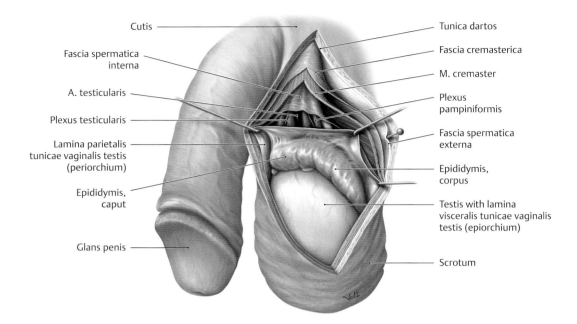

A The scrotum and coverings of the testis in situ

Left lateral view with the scrotum opened in layers. The testis is a paired organ having the approximate size and shape of a plum (see **D**). It is divided by fibrous septa into approximately 350 lobuli. The layers of the scrotum and coverings of the testis are formed by the layers of the anterior abdominal wall during the developmental descent of the testis (see **E**). As the testis descends, it carries with it a finger-shaped process of peritoneum (processus vaginalis peritonei) through the canalis inguinalis; normally this process becomes obliterated and separated from the cavitas peritonealis at the anulus inguinalis profundus. Thus the peritoneum forms a closed sac within the scrotum (tunica vaginalis) composed of a lamina visceralis and a lamina parietalis. An abnormal collection of serous fluid in the space between the two peritoneal layers (hydrocele) may exert pressure on the testis, causing clinical complaints. Occasionally, however, the peritoneal process remains patent and gives rise to a congenital indirect inguinal hernia.

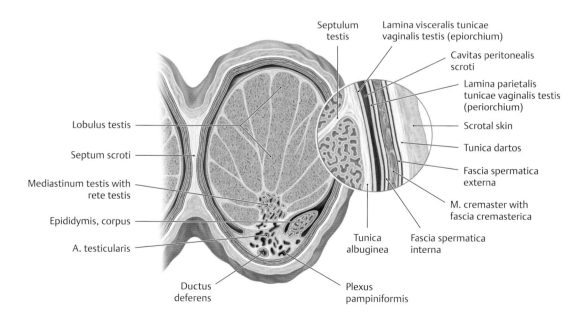

B Scrotum and coverings of the testis in cross-section

Transverse section through the right testis, viewed from above. The magnified view shows the various layers that make up the coverings of the testis. The testis is surrounded by a firm fibrous capsule, the tunica albuginea. Fine connective-tissue septa radiate inward from the tunica albuginea to the mediastinum testis, subdividing the testis into approximately 350–370 lobules that contain the tubuli seminiferi (see **C**). The tubuli seminiferi are the sites where the spermatocytes develop (spermatogenesis). Groups of cells embedded in the interstitial connective tissue produce testosterone.

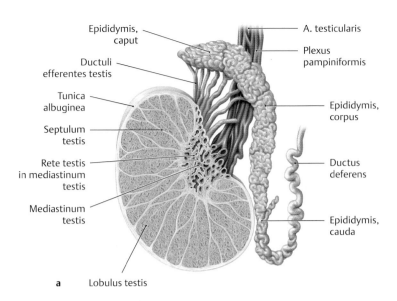

a Lobulus testis

b

Lobulus testis with ductuli seminiferi contorti

Ductus epididymis with cauda epididymidis

C Structure of the testis and epididymis

Left lateral view of the left testis and epididymis. The testis has been sectioned in the sagittal plane, and the epididymis has been elevated from the testis. The wedge-shaped lobuli of the testis contain the **tubuli seminiferi** (tubuli seminiferi contorti, approximately 3 cm long coiled, 20 cm long uncoiled), where the sperm develop. The tissue between the tubuli seminiferi contorti contains the interstitial (Leydig) cells, which produce androgens, principally testosterone. The tubuli semi-niferi contorti continue into the tubuli seminiferi *recti*, which continue into the rete testis, a network of anastomosing epithelium-lined chan-nels. The rete testis is connected to approximately 12 ductuli efferentes testis, which open into the epididymis. Attached to the posterior aspect of the testis, the epididymis is the organ of storage and maturation for the spermatozoa. The caput epididymidis consists mostly of the ductuli

efferentes testis, while its corpus and cauda consist of the highly convo-luted ductus epididymidis (approximately 6 m long when unraveled). In the caput epididymidis, the ductuli efferentes testis open into the duc-tus epididymidis, which is continuous at its caudal end with the ductus deferens.

Note: The testis and epididymis lie inside the scrotum and *outside* the cavitas abdominalis because the temperature within the body cavity is too high for normal spermatogenesis. Thus, failure of the testis to descend normally into the scrotum (i.e., an inguinal testis) is frequently associated with infertility.

The formation and maturation of spermatocytes in the testis, the migra-tion of spermatozoa in the epididymis, and their final storage in the cau-dal part of the epididymal duct takes approximately 80 days.

D Normal values for the testis and epididymis

Testis		Epididymis	
Weight	ca. 20 g	Length of ductus epididymidis	
Length	ca. 4 cm	– Uncoiled	ca. 6 m
Width	ca. 2 cm	– Coiled	ca. 6 cm
350–370 lobuli testis			
Approximately 12 ductuli efferentes testis			

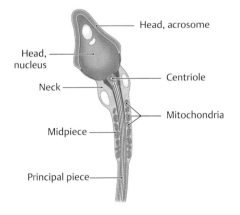

E Coverings of the testis and layers of the abdominal wall

The canalis inguinalis is an evagination of the abdominal wall. As a result, the anatomical layers of the abdominal wall have their counter-parts in the layers of the scrotum and testicular coverings.

Layers of the abdominal wall	Coverings of the funiculus spermaticus and testis
• Abdominal skin and funiculus spermaticus of superficial fascia	→ Scrotal skin with tunica dartos
• Aponeurosis musculi obliqui externi abdominis	→ Fascia spermatica externa
• M. obliquus internus abdominis and its aponeurosis	→ M. cremaster and its fascia
• Fascia transversalis	→ Fascia spermatica interna
• Peritoneum	→ Tunica vaginalis: lamina parietalis and lamina visceralis

F Ultrastructure of a mature spermatozoon

It takes approximately 80 days for a spermatic stem cell (spermatogo-nium) to develop into a mature spermatozoon. The spermatogonia are formed in the convoluted seminiferous tubules, while final maturation takes place in the epididymis. The ultrastructural features of the sper-matozoon, which is approximately 60 μm long (with tail), include the following:

• The *head* with the acrosome and nucleus
• The *tail* (flagellum), which contains the axonema (axial filament) and consists of several parts:
  – Neck
  – Midpiece
  – Principal piece
  – End piece (not shown here)

341

5.13 Male Genitalia: Seminiferous Structures and Ejaculate

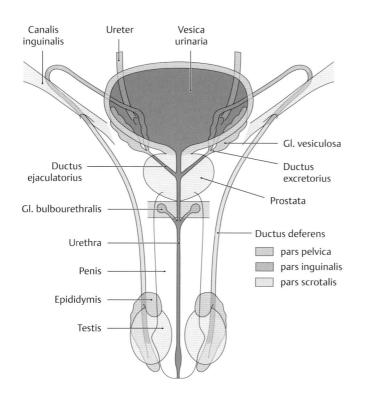

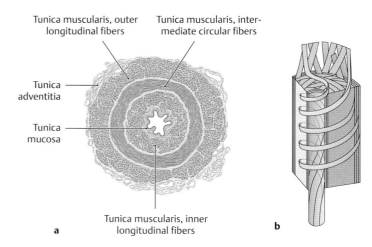

A Overview of the seminiferous structures

Anterior view of the male reproductive tract. The vesica urinaria is also shown to aid orientation.

Note: The urethra masculina serves as a common urinary and genital passage.

The ductus deferens and the ductus excretorius of the gl. vesiculosa join to form the ductus ejaculatorius, which opens into the urethra (see **C**).

B Wall structure and musculature of the ductus deferens

a Wall structure of the ductus deferens, cross-section through the lumen. The ductus deferens (vas deferens) is approximately 40 cm long and 3 mm in diameter. It arises in continuity with the ductus epididymidis at the caudal end of the epididymis. Its function is to transport the sperm suspension rapidly toward the urethra during ejaculation. It is equipped for this task with powerful smooth muscle fibers that appear to be arranged in three layers (longitudinal, circular, and longitudinal; see **b**). Facing the lumen of the ductus deferens is a simple columnar epithelium. Close to the epididymis the epithelium becomes pseudostratified, and many cells bear stereocilia (non-motile cellular projections).

b Musculature of the ductus deferens, three-dimensional representation of the muscle fiber pattern (after Rauber and Kopsch). The smooth muscle of the ductus deferens appears to have a three-layered arrangement when viewed in cross-section. Actually, however, the muscle fibers are arranged in a continuous pattern that spirals around the duct lumen in turns of varying obliquity. The smooth-muscle fibers of the ductus deferens have an extremely rich sympathetic innervation, as ejaculation is triggered by the sympathetic nervous system.

C Site of spermatogenesis and pathway of sperm transport

The seminiferous structures in the strict sense consist of the ductuli efferentes testis, ductus epididymidis, and ductus deferens.

Testis	• Tubuli seminiferi contorti (spermatogenesis) • Tubuli seminiferi recti • Rete testis • Ductuli efferentes testis
Epididymis • Caput	• Ductuli efferentes testis (open into ductus epididymidis)
• Corpus • Cauda	• Ductus epididymidis • Ductus epididymidis (opens into ductus deferens)
Canalis inguinalis and cavitas pelvis	• Ductus deferens
Prostata	• Ductus ejaculatorius (union of ductus deferens and ductus excretorius of gl. vesiculosa)
Diaphragma pelvis and penis (corpus spongiosum)	• Urethra

D The ejaculate (normal values and terminology)

The ejaculate consists of spermatozoa and seminal fluid, which comes mainly from the gll. vesiculosae (approximately 70%) and prostata (approximately 30%).

Quantity pH	2–6 ml 7.0–7.8
Sperm count	ca. 40 million spermatozoa/mL (40–50% of which show vigorous motility; at least 60% are structurally normal)
Length of spermatozoa	ca. 60 μm
Normospermia Aspermia Hypospermia	Normal ejaculate No ejaculate <2 mL of ejaculate
Normozoospermia Azoospermia Oligozoospermia	Normal sperm count (see above) No spermatozoa <20 million spermatozoa/mL
Necrozoospermia Teratozoospermia	All spermatozoa are motionless >60% of spermatozoa are structurally abnormal

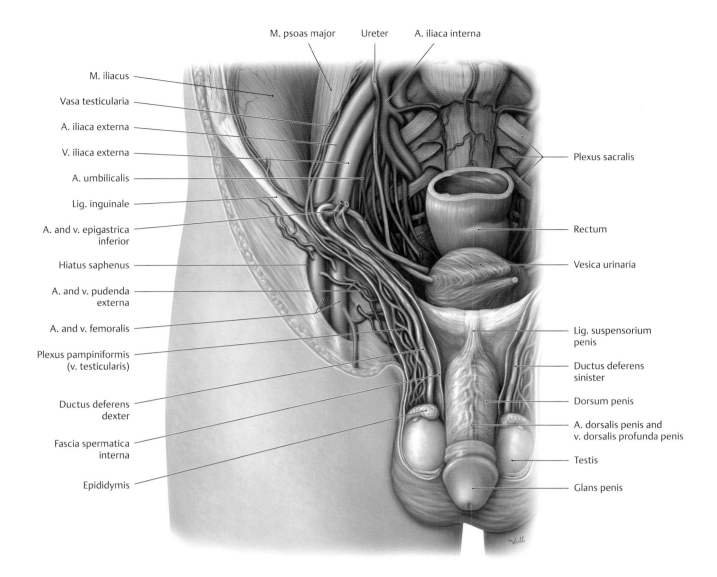

M. psoas major Ureter A. iliaca interna

M. iliacus

Vasa testicularia

A. iliaca externa

V. iliaca externa

A. umbilicalis

Lig. inguinale

A. and v. epigastrica inferior

Hiatus saphenus

A. and v. pudenda externa

A. and v. femoralis

Plexus pampiniformis (v. testicularis)

Ductus deferens dexter

Fascia spermatica interna

Epididymis

Plexus sacralis

Rectum

Vesica urinaria

Lig. suspensorium penis

Ductus deferens sinister

Dorsum penis

A. dorsalis penis and v. dorsalis profunda penis

Testis

Glans penis

E The funiculus spermaticus in situ

Anterior view. The canalis inguinalis has been opened on both sides, and the coverings of the funiculus spermaticus have been opened anteriorly to show the course of the ductus deferens. The canalis inguinalis is markedly larger in the male than in the female due to the presence of the funiculus spermaticus. This larger canal and the larger inguinal ring predispose the male to the herniation of abdominal viscera through the canalis inguinalis (inguinal hernia).

Note: The ductus deferens passes lateral to the a. and v. epigastrica inferior. This relationship should be noted in operations on the inguinal ring to avoid vascular injury.

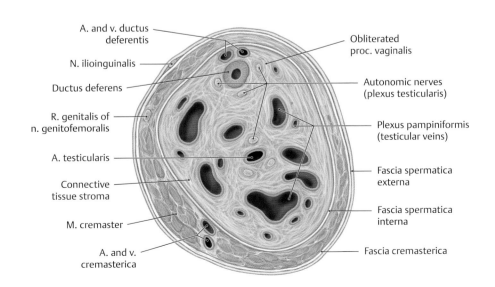

A. and v. ductus deferentis

N. ilioinguinalis

Ductus deferens

R. genitalis of n. genitofemoralis

A. testicularis

Connective tissue stroma

M. cremaster

A. and v. cremasterica

Obliterated proc. vaginalis

Autonomic nerves (plexus testicularis)

Plexus pampiniformis (testicular veins)

Fascia spermatica externa

Fascia spermatica interna

Fascia cremasterica

F Contents of the funiculus spermaticus

Transverse section through the funiculus spermaticus to display the wall layers of the cord and the arrangement of its contents. Even a normally developed venous network (plexus pampiniformis) may be affected by abnormal varicose dilation about the testis (varicocele, due for example to a venous outflow obstruction) and may raise the temperature of the testis, leading to decreased fertility.

Note: The plexus pampiniformis drains into the v. testicularis. The v. testicularis dextra opens into the v. cava inferior, while the v. testicularis sinistra runs close to the polus inferior of the ren and enters the v. renalis at almost a 90° angle. Thus, it is more common for varicoceles to develop on the left side than on the right side in response to a condition that obstructs testicular venous flow (mass on the polus inferior renis, vein entering at a hemodynamically unfavorable angle).

343

5.14 Branches of the Arteria Iliaca Interna: Overview of Arteries Supplying the Pelvic Organs and Pelvic Wall

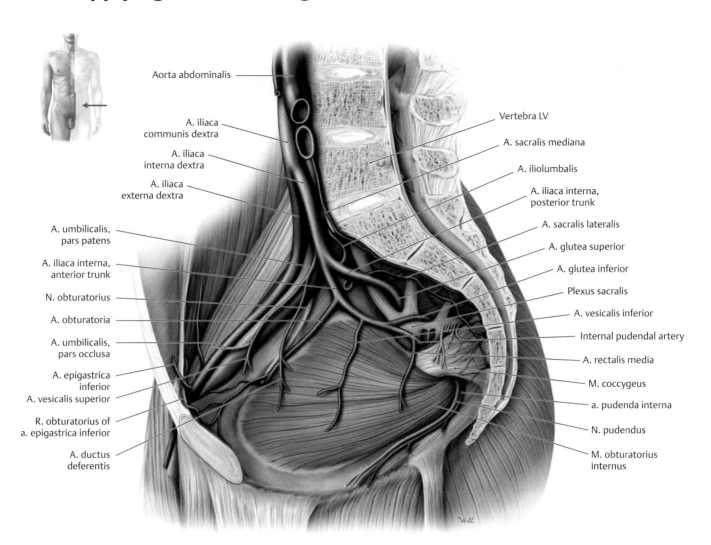

Aorta abdominalis

A. iliaca communis dextra

A. iliaca interna dextra

A. iliaca externa dextra

A. umbilicalis, pars patens

A. iliaca interna, anterior trunk

N. obturatorius

A. obturatoria

A. umbilicalis, pars occlusa

A. epigastrica inferior

A. vesicalis superior

R. obturatorius of a. epigastrica inferior

A. ductus deferentis

Vertebra LV

A. sacralis mediana

A. iliolumbalis

A. iliaca interna, posterior trunk

A. sacralis lateralis

A. glutea superior

A. glutea inferior

Plexus sacralis

A. vesicalis inferior

Internal pudendal artery

A. rectalis media

M. coccygeus

a. pudenda interna

N. pudendus

M. obturatorius internus

A Branches of the right arteria iliaca interna in the male pelvis
Sagittal section viewed from the left side, idealized, the pelvic organs have been removed.
The a. iliaca interna arises from the a. iliaca communis. In 60% of cases it divides anterior to the m. piriformis (see **D**) into an anterior and posterior trunk. The anterior trunk gives off visceral branches and also parietal

branches to the pelvic wall, while the posterior trunk gives off branches only to the pelvic wall. The sequence of the branches is shown in **C**.
Note the relationship of the a. iliaca interior and its branches to the plexus sacralis. Several branches of the a. iliaca interna "disappear" behind this nerve plexus.

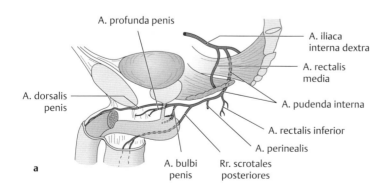

A. profunda penis

A. dorsalis penis

a

A. iliaca interna dextra

A. rectalis media

A. pudenda interna

A. rectalis inferior

A. perinealis

A. bulbi penis   Rr. scrotales posteriores

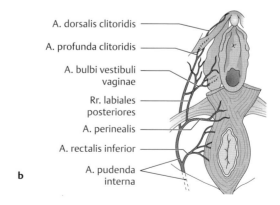

A. dorsalis clitoridis

A. profunda clitoridis

A. bulbi vestibuli vaginae

Rr. labiales posteriores

A. perinealis

A. rectalis inferior

A. pudenda interna

b

B Course and branches of the right arteria pudenda interna on the pelvic floor
The a. pudenda interna is only partially visible in **A**. This diagram illustrates its further course.

a Course of the artery in the male (same perspective as in **A**);
b Course of the artery in the female. The course of the a. pudenda interna is analogous to its course in the male pelvis. An inferior view is shown to supplement the lateral view in **a**, and because this view is important in surgical procedures on the female diaphragma pelvis.

C Sequence of branches of the arteria iliaca interna

Each a. iliaca interna supplies the walls and organs of the pelvis with five parietal branches and five or six visceral branches (→ = "gives off").

Parietal branches (pelvic walls)

A. iliolumbalis to the lateral pelvic wall	→ *R. lumbalis* → *R. spinalis* → *R. iliacus*
Aa. sacrales laterales to the posterior pelvic wall	→ *Rr. spinales*
A. obturatoria to the medial thigh and lateral pelvic wall	→ *R. pubicus* → *R. acetabularis* → *R. anterior* → *R. posterior*
A. glutea superior to the gluteal region	→ *R. superficialis* → *R. profundus*
A. glutea inferior to the gluteal region	→ *A. comitans nervi ischiadici*

Visceral branches (pelvic organs)

A. umbilicalis pars patens gives off	→ *A. ductus deferentis* → *Aa. vesicales superiores (to the vesica urinaria)*
A. vesicalis inferior to the fundus vesicae urinariae	→ *Rr. prostatici*
A. uterina to the uterus, tubae uterinae, vagina, and ovaria	→ *Rr. helicini* → *Rr. vaginales* → *R. ovaricus* → *R. tubarius*

A. vaginalis
May arise as a separate branch from the a. iliaca interna (as noted here) or, more commonly, from the a. vesicalis inferior or a. uterina ("vaginal azygos artery")

A. rectalis media to the ampulla recti and m. levator ani	→ *Rr. vaginales (f)* → *Rr. prostatici (m)*
A. pudenda interna (included with the visceral branches because it gives off the a. rectalis inferior)	→ *A. rectalis inferior (to the terminal rectum, etc.)* → *A. perinealis* → *Rr. scrotales posteriores (m),* *rr. labiales posteriores (f)* → *A. urethralis* → *A. bulbi vestibuli (f), a. bulbi penis (m)* → *A. dorsalis clitoridis (f), a. dorsalis penis (m)* → *A. profunda clitoridis (f), a. profunda penis (m)* → *Aa. perforantes penis*

D Arterial pathways in the pelvic wall

Medial view of right hemipelvis showing the pelvic apertures that transmit the arteries and corresponding veins. There are a total of six pathways, whose landmarks are the m. piriformis, lig. sacrospinale, lig. sacrotuberale, lig. inguinale, and membrana obturatoria (see also **E**).

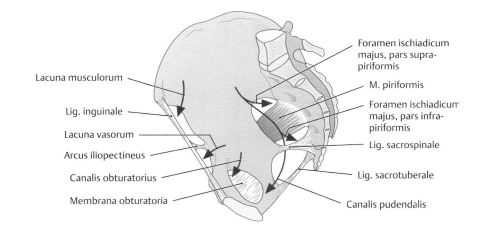

Lacuna musculorum
Lig. inguinale
Lacuna vasorum
Arcus iliopectineus
Canalis obturatorius
Membrana obturatoria

Foramen ischiadicum majus, pars suprapiriformis
M. piriformis
Foramen ischiadicum majus, pars infrapiriformis
Lig. sacrospinale
Lig. sacrotuberale
Canalis pudendalis

E Neurovascular tracts on the pelvic wall

There are six major neurovascular tracts on the pelvic walls, four of which (*) contain branches from the a. iliaca interna.

Tract	Neurovascular structures transmitted
Posterior ① Foramen ischiadicum majus, suprapiriform part* (above the piriformis)	A. and v. glutea superior, n. gluteus superior
② Foramen ischiadicum minus, infrapiriform part* (below the piriformis)	A. and v. glutea inferior, n. gluteus inferior, n. ischiadicus, a. and v. pudenda interna, n. pudendus, n. cutaneus femoris posterior
On pelvic floor ③ Canalis pudendalis*	A. and v. pudenda interna, n. pudendus
Lateral ④ Canalis obturatorius*	A. and v. obturatoria, n. obturatorius
Anterior ⑤ Lacuna musculorum (posterior to lig. inguinale, lateral to arcus iliopectineus)	N. femoralis, n. cutaneus femoris lateralis
⑥ Lacuna vasorum (posterior to lig. inguinale, medial to arcus iliopectineus)	A. and v. femoralis, lymphatic vessels (the a. femoralis is a branch of the a. iliaca externa), r. femoralis of n. genitofemoralis

5.15 Vascularization of the Male Pelvic Organs

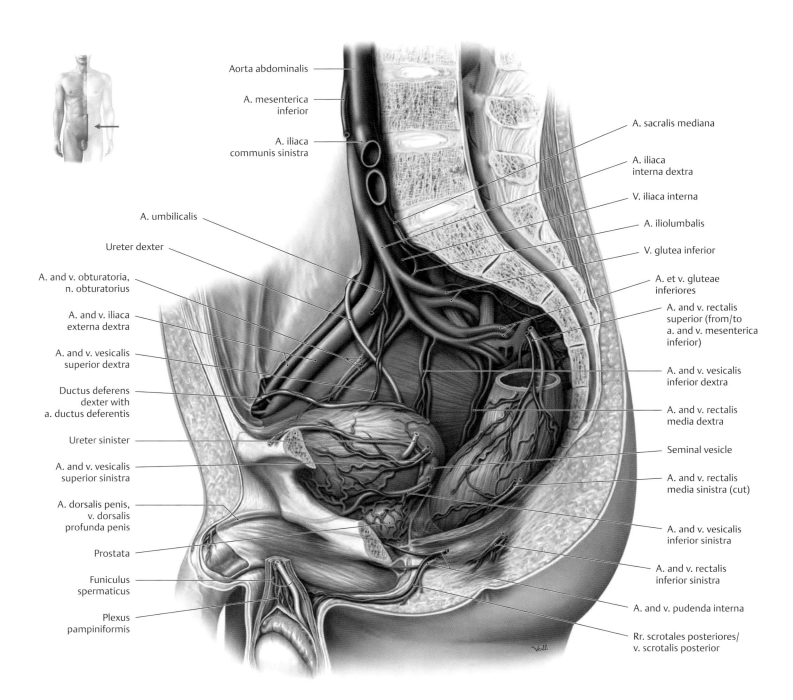

Aorta abdominalis

A. mesenterica inferior

A. iliaca communis sinistra

A. umbilicalis

Ureter dexter

A. and v. obturatoria, n. obturatorius

A. and v. iliaca externa dextra

A. and v. vesicalis superior dextra

Ductus deferens dexter with a. ductus deferentis

Ureter sinister

A. and v. vesicalis superior sinistra

A. dorsalis penis, v. dorsalis profunda penis

Prostata

Funiculus spermaticus

Plexus pampiniformis

A. sacralis mediana

A. iliaca interna dextra

V. iliaca interna

A. iliolumbalis

V. glutea inferior

A. et v. gluteae inferiores

A. and v. rectalis superior (from/to a. and v. mesenterica inferior)

A. and v. vesicalis inferior dextra

A. and v. rectalis media dextra

Seminal vesicle

A. and v. rectalis media sinistra (cut)

A. and v. vesicalis inferior sinistra

A. and v. rectalis inferior sinistra

A. and v. pudenda interna

Rr. scrotales posteriores/ v. scrotalis posterior

A Arterial supply and venous drainage of the pelvic organs in the male (overview)

Right hemipelvis (compiled from multiple sagittal sections) viewed from the left side, idealized. The pelvic organs derive their **arterial supply** from the visceral branches of the a. iliaca interna. Their **venous drainage** is by corresponding veins (often running parallel to the arteries), which drain to the v. iliaca interna. The veins, unlike the arteries, are frequently multiple on each side of the pelvis and are often expanded near the organs to form large plexuses. The main differences in the arterial supply and venous drainage of the pelvic organs in the male and female are based on the copious blood supply to the uterus and vagina in the female: The uterus and vagina are supplied by *their own* major vessels. In the male, however, the accessory sex glands are supplied by smaller branches arising from the vessels of nearby organs (vesica urinaria, rectum).

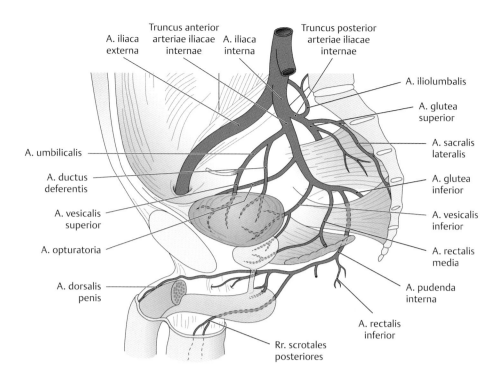

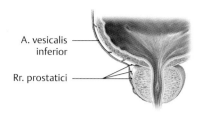

D Arterial supply of the prostata
Coronal section, anterior view. Most rr. prostatici arise from the a. vesicalis inferior, and a smaller number arise from the a. rectalis media (not shown here). The rr. prostatici ramify into a great many branchlets outside the capsula prostatica.

B Sequence of branches of the right arteria iliaca interna and their projection onto the male pelvis

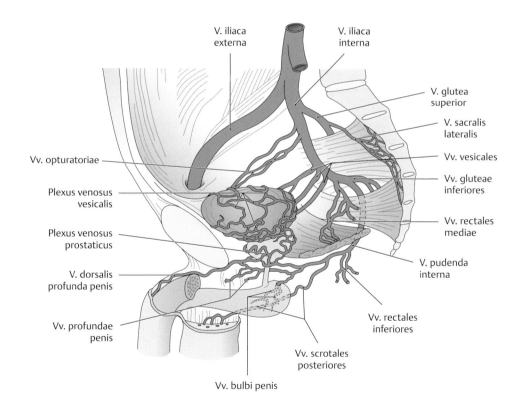

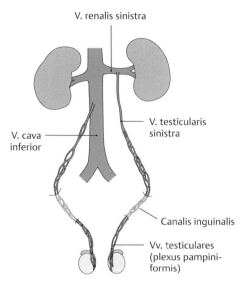

E Asymmetric venous drainage of the right and left testes
Venous blood from the testis and epididymis flows into the vv. testiculares in the area of the mediastinum testis. Especially distally, these veins form an elongated venous network called the plexus pampiniformis. The plexus surrounds branches of the a. testicularis and runs with it through the canalis inguinalis into the retroperitoneum where the v. testicularis dextra opens into the v. cava inferior and the v. testicularis sinistra empties into the left v. renalis. The asymmetric venous drainage is of clinical significance: The v. testicularis sinistra opens into the left v. renalis at a right angle. This creates a physiological constriction that can obstruct outflow from the v. testicularis sinistra, which can result in enlargements called varicoceles (see p. 343) of the v. testicularis sinistra and thus of the plexus pampiniformis. As a result, the plexus pampiniformis can no longer perform its "thermostat" function (cooling of blood to the testis in the a. testicularis) leading to hyperthermia, which affects the fertility of the left testis.

C Venous drainage of the vesica urinaria and male genitalia
Large venous plexuses around the vesica urinaria (plexus venosus vesicalis) and prostata (plexus venosus prostaticus) drain through the vv. vesicales to the v. iliaca interna. An anastomotic connection between the plexus venosus prostaticus and plexus venosus vertebralis (not shown here, aids venous drainage of the columna vertebralis and canalis spinalis) creates a route by which tumor cells from a prostatic carcinoma may metastasize to the spine (which may first come to clinical attention as back pain).

5.16 Vascularization of the Female Pelvic Organs

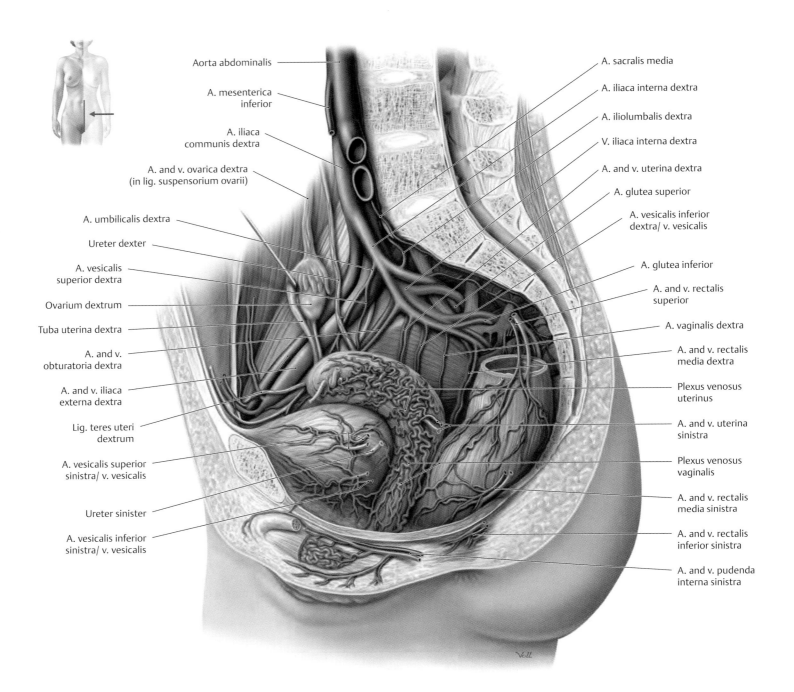

Aorta abdominalis

A. mesenterica inferior

A. iliaca communis dextra

A. and v. ovarica dextra (in lig. suspensorium ovarii)

A. umbilicalis dextra

Ureter dexter

A. vesicalis superior dextra

Ovarium dextrum

Tuba uterina dextra

A. and v. obturatoria dextra

A. and v. iliaca externa dextra

Lig. teres uteri dextrum

A. vesicalis superior sinistra/ v. vesicalis

Ureter sinister

A. vesicalis inferior sinistra/ v. vesicalis

A. sacralis media

A. iliaca interna dextra

A. iliolumbalis dextra

V. iliaca interna dextra

A. and v. uterina dextra

A. glutea superior

A. vesicalis inferior dextra/ v. vesicalis

A. glutea inferior

A. and v. rectalis superior

A. vaginalis dextra

A. and v. rectalis media dextra

Plexus venosus uterinus

A. and v. uterina sinistra

Plexus venosus vaginalis

A. and v. rectalis media sinistra

A. and v. rectalis inferior sinistra

A. and v. pudenda interna sinistra

A Arterial supply and venous drainage of the pelvic organs in the female (overview)

Female pelvic organs viewed from the left side.

Arterial supply: The uterus is supplied by the a. uterina, which gives off a r. tubarius and a r. ovaricus. The vesica urinaria receives its blood supply from the aa. vesicales superiores and a. vesicalis inferior. The rectum receives supply from the a. rectalis media, a branch of the a. iliaca interna, and from the a. rectalis inferior, which arises from the a. pudenda interna. The a. pudenda interna also supplies the diaphragma pelvis and the external female genital organs. A characteristic of the ovarium is that it has two sources of blood supply: because the ovaria descend during embryonic development, they drag their vascular structures (a. and v. ovarica) with them from the upper abdomen into the pelvic region (there the a. ovarica gives off a r. tubae to the tuba uterina) where the a. ovarica anastomoses with the a. uterina. The

a. uterina runs in the lig. latum uteri to the uterus where it crosses the ureter (see p. 351). The a. uterina reaches the uterus at the junction of the corpus and cervix uteri. There it often gives off a r. vaginalis and from this point ascends in a torturous manner to the uteri. This torturous course enables the a. uterina to elongate during pregnancy when the uterus enlarges.

Venous drainage: The uterus is drained by the plexus venosus uterinus into the v. uterina, which runs a course analogous to the artery. The v. uterina empties into the v. iliaca interna. The v. ovarica dextra carries blood from its corresponding ovarium directly to the v. cava inferior while the v. ovarica sinistra drains into the left v. renalis before reaching the v. cava inferior. The vesica urinaria drains through the vv. vesicales. Parts of the rectum that are supplied by branches of the a. iliaca interna drain through same-named veins into the v. illiaca interna.

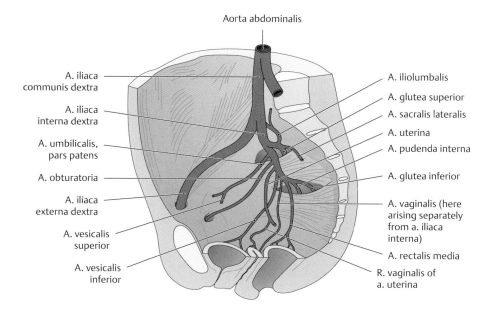

Aorta abdominalis

A. iliaca communis dextra

A. iliaca interna dextra

A. umbilicalis, pars patens

A. obturatoria

A. iliaca externa dextra

A. vesicalis superior

A. vesicalis inferior

A. iliolumbalis

A. glutea superior

A. sacralis lateralis

A. uterina

A. pudenda interna

A. glutea inferior

A. vaginalis (here arising separately from a. iliaca interna)

A. rectalis media

R. vaginalis of a. uterina

B Sequence of branches of the arteria iliaca interna in the female pelvis

Left lateral view. The vessels to the uterus and vagina mark the principal difference from the vasculature of the male pelvis (see also **B**, p.347). The **uterus** receives a large vessel, the a. uterina, which usually arises separately from the a. iliaca interna (the analogous vessel in the male, the a. ductus deferentis, usually branches from the a. umbilicalis). The a. uterina may also arise from the a. rectalis media, which is larger in those cases. The arterial supply to the **vagina** is also subject to variation. The vagina may be supplied by a separate a. vaginalis branching from the a. iliaca interna or by a r. vaginalis arising from either the a. uterina or the a. vesicalis inferior.

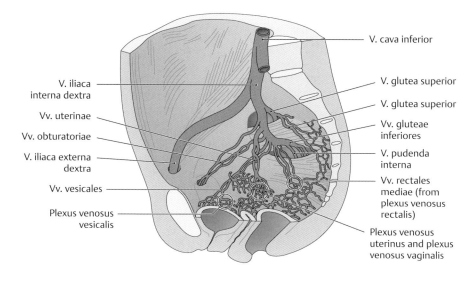

V. cava inferior

V. iliaca interna dextra

Vv. uterinae

Vv. obturatoriae

V. iliaca externa dextra

Vv. vesicales

Plexus venosus vesicalis

V. glutea superior

V. glutea superior

Vv. gluteae inferiores

V. pudenda interna

Vv. rectales mediae (from plexus venosus rectalis)

Plexus venosus uterinus and plexus venosus vaginalis

C Venous drainage of the organs of the female pelvis

Left lateral view showing the right v. iliaca interna. The female pelvic organs are generally drained by four plexuses (see also **Ac**, p. 350):

- Plexus venosus vesicalis (vv. vesicales)
- Plexus venosus vaginalis (vaginal veins)
- Plexus venosus uterinus (vv. uterinae)
- Plexus venosus rectalis (vv. rectales mediae).

The vv. rectales mediae and inferiores drain to the v. iliaca interna. The v. rectalis superior drains into the v. mesenterica inferior. (The vv. rectales superior and inferiores are not shown here.)

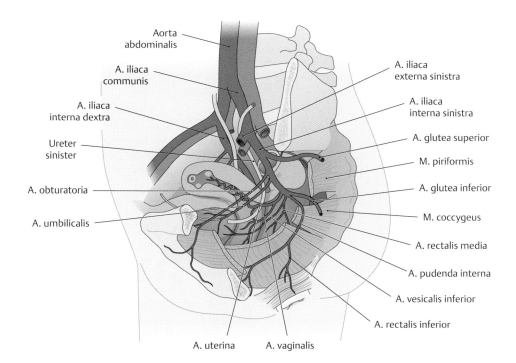

Aorta abdominalis

A. iliaca communis

A. iliaca interna dextra

Ureter sinister

A. obturatoria

A. umbilicalis

A. iliaca externa sinistra

A. iliaca interna sinistra

A. glutea superior

M. piriformis

A. glutea inferior

M. coccygeus

A. rectalis media

A. pudenda interna

A. vesicalis inferior

A. rectalis inferior

A. uterina   A. vaginalis

D Arterial supply of the uterus, vagina, and vesica urinaria

View into the pelvis from the left side. The lig. latum uteri has been cut open to display the branches of the left a. iliaca interna.
Note: The serpentine course of the a. uterina along the corpus uteri is particularly well demonstrated in this lateral view (see also **A**). The origins of the a. uterina and a. vaginalis are subject to considerable variation.

5.17 Vascularization of the Female Internal Genitalia and Vesica Urinaria

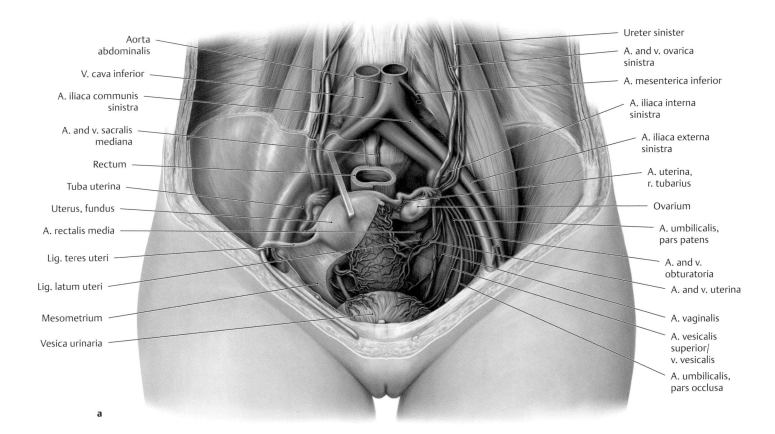

Aorta abdominalis
V. cava inferior
A. iliaca communis sinistra
A. and v. sacralis mediana
Rectum
Tuba uterina
Uterus, fundus
A. rectalis media
Lig. teres uteri
Lig. latum uteri
Mesometrium
Vesica urinaria

Ureter sinister
A. and v. ovarica sinistra
A. mesenterica inferior
A. iliaca interna sinistra
A. iliaca externa sinistra
A. uterina, r. tubarius
Ovarium
A. umbilicalis, pars patens
A. and v. obturatoria
A. and v. uterina
A. vaginalis
A. vesicalis superior/ v. vesicalis
A. umbilicalis, pars occlusa

a

A Vascularization of the female internal genital organs

a Overview; all of the peritoneum has been removed on the left side and most has been removed on the right side; the uterus has been straightened and tilted to the right; **b** Arterial supply; **c** Venous drainage.

The female internal genital organs are supplied by two large arteries or their branches:

- Ovarium: receives its arterial supply from two sources: predominantly from the a. ovarica as well as from the r. ovaricus of the a. uterina (see ovarian arcade below);
- Uterus: from the a. uterina,
- Tuba uterina: from one branch each of the aa. ovarica and uterina.

The two large arteries arise from different trunks: the a. ovarica usually originates from the aorta abdominalis (for variants see **C**), the a. uterina from the a. iliaca interna (visceral branch).
Note the ovarian arcade (see **b**), which needs to be noted during surgery: It is formed by the a. ovarica and the r. ovaricus of the a. uterina.

The female genital organs are drained by two large veins or venous plexuses:

- Uterus: by the plexus venosus uterinus and partially by the plexus venosus vaginalis that empty into the v. iliaca interna
- Ovaria: on the right side by the v. ovarica dextra directly into the v. cava interna, and on the left side into the left v. renalis before reaching the v. cava inferior; by the plexus venosus ovaricus: venous anastomosis between v. ovarica and v. uterina (plexus drains into both veins)

Arteries and veins run within the peritoneum: the a. and v. ovarica in the lig. suspensorium ovarii, and the a. and v. uterina in the lig. latum uteri.

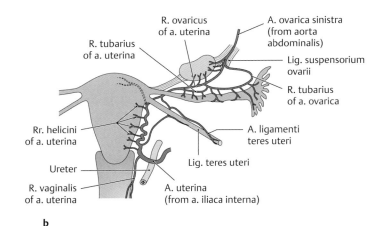

R. ovaricus of a. uterina
A. ovarica sinistra (from aorta abdominalis)
R. tubarius of a. uterina
Lig. suspensorium ovarii
R. tubarius of a. ovarica
Rr. helicini of a. uterina
A. ligamenti teres uteri
Ureter
Lig. teres uteri
R. vaginalis of a. uterina
A. uterina (from a. iliaca interna)

b

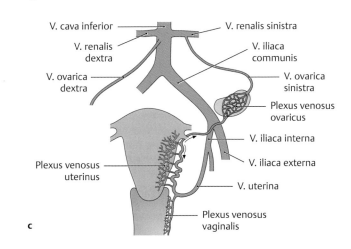

V. cava inferior
V. renalis sinistra
V. renalis dextra
V. iliaca communis
V. ovarica dextra
V. ovarica sinistra
Plexus venosus ovaricus
V. iliaca interna
V. iliaca externa
V. uterina
Plexus venosus uterinus
Plexus venosus vaginalis

c

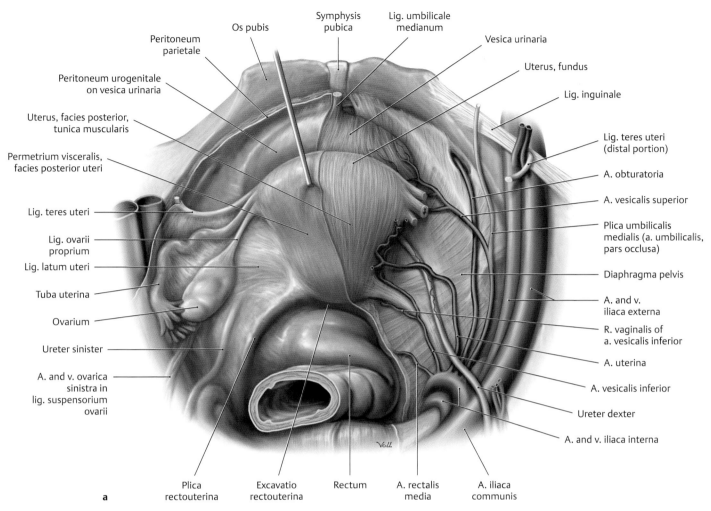

Symphysis pubica
Os pubis
Peritoneum parietale
Lig. umbilicale medianum
Vesica urinaria
Peritoneum urogenitale on vesica urinaria
Uterus, fundus
Uterus, facies posterior, tunica muscularis
Lig. inguinale
Permetrium visceralis, facies posterior uteri
Lig. teres uteri (distal portion)
A. obturatoria
A. vesicalis superior
Lig. teres uteri
Lig. ovarii proprium
Plica umbilicalis medialis (a. umbilicalis, pars occlusa)
Lig. latum uteri
Diaphragma pelvis
Tuba uterina
A. and v. iliaca externa
Ovarium
R. vaginalis of a. vesicalis inferior
Ureter sinister
A. uterina
A. and v. ovarica sinistra in lig. suspensorium ovarii
A. vesicalis inferior
Ureter dexter
A. and v. iliaca interna
Plica rectouterina
Excavatio rectouterina
Rectum
A. rectalis media
A. iliaca communis

a

B Relationship of the arteria uterina and ureter
a superior view looking into the pelvis, most of the peritoneum has been removed on the right side, the intestinum crassum has been detached so that only a rectal stump is visible; **b** left lateral view of left a. uterina and left ureter.
The a. uterina runs in the lig. latum uteri (in **a** removed on the right side and left in situ on the left side for clarity) to the uterus. There the ureter crosses inferior to the a. uterina (the ureter is thus susceptible to injury during operations on the uterus).

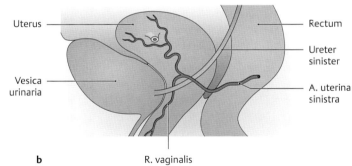

Uterus
Rectum
Ureter sinister
Vesica urinaria
A. uterina sinistra
b
R. vaginalis

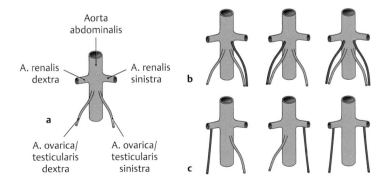

Aorta abdominalis
A. renalis dextra
A. renalis sinistra
b
a
A. ovarica/ testicularis dextra
A. ovarica/ testicularis sinistra
c

C Variants in the origin of the aa. ovaricae and testiculares
(after Lippert and Pabst)
a Typical case: The aa. ovaricae or testiculares arise from the aorta abdominalis (approximately 70 % of cases).
b Accessory vessels are present (approximately 15 %).
c The arteries arise from the a. renalis (approximately 15 %).

351

5.18 Lymphatic Drainage of the Male and Female Genitalia

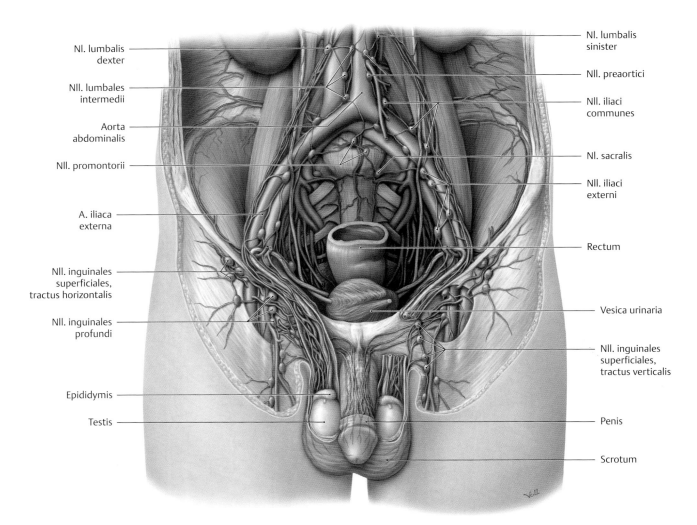

A Nodi lymphoidei and vasa lymphatica of the male internal and external genitalia

Anterior view. All portions of the gastrointestinal tract have been removed except for a rectal stump. The peritoneum has been removed, and the vesica urinaria has been pulled slightly to the left. The *external genitalia* consist of the penis and scrotum, while the testis and epididymis (despite their location) are included with the *internal genitalia* because of their embryonic origin, along with the prostata and gll. vesiculosae. (The lymphatic drainage of the prostata, testis, and epididymis is described in **B**.)

Note: The nll. lumbales that drain the *testis and epididymis* are located farther from these organs than most "visceral lymph nodes." As with the ovarium, this results in a long drainage pathway from the testis and epididymis to the nll. lumbales. Metastases from a testicular malignancy are most frequently encountered in the nll. lumbales. The *external genitalia* are drained by the nll. inguinales superficiales and profundi. The vasa lymphatica on the dorsum of the penis are connected by anastomoses that allow for bilateral lymphatic drainage. Because of this bilateral arrangement, a malignant tumor on the right side of the penis may metastasize to the right *and* left nll. inguinales.

B Lymphatic drainage of the testis, epididymis, and accessory sex glands

All lymph from the male genitalia is ultimately channeled by various groups of nll. parietales to nodi lumbales distributed around the aorta abdominalis and v. cava inferior (see pp. 221 and 223). The following specific drainage pathways are available:

Testis and epididymis: long, direct drainage pathway along the testicular vessels to the right and left nll. lumbales

Ductus deferens: to the nll. iliaci (the external more than the internal)

Gl. vesiculosa: nll. iliaci interni and externi (same pathway as the ductus deferens)

Prostata (multiple pathways): nll. iliaci externi; along the vesicular vessels to the nll. iliaci interni; nll. sacrales (and on to the nll. lumbales).

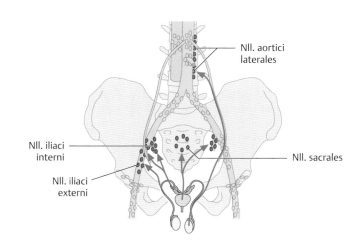

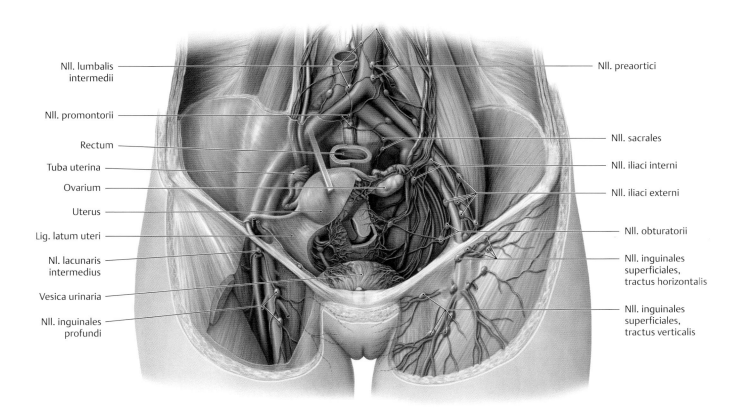

C Lymph nodes and lymphatic pathways of the female internal and external genitalia

Anterior view. The uterus is retracted to the right. The lig. latum uteri (see p. 322) has been removed on the left side and partially opened on the right side to display the numerous lymphatic vessels that traverse the ligament. For clarity, the drawing shows only isolated nodi lymphoidei within certain groups of nodes. *Lymph from the internal genitalia* in the female pelvis drains principally to the nll. iliaci and lumbales, while *lymph from the external genitalia* drains mainly to the nll. inguinales. The

nll. inguinales are divided by clinical criteria into a horizontal tract and vertical tract. It is believed that the *external* genitalia are drained mainly by the vertical tract.

Note: The ovarium, though located in the pelvis, drains to the nll. lumbales. A large portion of the vasa lymphatica of the uterus course within the lig. latum uteri. Consequently the lymphogenous spread of malignant uterine tumors takes place along that ligament, proceeding laterally toward the pelvic wall.

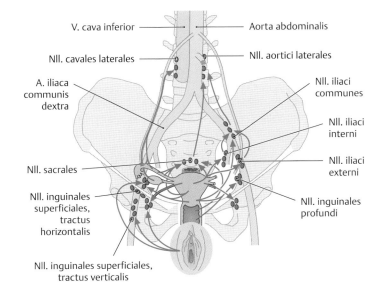

D Lymphatic drainage of the female genitalia

All of the genitalia are drained by various groups of nll. parietales, which ultimately drain to nll. lumbales distributed around the aorta abdominalis and v. cava inferior (see pp. 221 and 223).

External genitalia (and lowest portions of the vagina): nll. inguinales superficiales and profundi, plus an accessory route (not shown) directly to the nll. iliaci

Internal genitalia:

- Ovarium, fundus uteri, and (mainly distal) portions of the tuba uterina: long drainage pathway to the nll. lumbales around the aorta abdominalis and v. cava inferior
- Fundus and corpus uteri and (mainly proximal) portions of the tuba uterina: nll. sacrales, nll. iliaci interni and externi
- Uterus (cervix) and middle and upper portions of vagina: nll. inguinales profundi

Note: Small nll. viscerales for the uterus and vagina (nodi parauterini and paravaginales, not shown here) are embedded in regional pelvic connective tissue close to the organs they serve.

5.19 Autonomic Innervation of the Male Genitalia

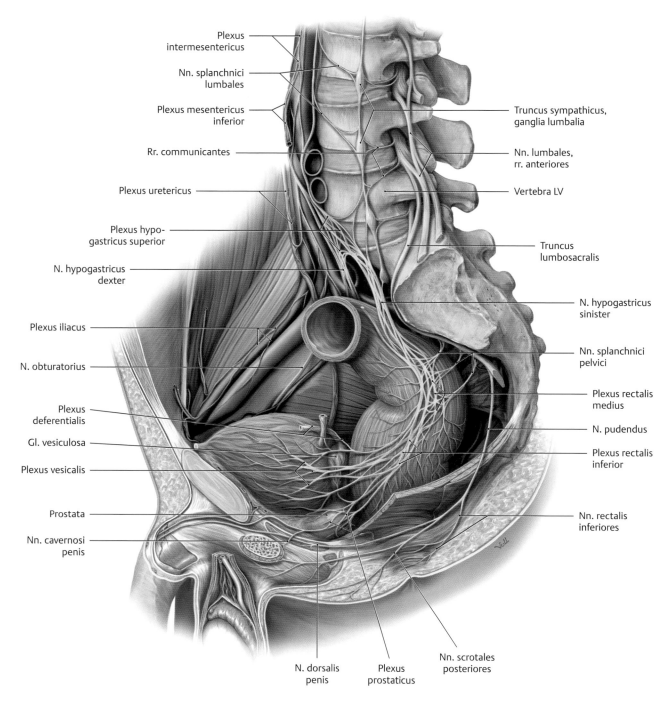

Plexus intermesentericus

Nn. splanchnici lumbales

Plexus mesentericus inferior

Rr. communicantes

Plexus uretericus

Plexus hypogastricus superior

N. hypogastricus dexter

Plexus iliacus

N. obturatorius

Plexus deferentialis

Gl. vesiculosa

Plexus vesicalis

Prostata

Nn. cavernosi penis

Truncus sympathicus, ganglia lumbalia

Nn. lumbales, rr. anteriores

Vertebra LV

Truncus lumbosacralis

N. hypogastricus sinister

Nn. splanchnici pelvici

Plexus rectalis medius

N. pudendus

Plexus rectalis inferior

Nn. rectalis inferiores

N. dorsalis penis

Plexus prostaticus

Nn. scrotales posteriores

A Overview of the autonomic innervation of the male genitalia
Opened male pelvis viewed from the left side. This drawing is a composite from many planes of section to show the three-dimensional relationships more clearly. The *sympathetic* fibers that supply the testis and epididymis form the nn. splanchnici minor, imus, and lumbales. Those that supply the accessory sex glands (prostata, gl. vesiculosa, and gll. bulbourethrales), penis, and ductus deferens arise from the nn. splanchnici lumbales and sacrales. The *parasympathetic* supply to the male genitalia is much more modest than the sympathetic supply; it arises predominantly from the nn. splanchnici pelvici (see **B**). Sympathetic and parasympathetic fibers join to form the *plexus hypogastricus inferior*, which also receives the nn. hypogastrici (arise from the division of the plexus hypogastricus superior). The paired plexus hypogastrici inferiores, which give origin to the plexuses that supply the urinary organs (see p. 225), then divide into multiple plexuses that innervate the genital organs (see **C**).

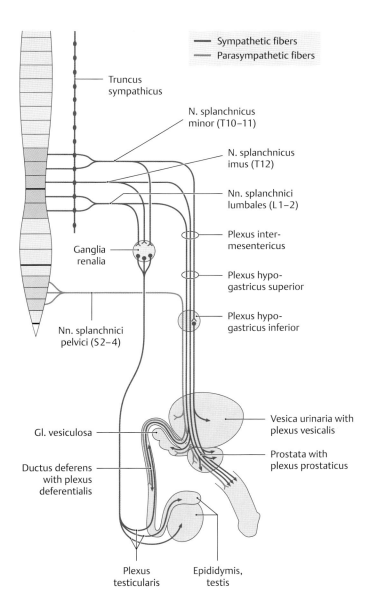

— Sympathetic fibers
— Parasympathetic fibers

Truncus sympathicus

N. splanchnicus minor (T10–11)

N. splanchnicus imus (T12)

Nn. splanchnici lumbales (L1–2)

Plexus inter-mesentericus

Ganglia renalia

Plexus hypo-gastricus superior

Plexus hypo-gastricus inferior

Nn. splanchnici pelvici (S2–4)

Vesica urinaria with plexus vesicalis

Gl. vesiculosa

Prostata with plexus prostaticus

Ductus deferens with plexus deferentialis

Plexus testicularis

Epididymis, testis

C Autonomic innervation of the male genitalia

First neuron	Peripheral course (sympathetic and parasympathetic)	Target organ	Effect
Sympathetic:			
T10–T12 (nn. splanchnici minor and imus)	Via ganglia renalia to plexus testicularis	• Testis • Epididymis	• Vasocon-striction
L1–L2 (nn. splanchnici lumbales and sacrales)	Via plexus hypogas-tricus superior and plexus hypogastri-cus inferior to plexus prostaticus and to	• Prostata • Gll. bulboure-thrales and vesiculosa • Penis (partly)	• Stimulate secretions
	Plexus deferentialis	• Ductus deferens	• Ejaculation • Contraction
Parasympathetic:			
S2–S4 (nn. splanchnici pelvici)	Via plexus hypogas-tricus inferior to plexus prostaticus, continuing to the nn. cavernosi penis	• Penis, erectile tissues	• Erection

B Details of the autonomic innervation of the male genitalia

- The **accessory sex glands (prostata, gl. vesiculosa, and gll. bulbourethralis)** receive their autonomic innervation from the plexus prostaticus, which branches from the plexus hypogastricus inferior (also believed to carry pain fibers).
- The **penis** also receives its autonomic innervation from branches of the plexus prostaticus and from the nn. cavernosi penis (see **A**). In both cases the synapse with the postsynaptic neuron occurs in the ganglion cells of the plexus hypogastricus inferior.
- The **ductus deferens** is supplied mainly by the plexus deferentialis, which also branches from the plexus hypogastricus inferior and to a lesser degree from the plexus testicularis that runs along the a. testicularis.
- The **testis**, because of its developmental descent, receives most of its autonomic innervation from the plexus testicularis (sympathetic fibers along the a. testicularis, which synapse in the ganglia renalia). The plexus testicularis also gives off fibers to the epididymis. Both organs receive a smaller amount of autonomic innervation from the plexus hypogastricus inferior (not included in **C**).

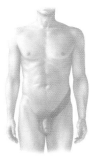

D Referred pain from the male gonadae

The pain associated with diseases of the testis (e.g., inflammation) may be referred to this skin area. Gonadal pain, like intestinal pain, is not perceived at the anatomical location of the organ.

5.20 Autonomic Innervation of the Female Genitalia

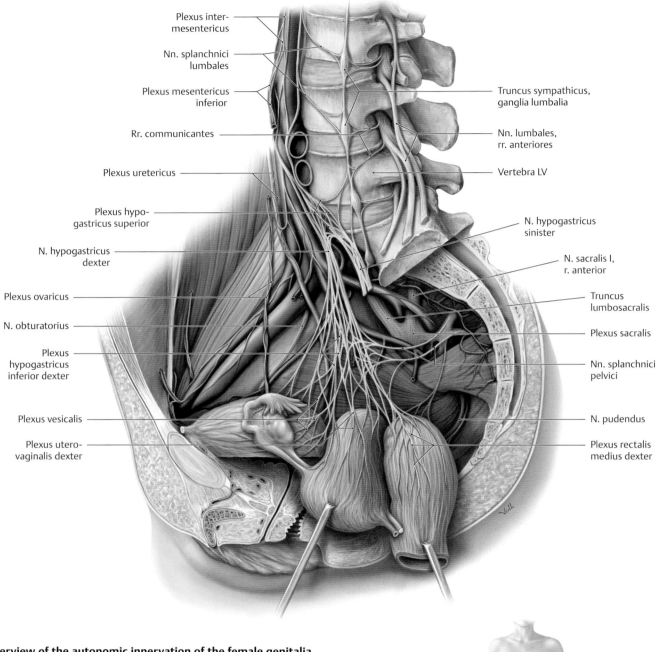

Plexus inter-mesentericus

Nn. splanchnici lumbales

Plexus mesentericus inferior

Rr. communicantes

Plexus uretericus

Plexus hypogastricus superior

N. hypogastricus dexter

Plexus ovaricus

N. obturatorius

Plexus hypogastricus inferior dexter

Plexus vesicalis

Plexus utero-vaginalis dexter

Truncus sympathicus, ganglia lumbalia

Nn. lumbales, rr. anteriores

Vertebra LV

N. hypogastricus sinister

N. sacralis I, r. anterior

Truncus lumbosacralis

Plexus sacralis

Nn. splanchnici pelvici

N. pudendus

Plexus rectalis medius dexter

A Overview of the autonomic innervation of the female genitalia
An opened female pelvis viewed from the left side, with the rectum and uterus reflected. This drawing is a composite from multiple planes of section to show the three-dimensional relationships more clearly. The *sympathetic* fibers for the uterus, tubae uterinae, and ovaria arise predominantly from the nn. splanchnici minor, imus, and lumbales. The *parasympathetic* fibers arise from the nn. splanchnici pelvici.
Note: The fibers that are distributed to the ovarium synapse mainly in the ganglia renalia because as the ovarium undergoes its developmental descent, it carries its autonomic supply from the abdomen with it. The fibers then continue on to the plexus ovaricus, which also receives fibers from the plexus mesentericus superior. This is analogous to the innervation of the testis via the ganglia renalia and the plexus mesenterici superior and inferior and testicularis in the male.

B Referred pain from the female gonadae
The pain associated with ovarian diseases (e.g., inflammation) may project to these skin areas and may not be perceived within the organ itself.

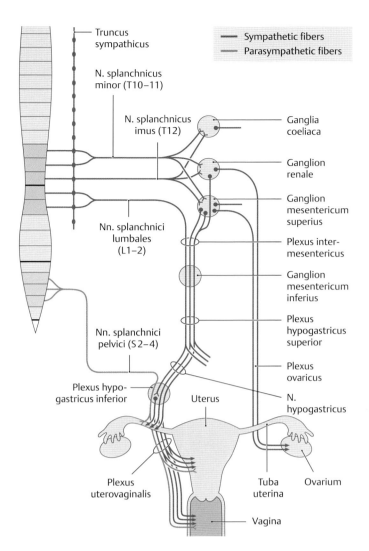

D Autonomic innervation of the female genitalia

First neuron	Peripheral course (sympathetic and parasympathetic)	Target organ	Effect
Sympathetic:			
T10–T12 (nn. splanchnici minor and imus)	Via ganglia renalia and ganglion mesentericum superius to plexus ovaricus	• Ovarium	• Vasoconstriction
L1–L2 (nn. splanchnici lumbales)	Via plexus hypogastricus superior, nn. hypogastrici, and plexus hypogastricus inferior to plexus uterovaginalis	• Uterus • Tuba uterina • Vagina • Vagina	• Contraction (in uterus, depends on hormone status) • Vasoconstriction
Parasympathetic:			
S2–S4 (nn. splanchnici pelvici)	Plexus hypogastricus inferior to plexus uterovaginalis, continuing to nn. cavernosi clitoridis	• Uterus, tuba uterina • Vagina • Clitoris	• Vasodilation • Transudation • Erection

C Autonomic innervation of the female genitalia

Because of the developmental descent of the **ovarium**, its nerve supply extends a considerable distance along the a. ovarica in the lig. suspensorium ovarii (the plexus ovaricus, which arises from the plexus aorticus abdominalis via the ganglia renalia — analogous to the innervation of the testis via the plexus testicularis).

The **uterus, tuba uterina,** and **vagina** receive their autonomic innervation from the plexus hypogastricus inferior. The *sympathetic* portion is derived from the nn. splanchnici minor, imus, and lumbales, which synapse partly in the ganglia mesenterica and partly in the ganglion cells of the plexus hypogastricus inferior. The *parasympathetic* fibers are derived from the nn. splanchnici pelvici (S2–S4), which synapse in the plexus hypogastricus inferior or in/on the organ wall. Branches from the plexus hypogastricus inferior form the prominent plexus uterovaginalis (of Frankenhäuser) located on both sides of the uterus. The ovarium may receive additional autonomic innervation along the tuba uterina from the plexus hypogastricus inferior.

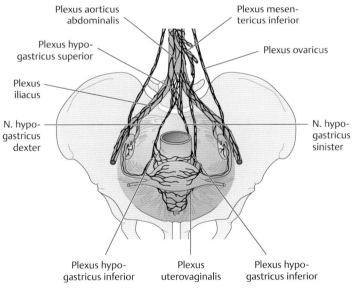

E Overview of the autonomic plexuses in the female pelvis

Anterior view.

Note the division of the of the plexus hypogastricus superior into *two nn. hypogastrici*, which are continuous with *both plexus hypogastrici inferiores.* The latter then give off individual visceral plexuses to the rectum, uterus, vagina, and vesica urinaria (see **A**).

The ovarium is supplied chiefly by the plexus ovaricus, which runs along the a. ovarica in the lig. suspensorium ovarii. Thus, the autonomic supply of the female pelvis corresponds to that in the male, although the plexuses in the female pelvis are more strongly developed due to the very rich nerve supply of the uterus.

6.1 Surface Anatomy, Topographic Regions, and Palpable Bony Landmarks

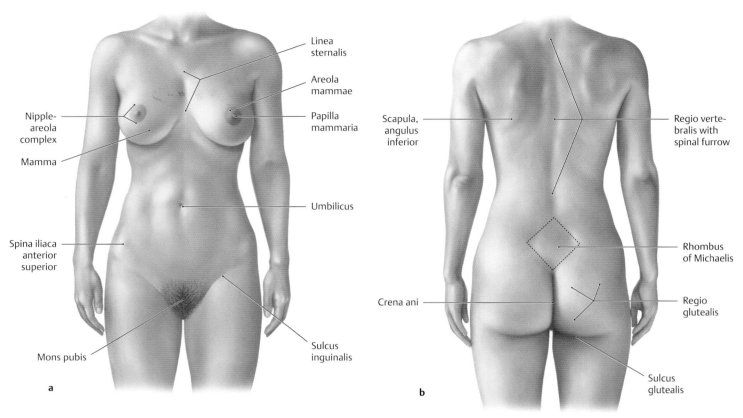

A Surface anatomy of the female
a Anterior view; **b** Posterior view.

Labels (left image, anterior view):
- Linea sternalis
- Areola mammae
- Papilla mammaria
- Nipple-areola complex
- Mamma
- Umbilicus
- Spina iliaca anterior superior
- Mons pubis
- Sulcus inguinalis

Labels (right image, posterior view):
- Scapula, angulus inferior
- Regio vertebralis with spinal furrow
- Rhombus of Michaelis
- Crena ani
- Regio glutealis
- Sulcus glutealis

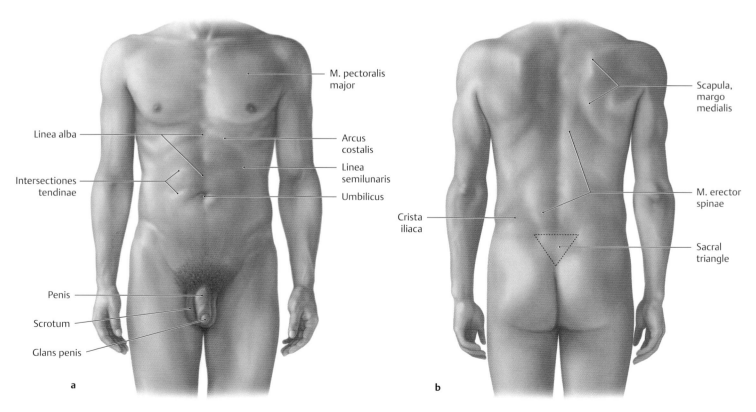

B Surface anatomy of the male
a Anterior view; **b** Posterior view.

Labels (left image, anterior view):
- M. pectoralis major
- Linea alba
- Arcus costalis
- Linea semilunaris
- Intersectiones tendinae
- Umbilicus
- Penis
- Scrotum
- Glans penis

Labels (right image, posterior view):
- Scapula, margo medialis
- M. erector spinae
- Crista iliaca
- Sacral triangle

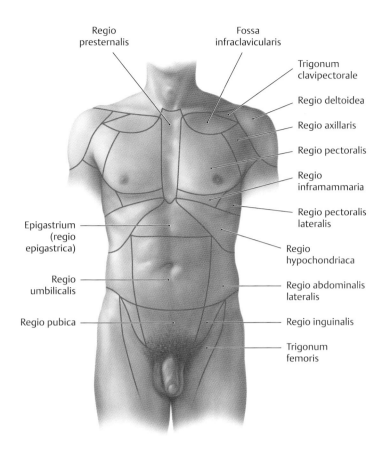

Regio presternalis

Fossa infraclavicularis

Trigonum clavipectorale

Regio deltoidea

Regio axillaris

Regio pectoralis

Regio inframammaria

Regio pectoralis lateralis

Regio hypochondriaca

Regio abdominalis lateralis

Regio inguinalis

Trigonum femoris

Epigastrium (regio epigastrica)

Regio umbilicalis

Regio pubica

C Thoracic and abdominal regions
Anterior view.

Regio vertebralis

Regio suprascapularis

Regio deltoidea

Regio scapularis

Regio interscapularis

Regio pectoralis lateralis

Regio infrascapularis

Trigonum lumbale

Regio sacralis

Regio glutealis

Regio analis

D Back and gluteal regions
Posterior view.

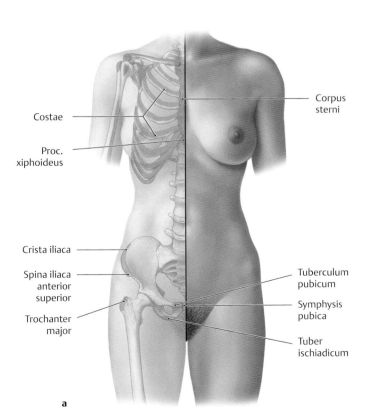

Costae

Proc. xiphoideus

Crista iliaca

Spina iliaca anterior superior

Trochanter major

Corpus sterni

Tuberculum pubicum

Symphysis pubica

Tuber ischiadicum

a

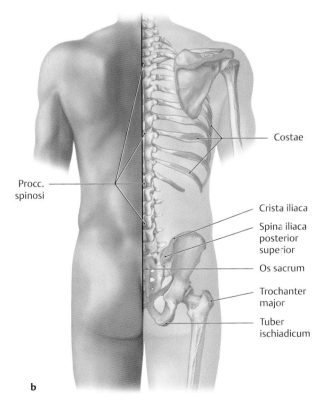

Procc. spinosi

Costae

Crista iliaca

Spina iliaca posterior superior

Os sacrum

Trochanter major

Tuber ischiadicum

b

E Body surface contours and palpable bony landmarks of the trunk
a Anterior view; **b** Posterior view.

359

6.2 Location of the Abdominal and Pelvic Organs and their Projection onto the Trunk Wall

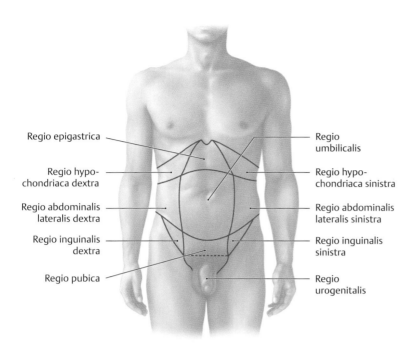

Regio epigastrica

Regio hypo-chondriaca dextra

Regio abdominalis lateralis dextra

Regio inguinalis dextra

Regio pubica

Regio umbilicalis

Regio hypo-chondriaca sinistra

Regio abdominalis lateralis sinistra

Regio inguinalis sinistra

Regio urogenitalis

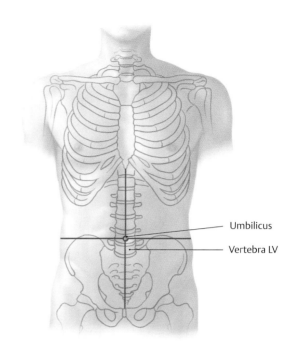

Umbilicus

Vertebra LV

A Regions of the anterior trunk wall
Three levels can be identified on the abdominal wall from above downward: the epigastrium, mesogastrium, and hypogastrium. Each level consists of three regions:

- The median region of the epigastrium is the *regio epigastrica*. It is flanked laterally by the right and left regiones hypochondriacae.
- The median region of the mesogastrium is the *regio umbilicalis*, which is bounded laterally by the right and left regiones abdominales laterales.
- The median region of the hypogastrium is the regio pubica, which is flanked by the right and left *regiones inguinales*.

The levels of the abdomen are defined by horizontal planes that are determined by palpable bony landmarks (see **C**).

B Quadrants of the anterior trunk wall
The quadrants of the anterior trunk wall are centered on the umbilicus, which lies at the level of the corpora vertebrarum L 3–4 and are named right and left upper and lower quadrant (RUQ, LUQ, RLQ, LLQ).

C Horizontal (transverse) planes in the anterior trunk wall
The anterior trunk wall is divided transversely by the following imaginary planes of section:

- **Planum xiphosternale:** passes through the synchondrosis between the processus *xiphoideus* and corpus *sterni*.
- **Planum transpyloricum:** plane midway between the incisura jugularis of the sternum and the superior border of the symphysis pubica. Located at the level of the L 1 vertebra, it divides the anterior trunk wall into upper and lower halves. The pylorus of the gaster is generally located slightly *below* this plane.
- **Planum subcostale:** passes through the *lowest points of the arcus costalis* of the tenth rib at the level of the corpus vertebrae L2. It marks the boundary between the epigastrium and mesogastrium (see **A**).
- **Planum supracristale:** usually passes through the corpus vertebrae L4, connecting the *highest points on the cristae iliacae*.
- **Planum intertuberculare:** connects the tubercula iliaca and passes through the corpus vertebrae L 5. The planum intertuberculare marks the boundary between the mesogastrium and hypogastrium.
- **Planum interspinale:** connects the two *spinae iliacae anteriores superiores*.

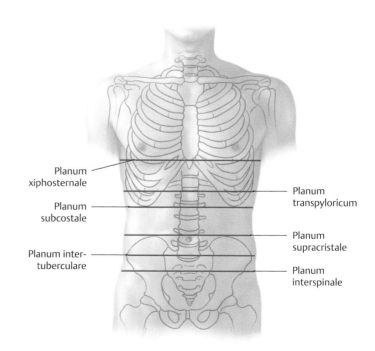

Planum xiphosternale

Planum subcostale

Planum inter-tuberculare

Planum transpyloricum

Planum supracristale

Planum interspinale

Note: The three upper planes are variable in their location, which depends on the position and shape of the cavea thoracis. The key variables are respiratory position, age, sex, and constitutional type.

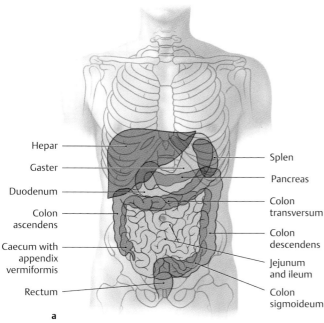

Hepar
Gaster
Duodenum
Colon ascendens
Caecum with appendix vermiformis
Rectum

Splen
Pancreas
Colon transversum
Colon descendens
Jejunum and ileum
Colon sigmoideum

a

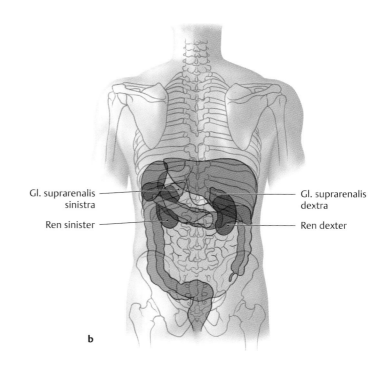

Gl. suprarenalis sinistra
Ren sinister

Gl. suprarenalis dextra
Ren dexter

b

D Projection of the abdominal and pelvic organs onto the trunk wall

a Anterior trunk wall; **b** Posterior trunk wall.

The surface projection of organs on the trunk wall depends on body posture, age, constitutional type, sex, nutritional state, and respiratory position.

Note the overlap of the cavitates abdominis and thoracica: Perforating injuries of the cavitas abdominis that involve the hepar, for example, may also involve the cavitas pleuralis ("multicavity injury"). The projections of individual organs are shown in **E**.

E Projection of anatomical structures in the abdomen and pelvis onto the columna vertebralis

The spinal notation refers to corpora vertebrarum.

T 7	Superior border of the hepar
T 12	Hiatus aorticus
L 1	• Planum transpyloricum (generally the pylorus is at or below this plane) • Fundus vesicae biliaris • Hilum renale • Pars superior duodeni • Collum pancreatis • Origin of the truncus coeliacus • Origin of the a. mesenterica superior • Attachment of the mesocolon transversum • Hilum splenicum
L 1/2	• Origin of the aa. renales
L 2	Flexura duodenojejunalis
L 3	Origin of the a. mesenterica inferior
L 3/4	Umbilicus
L 4	Bifurcatio aortae
L 5	Origin of the v. cava inferior from the vv. iliacae communes
S 3	Upper (cranial) border of the rectum

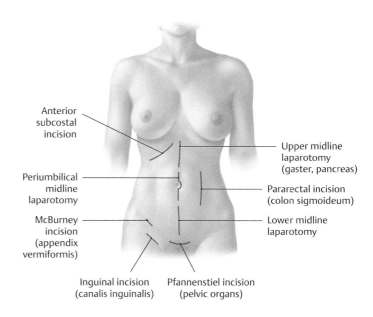

Anterior subcostal incision

Periumbilical midline laparotomy

McBurney incision (appendix vermiformis)

Upper midline laparotomy (gaster, pancreas)

Pararectal incision (colon sigmoideum)

Lower midline laparotomy

Inguinal incision (canalis inguinalis)

Pfannenstiel incision (pelvic organs)

F Placement of surgical skin incisions in the anterior abdominal wall

Note: The periumbilical midline incision passes around the *left* side of the umbilicus to avoid cutting the remnant of the v. umbilicalis on the *right* side (the ligamentum teres hepatis, see p. 253). This v. umbilicalis remnant is generally but not always obliterated, and injury to the vessel, if it is still patent, may cause significant bleeding.

The McBurney incision is also called the *gridiron incision* because it changes direction in different planes of the trunk wall. The muscles of the trunk wall can be divided less traumatically by tailoring the direction of the cut to the prevailing fiber direction of the various muscle layers.

361

6.3 Topography of the Opened Cavitas Peritonealis (Supracolic Part and Infracolic Part)

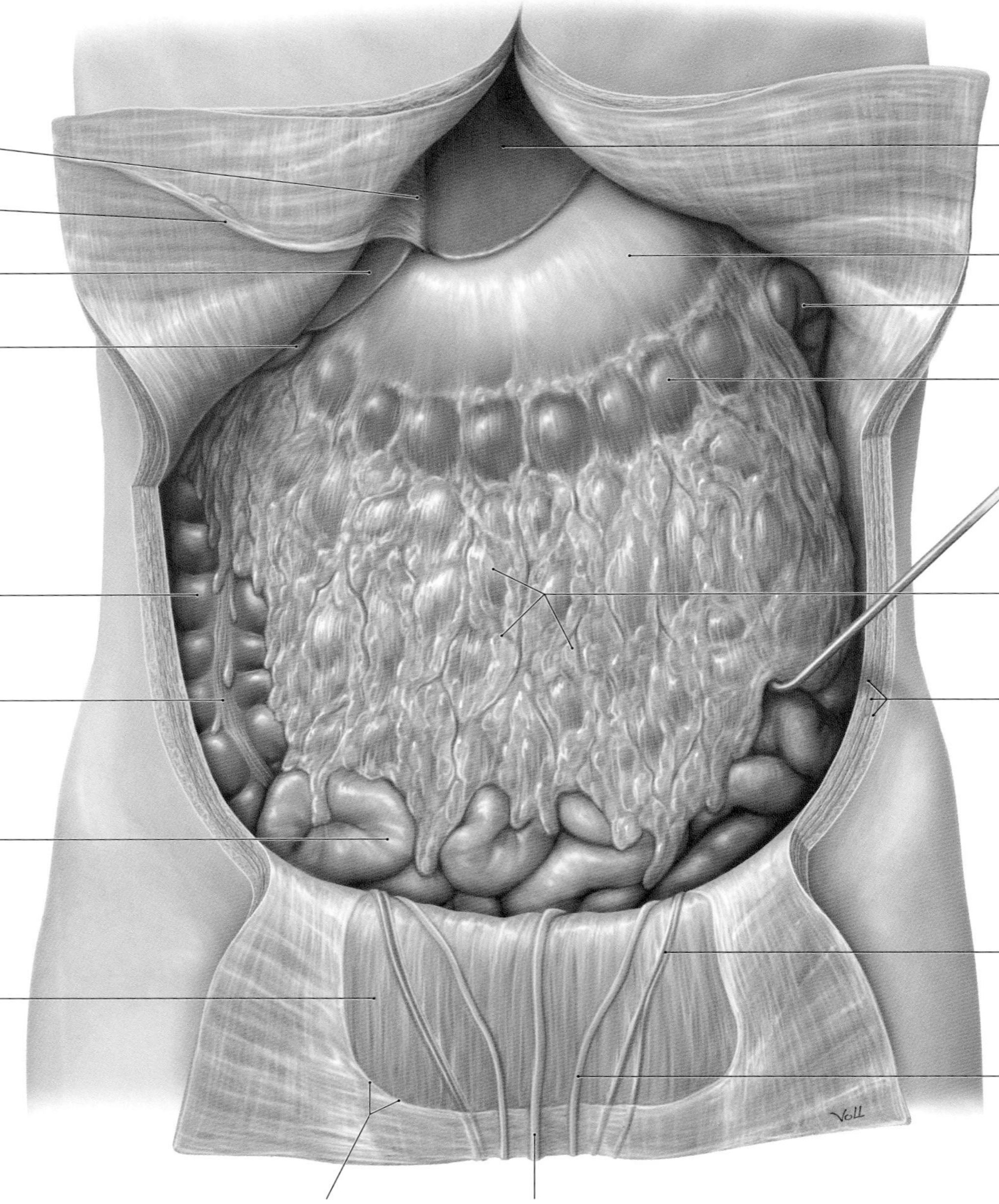

Lig. falciforme hepatis
Lig. teres hepatis
Lobus heparis dexter
Vesica biliaris
Colon ascendens
Taenia coli
Ileum
M. rectus abdominis
Linea arcuata
Plica umbilicalis mediana (with obliterated urachus)
Lobus heparis sinister
Gaster
Flexura coli sinistra
Colon transversum
Omentum majus
Mm. obliqui externus and internus abdominis, m. transversus abdominis
Plica umbilicalis lateralis (plica epigastrica with a. and v. epigastrica inferior)
Plica umbilicalis medialis (with obliterated a. umbilicalis)
Voll

A The omentum majus in situ
Anterior view. The layers of the abdominal wall have been opened and retracted to display the omentum majus in its normal anatomical position. The omentum majus is draped over the loops of intestinum tenue, which are visible only at the inferior border of the omentum. The omentum majus is an apronlike fold of peritoneum suspended from the curvatura major of the gaster and covering the anterior surface of the colon transversum. It develops from the embryonic mesogastrium dorsalis, which becomes greatly enlarged to form a peritoneal sac suspended from the curvatura major. The omentum majus is relatively mobile, and is subject to considerable variation. Not infrequently, adhesions form between the omentum majus and the peritoneal covering of organs, especially as a result of local inflammation. While these adhesions help contain the spread of inflammation, they also limit the mobility of the organ to which the omentum is adherent. Peritoneal adhesions may undergo fibrotic changes over time, forming tough bands of scar tissue that may cause extrinsic narrowing and obstruction of organs such as the intestinum tenue. In many cases the omentum majus also assumes importance as a lymphoid organ through the secondary acquisition of nodi lymphoidei. The omentum minus is described on p. 364.

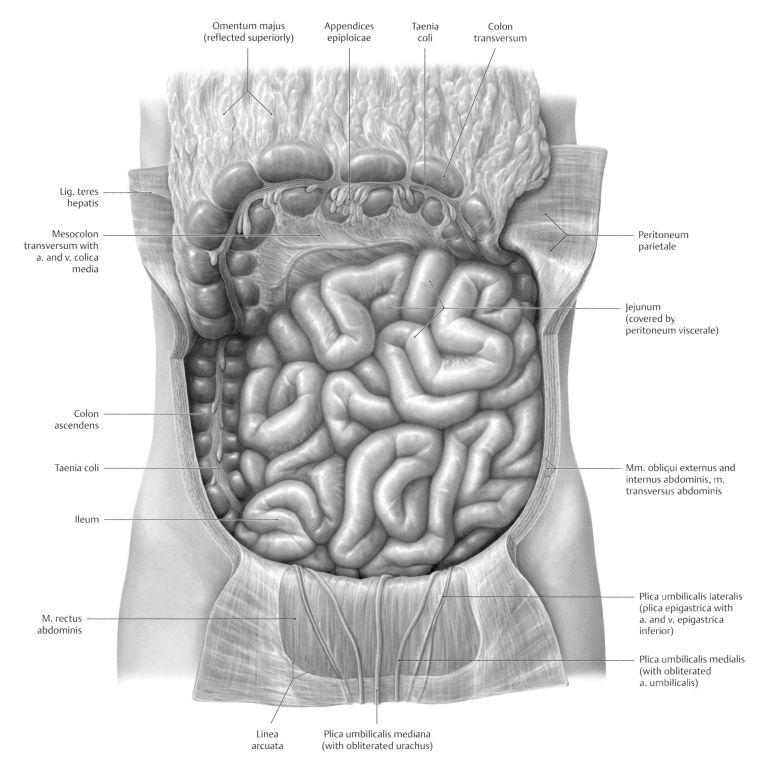

Omentum majus (reflected superiorly)

Appendices epiploicae

Taenia coli

Colon transversum

Lig. teres hepatis

Mesocolon transversum with a. and v. colica media

Peritoneum parietale

Jejunum (covered by peritoneum viscerale)

Colon ascendens

Taenia coli

Mm. obliqui externus and internus abdominis, m. transversus abdominis

Ileum

M. rectus abdominis

Plica umbilicalis lateralis (plica epigastrica with a. and v. epigastrica inferior)

Plica umbilicalis medialis (with obliterated a. umbilicalis)

Linea arcuata

Plica umbilicalis mediana (with obliterated urachus)

B Dissection with the omentum majus reflected superiorly and the intestinum tenue in situ

Anterior view. The omentum majus has been reflected superiorly, carrying with it the colon transversum, to demonstrate how the intraperitoneal part of the intestinum tenue is framed by the colon segments. The mesocolon transversum divides the cavitas peritonealis into a supracolic part and an infracolic part (see **B**, p. 208).

The large epithelial surface area of the peritoneum is important clinically:

• With bacterial infection (caused by external trauma or the seepage of septic material from an inflamed appendix), pathogenic microorganisms can easily spread within the cavitas peritonealis, where bacterial toxins are readily absorbed and carried into the bloodstream. As a result, bacterial peritonitis (inflammation of the peritoneum) generally constitutes a very serious and life-threatening condition.

• Localized inflammations may result in peritoneal adhesions and scar tissue bands (see **A**).

• The large surface area can be utilized for peritoneal dialysis in patients with renal failure: A dialysis solution instilled into the cavitas peritonealis can absorb waste products from the blood through the peritoneum, allowing them to be removed from the body.

6.4 Drainage Spaces and Recesses within the Cavitas Peritonealis

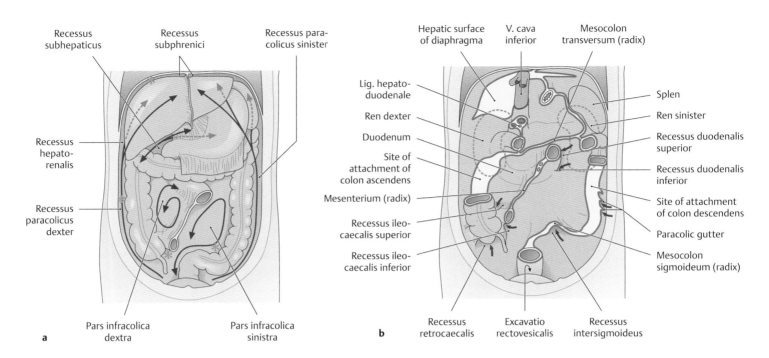

A Drainage spaces and recesses within the cavitas peritonealis

a Anterior view with the omentum majus and intestinum tenue removed; preferred metastatic sites (see blue stars);

b Posterior wall of the cavitas peritonealis, anterior view. The mesenteric roots and sites of organ attachment create partially bounded spaces (recesses or sulci). Peritoneal fluid released by the peritoneal epithelium (transudate) can flow freely within these spaces.

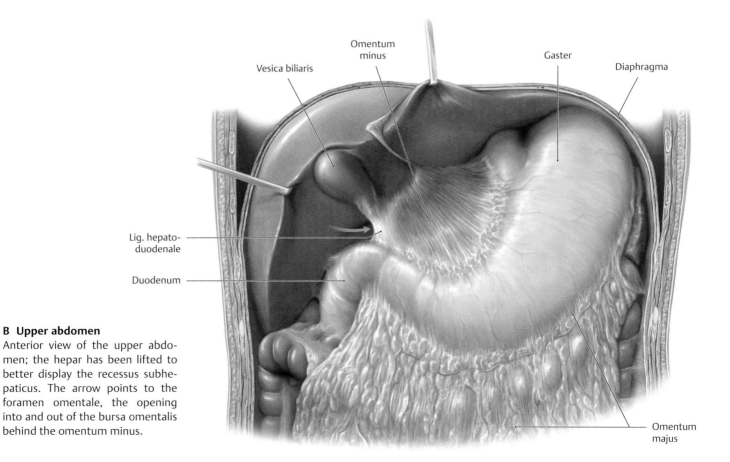

B Upper abdomen

Anterior view of the upper abdomen; the hepar has been lifted to better display the recessus subhepaticus. The arrow points to the foramen omentale, the opening into and out of the bursa omentalis behind the omentum minus.

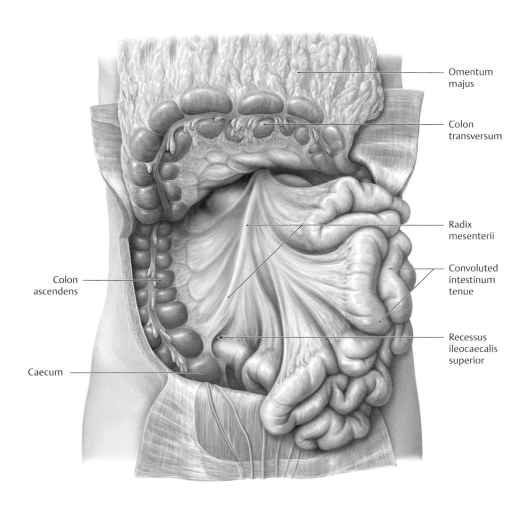

Omentum
majus

Colon
transversum

Radix
mesenterii

Convoluted
intestinum
tenue

Colon
ascendens

Recessus
ileocaecalis
superior

Caecum

**C Recesses in the posterior wall of the peri-
toneal cavity**

Anterior view of a male abdomen and pelvis.
Because the peritoneum extends between
organs, it forms recesses and sulci (see also **A**).
In a sense, the bursa omentalis may be considered the largest recess in the cavitas peritonealis (see p. 368).

Note: The individual recesses are located
between an organ and the wall of the cavitas
peritonealis or between organs. Freely mobile
loops of the intestinum tenue may become
entrapped in these recesses ("internal hernia")
hindering the passage of the intestinal contents and potentially causing a life-threatening
bowel obstruction ("mechanical ileus").

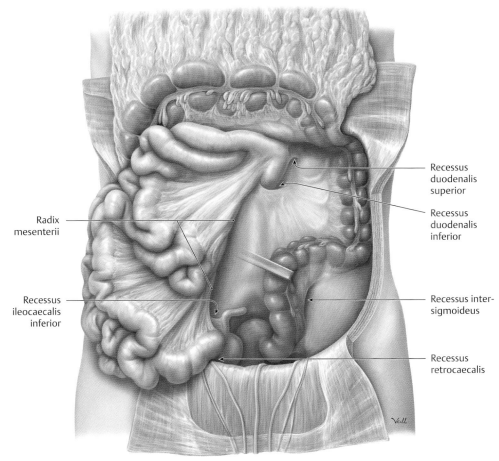

Radix
mesenterii

Recessus
ileocaecalis
inferior

Recessus
duodenalis
superior

Recessus
duodenalis
inferior

Recessus inter-
sigmoideus

Recessus
retrocaecalis

6.5   Overview of the Mesenteria

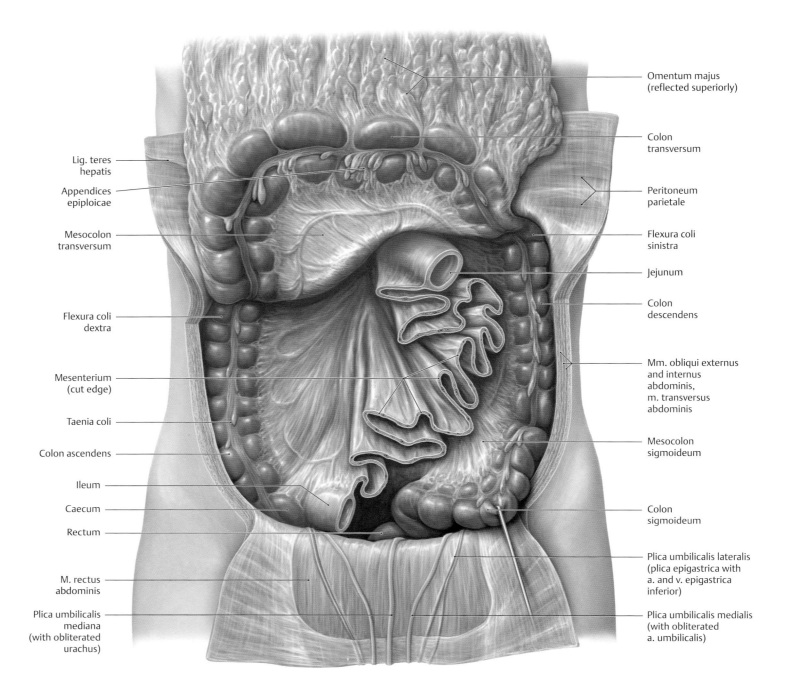

A Overview of the mesenteries with the greater omentum reflected superiorly and the small intestine removed

Anterior view. The colon transversum and omentum majus have been reflected superiorly and the intraperitoneal intestinum tenue has been removed, leaving short stumps of jejunum and ileum. Three principal mesenteria are distinguishable in relation to the intestina tenue and crassum (the formation of the mesenteria is described on p. 42):

- The mesenterium of the intestinum tenue (the mesenterium proper)
- The mesocolon transversum
- The mesocolon sigmoideum (called also the mesosigmoid)

The origins of the mesenterium are shown in **B**. *Smaller mesenteria* are found on the appendix vermiformis (*mesoappendix vermiformis*) and rarely the upper part of the rectum (*mesorectum*, see **C**).

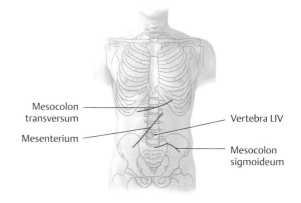

B Projection of the mesenteric roots onto the skeleton

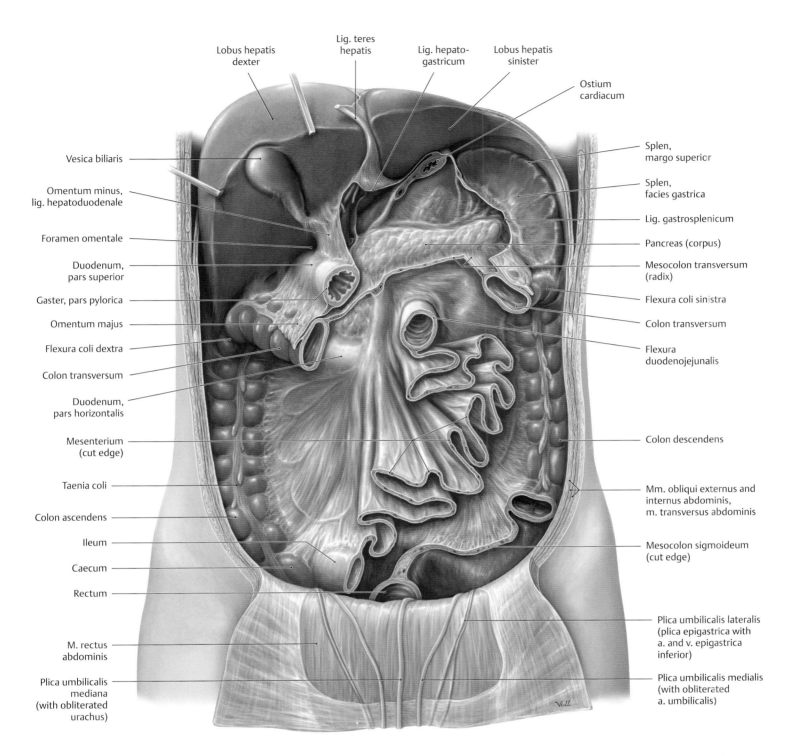

Lobus hepatis
dexter

Lig. teres
hepatis

Lig. hepato-
gastricum

Lobus hepatis
sinister

Ostium
cardiacum

Vesica biliaris

Omentum minus,
lig. hepatoduodenale

Foramen omentale

Duodenum,
pars superior

Gaster, pars pylorica

Omentum majus

Flexura coli dextra

Colon transversum

Duodenum,
pars horizontalis

Mesenterium
(cut edge)

Taenia coli

Colon ascendens

Ileum

Caecum

Rectum

M. rectus
abdominis

Plica umbilicalis
mediana
(with obliterated
urachus)

Splen,
margo superior

Splen,
facies gastrica

Lig. gastrosplenicum

Pancreas (corpus)

Mesocolon transversum
(radix)

Flexura coli sinistra

Colon transversum

Flexura
duodenojejunalis

Colon descendens

Mm. obliqui externus and
internus abdominis,
m. transversus abdominis

Mesocolon sigmoideum
(cut edge)

Plica umbilicalis lateralis
(plica epigastrica with
a. and v. epigastrica
inferior)

Plica umbilicalis medialis
(with obliterated
a. umbilicalis)

C Overview of the mesenteria* with the omentum majus removed
Anterior view. The mesenteria have been exposed by removing the gaster, jejunum, and ileum, leaving short stumps of intestinum tenue. The hepar has been reflected superiorly to display one part of the omentum minus: the lig. hepatoduodenale, which connects the hepar to the pylorus and duodenum. The other part of the omentum minus, the lig. hepatogastricum (peritoneal fold between the hepar and curvatura minor of the gaster), has been removed with the gaster, opening the anterior wall of the bursa omentalis. Most of the colon transversum and colon sigmoideum have been removed to display the roots of the mesocolon transversum and mesocolon sigmoideum.
Note: The cola ascendens and descendens become attached to the posterior wall of the cavitas peritonealis during the fourth month of embryonic development. The mesenteria of the cola ascendens and descendens become fused to the posterior wall of the cavitas

peritonealis. The mesocolon transversum crosses over the duodenum, whose mesenterium also fuses to the posterior wall of the mesocolon transversum during embryonic development (see p. 46). The mesocolon transversum necessarily passes over this "retroperitoneal portion" of the duodenum because of its attachment to the posterior wall of the cavitas peritonealis. Developmentally, almost all of the mesenteria are mesenteria dorsalia. Only upper abdominal organs like the gaster and hepar have mesenteria ventralia.

* "Mesenterium" in the broad sense refers to any of the peritoneal folds attached to the intestina tenue and crassum. "Mesenterium" in the strict sense refers specifically to the mesenterium of the jejunum and ileum, and consequently the terms "mesojejunum" and "mesoileum" are not used.

6.6   Topography of the Bursa Omentalis

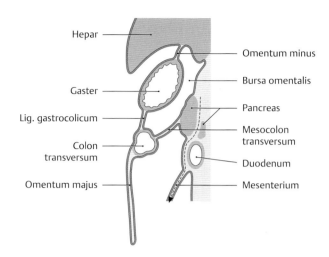

A Shape and location of the bursa omentalis in sagittal section

Left lateral view. The bursa omentalis is the largest potential space in the cavitas peritonealis. It is located behind the omentum minus and gaster.

Note: As the gaster rotates during embryonic development, the bursa omentalis comes to lie posterior to the gaster. The pancreas, which migrates into the retroperitoneum secondarily, thus forms part of the posterior wall of the bursa, which provides a route for gaining surgical access to that organ. As the gaster rotates in the clockwise direction (viewed from the front), its curvatura minor points to the right and also superiorly, simultaneously displacing the hepar superiorly and to the right. As a result of this, the bursa omentalis comes to lie partially posterior to the hepar.

B Boundaries of the bursa omentalis

Anterior	Omentum minus, lig. gastrocolicum
Posterior	Pancreas, aorta (pars abdominalis), truncus coeliacus, a. and v. splenica, plica gastropancreatica, left gl. suprarenalis, polus superior of left kidney
Superior	Hepar (with lobus caudatus), recessus superior of bursa omentalis
Inferior	Mesocolon transversum, recessus inferior of bursa omentalis
Left	Splen, lig. gastrosplenicum, recessus splenicus of bursa omentalis
Right	Hepar, bulbus duodeni

C Surgical approaches to the bursa omentalis (see A)

- Through the foramen omentale (natural opening, see **E**)
- Between the curvatura major of the gaster and the colon transversum through the lig. gastrocolicum
- Through the mesocolon transversum after elevating the colon transversum (inferior approach)
- Between the curvatura minor of the gaster and the hepar (through the omentum minus)

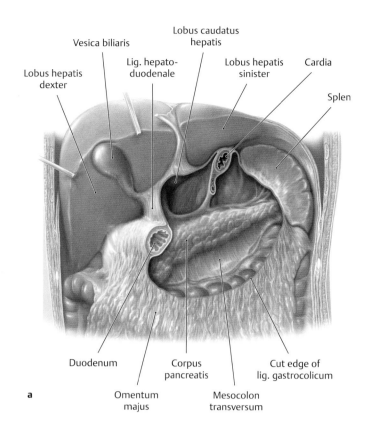

a

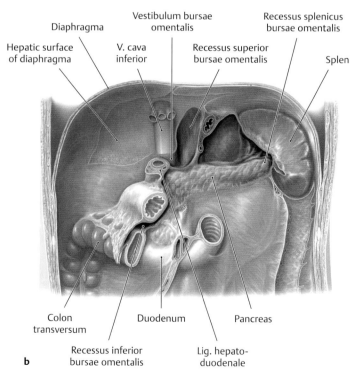

b

D Bursa omentalis, anterior view

a Boundaries of the bursa omentalis, also the shape and location of the gastric bed

b Structure of the posterior wall of the bursa omentalis

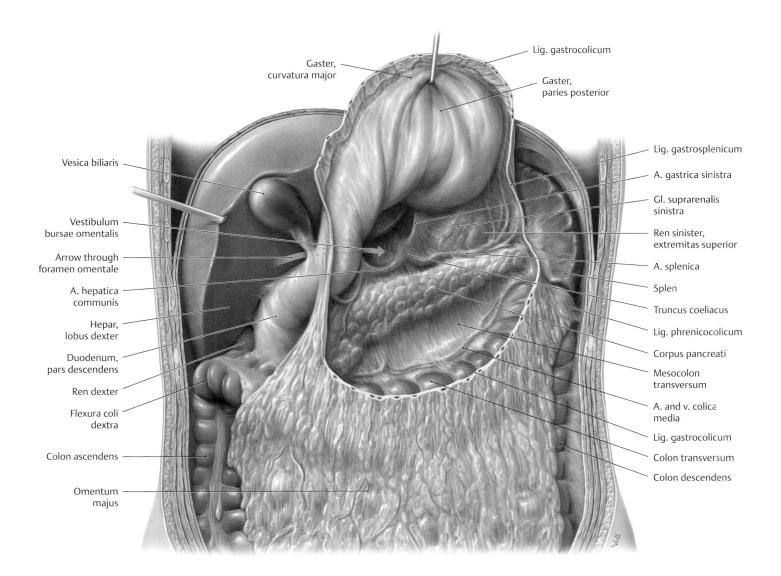

Gaster, curvatura major

Lig. gastrocolicum

Gaster, paries posterior

Lig. gastrosplenicum

A. gastrica sinistra

Gl. suprarenalis sinistra

Ren sinister, extremitas superior

A. splenica

Splen

Truncus coeliacus

Lig. phrenicocolicum

Corpus pancreati

Mesocolon transversum

A. and v. colica media

Lig. gastrocolicum

Colon transversum

Colon descendens

Vesica biliaris

Vestibulum bursae omentalis

Arrow through foramen omentale

A. hepatica communis

Hepar, lobus dexter

Duodenum, pars descendens

Ren dexter

Flexura coli dextra

Colon ascendens

Omentum majus

E Bursa omentalis in the upper abdomen

Anterior view. The lig. gastrocolicum has been divided, the gaster has been reflected superiorly (surgical approach), and the hepar has been retracted superolaterally. The foramen omentale (arrow) is the only natural orifice of the bursa omentalis (opens posterior to the lig. hepatoduodenale). The vestibulum of the bursa omentalis lies just past the foramen and forms the initial portion of the bursa cavity.

F Transverse section through the bursa omentalis

Schematic section through the abdomen at the T 12/L 1 level, viewed from below.

Note the walls and recesses that result from the formation of the bursa during the embryonic rotation of the gaster. Because the initial upper right portion of the embryonic body cavity moves posteriorly as part of the 90° rotation of the gaster, structures that were formerly posterior (splen) move to the left side while structures that were formerly anterior (hepar) move to the right side. Recesses in the bursa omentalis extend close to these organs **B**).

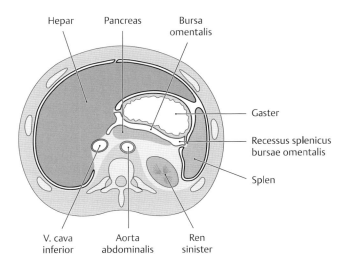

Hepar   Pancreas   Bursa omentalis

Gaster

Recessus splenicus bursae omentalis

Splen

V. cava inferior   Aorta abdominalis   Ren sinister

6.7 Topography of the Upper Abdominal Organs: Hepar, Vesica Biliaris, Duodenum, and Pancreas

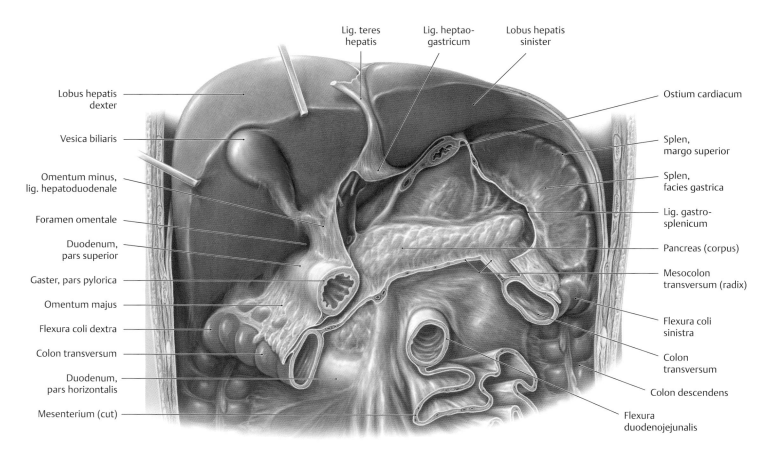

Lig. teres hepatis
Lig. heptaogastricum
Lobus hepatis sinister
Lobus hepatis dexter
Vesica biliaris
Omentum minus, lig. hepatoduodenale
Foramen omentale
Duodenum, pars superior
Gaster, pars pylorica
Omentum majus
Flexura coli dextra
Colon transversum
Duodenum, pars horizontalis
Mesenterium (cut)
Ostium cardiacum
Splen, margo superior
Splen, facies gastrica
Lig. gastrosplenicum
Pancreas (corpus)
Mesocolon transversum (radix)
Flexura coli sinistra
Colon transversum
Colon descendens
Flexura duodenojejunalis

A Location of the hepar and vesica biliaris
Anterior view. The gaster and intestinum tenue have been removed, leaving a short stump of the jejunum. Most of the colon transversum has been removed. The hepar has been lifted for better exposure of parts of the omentum minus, lig. hepatoduodenale and pancreas (for the contents of the lig. hepatoduodenale see **Eb**).

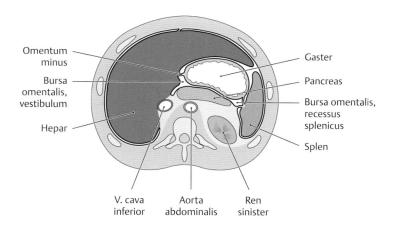

Omentum minus
Bursa omentalis, vestibulum
Hepar
Gaster
Pancreas
Bursa omentalis, recessus splenicus
Splen
V. cava inferior
Aorta abdominalis
Ren sinister

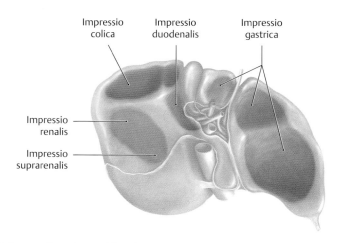

Impressio colica
Impressio duodenalis
Impressio gastrica
Impressio renalis
Impressio suprarenalis

B Position of the hepar
Transverse section through the abdomen at approximately the T 12/L 1 level, viewed from below. The hepar is intraperitoneal except for the area nuda, which is not visible here. The lobus hepatis sinister Aextends into the LUQ, where it is anterior to the gaster. The peritoneal fold between the hepar and the curvatura minor of the gaster (omentum minus) can be seen. Portions of the hepar form the right boundary of the bursa omentalis.

C Areas of contact with other organs
View of the visceral surface of the hepar.
Note: Impressions from organs that are in direct contact with the hepar are visible only on a liver that has been hardened in place by a chemical preservative ("fixation"). An unfixed hepar from a cadaver that has not been chemically preserved is so soft that generally it will not show organ impressions. Diseases of the hepar may easily spread to other organs, and vice versa, at areas of contact with adjacent organs (extensive owing to the size and topography of the hepar).

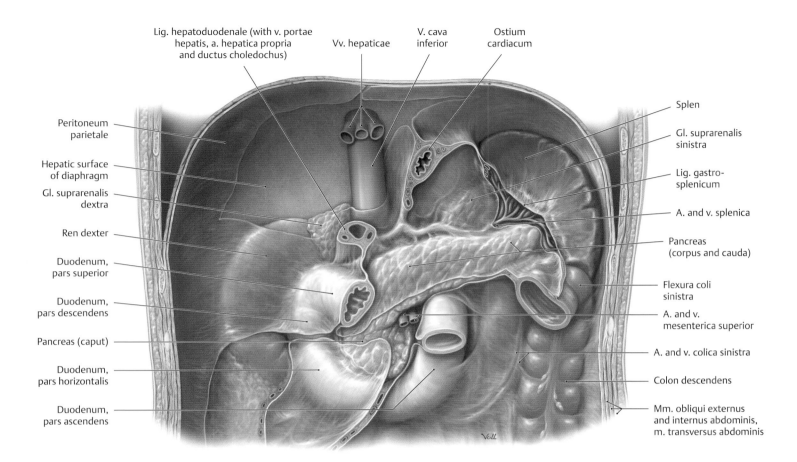

Lig. hepatoduodenale (with v. portae hepatis, a. hepatica propria and ductus choledochus)

Vv. hepaticae

V. cava inferior

Ostium cardiacum

Peritoneum parietale

Hepatic surface of diaphragm

Gl. suprarenalis dextra

Ren dexter

Duodenum, pars superior

Duodenum, pars descendens

Pancreas (caput)

Duodenum, pars horizontalis

Duodenum, pars ascendens

Splen

Gl. suprarenalis sinistra

Lig. gastro-splenicum

A. and v. splenica

Pancreas (corpus and cauda)

Flexura coli sinistra

A. and v. mesenterica superior

A. and v. colica sinistra

Colon descendens

Mm. obliqui externus and internus abdominis, m. transversus abdominis

D Location of duodenum and pancreas

Anterior view. The hepar, gaster and intestinum tenue have been removed, leaving the duodenum and a very small stump of the jejunum. The cola ascendens and transversum have been removed to expose the right kidney, pancreas, and duodenal loop. The secondarily retroperitoneal colon descendens is left in situ. The pancreas and duodenum are also secondarily retroperitoneal (for peritoneal relationships see p. 209).

Both kidneys and gll. suprarenales, located in the spatium retroperitoneale, are visible through the peritoneum parietale. The kidneys and gll. suprarenales are primarily retroperitoneal. The intraperitoneal splen is located in the left upper quadrant in a compartment called the splenic niche.

Note: The root of the (intraperitoneal) colon transversum crosses anterior to the duodenum and pancreas.

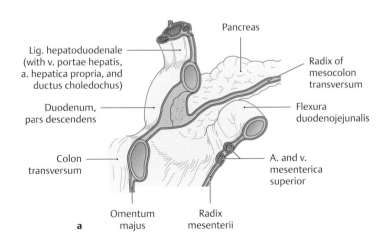

Pancreas

Lig. hepatoduodenale (with v. portae hepatis, a. hepatica propria, and ductus choledochus)

Duodenum, pars descendens

Colon transversum

Radix of mesocolon transversum

Flexura duodenojejunalis

A. and v. mesenterica superior

Omentum majus

Radix mesenterii

a

Vesica biliaris

A. cystica

Ductus choledochus

V. portae hepatis

Calot's triangle (p. 248)

A. hepatica propria

Lig. hepatoduodenale

b

E Peritoneal relationships of the duodenum and pancreas; contents of the ligamentum hepatoduodenale

a Peritoneal relationships of the duodenum and pancreas, anterior view. The root of the mesocolon transversum crosses over the pars descendens of the duodenum and the pancreas.

b Contents of the ligamentum hepatoduodenale. The lig. hepatoduodenale is part of the omentum minus and connects the hepar with the pylorus and pars superior of the duodenum. It contains the v. portae hepatis, the a. hepatica propria, and the ductus choledochus.

371

6.8 Topography of the Upper Abdominal Organs: Gaster and Splen

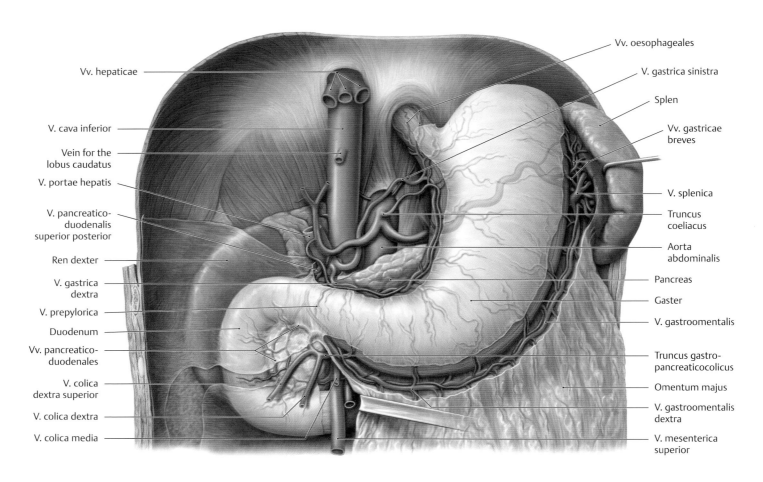

Vv. hepaticae

V. cava inferior

Vein for the lobus caudatus

V. portae hepatis

V. pancreatico- duodenalis superior posterior

Ren dexter

V. gastrica dextra

V. prepylorica

Duodenum

Vv. pancreatico- duodenales

V. colica dextra superior

V. colica dextra

V. colica media

Vv. oesophageales

V. gastrica sinistra

Splen

Vv. gastricae breves

V. splenica

Truncus coeliacus

Aorta abdominalis

Pancreas

Gaster

V. gastroomentalis

Truncus gastro- pancreaticocolicus

Omentum majus

V. gastroomentalis dextra

V. mesenterica superior

A Location of the gaster and splen

Anterior view. The hepar and omentum minus have been removed, the omentum majus has been opened and retracted to the left, and the gaster pulled slightly downward for better exposure. At several sites, the peritoneum has been removed or windowed for better exposure of the opening of the vv. hepaticae into the v. cava inferior and the opening of the vv. gastricae into the v. portae hepatis at the margin of the lig. hepatoduodenale (here completely opened). The splen is retracted from its "niche" and lies close to the fundus and curvatura major of the gaster. The intraperitoneal gaster covers most of the retroperitoneal pancreas. The omentum majus, a remnant of the mesogastrium dorsale, is suspended from the curvatura major of the gaster. The gaster is partially shown transparent to display the a. splenica that extends behind the gaster from the truncus coeliacus to the splen.

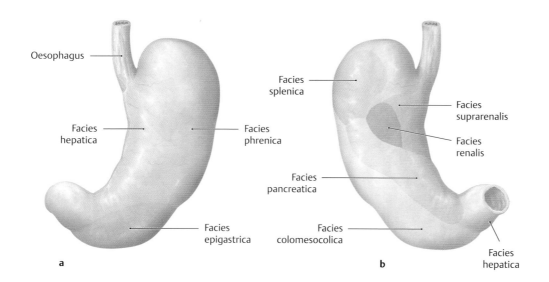

Oesophagus

Facies hepatica

Facies epigastrica

Facies splenica

Facies phrenica

Facies colomesocolica

Facies suprarenalis

Facies renalis

Facies pancreatica

Facies hepatica

a

b

B Areas of contact with adjacent organs

a, b Anterior and posterior views of the parietes gastrici. Because the gaster is intraperitoneal, it is very mobile relative to adjacent organs. But since the gaster is in close contact with other organs, lesions that penetrate the paries gastri (ulcers, malignant tumors) may spread to nearby organs or may cause adhesions to develop between the gaster and adjacent organs.

Vv. hepaticae

Vv. oesophageales

V. cava inferior

V. gastrica sinistra

Truncus coeliacus

V. portae hepatis

V. pancreatico-
duodenalis
superior posterior

V. gastrica dextra

Truncus gastro-
pancreaticocolicus

Vv. pancreatico-
duodenales

V. colica
dextra superior

V. colica dextra

Vv. gastricae
breves

V. splenica

V. gastroomentalis
sinistra

V. suprarenalis
sinistra

V. renalis sinistra

A. mesenterica
superior

V. gastroomentalis

V. testicularis/
ovarica sinistra

V. colica
media

V. mesenterica
superior

V. mesenterica
inferior

C Location of the pancreas, spleen, and major vessels

Anterior view. The gaster has been partially removed and pulled slightly downward, and most of the intestina have been removed leaving only the duodenum. The splen has been lifted from its bed and retracted anterolaterally toward the fundus gastricus. Part of the corpus pancreatis has been resected. Most of the peritoneum has been removed, and retroperitoneal fat and connective tissue have been cleared away.

The secondarily retroperitoneal pancreas crosses over the polus superior of the left kidney that also lies in the spatium retroperitoneale.

The diagram shows that the displayed retroperitoneal organs are not arranged in a coronal plane but oriented anterior to posterior. The most anterior organ in the right upper quadrant is the duodenum. Posterior to the duodenum lies the pancreas that is oriented transversely in the right and left upper quadrants. The most posterior organs are the two kidneys (here only the left kidney is clearly visible, the right kidney is covered by the duodenum and the caput pancreatis).

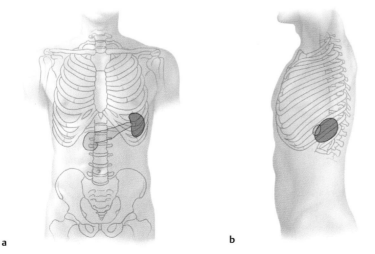

a   b

D Projection of the pancreas and splen onto the skeleton

Anterior (a) and left lateral (b) views. The corpus pancreatis is located at the L 1/L 2 level, its caput extends a little lower. The corpus, along with the cauda pancreatis, is directed upward and to the left (almost to T 12). The splen is located in the left upper quadrant. Its longitudinal axis follows the line of the tenth rib. The cauda pancreatis seems to touch the splen. It only "seems" to touch it because the pancreas lies retroperitoneal and the splen lies intraperitoneal. Thus, they are separated by the peritonea parietale and viscerale (i.e., by the cavitas peritonealis).

Note in particular how far posterior the splen is located as shown in (b). Just like the hepar, the splen touches the posterior wall of the cavitas peritonealis.

6.9 Cross-Sectional Anatomy of the Upper Abdominal Organs

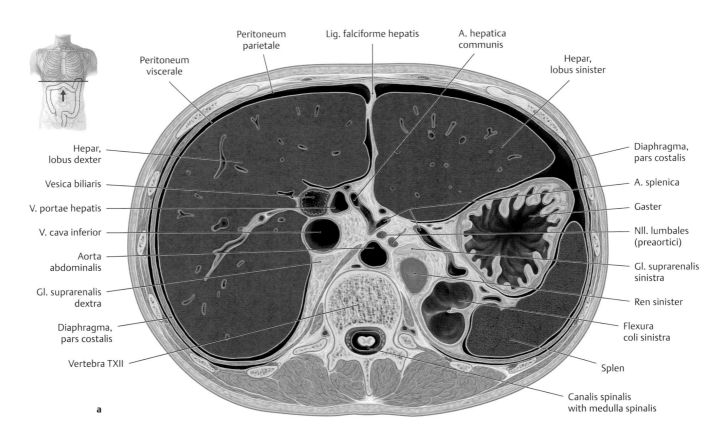

Peritoneum parietale

Lig. falciforme hepatis

A. hepatica communis

Hepar, lobus sinister

Peritoneum viscerale

Diaphragma, pars costalis

Hepar, lobus dexter

A. splenica

Vesica biliaris

Gaster

V. portae hepatis

Nll. lumbales (preaortici)

V. cava inferior

Aorta abdominalis

Gl. suprarenalis sinistra

Gl. suprarenalis dextra

Ren sinister

Diaphragma, pars costalis

Flexura coli sinistra

Vertebra TXII

Splen

Canalis spinalis with medulla spinalis

a

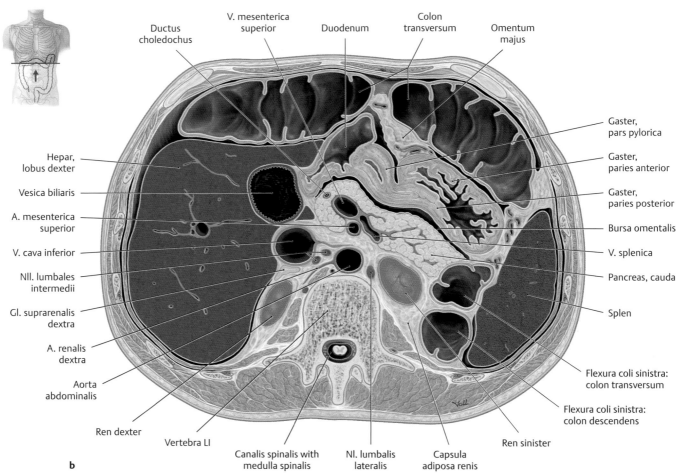

Ductus choledochus

V. mesenterica superior

Duodenum

Colon transversum

Omentum majus

Gaster, pars pylorica

Hepar, lobus dexter

Gaster, paries anterior

Vesica biliaris

Gaster, paries posterior

A. mesenterica superior

Bursa omentalis

V. cava inferior

V. splenica

Nll. lumbales intermedii

Pancreas, cauda

Gl. suprarenalis dextra

Splen

A. renalis dextra

Flexura coli sinistra: colon transversum

Aorta abdominalis

Flexura coli sinistra: colon descendens

Ren dexter

Ren sinister

Vertebra LI

Canalis spinalis with medulla spinalis

Nl. lumbalis lateralis

Capsula adiposa renis

b

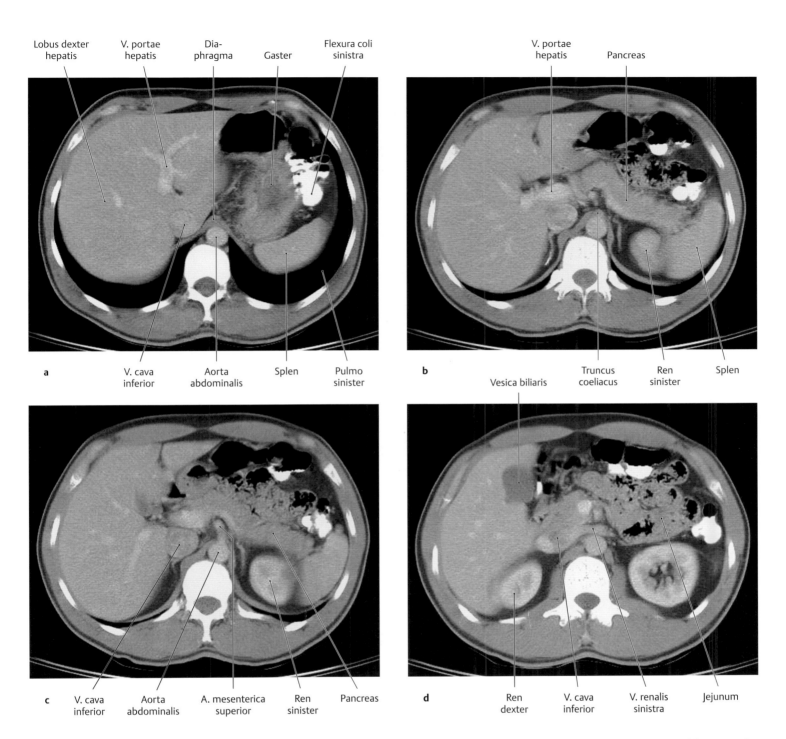

Lobus dexter hepatis | V. portae hepatis | Dia-phragma | Gaster | Flexura coli sinistra

a   V. cava inferior   Aorta abdominalis   Splen   Pulmo sinister

V. portae hepatis | Pancreas

b   Vesica biliaris   Truncus coeliacus   Ren sinister   Splen

c   V. cava inferior   Aorta abdominalis   A. mesenterica superior   Ren sinister   Pancreas

d   Ren dexter   V. cava inferior   V. renalis sinistra   Jejunum

B Abdominal computed tomography

Axial scans of the upper abdominal organs at the T 12 level (**a**), L 1 level (**b** and **c**), and L 2 level (**d**). Inferior views (from: Möller, T.B., E. Reif: Taschenatlas der Schnittbildanatomie, Band II: Thorax, Abdomen, Becken, 2. Aufl, Thieme, Stuttgart 2000).

Note: The pancreas is normally located at the L 1/2 level between the exit of the truncus coeliacus (see **b**) and the a. mesenterica superior (see **c**) from the aorta abdominalis.

A Transverse sections through the abdomen

a At the T 12 level; b At the L 1 level, inferior views.

The level that most organs occupy in the body is dependent on age, posture, constitutional type, nutritional state, and respiration. Thus, a section at a certain level may show considerable variation, especially in the organs that just border the plane of section. A section at the T 12 level

(**a**) passes only through the left kidney, which is more superior than the right kidney (the right kidney is more inferior because of the hepar and is below the plane of section). However, both gll. suprarenales are visible, and the position of the right kidney can be inferred at the T 12 level from the location of the right gl. suprarenalis. At the L 1 level, the section almost always passes through both kidneys (see **b**).

375

6.10 Topography of the Intestina Tenue and Crassum

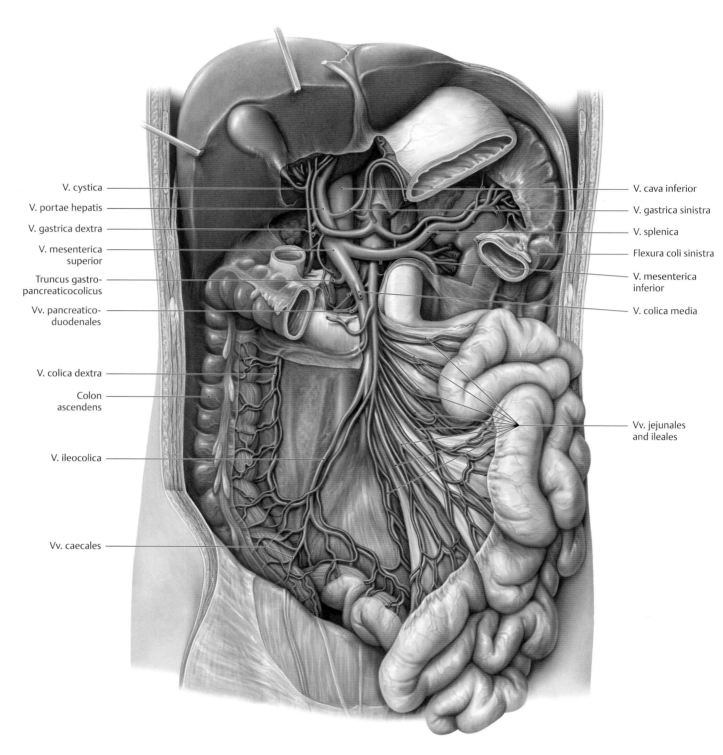

V. cystica

V. portae hepatis

V. gastrica dextra

V. mesenterica superior

Truncus gastro-pancreaticocolicus

Vv. pancreatico-duodenales

V. colica dextra

Colon ascendens

V. ileocolica

Vv. caecales

V. cava inferior

V. gastrica sinistra

V. splenica

Flexura coli sinistra

V. mesenterica inferior

V. colica media

Vv. jejunales and ileales

A Location of the intestinum tenue

Anterior view of the opened abdomen. The hepar has been lifted, most of the gaster and the colon transversum have been removed, and the pancreas has been largely resected.

The intestinum tenue is the longest individual organ. Its location varies to such a degree that pointing out its relation to palpable bony landmarks is not useful. Reference points are useful only for the initial and terminal segments of the intestinum tenue. The initial segment is the duodenum, a C-shaped loop that lies secondarily retroperitoneal in the right topper quadrant inferior (and slightly posterior) to the hepar, approximately at the L 1-3 level. The duodenum is crossed by the mesocolon transversum. The terminal part of the intestinum tenue is the ileum at the junction of the caecum with the colon ascendens. The ileum is located in the right lower quadrant slightly inferior to the crista iliaca. Most of the jejunum and ileum (both completely intraperitoneal) lie in the form of coils in the lower abdomen between the mesocolon transversum and the apertura pelvis superior within a "frame" formed by the colon. The jejunum and ileum are covered by the omentum majus (here removed) and are located more anterior than the duodenum (anterior layer of the abdomen). In this view, the mesenterium has been largely removed to expose the numerous aa. and vv. jejunales and ileales.

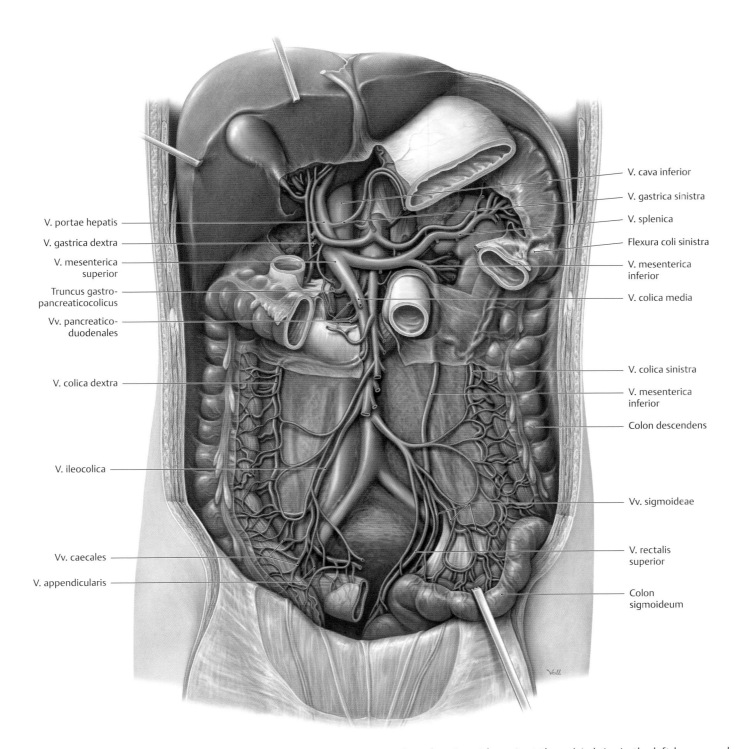

V. portae hepatis

V. gastrica dextra

V. mesenterica superior

Truncus gastro-pancreaticocolicus

Vv. pancreatico-duodenales

V. colica dextra

V. ileocolica

Vv. caecales

V. appendicularis

V. cava inferior

V. gastrica sinistra

V. splenica

Flexura coli sinistra

V. mesenterica inferior

V. colica media

V. colica sinistra

V. mesenterica inferior

Colon descendens

Vv. sigmoideae

V. rectalis superior

Colon sigmoideum

B Location of the large intestine

Anterior view of the opened abdomen. The hepar has been lifted, most of the gaster and the colon transversum have been removed, the pancreas has been largely resected, and the intestinum tenue has been removed leaving only the duodenum and a small stump of the jejunum and ileum. By removing a large area of the peritoneum, the neurovascular structures running to the cola ascendens and descendens are made visible.

The intestinum crassum forms a frame around the intestinum tenue. Its location also varies, but to a lesser degree than the intestinum tenue:

- The cola ascendens and descendens (both secondarily retroperitoneal) are along the right and left sides,
- The colon transversum (intraperitoneal) runs horizontally across the border between the upper and lower abdomen,

- The colon sigmoideum is at the pelvic brim in the left lower quadrant, and
- The rectum and canalis analis (retro or subperitoneal) are in the pelvis anterior to the os sacrum.

Using bony landmarks makes sense only as reference points to define the location of the rectum that extends in front of the os sacrum from the junction between S 2 and S 3 to the diaphragma pelvis. Because of the colon's proximity to the hepar (flexura coli dextra, or flexura coli hepatica) and splen (flexura coli sinistra, or flexura coli splenica) they also serve as topographic reference points. If the abdomen is divided into layers from anterior to posterior, the intraperitoneal colon transversum is located in the anterior layer, and the retroperitoneal portions of the cola ascendens and descendens are located in the middle layer. However, the colon descendens lies significantly more posterior than the colon ascendens.

6.11 Radiography of the Intestina Tenue and Crassum

A Standing abdominal radiograph

Depending on the medical problem, images of the gastrointestinal tract may be obtained using conventional X-rays (with or without the administration of a contrast medium), computerized tomography (CT and MRI) or sonography. Left lateral decubitus or standing abdominal radiographs are employed to detect the presence of free gas within the cavitas peritonealis, which may indicate perforation of a hollow organ, or to look for fluid levels in the intestinal lumen if ileus is suspected.

a Standing abdominal image–normal findings: the diaphragma is clearly defined (arrows) with no evidence of free gas under the domes of the diaphragma. Under normal physiologic conditions, small quantities of gas are present (intestinal gases or gastric bubble);

b Mechanical ileus after right hemicolectomy: proximal to the site of stenosis, greatly distended coils of the ileum are visible as well as airfluid levels at different heights in the remaining colon. The pattern of distribution of the airfluid levels may indicate the site of obstruction (see **c**);

c Schematic representation of radiologic findings in cases of mechanical ileus showing the different levels at which the obstruction has occurred: **I** duodenal ileus demonstrating the 'double-bubble' characteristic, **II** high and **III** deep intestinum tenue ileus (no presence of gas in colonic frame), **IV** intestinum crassum ileus with airfluid levels located along the course of the colon (from Reiser, M. et al.: Radiologie [Duale Reihe], 2nd edition, Thieme, Stuttgart 2006).

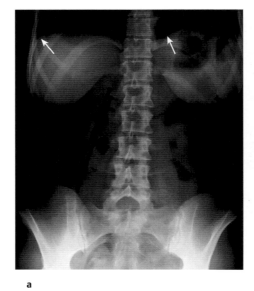
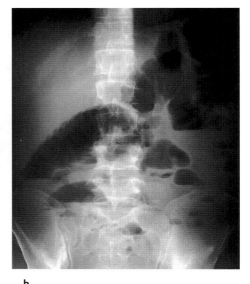

a   b

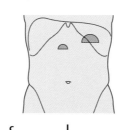
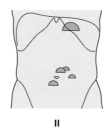
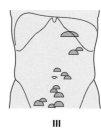
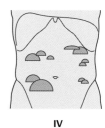

c   I   II   III   IV

Plicae circulares   Jejunum

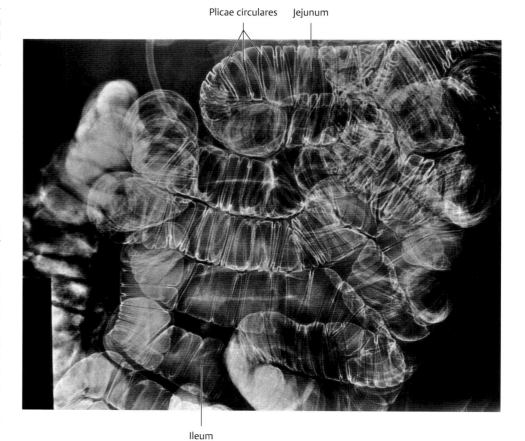
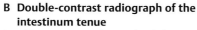

Ileum

B Double-contrast radiograph of the intestinum tenue

Double-contrast radiograph of the intestinum tenue in the anteroposterior projection (X-ray source in front of the patient, film-screen combination behind the patient). Anterior view. In a double-contrast study, air is instilled into the bowel through a tube and a radiopaque liquid contrast medium (barium sulfate) is administered to provide an exceptionally high-contrast image. This technique guarantees high morphological resolution and is sensitive in detecting mucosal changes. The image to the right illustrates a normal double-contrast study. The transversely oriented plicae circulares of the intestinum tenue are defined with great clarity.

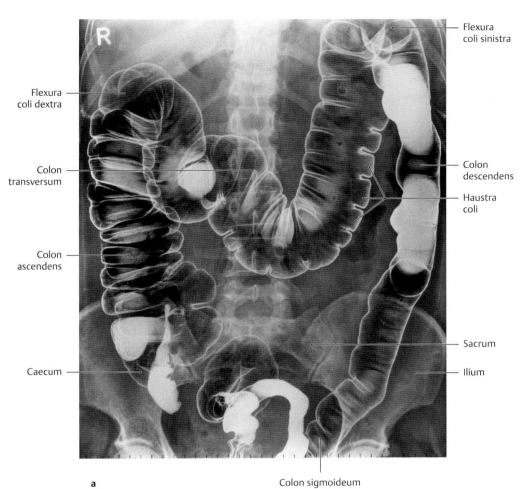

Flexura coli dextra

Colon transversum

Colon ascendens

Caecum

a

Flexura coli sinistra

Colon descendens

Haustra coli

Sacrum

Ilium

Colon sigmoideum

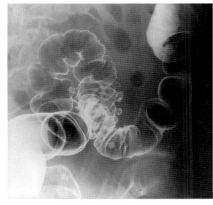

b

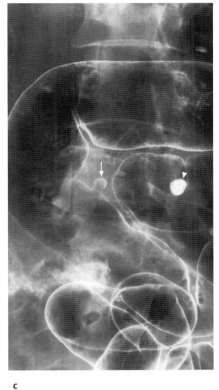

c

C Double-contrast radiograph of the intestinum crassum

(from: Reiser, M. et al.: Radiologie [Duale Reihe], 2. Aufl. Thieme, Stuttgart 2006)

Double-contrast radiograph of a normal intestinum crassum in the anteroposterior projection, anterior view; **a** Normal findings; **b** Multiple evaginations with sigmoid diverticulitis; **c** Colonic diverticula viewed in profile (arrow) and en face (tip of arrow); **d** Colon polyp; **e** Schematic diagram of criteria for the radiologic distinction between polyps and diverticula.

In **a** the different parts of the intestinum crassum and their haustra are clearly visible. The radiopaque contrast medium is not evenly distributed: the more opaque, white areas of variable size indicate sites where the contrast medium has pooled.

Note: Both colonic diverticula and colon polyps display characteristic pathological changes in the intestinum crassum. Whereas diverticula are evaginations of circumscribed wall portions of the intestinum crassum, polyps are initially benign, circumscribed, pedunculated or parietal mucosal protrusions. Their

radiological distinction is apparent in the double-contrast radiograph because of certain criteria when viewed both in profile and en face (see **e**). Inflammatory changes of the diverticula are called diverticulitis. An acute episode can lead to severe stenosis with an increased risk of perforation. As the colonic diverticula increase in size they carry a higher risk of malignant transformation (colonic carcinoma see p. 248).

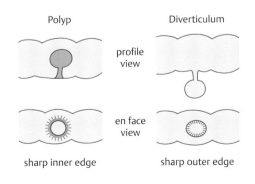

Polyp

Diverticulum

profile view

en face view

sharp inner edge

sharp outer edge

e

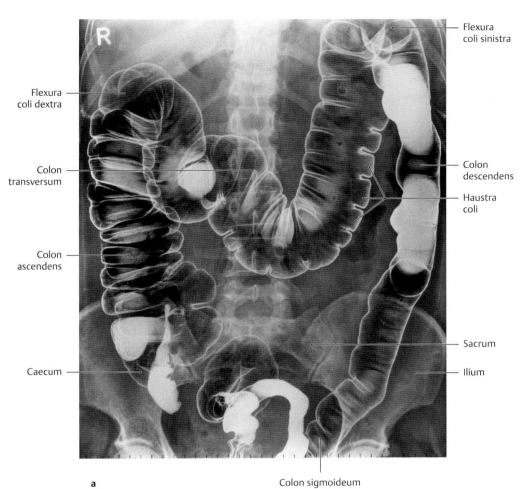

d

379

6.12   Topography of the Rectum

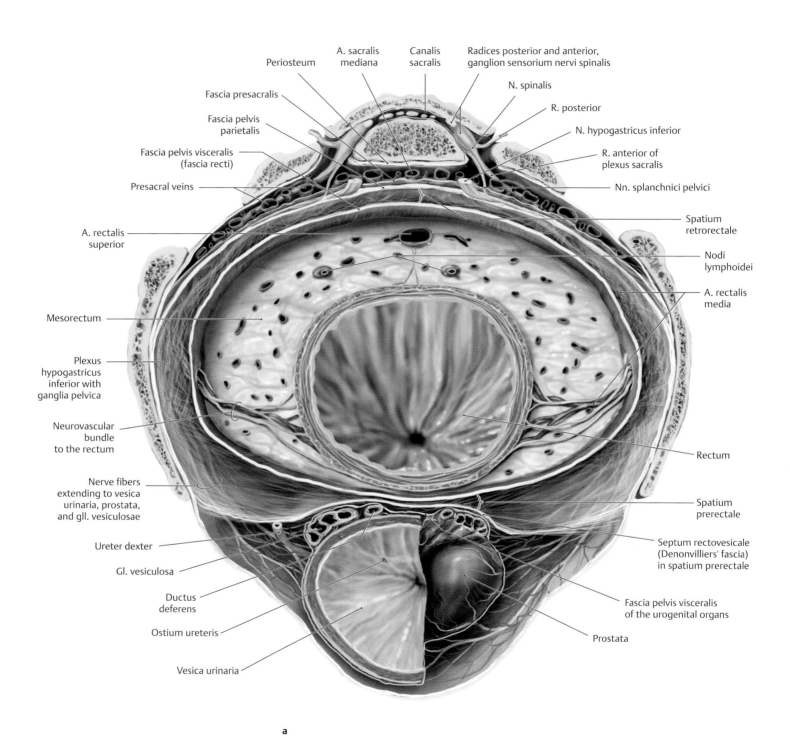

Periosteum
A. sacralis mediana
Canalis sacralis
Radices posterior and anterior, ganglion sensorium nervi spinalis
Fascia presacralis
N. spinalis
Fascia pelvis parietalis
R. posterior
Fascia pelvis visceralis (fascia recti)
N. hypogastricus inferior
R. anterior of plexus sacralis
Presacral veins
Nn. splanchnici pelvici
A. rectalis superior
Spatium retrorectale
Nodi lymphoidei
A. rectalis media
Mesorectum
Plexus hypogastricus inferior with ganglia pelvica
Neurovascular bundle to the rectum
Rectum
Nerve fibers extending to vesica urinaria, prostata, and gll. vesiculosae
Spatium prerectale
Septum rectovesicale (Denonvilliers' fascia) in spatium prerectale
Ureter dexter
Gl. vesiculosa
Fascia pelvis visceralis of the urogenital organs
Ductus deferens
Ostium ureteris
Prostata
Vesica urinaria

a

A Perirectal area with mesorectal fascial envelope
(after Wedel and Stelzner)

Male pelvis; **a** Transverse section at the level of the lower third of the vesica urinaria, viewed from above; **b** Midsagittal section, viewed from the left side.

Continence-maintaining operations, for example, total mesorectal excision (TME), play an increasingly important role in rectal cancer surgery (see p. 249). Of particular significance for the surgical treatment of rectal carcinoma are the mesorectal fascial envelopes, which divide the perirectal area and protect the neurovascular structures supplying the rectum and other pelvic organs. These fascial envelopes are derived from the fascia transversalis that continues into the pelvis as the fascia pelvis. Its visceral layer covers the pelvic organs and its parietal layer covers the bony and muscular pelvic wall.

At the sites where the organs are attached to the diaphragma pelvis, the fascial layers merge. One important compartment is the mesorectum, consisting of perirectal connective tissue and fat (also known as the rectal adventitia). It contains the superior rectal vessels and the rectal vasa lymphatica and their nodi lymphoidei. Thus, the mesorectum is an area where rectal cancer can typically spread. The fascia pelvis visceralis, which surrounds the mesorectum (and is commonly known as rectal fascia) abuts anteriorly and posteriorly against avascular and nerve-free

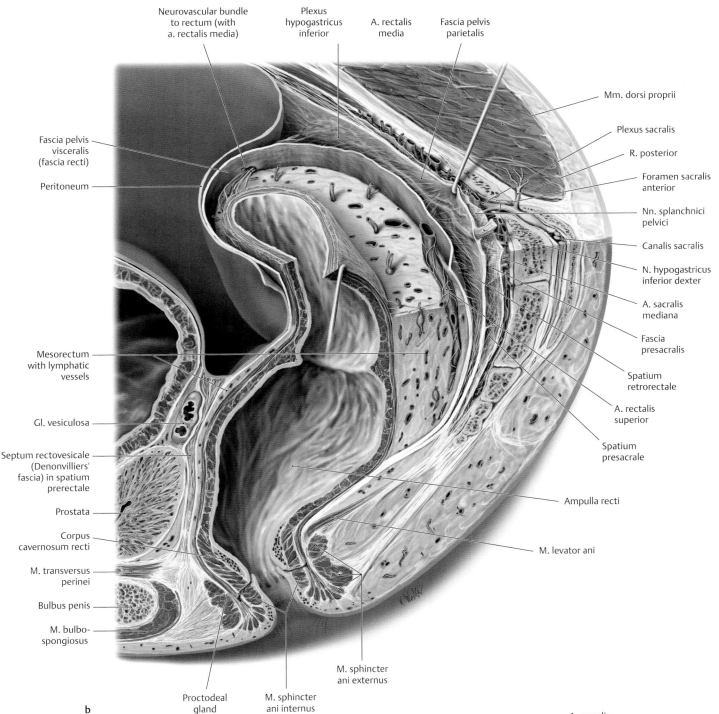

Neurovascular bundle to rectum (with a. rectalis media)

Plexus hypogastricus inferior

A. rectalis media

Fascia pelvis parietalis

Mm. dorsi proprii

Plexus sacralis

R. posterior

Foramen sacralis anterior

Nn. splanchnici pelvici

Canalis sacralis

N. hypogastricus inferior dexter

A. sacralis mediana

Fascia presacralis

Spatium retrorectale

A. rectalis superior

Spatium presacrale

Ampulla recti

M. levator ani

Fascia pelvis visceralis (fascia recti)

Peritoneum

Mesorectum with lymphatic vessels

Gl. vesiculosa

Septum rectovesicale (Denonvilliers' fascia) in spatium prerectale

Prostata

Corpus cavernosum recti

M. transversus perinei

Bulbus penis

M. bulbo-spongiosus

Proctodeal gland

M. sphincter ani internus

M. sphincter ani externus

b

slit-like spaces (spatia retrorectale and prerectale). Opening of these spaces allows for a posterior and anterior mobilization of the rectum during the TME procedure (see p. 249). Further posteriorly lies the fascia pelvis parietalis (also known as Waldeyer's fascia). It encloses two bundles of sympathetic nerves (the left and right nn. hypogastrici), which run laterally (see **c**). After receiving parasympathetic contributions from the nn. splanchnici pelvici, which arise from sacral nn. spinales in the area of the pararectal fascia, the nn. hypogastrici together with the a. rectalis media approach the lateral wall of the rectum. Prominent venous plexuses (presacral veins) run between the fascia pelvis parietalis and sacral periosteum in the presacral space. Anteriorly, the mesorectum is bounded by the fascia propria (Denonvilliers' fascia) of the urogenital organs, which particularly in males consists of a distinct plate of connective tissue at the level of the prostata and the gll. vesiculosae.

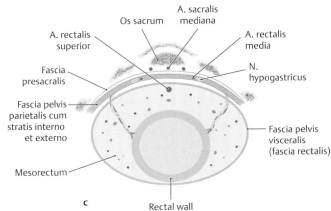

A. sacralis mediana

Os sacrum

A. rectalis superior

A. rectalis media

N. hypogastricus

Fascia presacralis

Fascia pelvis parietalis cum stratis interno et externo

Fascia pelvis visceralis (fascia rectalis)

Mesorectum

Rectal wall

c

6.13 Retroperitoneum: Overview and Divisions

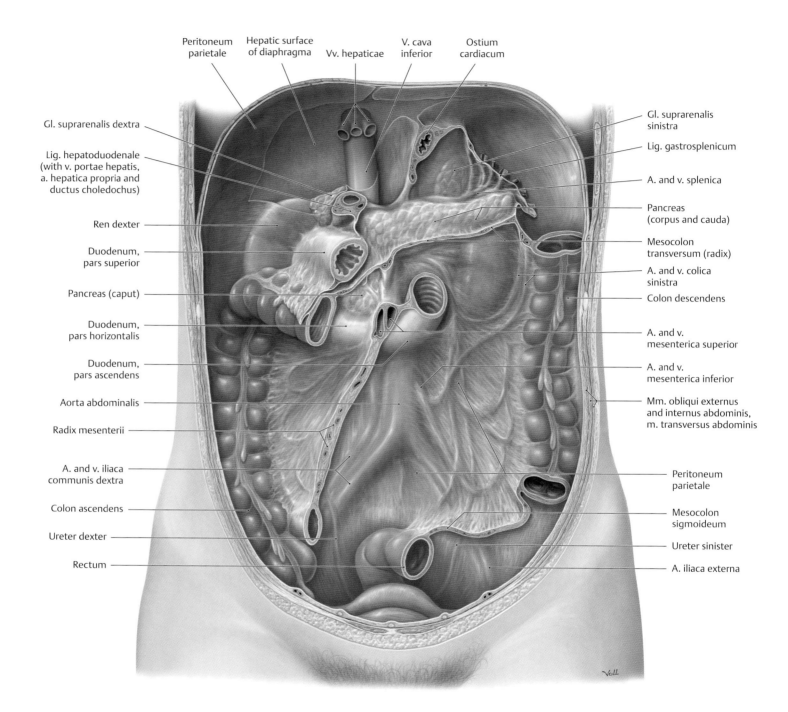

Peritoneum parietale | Hepatic surface of diaphragma | Vv. hepaticae | V. cava inferior | Ostium cardiacum

Gl. suprarenalis dextra

Lig. hepatoduodenale (with v. portae hepatis, a. hepatica propria and ductus choledochus)

Ren dexter

Duodenum, pars superior

Pancreas (caput)

Duodenum, pars horizontalis

Duodenum, pars ascendens

Aorta abdominalis

Radix mesenterii

A. and v. iliaca communis dextra

Colon ascendens

Ureter dexter

Rectum

Gl. suprarenalis sinistra

Lig. gastrosplenicum

A. and v. splenica

Pancreas (corpus and cauda)

Mesocolon transversum (radix)

A. and v. colica sinistra

Colon descendens

A. and v. mesenterica superior

A. and v. mesenterica inferior

Mm. obliqui externus and internus abdominis, m. transversus abdominis

Peritoneum parietale

Mesocolon sigmoideum

Ureter sinister

A. iliaca externa

A Overview of the retroperitoneum

Anterior view of a female abdomen and pelvis. Most of the gaster, splen, intestinum tenue, colon transversum, and colon sigmoideum (intraperitoneal organs) have been removed. The stump of the oesophagus at the ostium cardiacum is visible to provide an anatomical landmark.

Note: Some of the retroperitoneal organs are fully integrated in that space, having formed in the retroperitoneum: the kidneys, gll. suprarenales, great vessels, and nervi. Other structures form in the cavitas peritonealis and migrate to the retroperitoneum secondarily (the pancreas and duodenum, see **B**). Their peritoneum viscerale becomes fused to the peritoneum parietale of the posterior wall, and they retain a peritoneal covering on their anterior surface. The primary retroperitoneal organs do not have a peritoneal covering because they are fully integrated into the retroperitoneal connective tissue.

B Organs and neurovascular structures in the retroperitoneum

Organs	Vessels	Nerves
Primarily retroperitoneal (or extraperitoneal):	(all primarily retroperitoneal)	(all primarily retroperitoneal)
• Right and left renes • Right and left gll. suprarenales • Right and left ureteres *Secondarily retroperitoneal:* • Pancreas • Duodenum: partes descendens and horizontalis, some of the pars ascendens • Cola ascendens and descendens • Variable: portions of the caecum • Rectum to the flexura sacralis	• Aorta (pars abdominalis) and its branches • V. cava inferior and its tributaries • Vv. lumbales ascendentes • V. portae hepatis (before coursing in the lig. hepatoduodenale) and its tributaries • Nll. lumbales, sacrales, and iliaci, trunci lumbales, cisterna chyli	• Branches of the plexus lumbalis (nn. iliohypogastricus, ilioinguinalis, genitofemoralis, cutaneus femoralis lateralis, femoralis, and obturatorius) • Truncus sympathicus • Ganglia autonomica and plexus autonomici

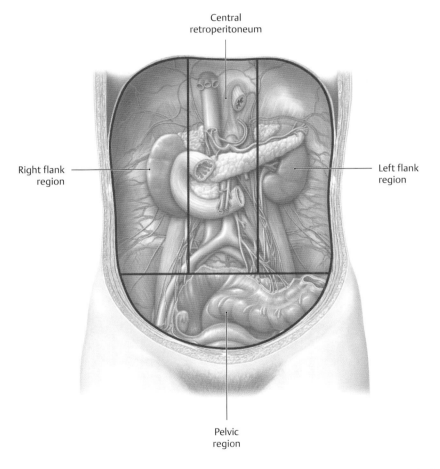

Central retroperitoneum

Right flank region

Left flank region

Pelvic region

C Zones of the retroperitoneum (after von Lanz and Wachsmuth)
The retroperitoneum, like other body cavities, can be divided into zones based on clinical criteria. This type of classification is useful for evaluating what organs may be jointly affected by disease or injury due to their proximity to each other, even if they belong to entirely different functional systems. The retroperitoneum is divided into three zones:

Zone 1: central retroperitoneum with the duodenum and great vessels
Zone 2: left and right flank regions with the kidneys, ureteres, colon ascendens, and colon descendens (omitted here to give a clearer view of the other organs)
Zone 3: pelvic region (corresponding to the hypogastrium) with the vesica urinaria, distal ureteres, rectum, and internal genitalia

6.14 Retroperitoneum: Peritoneal Relationships

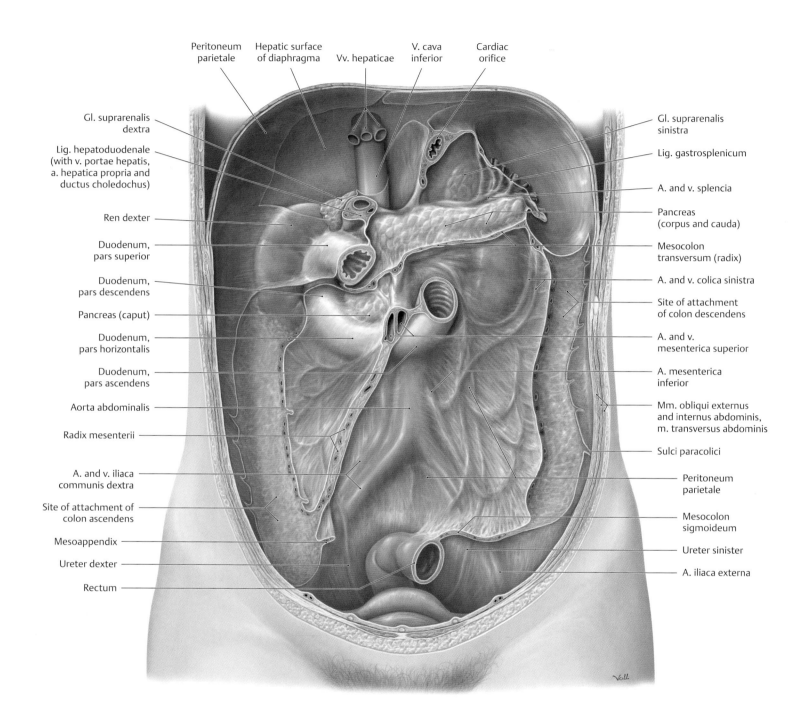

Peritoneum parietale · Hepatic surface of diaphragma · Vv. hepaticae · V. cava inferior · Cardiac orifice

Gl. suprarenalis dextra

Lig. hepatoduodenale (with v. portae hepatis, a. hepatica propria and ductus choledochus)

Ren dexter

Duodenum, pars superior

Duodenum, pars descendens

Pancreas (caput)

Duodenum, pars horizontalis

Duodenum, pars ascendens

Aorta abdominalis

Radix mesenterii

A. and v. iliaca communis dextra

Site of attachment of colon ascendens

Mesoappendix

Ureter dexter

Rectum

Gl. suprarenalis sinistra

Lig. gastrosplenicum

A. and v. splencia

Pancreas (corpus and cauda)

Mesocolon transversum (radix)

A. and v. colica sinistra

Site of attachment of colon descendens

A. and v. mesenterica superior

A. mesenterica inferior

Mm. obliqui externus and internus abdominis, m. transversus abdominis

Sulci paracolici

Peritoneum parietale

Mesocolon sigmoideum

Ureter sinister

A. iliaca externa

A Peritoneal relationships on the posterior wall of the cavitas peritonealis

Anterior view of the opened thorax and abdomen. All of the intraperitoneal organs have been removed to display the retroperitoneum (spatium retroperitoneale). The posterior wall of the cavitas peritonealis also forms the anterior wall of the retroperitoneum. Unlike the anterior wall of the cavitas peritonealis, which consists largely of muscles and fasciae, much of the posterior wall is formed by the organs in the retroperitoneum, which are visible through the peritoneum parietale in this dissection. For clarity, the retroperitoneal connective tissue and fat have been thinned out to display the course of the retroperitoneal vessels and the ureter (where it crosses in front of the iliac vessels). The hepatic surface of the diaphragma is devoid of peritoneum and corresponds to the area nuda of the hepar. The cola ascendens and descendens (removed here for clarity) are attached by connective tissue to the posterior wall of the cavitas peritonealis, so they are also located in the retroperitoneum (see p. 382). In this specimen, the area of attachment of the colon ascendens extends further inferiorly to the pelvis than usual. The mesocolon transversum, like the colon transversum, is located anterior to the duodenum (i.e., is intraperitoneal). The migration of these organs during embryonic development is described on p. 42 f. The mesocolon sigmoideum crosses anterior to the left iliac vessels and left ureter.

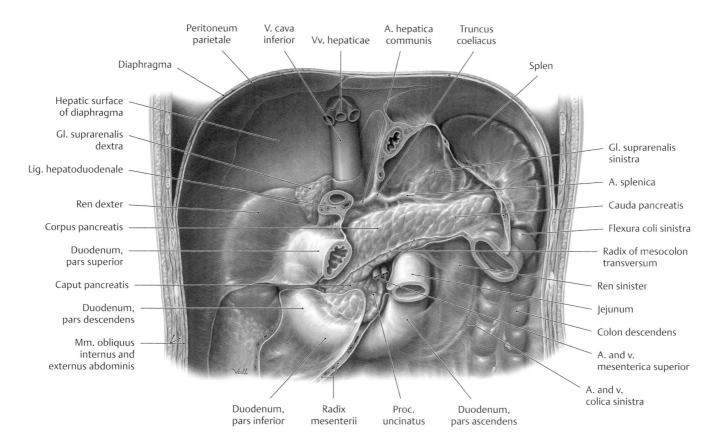

Diaphragma

Peritoneum parietale
V. cava inferior
Vv. hepaticae
A. hepatica communis
Truncus coeliacus
Splen

Hepatic surface of diaphragma

Gl. suprarenalis dextra

Lig. hepatoduodenale

Ren dexter

Corpus pancreatis

Duodenum, pars superior

Caput pancreatis

Duodenum, pars descendens

Mm. obliquus internus and externus abdominis

Gl. suprarenalis sinistra

A. splenica

Cauda pancreatis

Flexura coli sinistra

Radix of mesocolon transversum

Ren sinister

Jejunum

Colon descendens

A. and v. mesenterica superior

A. and v. colica sinistra

Duodenum, pars inferior
Radix mesenterii
Proc. uncinatus
Duodenum, pars ascendens

B Retroperitoneum

Anterior view. All intraperitoneal organs have been removed except for the splen and a short stump of the jejunum (both of which have been left in place to aid orientation). The retroperitoneal colon ascendens has also been removed; and to better display the kidneys, the retroperitoneal connective tissue is only hinted at.

The retroperitoneal organs "shine" through the peritoneum. The root of the mesocolon transversum crosses over the right kidney, duodenum

and pancreas. From a superior to inferior direction, the root of the mesenterium crosses the caput pancreatis. During retroperitonealization, the colon descendens migrates so far to the posterior body wall, that it comes to lie almost in a coronal plane with the left ren. The intraperitoneal splen lies in its own small compartment located in the upper quadrant in close vicinity to the cauda pancreatis, colon descendens, and left kidney. However, the splen is separated from these organs by the cavitas peritonealis.

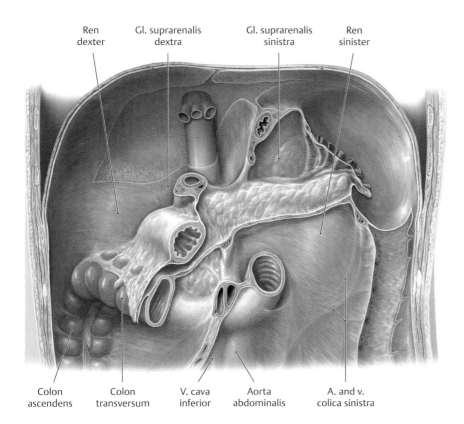

Ren dexter
Gl. suprarenalis dextra
Gl. suprarenalis sinistra
Ren sinister

Colon ascendens
Colon transversum
V. cava inferior
Aorta abdominalis
A. and v. colica sinistra

C Transperitoneal view of the retroperitoneum

Anterior view. The intraperitoneal organs have been removed except a small part of the colon transversum. The retroperitoneal colon descendens has also been removed. The connective tissue and fat in the retroperitoneum are of normal volume in this dissection. The kidneys form in the retroperitoneum during embryonic development and are embedded in the retroperitoneal fat and connective tissue. Thus the kidneys, like the great vessels, are obscured by the anterior wall of the retroperitoneum and are visible only as bulges behind the peritoneum parietale. Additionally, the anterior layer of the fascia renalis is interposed between the kidneys and the peritoneum parietale (see p. 292). Because the pancreas is secondarily retroperitoneal, it is not fully integrated into the retroperitoneal fat and connective tissue. Being attached to the posterior wall of the cavitas peritonealis "only" by fusion of the peritoneal layers, the pancreas can be seen with much greater clarity. Although its anterior surface is covered by peritoneum, that layer is more translucent than the retroperitoneal connective tissue and fat.

385

6.15 Retroperitoneum: Organs of the Retroperitoneum

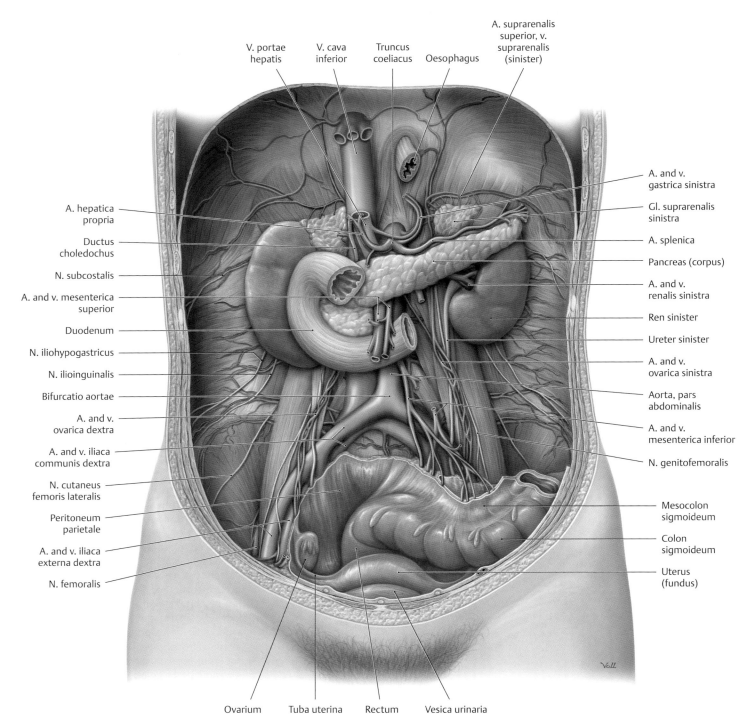

V. portae hepatis — V. cava inferior — Truncus coeliacus — Oesophagus — A. suprarenalis superior, v. suprarenalis (sinister)

A. hepatica propria

Ductus choledochus

N. subcostalis

A. and v. mesenterica superior

Duodenum

N. iliohypogastricus

N. ilioinguinalis

Bifurcatio aortae

A. and v. ovarica dextra

A. and v. iliaca communis dextra

N. cutaneus femoris lateralis

Peritoneum parietale

A. and v. iliaca externa dextra

N. femoralis

A. and v. gastrica sinistra

Gl. suprarenalis sinistra

A. splenica

Pancreas (corpus)

A. and v. renalis sinistra

Ren sinister

Ureter sinister

A. and v. ovarica sinistra

Aorta, pars abdominalis

A. and v. mesenterica inferior

N. genitofemoralis

Mesocolon sigmoideum

Colon sigmoideum

Uterus (fundus)

Ovarium — Tuba uterina — Rectum — Vesica urinaria

A Retroperitoneal organs, anterior view

Organs of the upper retroperitoneum, anterior view. Intraperitoneal organs except for the colon sigmoideum have been removed; the uterus and adnexa as well as the subperitoneal vesica urinaria have been left in place to aid orientation. Retroperitoneal segments of the colon, peritoneum parietale, and retroperitoneal connective tissue have been completely removed; thus leaving peritoneum only in the area of the mentioned pelvic organs. The posterior wall of the cavitas abdominalis with its neurovascular structures is visible. The most dominant structures are the major retroperitoneal vascular trunks, the aorta abdominalis and v. cava inferior, anterior or lateral to which the organs in the spatium retroperitoneale are located.

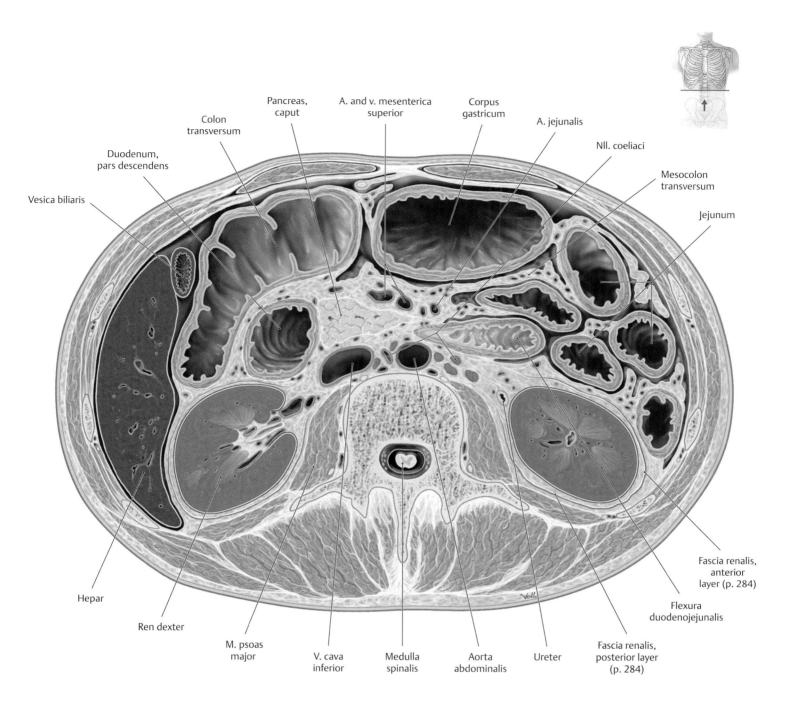

B Retroperitoneal organs in transverse section

Transverse section through the abdomen approximately at the L 1 level, inferior view.

This transverse section shows the relative positions of the organs in the spatium retroperitoneale from anterior to posterior:

- the duodenum with the caput pancreatis are located most anteriorly,
- the cauda pancreatis (not visible here because it is above the sectional plane) lies posterior to the caput pancreatis as the pancreas runs obliquely backward,
- the two kidneys are located most posteriorly.

Between the "duodenum-pancreas plane" and the plane of the kidneys lie the major retroperitoneal vascular trunks; the aorta is located anterior to the columna vertebralis and the v. cava inferior is situated anterior and slightly right of the columna vertebralis. It is clearly visible how the hepar with the cavitas peritonealis extends slightly behind the right kidney, and that the colon descendens and left kidney lie almost in the same horizontal plane. It is clear how the kidneys are embedded in the retroperitoneal fat and connective tissue of the capsula adiposa.

387

6.16 Retroperitoneum: Location of the Kidneys

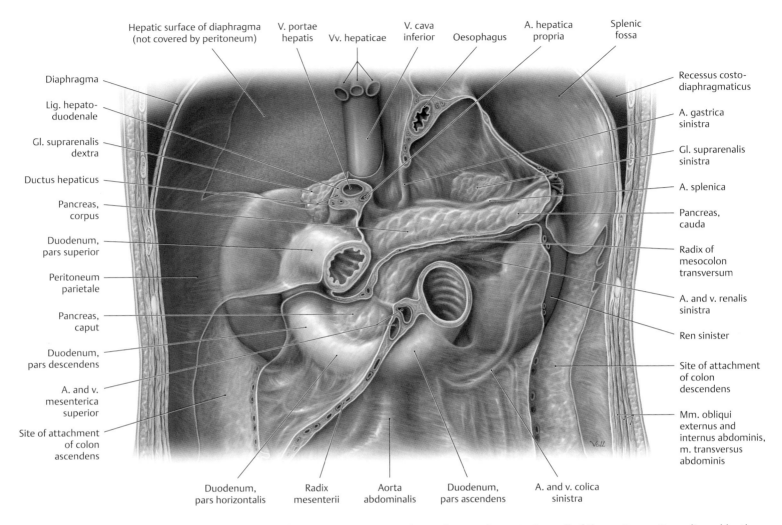

Hepatic surface of diaphragma (not covered by peritoneum)
V. portae hepatis
Vv. hepaticae
V. cava inferior
Oesophagus
A. hepatica propria
Splenic fossa

Diaphragma

Lig. hepato-duodenale

Gl. suprarenalis dextra

Ductus hepaticus

Pancreas, corpus

Duodenum, pars superior

Peritoneum parietale

Pancreas, caput

Duodenum, pars descendens

A. and v. mesenterica superior

Site of attachment of colon ascendens

Recessus costo-diaphragmaticus

A. gastrica sinistra

Gl. suprarenalis sinistra

A. splenica

Pancreas, cauda

Radix of mesocolon transversum

A. and v. renalis sinistra

Ren sinister

Site of attachment of colon descendens

Mm. obliqui externus and internus abdominis, m. transversus abdominis

Duodenum, pars horizontalis
Radix mesenterii
Aorta abdominalis
Duodenum, pars ascendens
A. and v. colica sinistra

A Topographical relations of the kidneys (renes) in the retroperitoneumm

Anterior view. All of the intraperitoneal organs and secondarily retroperitoneal portions of the colon (ascendens and descendens) have been removed, leaving the duodenum and pancreas in place. Most of the capsula adiposa anterior to the kidneys has also been removed. Both kidneys are overlapped by the attachments of the cola ascendens and descendens on the posterior wall of the cavitas peritonealis and by the root of the mesocolon transversum. Because the pancreas, parts of the duodenum, and the flexurae colicae sinistra and dextra are *secondarily* retroperitoneal, they are in close proximity to the *primarily* retroperitoneal kidneys but are still separated from them by the fat and connective tissue of the capsula adiposa (see **B**).

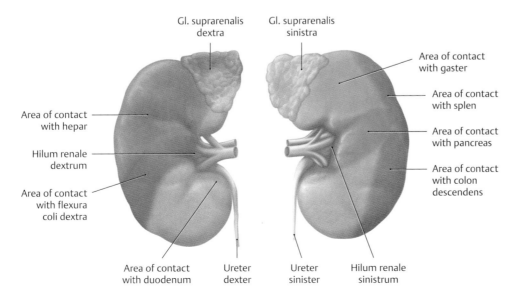

Gl. suprarenalis dextra

Gl. suprarenalis sinistra

Area of contact with gaster

Area of contact with splen

Area of contact with hepar

Area of contact with pancreas

Hilum renale dextrum

Area of contact with colon descendens

Area of contact with flexura coli dextra

Area of contact with duodenum
Ureter dexter
Ureter sinister
Hilum renale sinistrum

B Areas of renal contact with abdominal and pelvic organs

Anterior view. The gll. suprarenales (also shown for clarity) are very close to the kidneys but do not touch them, being separated from the renal surface by the capsula adiposa. The *facies anteriores* of the kidneys are related to numerous abdominal organs. The retroperitoneal organs are separated from the kidneys (also retroperitoneal) by the fasciae of the renal bed. The kidneys are additionally separated from the *intraperitoneal* organs by the peritoneum. As a result, surrounding organs do not form impressions on the kidneys, which are relatively firm and stable in their dimensions, and the areas of renal contact with other organs are important in terms of topographical anatomy but have little clinical importance.

C Proximity of the kidneys to the nervi iliohypogastrici and ilioinguinales

a Neurovascular structures on the anterior side of the posterior trunk wall. Lumbar fossa on the right side after removal of the anterior and lateral trunk wall, all the fasciae, the peritoneum and the intra- and retroperitoneal organs except for the right kidney. The v. cava inferior has been partially removed. Anterior view.

b Posterior view of the right kidney. The renal capsula adiposa and parts of the posterior trunk wall have been removed.

c Skin areas supplied by the nn. iliohypogastricus and ilioinguinalis to which pain is referred

After removal of trunk wall layers, the proximity of the kidneys to the nn. iliohypogastrici and ilioinguinales can be seen. Both are branches of the plexus lumbalis from T 12 and L 1, positioned lateral to the lumbar spine. These nerves supply motor innervation to the muscles of the trunk wall and sensory innervation to skin areas on the lateral and anterior abdominal wall. If an abnormally enlarged kidney exerts pressure on the nn. iliohypogastricus and ilioinguinalis, pain is referred to the skin areas shown in **c**. The distance between the kidney and n. subcostalis is usually large enough so that it is not compressed by renal enlargement.

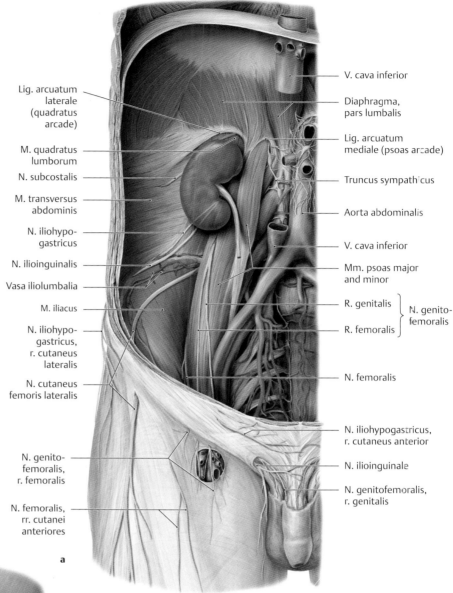

Lig. arcuatum laterale (quadratus arcade)
M. quadratus lumborum
N. subcostalis
M. transversus abdominis
N. iliohypogastricus
N. ilioinguinalis
Vasa iliolumbalia
M. iliacus
N. iliohypogastricus, r. cutaneus lateralis
N. cutaneus femoris lateralis
N. genitofemoralis, r. femoralis
N. femoralis, rr. cutanei anteriores

V. cava inferior
Diaphragma, pars lumbalis
Lig. arcuatum mediale (psoas arcade)
Truncus sympathicus
Aorta abdominalis
V. cava inferior
Mm. psoas major and minor
R. genitalis
R. femoralis } N. genitofemoralis
N. femoralis
N. iliohypogastricus, r. cutaneus anterior
N. ilioinguinale
N. genitofemoralis, r. genitalis

a

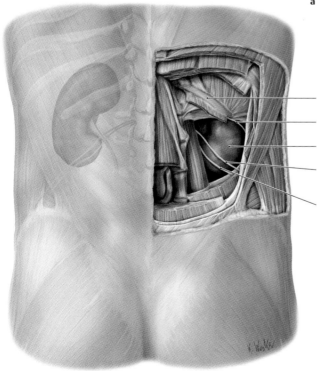

b

Costa XII
N. subcostalis
Ren dexter
N. iliohypogastricus
N. ilioinguinalis

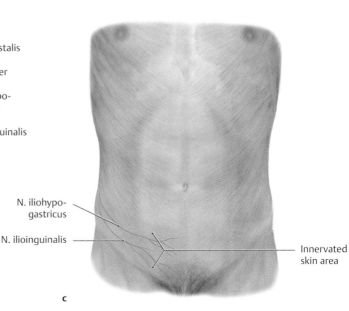

N. iliohypogastricus
N. ilioinguinalis
Innervated skin area

c

6.17 Peritoneal Relationships in the Anterior Abdominal Wall

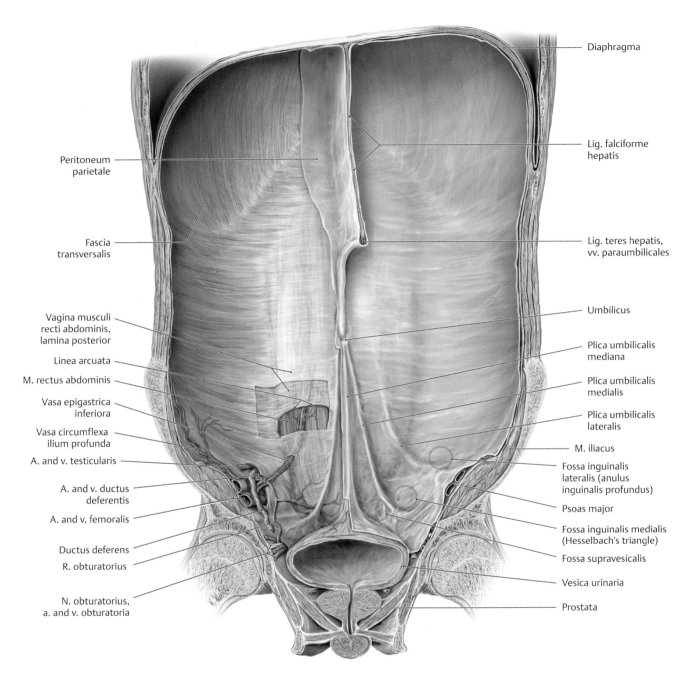

Diaphragma

Lig. falciforme hepatis

Peritoneum parietale

Lig. teres hepatis, vv. paraumbilicales

Fascia transversalis

Umbilicus

Vagina musculi recti abdominis, lamina posterior

Plica umbilicalis mediana

Linea arcuata

Plica umbilicalis medialis

M. rectus abdominis

Vasa epigastrica inferiora

Plica umbilicalis lateralis

Vasa circumflexa ilium profunda

M. iliacus

A. and v. testicularis

Fossa inguinalis lateralis (anulus inguinalis profundus)

A. and v. ductus deferentis

Psoas major

A. and v. femoralis

Fossa inguinalis medialis (Hesselbach's triangle)

Ductus deferens

Fossa supravesicalis

R. obturatorius

Vesica urinaria

N. obturatorius, a. and v. obturatoria

Prostata

A Peritoneal relationships on the posterior surface of the abdominal wall

Posterior surface of the anterior abdominal wall, viewed from the posterior aspect. The peritoneum on the left side has been removed to display the contents of the peritoneal folds (plicae umbilicales). They are formed by the peritoneum that covers structures on the posterior surface of the anterior trunk wall. The peritoneum parietale lying between the folds raised by these structures forms shallow depressions called fossae.

Peritoneal folds (plicae umbilicales):
• One plica umbilicalis mediana: This is where the peritoneum parietale covers the lig. umbilicale medianum, which is the obliterated urachus (remnant of the allantois that is obliterated during embryonic development).
  Note: Incomplete obliteration of the urachus may lead to umbilical fistulae in postnatal life.
• Two plicae umbilicales mediales: Sites where the peritoneum parietale covers the a. umbilicalis (the portion of the artery that becomes occluded at birth)

• Two plicae umbilicales laterales: Sites where the peritoneum parietale covers the a. and v. epigastrica inferior

Each of the paired *aa. umbilicales* consists of a proximal pars patens (which gives rise to the a. vesicalis superior and, in males, the a. ductus deferentis) and a distal pars occlusa. The unpaired *v. umbilicalis* is usually obliterated to form the lig. teres hepatis.

Peritoneal fossae:
• Two fossae supravesicales
• Two fossae inguinales mediales (posterior to the anulus inguinalis superficialis)
• Two fossae inguinales laterales (in which the anulus inguinalis profundus is located)

Note: The *anulus inguinalis profundus* (internal inguinal ring) is a structural weak point in the abdominal wall which forms the entrance to the canalis inguinalis. This canal provides a path for the descent of the testis during normal development, but also creates a potential route for the herniation of abdominal viscera (indirect inguinal hernia).

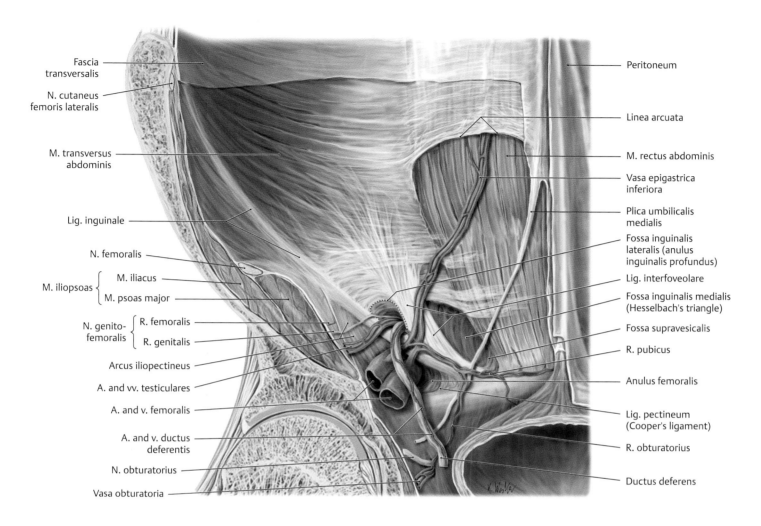

Fascia transversalis

N. cutaneus femoris lateralis

M. transversus abdominis

Lig. inguinale

N. femoralis

M. iliopsoas { M. iliacus
M. psoas major

N. genito-femoralis { R. femoralis
R. genitalis

Arcus iliopectineus

A. and vv. testiculares

A. and v. femoralis

A. and v. ductus deferentis

N. obturatorius

Vasa obturatoria

Peritoneum

Linea arcuata

M. rectus abdominis

Vasa epigastrica inferiora

Plica umbilicalis medialis

Fossa inguinalis lateralis (anulus inguinalis profundus)

Lig. interfoveolare

Fossa inguinalis medialis (Hesselbach's triangle)

Fossa supravesicalis

R. pubicus

Anulus femoralis

Lig. pectineum (Cooper's ligament)

R. obturatorius

Ductus deferens

B Internal hernial openings in the male inguinal and femoral region
Detail from **A**, posterior view. For better exposure of the hernial openings, the peritoneum and fascia transversalis have been partially removed. The internal hernia openings (see **C**) for indirect and direct inguinal hernias, femoral hernias and suprapubic (supravesical) hernias are color-coded.

C Overview of internal and external openings of abdominal hernias
Above the lig. inguinale, the plicae umbilicales mediana, mediales, and laterales (see A) form three weak spots on each side of the abdominal wall where indirect and direct inguinal hernias and suprapubic hernias typically occur. Another weak spot is located below the *lig. inguinale* and medial to the v. femoralis in the lacuna vasorum. There the anulus femoralis is covered only by compliant connective tissue, the septum femorale, which is permeated by numerous vasa lymphatica.

Internal opening	Hernia	External opening
Above the lig. inguinale:		
Fossa supravesicalis	Supravesical hernia	Anulus inguinalis superficialis
Fossa inguinalis medialis (Hesselbach's triangle)	Direct inguinal hernia	Anulus inguinalis superficialis
Fossa inguinalis lateralis (anulus inguinalis profundus)	Indirect inguinal hernia	Anulus inguinalis superficialis
Below the lig. inguinale:		
Anulus femoralis	Femoral hernia	Hiatus saphenus (fossa ovalis)

6.18 Peritoneal Relationships in the Pelvis Minor

A Paramedian section through the pelvis minor (= sectional plane slightly lateral from the midline)

a Female pelvis; **b** Male pelvis, both viewed from the right side.

Most of the connective tissue in the pelvic spatium extraperitoneale has been removed accounting for the apparently empty spaces between the organs. The vesica urinaria is well distended here so that the part of the vesica urinaria not covered by peritoneum is partially above the symphysis pubica (site of suprapubic bladder puncture).

Whereas the cavitas peritonealis in the male is completely closed, in the female the abdominal end of the patent tuba uterina creates a potential opening to the outside. The cervical mucus plug creates a germ-proof seal that protects the pelvis minor from ascending infections.

The peritoneum forms pouches in the pelvis minor of both males and females, the excavatio rectouterina (between the uterus and rectum) in the female and the excavatio rectovesicalis (deepest part in the pelvis between the vesica urinaria and rectum) in the male. Their specific shape depends on the degree of distention of the uterus and rectum or vesica urinaria and rectum. Generally, the excavatio rectouterina is deep and the excavatio rectovesicalis is shallow. The excavatio rectouterina (pouch of Douglas) is the deepest point in the female cavitas peritonealis (see **B**). This space is clinically significant because it can be accessed for puncture or ultrasound procedures by going through the vagina.

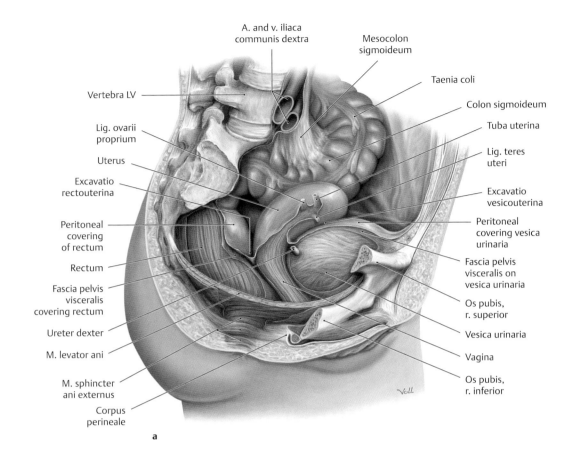

A. and v. iliaca communis dextra — Mesocolon sigmoideum — Taenia coli — Colon sigmoideum — Tuba uterina — Lig. teres uteri — Excavatio vesicouterina — Peritoneal covering vesica urinaria — Fascia pelvis visceralis on vesica urinaria — Os pubis, r. superior — Vesica urinaria — Vagina — Os pubis, r. inferior

Vertebra LV — Lig. ovarii proprium — Uterus — Excavatio rectouterina — Peritoneal covering of rectum — Rectum — Fascia pelvis visceralis covering rectum — Ureter dexter — M. levator ani — M. sphincter ani externus — Corpus perineale

a

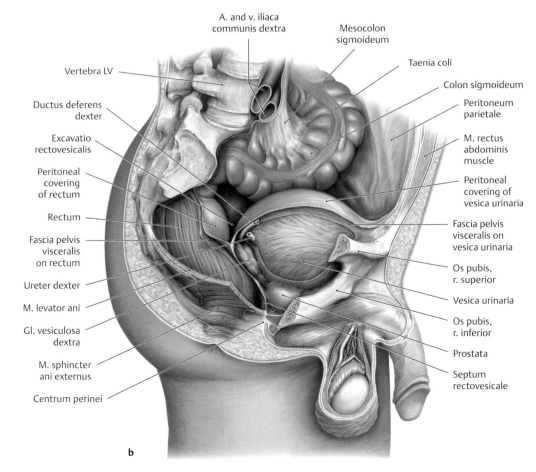

A. and v. iliaca communis dextra — Mesocolon sigmoideum — Taenia coli — Colon sigmoideum — Peritoneum parietale — M. rectus abdominis muscle — Peritoneal covering of vesica urinaria — Fascia pelvis visceralis on vesica urinaria — Os pubis, r. superior — Vesica urinaria — Os pubis, r. inferior — Prostata — Septum rectovesicale

Vertebra LV — Ductus deferens dexter — Excavatio rectovesicalis — Peritoneal covering of rectum — Rectum — Fascia pelvis visceralis on rectum — Ureter dexter — M. levator ani — Gl. vesiculosa dextra — M. sphincter ani externus — Centrum perinei

b

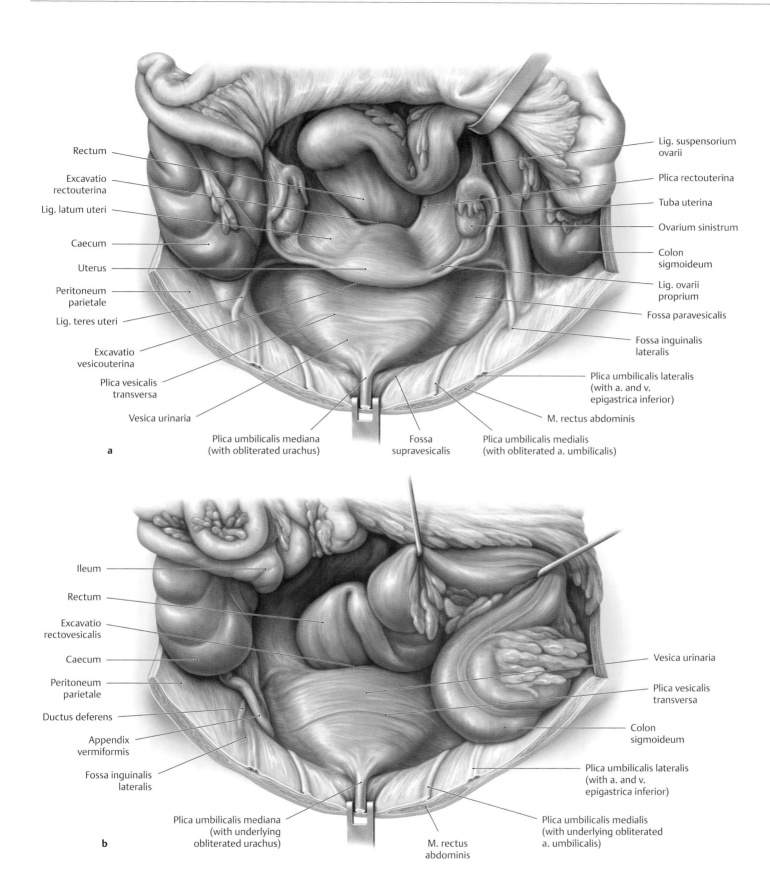

Rectum

Excavatio
rectouterina

Lig. latum uteri

Caecum

Uterus

Peritoneum
parietale

Lig. teres uteri

Excavatio
vesicouterina

Plica vesicalis
transversa

Vesica urinaria

Plica umbilicalis mediana
(with obliterated urachus)

Fossa
supravesicalis

Plica umbilicalis medialis
(with obliterated a. umbilicalis)

a

Lig. suspensorium
ovarii

Plica rectouterina

Tuba uterina

Ovarium sinistrum

Colon
sigmoideum

Lig. ovarii
proprium

Fossa paravesicalis

Fossa inguinalis
lateralis

Plica umbilicalis lateralis
(with a. and v.
epigastrica inferior)

M. rectus abdominis

Ileum

Rectum

Excavatio
rectovesicalis

Caecum

Peritoneum
parietale

Ductus deferens

Appendix
vermiformis

Fossa inguinalis
lateralis

Plica umbilicalis mediana
(with underlying
obliterated urachus)

M. rectus
abdominis

Plica umbilicalis medialis
(with underlying obliterated
a. umbilicalis)

Plica umbilicalis lateralis
(with a. and v.
epigastrica inferior)

Colon
sigmoideum

Plica vesicalis
transversa

Vesica urinaria

b

B Pelvis minor, anterosuperior view

a Female pelvis, **b** Male pelvis. Loops of the intestinum tenue and parts of the intestinum crassum have been retracted laterally to show the vesica urinaria and rectum.

The peritoneum parietale is reflected onto the surface of the vesica urinaria and then continues onto the anterior wall of the rectum, or in the female to the uterus and the anterior wall of the rectum (the upper part of which is covered by peritoneum). The posterior wall of the vesica urinaria and lower parts of the rectum are not covered by peritoneum. On the surface of the relatively empty vesica urinaria, as shown here, the peritoneum forms a transverse crease called the plica vesicalis transversa. It disappears when the vesica urinaria is full. For the plicae umbilicales see p. 390. In the female, the peritoneum covers most of the uterus and parametrial connective tissue (parametrium) except for the cervix uteri, not visible here. As intraperitoneal organs, the ovaria and tubae uterinae are covered by peritoneum. In the male, the peritoneum also covers the ductus deferens, which passes through the anterior wall via the canalis inguinalis.

6.19 Topography of Pelvic Connective Tissue, Levels of the Cavitas Pelvis, and the Diaphragma Pelvis

A Subdivision of the lesser pelvis by spaces and fasciae

Transverse (**a** and **b**) and midsagittal (**c** and **d**) sections through the (connective tissue of the) pelvis, anterosuperior and lateral views.

Spaces: The pelvis minor consists of the *pelvic cavitas peritonealis* and *pelvic spatium extraperitoneale* (see p. 9). The latter is further divided by the m. levator ani into an upper and lower part, creating the three levels of the pelvis minor (see **B**). The spaces are filled by connective tissue of variable density*. Topographically, based on the relationship to the peritoneum and pelvic wall, the spatium extraperitoneale can be subdivided into

- the spatium retropubicum: between the vesica urinaria and symphysis pubica;
- the spatium retroinguinale: behind the regio inguinalis and below the peritoneum;
- the spatium retroperitoneale: between the peritoneum and sacrum (the continuation of the retroperitoneum of the abdomen).

Fasciae: The *fascia pelvis* consists of fascia parietalis (covering the structures of the pelvic wall) and fascia visceralis (covering the pelvic organs). The connective tissue of the fascia visceralis is thickened at sites between and around the organs and is continuous with the adventitia or capsule of the pelvic organs:

- Fascia rectoprostatica: septum retrovesicale (Denonvilliers' fascia) (male pelvis, located between the rectum and vesica urinaria)
- Fascia rectovaginalis: septum rectovaginale (female pelvis, located between the rectum and vagina)

The *connective tissue* around the organs is also thickened and generally transmits the neurovascular bundles that supply the organs.

- Lig. recti laterale (in pararectal fascia)
- Lig. laterale vesicae (in paravesical fascia)
- Lig. pubovesicale
- Lig. transversum cervicis (in inferior parametrium)

* The spatium extraperitoneale is mostly filled by loose fatty connective tissue (sliding layer of connective tissue, mainly for the pelvic organs). At specific sites, the connective tissue is thickened and resembles dense, fibrous connective tissue (the entire fascia pelvis parietalis and parts of the fascia pelvis visceralis, as well as ligaments such as the lig. cardinale (lig. transversum cervicis), which differ in character from the ligaments of the musculoskeletal system).

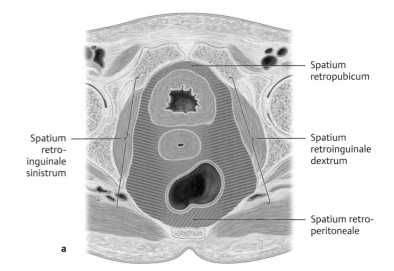

Spatium retropubicum

Spatium retroinguinale sinistrum

Spatium retroinguinale dextrum

Spatium retroperitoneale

a

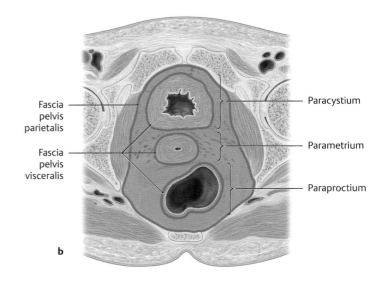

Fascia pelvis parietalis

Fascia pelvis visceralis

Paracystium

Parametrium

Paraproctium

b

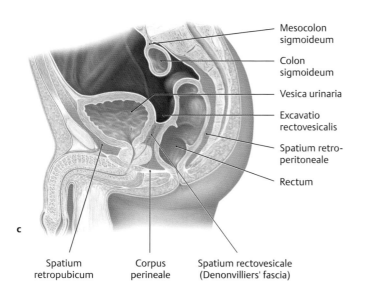

Mesocolon sigmoideum

Colon sigmoideum

Vesica urinaria

Excavatio rectovesicalis

Spatium retroperitoneale

Rectum

c

Spatium retropubicum

Corpus perineale

Spatium rectovesicale (Denonvilliers' fascia)

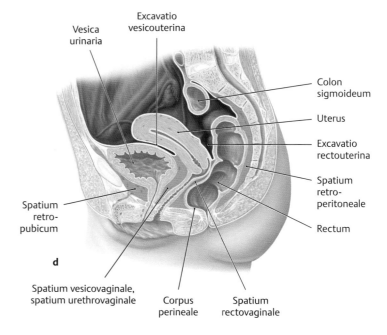

Excavatio vesicouterina

Vesica urinaria

Colon sigmoideum

Uterus

Excavatio rectouterina

Spatium retroperitoneale

Rectum

Spatium retropubicum

d

Spatium vesicovaginale, spatium urethrovaginale

Corpus perineale

Spatium rectovaginale

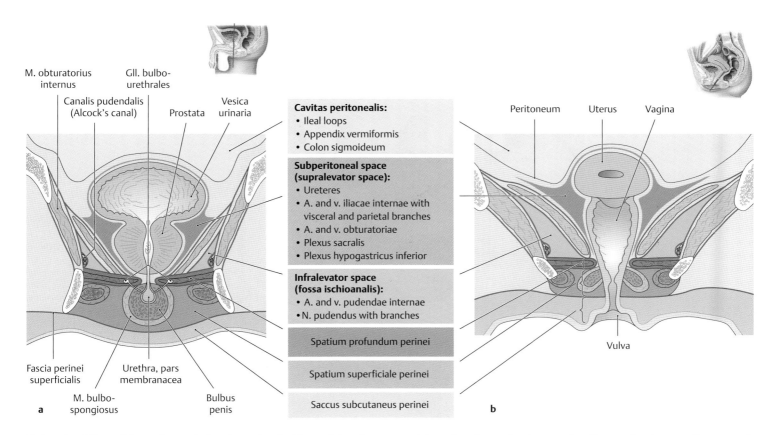

Cavitas peritonealis:
- Ileal loops
- Appendix vermiformis
- Colon sigmoideum

Subperitoneal space (supralevator space):
- Ureteres
- A. and v. iliacae internae with visceral and parietal branches
- A. and v. obturatoriae
- Plexus sacralis
- Plexus hypogastricus inferior

Infralevator space (fossa ischioanalis):
- A. and v. pudendae internae
- N. pudendus with branches

Spatium profundum perinei

Spatium superficiale perinei

Saccus subcutaneus perinei

B Levels of the pelvic region and structures located in each level

Coronal section (for exact location of sectional planes see insets above) through a male (**a**) and female (**b**) pelvis. In addition to the levels of the pelvic region, the perineal spaces (spatium profundum, spatium superficiale, and saccus subcutaneus) located below the pelvic region, are also outlined in color.

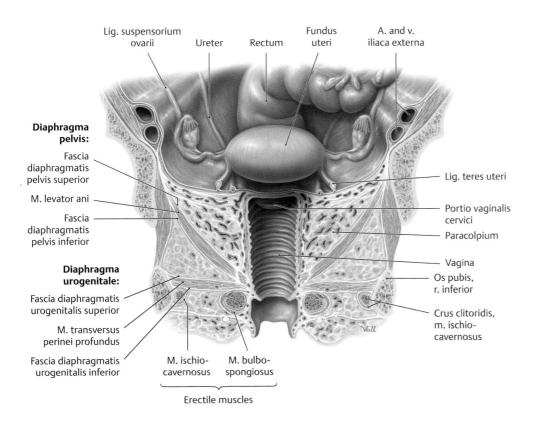

C Structure of the pelvic floor

The diaphragma pelvis is composed of three muscle and connective tissue plates that are also divided into three levels:

- **Upper layer:** diaphragma pelvis
- **Middle layer:** diaphragma urogenitale
- **Lower layer:** sphincters and erectile muscles of the urogenital and intestinal tracts

The funnel-shaped diaphragma pelvis is mainly formed by the m. levator ani and its superior and inferior muscular fasciae (fasciae superior and inferior diaphragmatis pelvis). The diaphragma urogenitale is a fibromuscular connective tissue sheet that stretches horizontally between the rr. ischiopubici and is mainly formed by the m. transversus perinei profundus and its superior and inferior muscular fasciae (superior and inferior fasciae of the diaphragma urogenitale). The sphincters and erectile muscles include the m. bulbospongiosus, m. ischiocavernosus, m. sphincter urethrae externus, m. sphincter ani externus, and their individual muscular fasciae.

395

6.20 Suspensory Apparatus of the Uterus

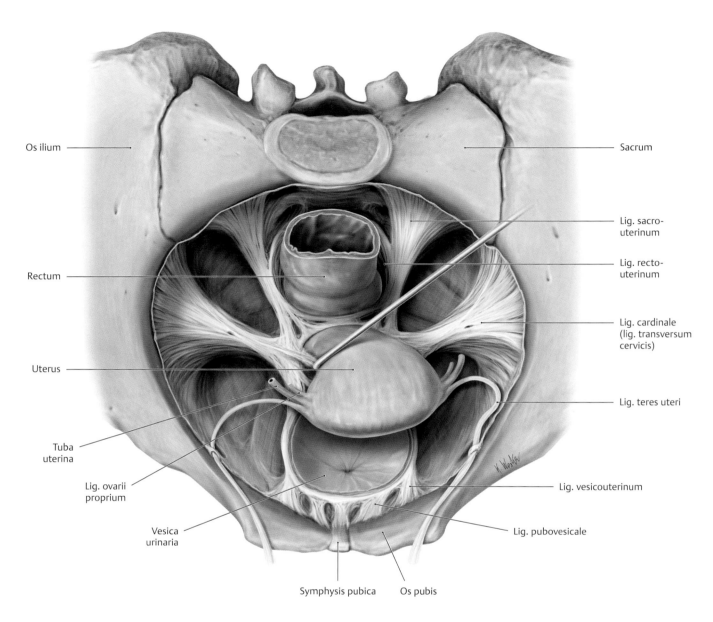

A Suspensory apparatus of the uterus

Location and function: The suspensory apparatus of the uterus is located in the subperitoneal connective tissue in the pelvis minor and consists of band-like structures of dense fibrous parts of the pelvic connective tissue (see p. 394). The uterus is mainly anchored at the cervix uteri by tissue strands that extend in both the sagittal and transverse directions. Like the neck of a bottle turned upside down, the isthmus uteri or portio supravaginalis cervicis is clasped and attached to the pelvis minor. In this way, the portio vaginalis cervicis lies on the interspinal line. This is referred to as the normal position of the uterus. Generally, the suspensory apparatus permits physiological mobility of the uterus so it can adjust to the distention of surrounding organs. When the vesica urinaria is full the uterus becomes more erect. When the rectum is full the uterus is pushed forward. If the vesica urinaria and rectum are both full the uterus is elevated.

Components: The strongest supporting structure is the *lig. cardinale* (Mackenrodt's ligament) also known as the lig. transversum cervicis, a fibrous layer in the parametrium. It fans out from the fascia of the

lateral pelvic wall to the portio supravaginalis cervicis. This fibrous apparatus keeps the uterus suspended in a position that is secured by the muscles of the diaphragma pelvis. In the sagittal direction, the uterus is anchored by band-like structures extending between the symphysis pubica and os sacrum. By running between vesica urinaria and cervix uteri as well as rectum and cervix uteri, these connective tissue fibers (*lig. pubovesicale, lig. vesicouterinum, lig. vesicouterinum*, and *lig. rectouterinum*) anchor the organs. The lig. teres uteri arises at the cornua uteri and runs along the canalis inguinalis to the labia majora where it is anchored. It has smooth muscle cells and holds the uterus forward in its typical position (anteversion–anteflexion, see p. 326).

Note: Intraperitoneal changes in uterine position are mostly congenital. However, tumors, inflammatory processes, and shortening of the suspensory ligaments can also influence uterine position. After childbirth, the uterus may assume a retroverted–retroflexed position (due to temporary overstretching of the uterine support system). As the body returns to its nonpregnant condition, the uterus returns to its normal position.

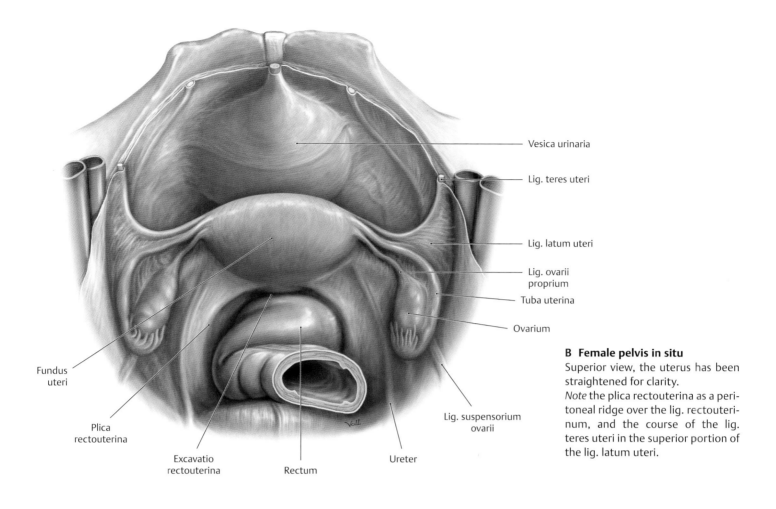

Vesica urinaria

Lig. teres uteri

Lig. latum uteri

Lig. ovarii proprium

Tuba uterina

Ovarium

Fundus uteri

Plica rectouterina

Excavatio rectouterina

Rectum

Ureter

Lig. suspensorium ovarii

B Female pelvis in situ
Superior view, the uterus has been straightened for clarity.
Note the plica rectouterina as a peritoneal ridge over the lig. rectouterinum, and the course of the lig. teres uteri in the superior portion of the lig. latum uteri.

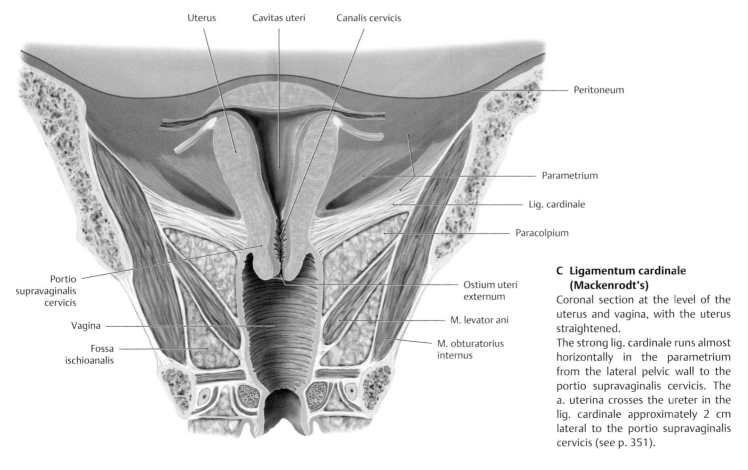

Uterus   Cavitas uteri   Canalis cervicis

Peritoneum

Parametrium

Lig. cardinale

Paracolpium

Portio supravaginalis cervicis

Vagina

Fossa ischioanalis

Ostium uteri externum

M. levator ani

M. obturatorius internus

C Ligamentum cardinale (Mackenrodt's)
Coronal section at the level of the uterus and vagina, with the uterus straightened.
The strong lig. cardinale runs almost horizontally in the parametrium from the lateral pelvic wall to the portio supravaginalis cervicis. The a. uterina crosses the ureter in the lig. cardinale approximately 2 cm lateral to the portio supravaginalis cervicis (see p. 351).

397

6.21 Female Pelvis in situ

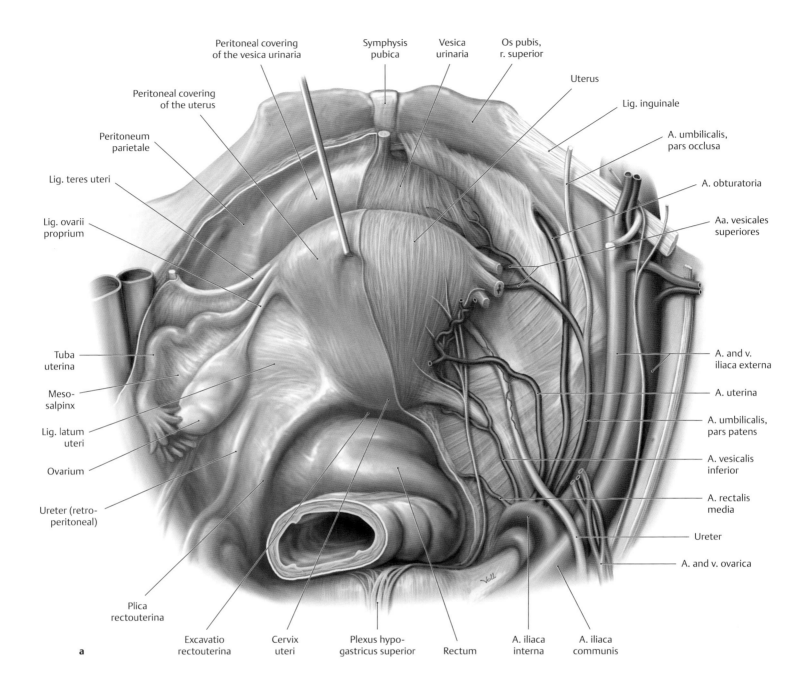

Peritoneal covering
of the vesica urinaria

Symphysis
pubica

Vesica
urinaria

Os pubis,
r. superior

Peritoneal covering
of the uterus

Uterus

Peritoneum
parietale

Lig. inguinale

Lig. teres uteri

A. umbilicalis,
pars occlusa

Lig. ovarii
proprium

A. obturatoria

Aa. vesicales
superiores

Tuba
uterina

A. and v.
iliaca externa

Meso-
salpinx

A. uterina

Lig. latum
uteri

A. umbilicalis,
pars patens

Ovarium

A. vesicalis
inferior

Ureter (retro-
peritoneal)

A. rectalis
media

Ureter

A. and v. ovarica

Plica
rectouterina

Excavatio
rectouterina

Cervix
uteri

Plexus hypo-
gastricus superior

Rectum

A. iliaca
interna

A. iliaca
communis

a

A Female pelvis in situ

a Posterosuperior view; the peritoneum covering the uterus, vesica urinaria, and lateral and posterior walls of the pelvis has been partially removed, and the uterus pulled slightly anteriorly. The lig. latum uteri (part of the parametrium, see p. 394), right ovarium, and tuba uterina have been removed. *Note:* The ureter crosses inferior to the a. uterina approximately 2 cm lateral to the cervix uteri.

b Schematic representation of the blood supply to the female urogenital tract, left-lateral view (after Platzer).

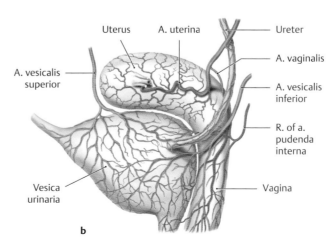

Uterus

A. uterina

Ureter

A. vesicalis
superior

A. vaginalis

A. vesicalis
inferior

R. of a.
pudenda
interna

Vesica
urinaria

Vagina

b

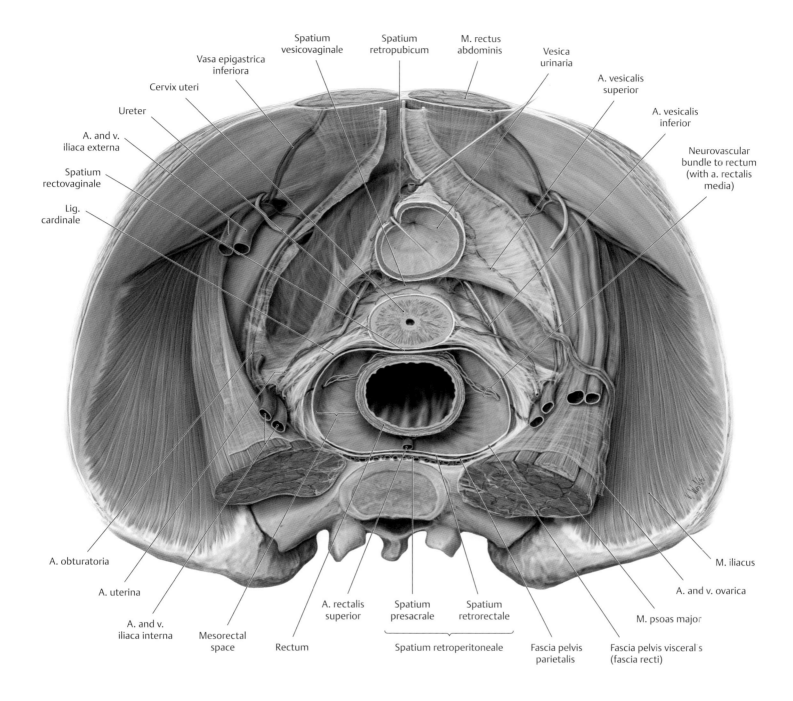

Spatium
vesicovaginale

Spatium
retropubicum

M. rectus
abdominis

Vasa epigastrica
inferiora

Vesica
urinaria

Cervix uteri

A. vesicalis
superior

Ureter

A. vesicalis
inferior

A. and v.
iliaca externa

Neurovascular
bundle to rectum
(with a. rectalis
media)

Spatium
rectovaginale

Lig.
cardinale

A. obturatoria

M. iliacus

A. uterina

A. and v. ovarica

A. and v.
iliaca interna

A. rectalis
superior

Spatium
presacrale

Spatium
retrorectale

M. psoas major

Mesorectal
space

Rectum

Spatium retroperitoneale

Fascia pelvis
parietalis

Fascia pelvis visceralis
(fascia recti)

B Female pelvis in situ, superior view

Transverse cut of cavitas pelvis; numerous structures have been removed for clarity. The uterus and adnexa have been removed, and the vesica urinaria and rectum have been opened superiorly. Vessels have been transected cranially so that the pelvic spaces are clearly visible:

- Spatium retropubicum in front of the vesica urinaria
- Spatium vesicovaginale between vesica urinaria and uterus
- Spatium rectovaginale between uterus and rectum
- Spatium retroperitoneale (with spatia retrorectale and presacrale) behind the rectum

For better exposure of the neurovascular bundle (a. rectalis media and nerve fibers of the plexus hypogastricus inferior) running to the rectum, the mesorectal adipose tissue (cf. p. 380) between the rectum and rectal fascia has been completely removed. It can be clearly seen that the a. uterina runs lateral to the cervix uteri in the lig. cardinale (see p. 396), at the base of the lig. latum uteri, and crosses the ureter 2 cm lateral to the cervix.

6.22 Male Pelvis in situ

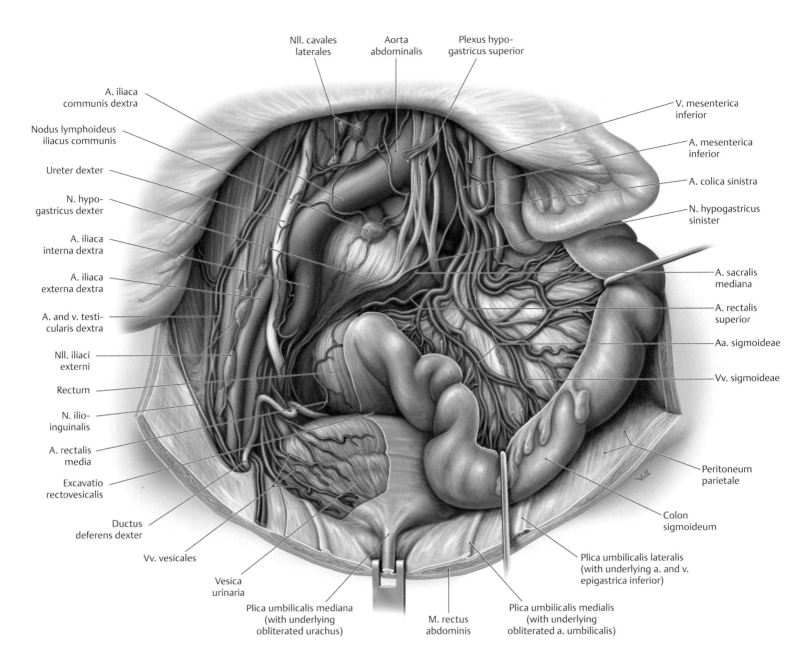

Nll. cavales laterales

Aorta abdominalis

Plexus hypo- gastricus superior

A. iliaca communis dextra

Nodus lymphoideus iliacus communis

Ureter dexter

N. hypo- gastricus dexter

A. iliaca interna dextra

A. iliaca externa dextra

A. and v. testi- cularis dextra

Nll. iliaci externi

Rectum

N. ilio- inguinalis

A. rectalis media

Excavatio rectovesicalis

Ductus deferens dexter

Vv. vesicales

Vesica urinaria

Plica umbilicalis mediana (with underlying obliterated urachus)

M. rectus abdominis

V. mesenterica inferior

A. mesenterica inferior

A. colica sinistra

N. hypogastricus sinister

A. sacralis mediana

A. rectalis superior

Aa. sigmoideae

Vv. sigmoideae

Peritoneum parietale

Colon sigmoideum

Plica umbilicalis lateralis (with underlying a. and v. epigastrica inferior)

Plica umbilicalis medialis (with underlying obliterated a. umbilicalis)

A Male pelvis in situ, anterosuperior view
he colon sigmoideum has been retracted anterolaterally and upward; and wide areas of peritoneum covering the mesocolon sigmoideum, rectum, vesica urinaria, and lateral and posterior pelvic walls have been removed to expose the underlying structures. Nodi lymphoidei and plexus autonomici are shown schematically for clarity. In the male pelvis, the peritoneum is reflected from the vesica urinaria to the rectum to form the excavatio rectovesicalis.

B Pelvic fasciae, mesorectum and course of the neurovascular bundle (see right page)
a Anterosuperior view of the male pelvis, the upper two-thirds of the rectum and vesica urinaria have been removed.
Clearly visible are the mesorectal adipose tissue together with the a. rectalis superior, which runs in it, and the fascial envelope (rectal fascia or fascia pelvis visceralis, cf. p. 380), which surrounds the mesorectum. Bilateral neurovascular bundles extend anteriorly between the fasciae pelvis visceralis and parietalis. Both form a plexus hypogastricus inferior, a network of sympathetic (inferior nn. hypogastrici) and parasympathetic (nn. splanchnici pelvici) nerves and ganglia (ganglia pelvica). The nerve fibers together with the a. rectalis media extend from the plexus to the rectum, and together with the aa. vesicales to the prostata, gll. vesiculosae, and vesica uterina.
b Sagittal section through male pelvis, pelvic connective tissue and most of the fascia pelvis have been removed; viewed from the left side.
The rectum and its mesorectal fascial envelope (rectal fascia/fascia pelvis visceralis) has been unfolded to show the location of the plexus hypogastricus inferior and the course of the neurovascular bundle on its lateral side between the fascial layers. Part of the septum rectovesicale has been left in place between the vesica urinaria, gll. vesiculosae, prostata, and rectum (cf. p. 380).

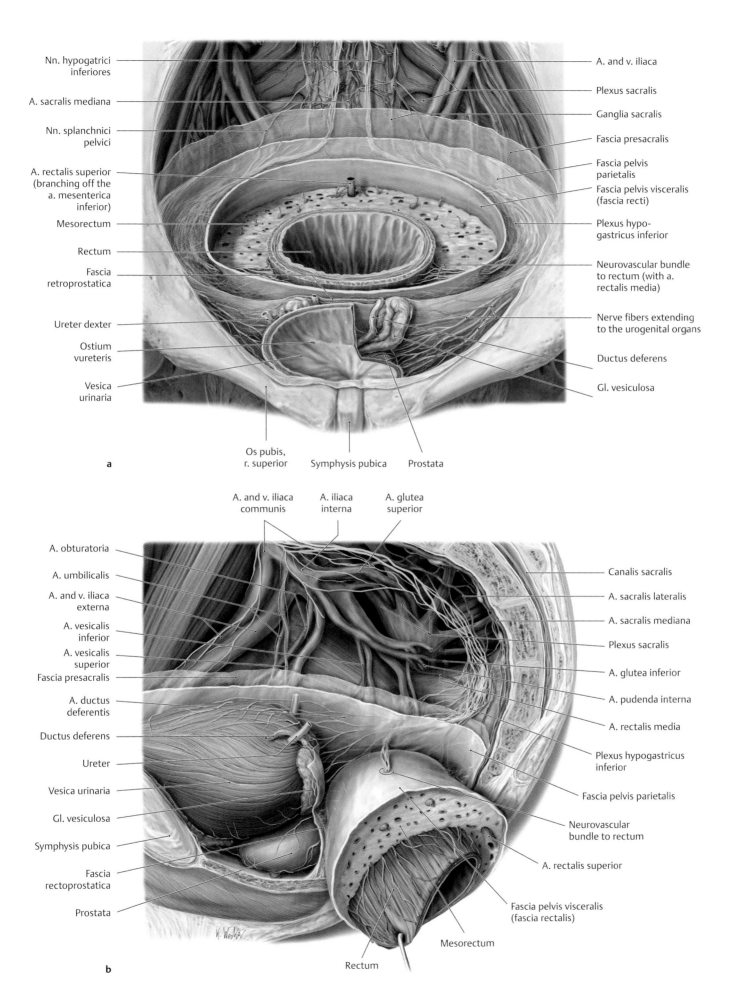

Nn. hypogatrici inferiores

A. sacralis mediana

Nn. splanchnici pelvici

A. rectalis superior (branching off the a. mesenterica inferior)

Mesorectum

Rectum

Fascia retroprostatica

Ureter dexter

Ostium vureteris

Vesica urinaria

A. and v. iliaca

Plexus sacralis

Ganglia sacralis

Fascia presacralis

Fascia pelvis parietalis

Fascia pelvis visceralis (fascia recti)

Plexus hypo-gastricus inferior

Neurovascular bundle to rectum (with a. rectalis media)

Nerve fibers extending to the urogenital organs

Ductus deferens

Gl. vesiculosa

Os pubis, r. superior

Symphysis pubica

Prostata

a

A. and v. iliaca communis

A. iliaca interna

A. glutea superior

A. obturatoria

A. umbilicalis

A. and v. iliaca externa

A. vesicalis inferior

A. vesicalis superior

Fascia presacralis

A. ductus deferentis

Ductus deferens

Ureter

Vesica urinaria

Gl. vesiculosa

Symphysis pubica

Fascia rectoprostatica

Prostata

Canalis sacralis

A. sacralis lateralis

A. sacralis mediana

Plexus sacralis

A. glutea inferior

A. pudenda interna

A. rectalis media

Plexus hypogastricus inferior

Fascia pelvis parietalis

Neurovascular bundle to rectum

A. rectalis superior

Fascia pelvis visceralis (fascia rectalis)

Mesorectum

Rectum

b

401

6.23 Cross-Sectional Anatomy of the Female Pelvis

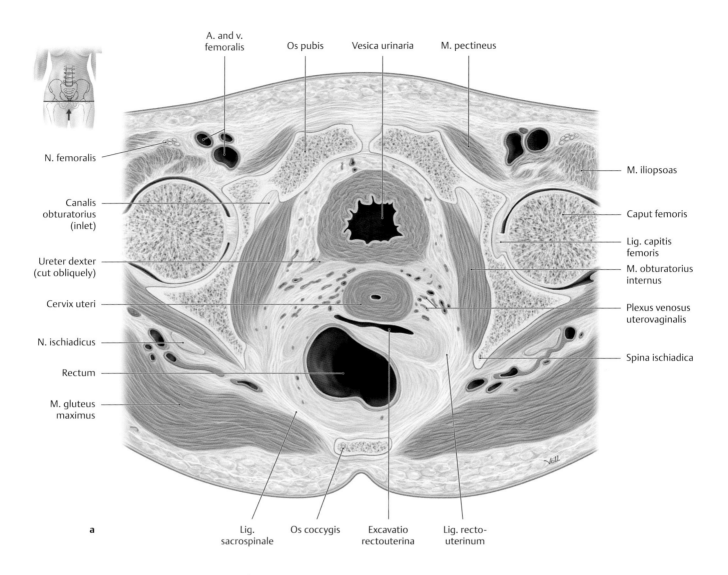

a

A. and v. femoralis — Os pubis — Vesica urinaria — M. pectineus

N. femoralis

M. iliopsoas

Canalis obturatorius (inlet)

Caput femoris

Lig. capitis femoris

Ureter dexter (cut obliquely)

M. obturatorius internus

Cervix uteri

Plexus venosus uterovaginalis

N. ischiadicus

Rectum

Spina ischiadica

M. gluteus maximus

Lig. sacrospinale — Os coccygis — Excavatio rectouterina — Lig. recto-uterinum

A Location of the female pelvic organs in transverse section

a Section through the female pelvis at the superior border of the symphysis pubica. The section cuts the vesica urinaria just below the ostia ureterum. Posterior to the vesica urinaria is a section of the cervix uteri, and behind that is the rectum (separated from the cervix uteri by the base of the excavatio rectouterina). As in the male pelvis, connective tissue is distributed around the vesica urinaria and rectum. Additional connective tissue is found around the cervix uteri, representing a downward prolongation of the lig. transversum cervicis. A venous network, the plexus venosi uterinus and vaginalis, is embedded in the connective tissue and is cut at numerous sites in the section above. This plexus provides venous drainage for the uterus and vagina.

Note: Peritoneal pouches exist in front of and behind the uterus: the excavatio vesicouterina anteriorly and the excavatio rectouterina posteriorly. The section shown here cuts the pelvis at the level of the excavatio rectouterina (culdesac). The excavatio vesicouterina does not extend as inferiorly and terminates above the plane of section. As a result, the area between the cervix and vesica urinaria in this section is occupied by connective tissue (formerly called the "vesicovaginal septum").

b **MRI of the pelvis, transverse scan** (from Hamm, B. et al.: MRT von Abdomen und Becken, 2. Aufl. Thieme, Stuttgart 2006). The image shows the low-signal intensity cervical stroma (arrows), which surrounds the narrow high-signal intensity canalis cervicis uteri.

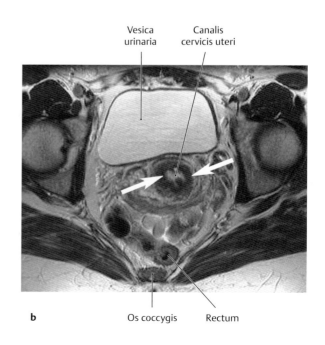

Vesica urinaria — Canalis cervicis uteri

b — Os coccygis — Rectum

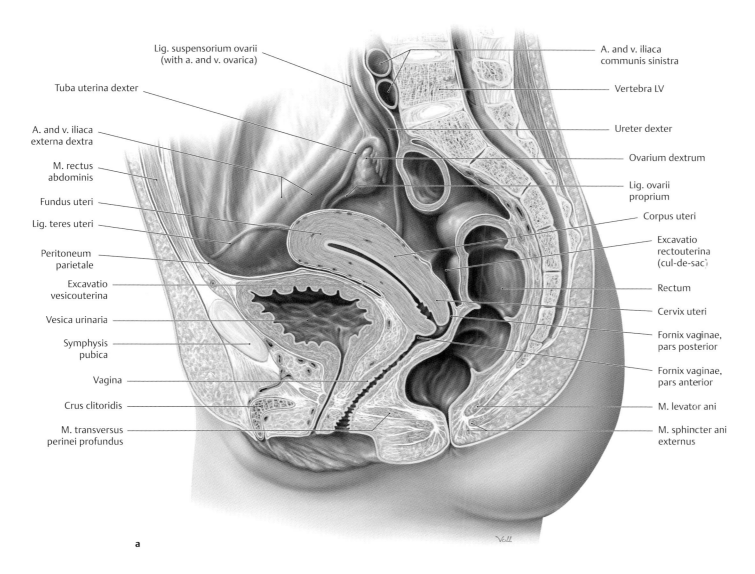

Lig. suspensorium ovarii
(with a. and v. ovarica)

A. and v. iliaca
communis sinistra

Tuba uterina dexter

Vertebra LV

A. and v. iliaca
externa dextra

Ureter dexter

M. rectus
abdominis

Ovarium dextrum

Fundus uteri

Lig. ovarii
proprium

Lig. teres uteri

Corpus uteri

Peritoneum
parietale

Excavatio
rectouterina
(cul-de-sac)

Excavatio
vesicouterina

Rectum

Vesica urinaria

Cervix uteri

Symphysis
pubica

Fornix vaginae,
pars posterior

Vagina

Fornix vaginae,
pars anterior

Crus clitoridis

M. levator ani

M. transversus
perinei profundus

M. sphincter ani
externus

a

B Location of the female pelvic organs in midsagittal section

a Viewed from the left side, the intestinum tenue and intestinum crassum, except for colon sigmoideum and rectum, have been removed.

Note: In the female, the uterus and its ligaments are interposed between the vesica urinaria and rectum. This leads to characteristic changes in the peritoneal relationships compared with the male pelvis. The peritoneum is reflected from the anterior wall of the cavitas peritonealis onto the vesica surface as in the male, but from there it is reflected onto the anterior wall of the uterus. Because the uterus typically occupies an anteflexed and anteverted position on the vesica urinaria (see p. 326), the peritoneum between the vesica urinaria and uterus forms a deep but narrow recess, the excavatio vesicouterina.

b **MRI of the pelvis,** sagittal section (from Hamm, B. et al.: MRT von Abdomen und Becken, 2. Aufl. Thieme, Stuttgart 2006). The image shows the uterus in the first half of the menstrual cycle (proliferative phase) with narrow endometrium and relatively low-signal intensity of the myometrium.

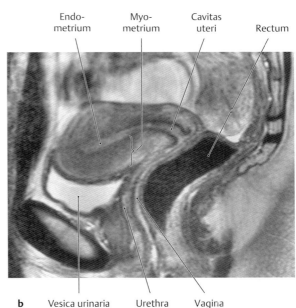

Endo-
metrium

Myo-
metrium

Cavitas
uteri

Rectum

b Vesica urinaria   Urethra   Vagina

6.24 Cross-Sectional Anatomy of the Male Pelvis

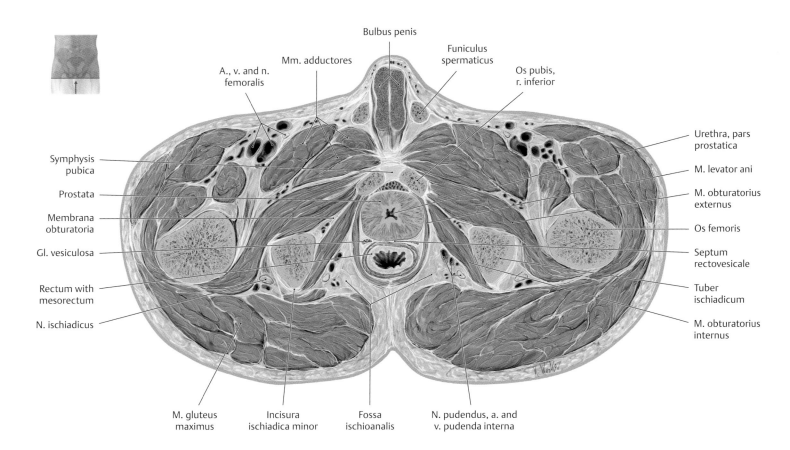

Bulbus penis

Mm. adductores

Funiculus spermaticus

A., v. and n. femoralis

Os pubis, r. inferior

Symphysis pubica

Urethra, pars prostatica

Prostata

M. levator ani

Membrana obturatoria

M. obturatorius externus

Gl. vesiculosa

Os femoris

Rectum with mesorectum

Septum rectovesicale

N. ischiadicus

Tuber ischiadicum

M. obturatorius internus

M. gluteus maximus

Incisura ischiadica minor

Fossa ischioanalis

N. pudendus, a. and v. pudenda interna

A Location of the male pelvic organs in transverse section

Section through the male pelvis at the level of the prostata, inferior view.

The diagram shows the location of the prostata posterior to the rr. inferiores ossis pubis and the symphysis pubica. Behind the prostata lie the sectioned gll. vesiculosae. The septum rectovesicale, an anteriorly oriented layer of connective tissue, extends between the prostata and rectum. It acts as a border between the mesorectum and the urogenital organs. Laterally and posteriorly, the m. levator ani borders the fossa ischioanalis.

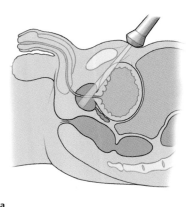

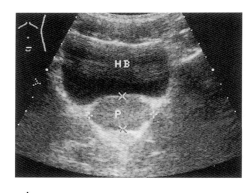

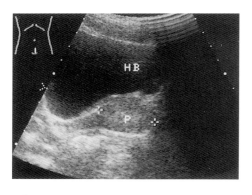

a

b

c

B Transvesical sonography of the prostate

a Schematic midsagittal section through the male pelvis to show suprapubic probe positioning, viewed from the left side; **b** Normal findings of the prostata imaged in the transverse plane; **c** Sagittal section through the prostata (from: Reiser, M et al.: Radiologie [Duale Reihe], 2. Aufl. Thieme, Stuttgart 2006).

Transvesical imaging of the prostata (P) is possible only when the vesica (HB) is sufficiently distended. Unlike transrectal sonography of the prostata, which allows for a differentiated assessment of the organ structure and facilitates proof that cancer has started to spread (see p. 338), suprapubic transvesical sonography provides a three-dimensional image of the organ (transverse, sagittal and frontal planes) and measurement of the volume by using the formula V=0.523 x a x b x c.

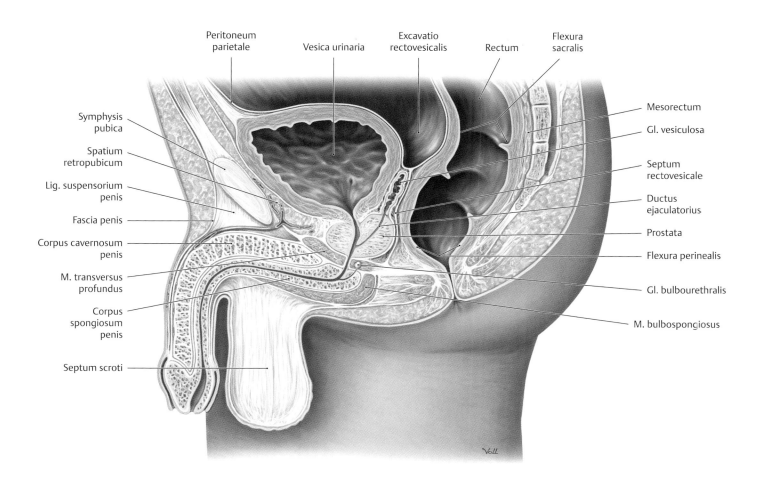

C Location of the male pelvic organs in sagittal section

Midsagittal section, viewed from the left.

The diagram shows the size and location of the vesica urinaria when it is significantly distended. When the vesica urinaria is empty, it is considerably smaller and lies behind the symphysis pubica and the peritoneum forms a transverse ridge on the surface of the vesica urinaria called the plica vesicalis transversa. The peritoneum extends from the vesica

urinaria to the anterior wall of the rectum and forms a small recess, the exavatio rectovesicalis (lowest part of the male cavitas peritonealis). The peritoneum does not reach the prostata.

Note the two curvatures of the rectum in the sagittal plane (flexura sacralis and flexura perinealis) and the septum rectovesicale along the posterior border of the prostata and gll. vesiculosae.

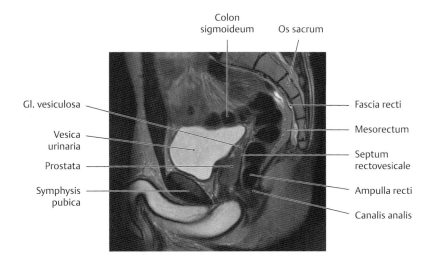

D Sagittal MRI scan of the male pelvis (T2-weighted TSE sequence)

Note: On T2-weighted MRI scans, the perirectal fat tissue of the rectum (mesorectum) is hyperintense. The mesorectal fascia (rectal fascia = fascia pelvis visceralis), which surrounds the mesorectum can be demonstrated as a fine low-signal intensity line (from Hamm, B. et al.: MRT von Abdomen und Becken, 2. Aufl. Thieme, Stuttgart 2006).

D Neurovascular Supply to the Organs

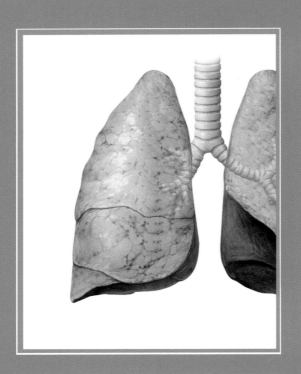

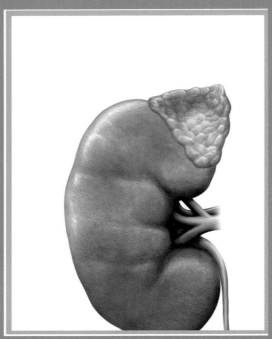

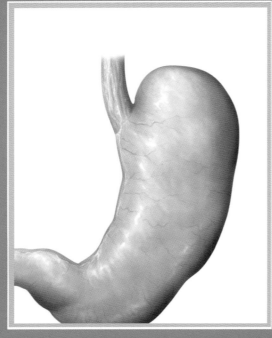

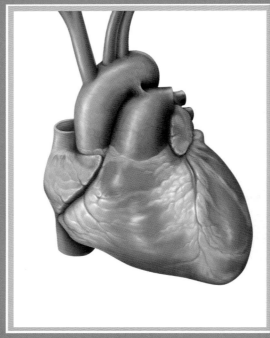

How to Use this Chapter

Each of the sections in this chapter reviews the neurovascular supply to an organ or group of organs in a schematized form. The following **subgroups** are distinguished in the diagrams:
- Arterial supply (red)
- Venous drainage (blue)
- Lymphatic drainage (green)
- Innervation (yellow)

The schematics can be used in various ways:
- *Reviewing* for a test: The student can quickly obtain a basic grasp of neurovascular structures and pathways.
- *Looking up* a specific structure: The diagrams make it easy to locate and identify a particular neurovascular supply.
- *Understanding* complex anatomy by appreciating the basic neurovascular supply to an organ in the diagrams and then referring back to the more complex anatomical relationships shown in earlier chapters.

Points to keep in mind when using the schematics:
- They reflect a simplified, idealized view.
- Topographical anatomy is ignored, and the structures are not drawn to scale.
- Organs that are in close proximity to each other but are supplied by different groups of neurovascular structures are shown in separate diagrams.
- By and large, variants are disregarded.
- In cases where the neurovascular supply is bilaterally symmetrical, only one side is shown.

1.1 Thymus

Arteries

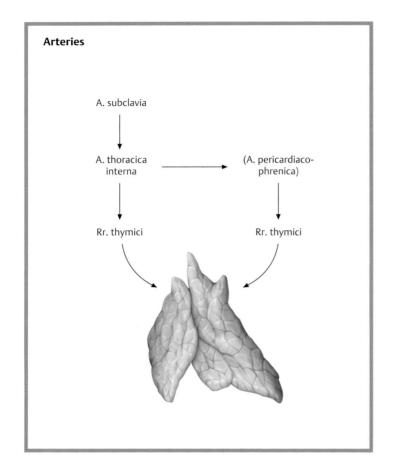

A. subclavia

↓

A. thoracica interna → (A. pericardiaco-phrenica)

↓ ↓

Rr. thymici   Rr. thymici

Veins

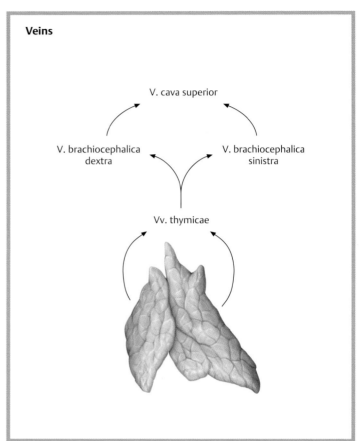

V. cava superior

V. brachiocephalica dextra   V. brachiocephalica sinistra

Vv. thymicae

Lymph nodes

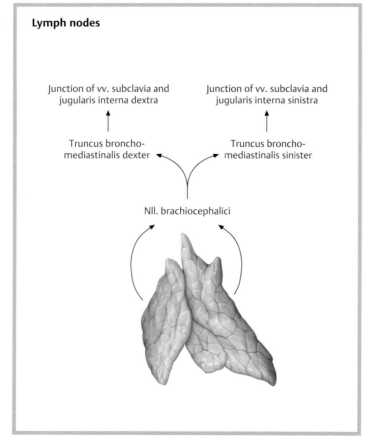

Junction of vv. subclavia and jugularis interna dextra

Junction of vv. subclavia and jugularis interna sinistra

Truncus broncho-mediastinalis dexter   Truncus broncho-mediastinalis sinister

Nll. brachiocephalici

Innervation

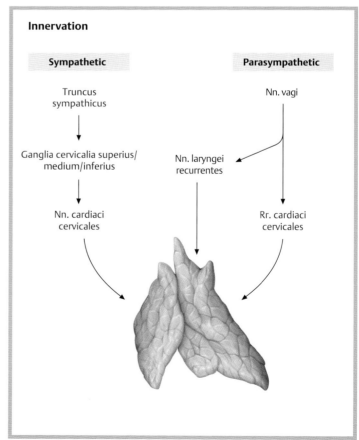

Sympathetic	Parasympathetic

Truncus sympathicus

Nn. vagi

↓

Ganglia cervicalia superius/medium/inferius

Nn. laryngei recurrentes

↓

Nn. cardiaci cervicales

Rr. cardiaci cervicales

1.2 Oesophagus

Arteries

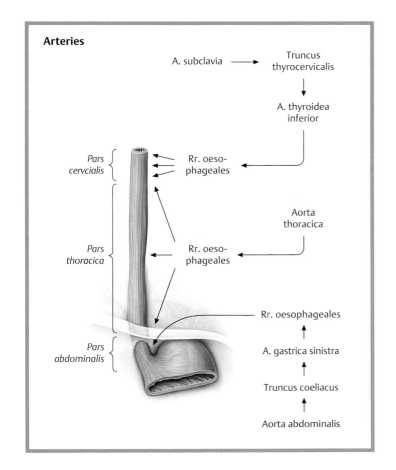

A. subclavia → Truncus thyrocervicalis

A. thyroidea inferior

Pars cervcialis — Rr. oeso-phageales

Aorta thoracica

Pars thoracica — Rr. oeso-phageales

Rr. oesophageales

Pars abdominalis — A. gastrica sinistra

Truncus coeliacus

Aorta abdominalis

Veins

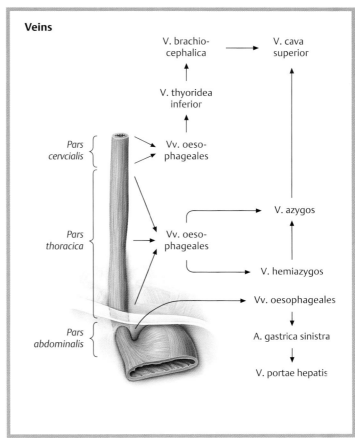

V. brachio-cephalica → V. cava superior

V. thyoridea inferior

Pars cervcialis — Vv. oeso-phageales

Pars thoracica — Vv. oeso-phageales → V. azygos

V. hemiazygos

Vv. oesophageales

Pars abdominalis — A. gastrica sinistra

V. portae hepatis

Lymph nodes

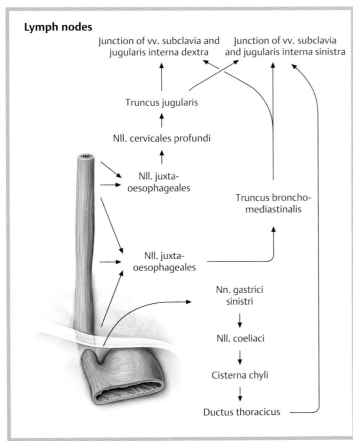

Junction of vv. subclavia and jugularis interna dextra

Junction of vv. subclavia and jugularis interna sinistra

Truncus jugularis

Nll. cervicales profundi

Nll. juxta-oesophageales

Truncus broncho-mediastinalis

Nll. juxta-oesophageales

Nn. gastrici sinistri

Nll. coeliaci

Cisterna chyli

Ductus thoracicus

Innervation

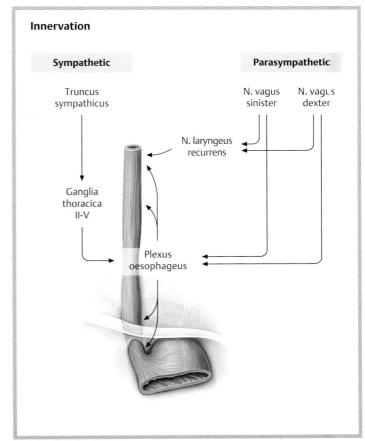

Sympathetic	Parasympathetic

Truncus sympathicus

N. vagus sinister — N. vagus dexter

N. laryngeus recurrens

Ganglia thoracica II–V

Plexus oesophageus

1.3 Heart

Arteries

Ventriculus
sinister

↓

Aorta ascendens

A. coronaria
dextra

A. coronaria
sinistra

R. inter-
ventricularis
posterior

R. inter-
ventricularis
anterior

R. circum-
flexus

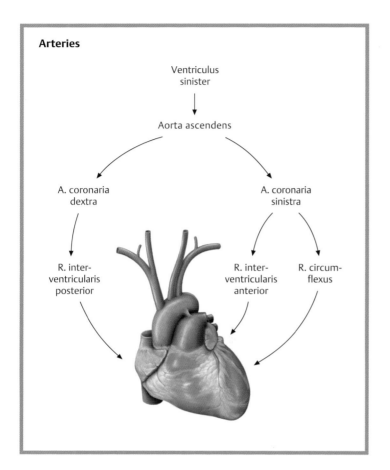

Veins

Atrium
dextrum

↑

Sinus coronarius

V. cardiaca
media

V. cardiaca
magna

V. cardiaca
parva

V. ventriculi
sinistri
posterior

V. inter-
ventricularis
anterior

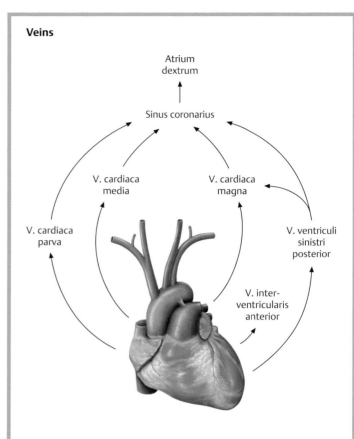

Lymph nodes

Truncus bronchomediastinalis

↑

Nll. brachiocephalici,
nll. tracheobronchiales

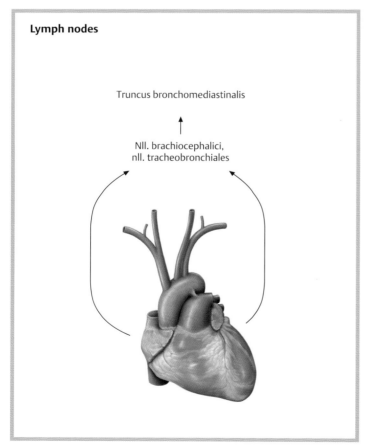

Innervation

| Sympathetic | Parasympathetic |

Truncus
sympathicus

Nn. vagi

Ganglia
thoracica
II–IV (V)

Ganglia
cervicalia

Nn. cardiaci
cervicales

Rr. cardiaci
cervicales

Rr. cardiaci
thoracici

Rr. cardiaci
thoracici

Plexus cardiacus

Myocardium

Aa.
coronariae

Nodus
sinuatrialis

Nodus atrio-
ventricularis

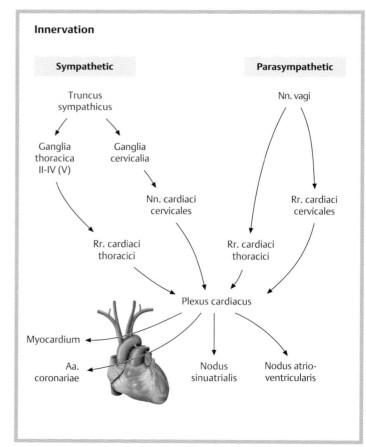

1.4 Pericardium

Arteries

A. subclavia
↓
A. thoracica
interna
↓
A. pericardiaco-
phrenica

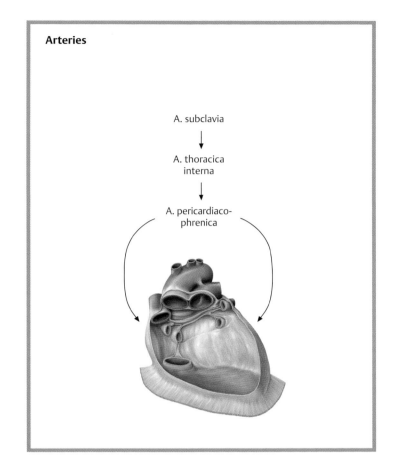

Veins

V. cava superior
↑
V. brachio-
cephalica
↑
V. thoracica
interna
↑
V. pericardiaco-
phrenica

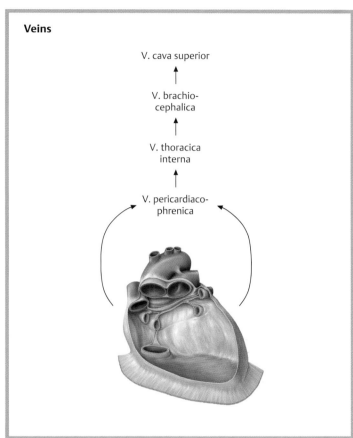

Lymph nodes

Truncus broncho-
mediastinalis
↑
Nll. parasternales
↑
Nll.
prepericardiaci

Nll. pericardiaci
laterales

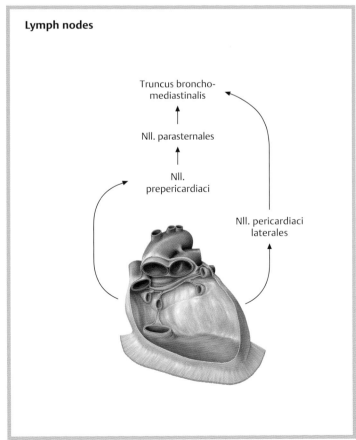

Innervation

Segmenta medullae
spinalis C(3) – 4 – (5)
↑
Plexus cervicalis
↑
N. phrenicus

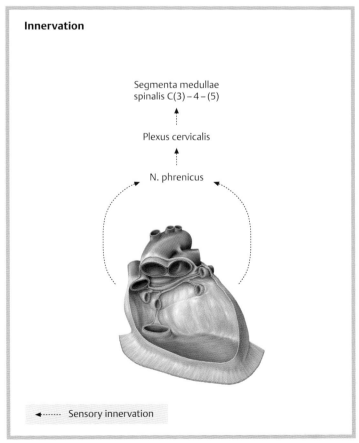

◄······ Sensory innervation

411

1.5   Lung and Trachea

Arteries

Pulmonary vessels	Bronchial vessels
Ventriculus dexter	Ventriculus sinister
↓	↓
Truncus pulmonalis	Aorta thoracica
	↓
A. pulmonalis dextra/sinistra	Rr. bronchiales

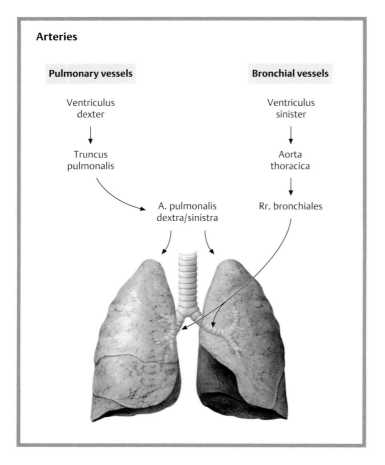

Veins

Pulmonary vessels	Bronchial vessels
Atrium sinistrum	Atrium dextrum
↑	↑
Truncus pulmonalis	V. cava superior
	↑
V. pulmonales dextrae/sinistrae	V. azygos ←
	V. hemiazygos (accessoria)
	Vv. bronchiales

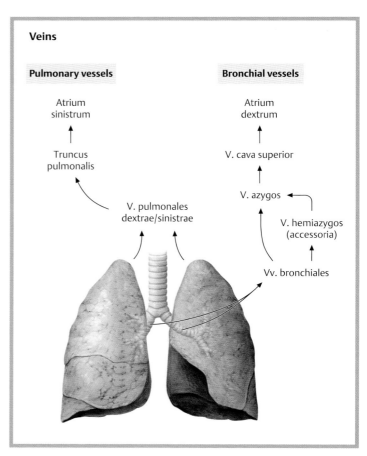

Lymph nodes

Junction of vv. subclavia and jugularis interna dextra   Junction of vv. subclavia and jugularis interna sinistra

Truncus bronchomediastinalis dexter/sinister

Nll. paratracheales

Nll. tracheobronchiales superiores/inferiores

Nll. broncho-pulmonales

Nll. intra-pulmonales

Nll. phrenici superiores

Nll. phrenici inferiores

Truncus lumbalis

Cisterna chyli ⟶ Ductus thoracicus

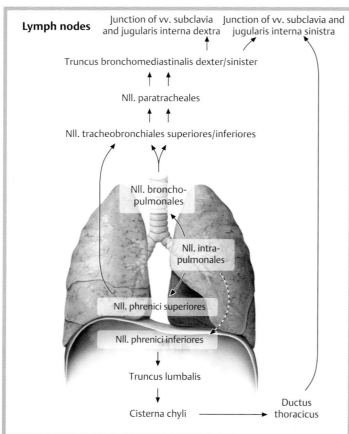

Innervation

Sympathetic	Parasympathetic
Truncus sympathicus	N. vagus sinister N. vagus dexter
↓	
Ganglia throacica III-IV	N. laryngeus recurrens
	Rr. tracheales
Rr. pulmonales	Rr. bronchiales

Plexus pulmonalis

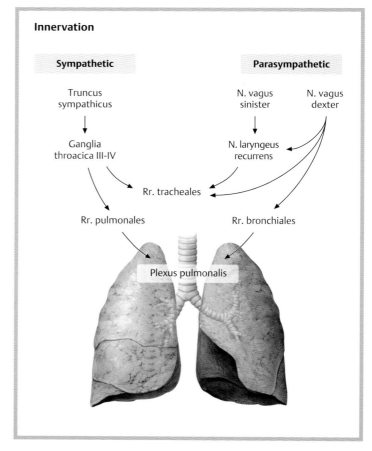

1.6 Diaphragma

Arteries

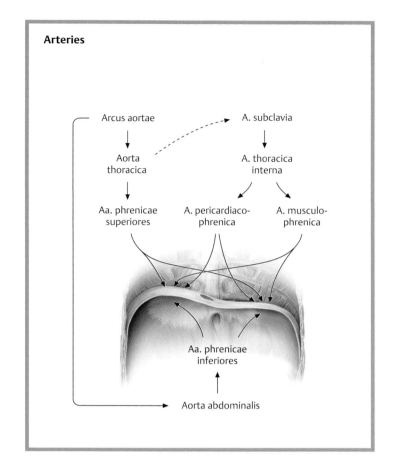

Arcus aortae → A. subclavia

Aorta thoracica

A. thoracica interna

Aa. phrenicae superiores

A. pericardiaco-phrenica

A. musculo-phrenica

Aa. phrenicae inferiores

Aorta abdominalis

Veins

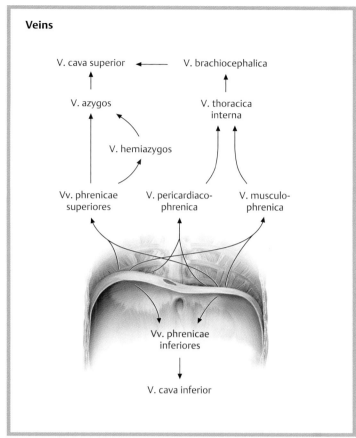

V. cava superior ← V. brachiocephalica

V. azygos

V. thoracica interna

V. hemiazygos

Vv. phrenicae superiores

V. pericardiaco-phrenica

V. musculo-phrenica

Vv. phrenicae inferiores

V. cava inferior

Lymph nodes

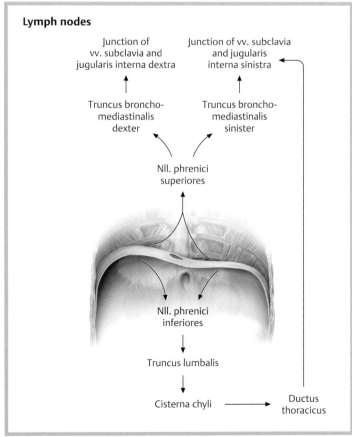

Junction of vv. subclavia and jugularis interna dextra

Junction of vv. subclavia and jugularis interna sinistra

Truncus broncho-mediastinalis dexter

Truncus broncho-mediastinalis sinister

Nll. phrenici superiores

Nll. phrenici inferiores

Truncus lumbalis

Cisterna chyli → Ductus thoracicus

Innervation

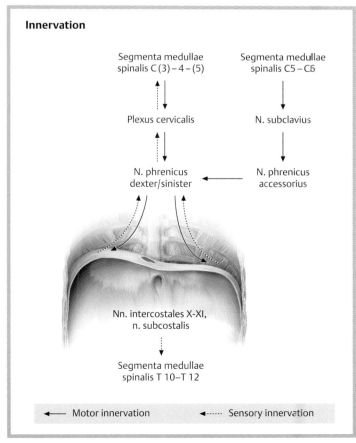

Segmenta medullae spinalis C (3) – 4 – (5)

Segmenta medullae spinalis C5 – C6

Plexus cervicalis

N. subclavius

N. phrenicus dexter/sinister ← N. phrenicus accessorius

Nn. intercostales X-XI, n. subcostalis

Segmenta medullae spinalis T 10–T 12

← Motor innervation   ◀······ Sensory innervation

413

1.7 Hepar, Vesica Biliaris, and Splen

Arteries

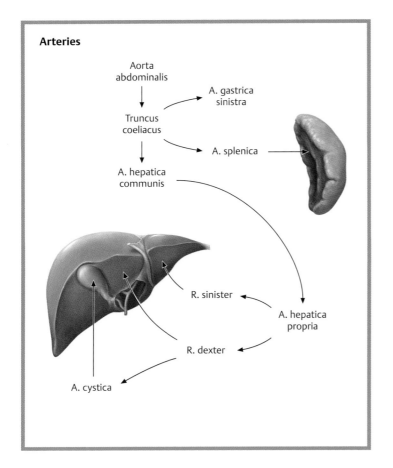

Veins

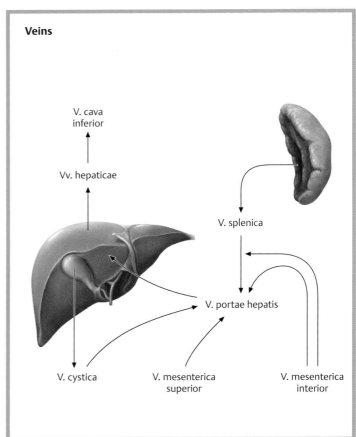

Lymph nodes

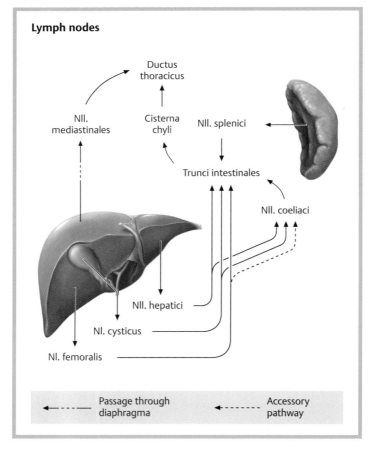

Innervation

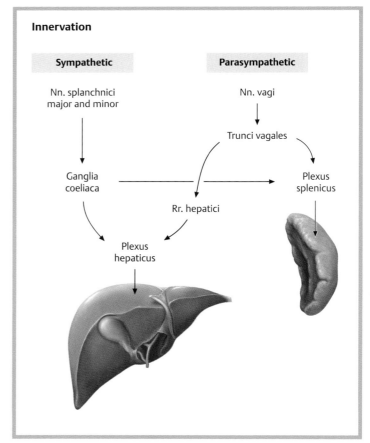

1.8   Gaster

Arteries

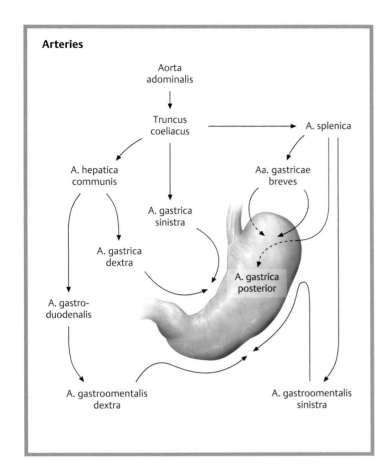

Aorta adominalis

↓

Truncus coeliacus → A. splenica

A. hepatica communis

Aa. gastricae breves

A. gastrica sinistra

A. gastrica dextra

A. gastrica posterior

A. gastro-duodenalis

A. gastroomentalis dextra

A. gastroomentalis sinistra

Veins

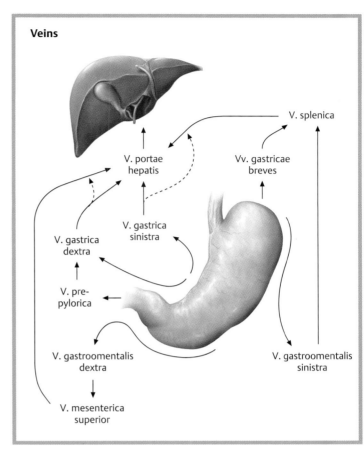

V. splenica

V. portae hepatis

Vv. gastricae breves

V. gastrica dextra

V. gastrica sinistra

V. pre-pylorica

V. gastroomentalis dextra

V. gastroomentalis sinistra

V. mesenterica superior

Lymph nodes

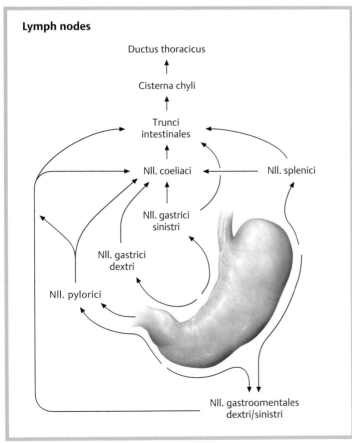

Ductus thoracicus

↑

Cisterna chyli

↑

Trunci intestinales

Nll. coeliaci ← Nll. splenici

Nll. gastrici sinistri

Nll. gastrici dextri

Nll. pylorici

Nll. gastroomentales dextri/sinistri

Innervation

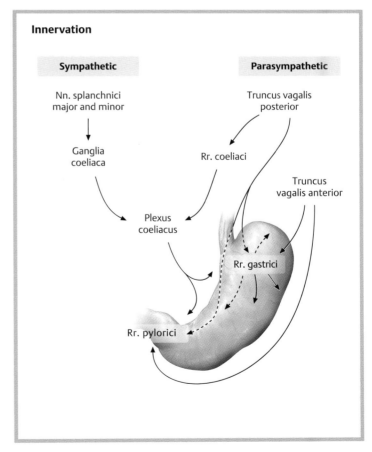

Sympathetic	**Parasympathetic**

Nn. splanchnici major and minor

Truncus vagalis posterior

Ganglia coeliaca

Rr. coeliaci

Truncus vagalis anterior

Plexus coeliacus

Rr. gastrici

Rr. pylorici

1.9 Duodenum and Pancreas

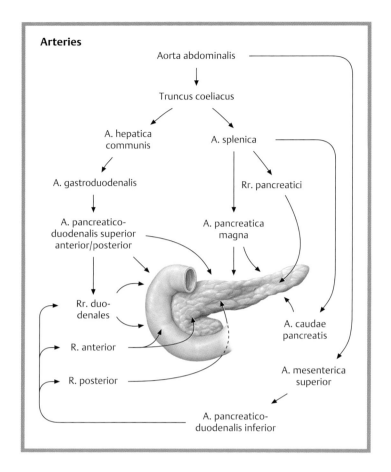

Arteries

Aorta abdominalis

Truncus coeliacus

A. hepatica communis

A. splenica

A. gastroduodenalis

Rr. pancreatici

A. pancreatico-duodenalis superior anterior/posterior

A. pancreatica magna

Rr. duo-denales

R. anterior

A. caudae pancreatis

R. posterior

A. mesenterica superior

A. pancreatico-duodenalis inferior

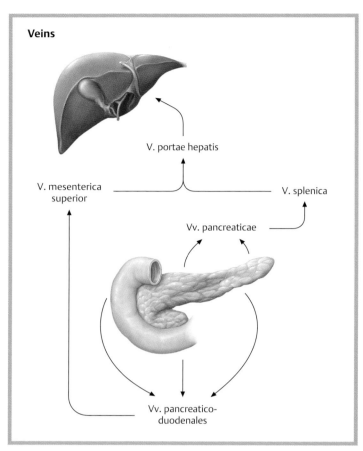

Veins

V. portae hepatis

V. mesenterica superior

V. splenica

Vv. pancreaticae

Vv. pancreatico-duodenales

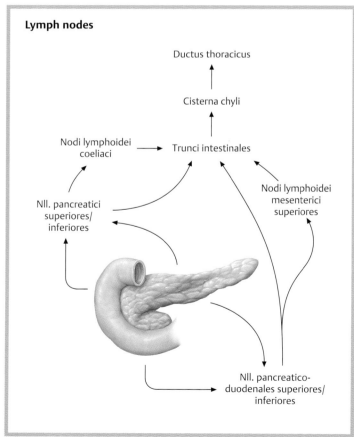

Lymph nodes

Ductus thoracicus

Cisterna chyli

Nodi lymphoidei coeliaci

Trunci intestinales

Nodi lymphoidei mesenterici superiores

Nll. pancreatici superiores/inferiores

Nll. pancreatico-duodenales superiores/inferiores

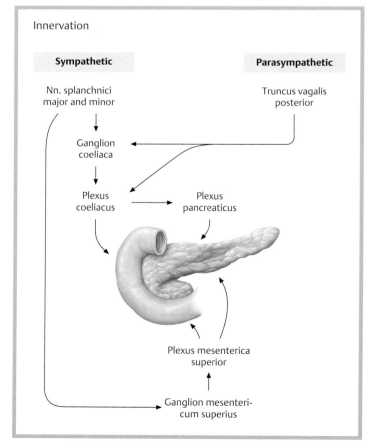

Innervation

Sympathetic	**Parasympathetic**

Nn. splanchnici major and minor

Truncus vagalis posterior

Ganglion coeliaca

Plexus coeliacus

Plexus pancreaticus

Plexus mesenterica superior

Ganglion mesentericum superius

1.10 Jejunum and Ileum

Arteries

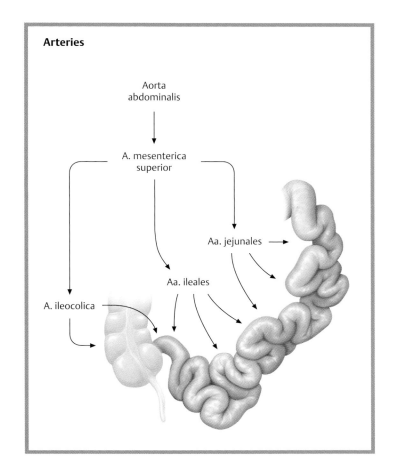

```
        Aorta
      abdominalis
          │
          ▼
    A. mesenterica
       superior
          │
   ┌──────┼──────┐
   │      │      │
   │      ▼      ▼
   │           Aa. jejunales ──▶
   │      │
   │      ▼
   │   Aa. ileales
   ▼
A. ileocolica
```

Veins

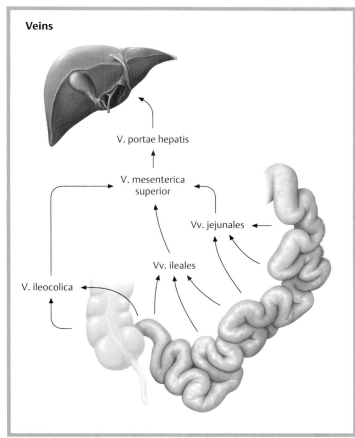

```
   V. portae hepatis
          ▲
          │
    V. mesenterica
       superior
   ▲      ▲      ▲
   │      │      │
   │      │   Vv. jejunales ◀──
   │      │
   │   Vv. ileales
   │
V. ileocolica ◀──
```

Lymph nodes

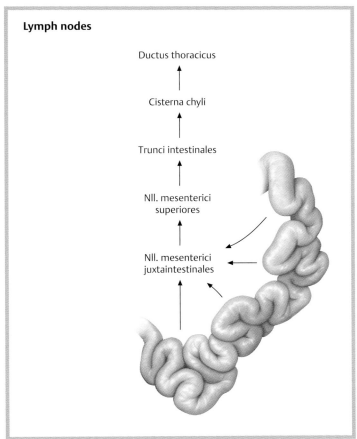

```
   Ductus thoracicus
          ▲
          │
     Cisterna chyli
          ▲
          │
  Trunci intestinales
          ▲
          │
   Nll. mesenterici
      superiores
          ▲
          │
   Nll. mesenterici
   juxtaintestinales
```

Innervation

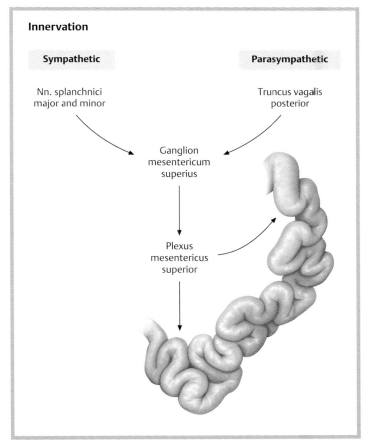

Sympathetic	Parasympathetic
Nn. splanchnici major and minor	Truncus vagalis posterior

```
         Ganglion
       mesentericum
         superius
            │
            ▼
          Plexus
       mesentericus
         superior
```

1.11 Caecum, Appendix Vermiformis, Colon Ascendens and Transversum

Arteries

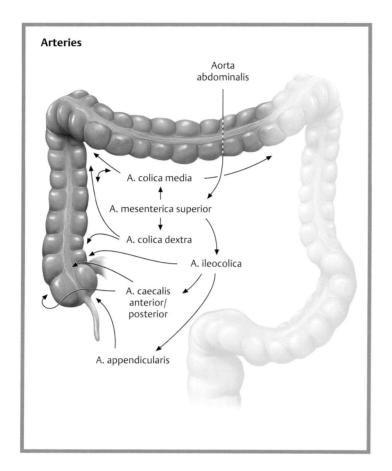

Aorta abdominalis
A. colica media
A. mesenterica superior
A. colica dextra
A. ileocolica
A. caecalis anterior/posterior
A. appendicularis

Veins

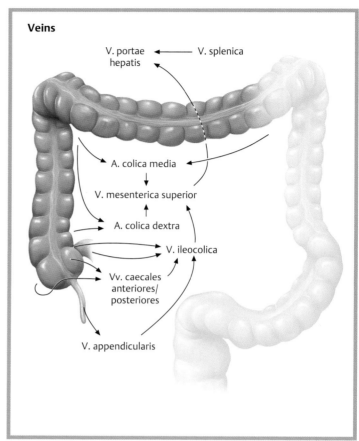

V. portae hepatis ← V. splenica
A. colica media
V. mesenterica superior
A. colica dextra
V. ileocolica
Vv. caecales anteriores/posteriores
V. appendicularis

Lymph nodes

Trunci intestinales → Cisterna chyli → Ductus thoracicus

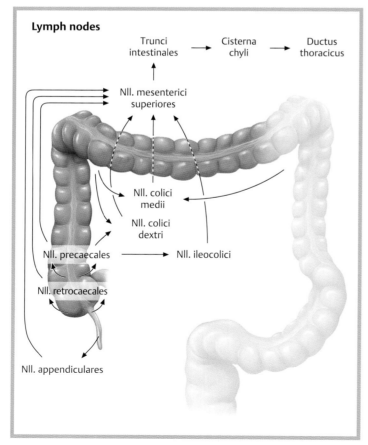

Nll. mesenterici superiores
Nll. colici medii
Nll. colici dextri
Nll. precaecales → Nll. ileocolici
Nll. retrocaecales
Nll. appendiculares

Innervation

Sympathetic	Parasympathetic
Nn. splanchnici major and minor	Truncus vagalis posterior
↓	
Ganglion mesentericum superius	
↓	
Plexus mesentericus superior	

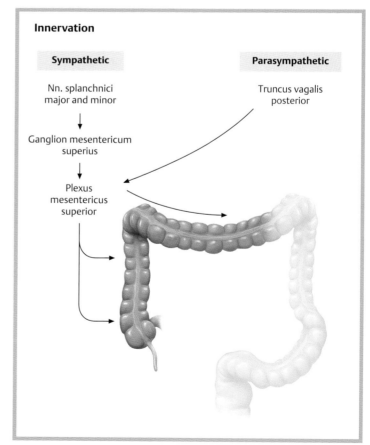

1.12 Colon Descendens and Colon Sigmoideum

Arteries

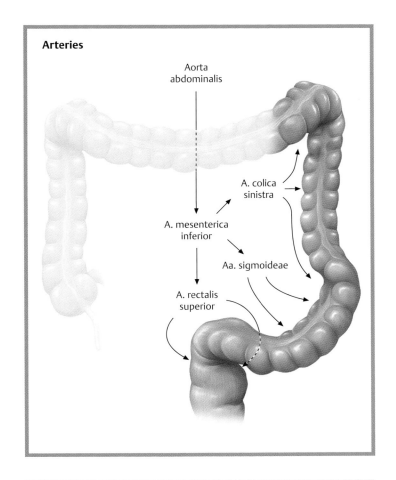

- Aorta abdominalis
- A. colica sinistra
- A. mesenterica inferior
- Aa. sigmoideae
- A. rectalis superior

Veins

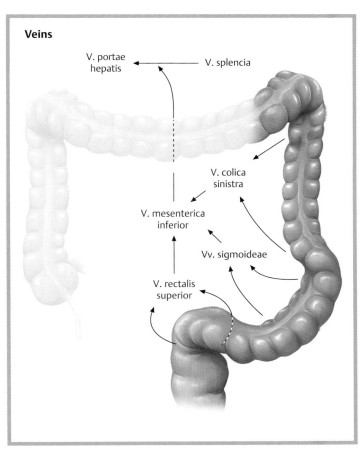

- V. portae hepatis
- V. splenica
- V. colica sinistra
- V. mesenterica inferior
- Vv. sigmoideae
- V. rectalis superior

Lymph nodes

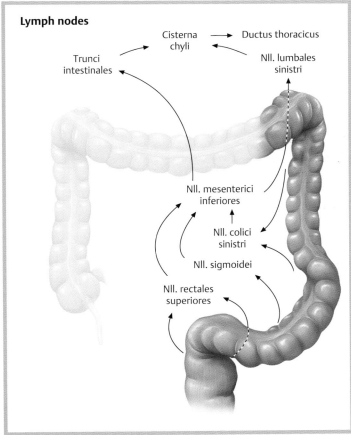

- Cisterna chyli
- Ductus thoracicus
- Trunci intestinales
- Nll. lumbales sinistri
- Nll. mesenterici inferiores
- Nll. colici sinistri
- Nll. sigmoidei
- Nll. rectales superiores

Innervation

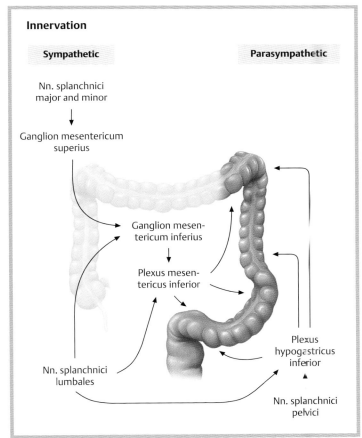

Sympathetic | **Parasympathetic**

- Nn. splanchnici major and minor
- Ganglion mesentericum superius
- Ganglion mesentericum inferius
- Plexus mesentericus inferior
- Nn. splanchnici lumbales
- Plexus hypogastricus inferior
- Nn. splanchnici pelvici

1.13 Rectum

Arteries

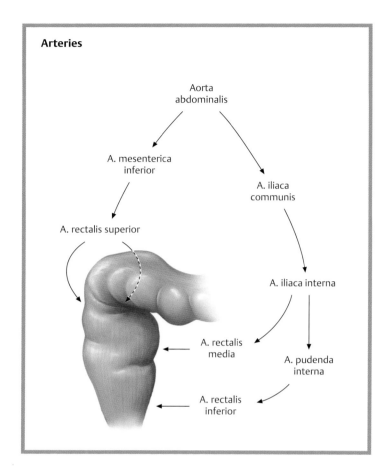

Aorta
abdominalis

A. mesenterica inferior

A. iliaca communis

A. rectalis superior

A. iliaca interna

A. rectalis media

A. pudenda interna

A. rectalis inferior

Veins

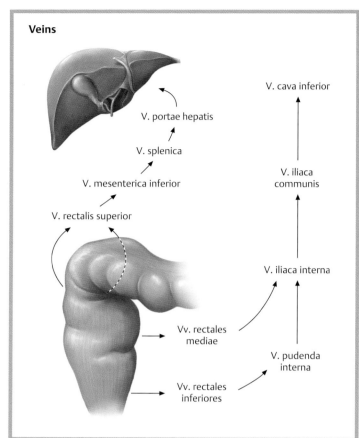

V. cava inferior

V. portae hepatis

V. splenica

V. mesenterica inferior

V. rectalis superior

V. iliaca communis

V. iliaca interna

Vv. rectales mediae

V. pudenda interna

Vv. rectales inferiores

Lymph nodes

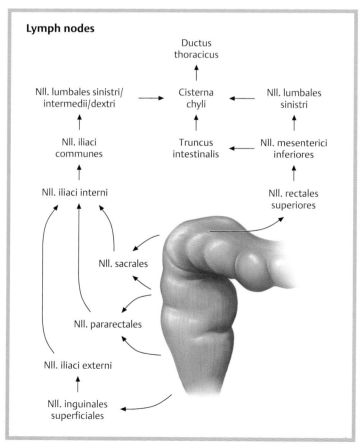

Ductus thoracicus

Nll. lumbales sinistri/ intermedii/dextri

Cisterna chyli

Nll. lumbales sinistri

Nll. iliaci communes

Truncus intestinalis

Nll. mesenterici inferiores

Nll. iliaci interni

Nll. rectales superiores

Nll. sacrales

Nll. pararectales

Nll. iliaci externi

Nll. inguinales superficiales

Innervation

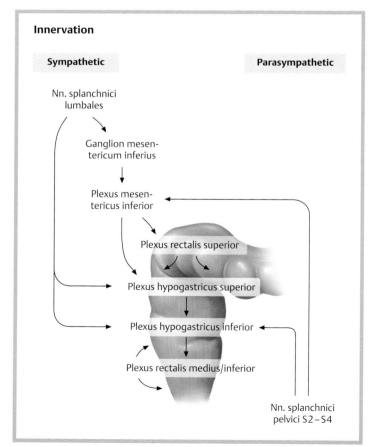

Sympathetic	Parasympathetic

Nn. splanchnici lumbales

Ganglion mesentericum inferius

Plexus mesentericus inferior

Plexus rectalis superior

Plexus hypogastricus superior

Plexus hypogastricus inferior

Plexus rectalis medius/inferior

Nn. splanchnici pelvici S2–S4

1.14 Kidney, Ureter, and Glandula Suprarenalis

Arteries

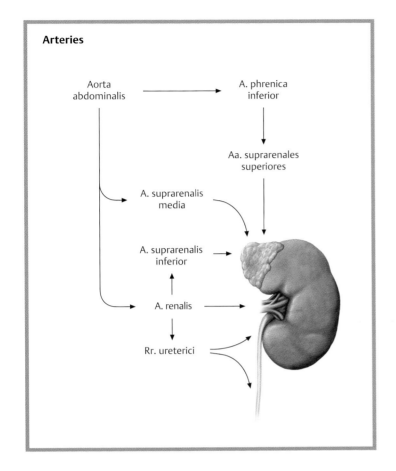

Veins

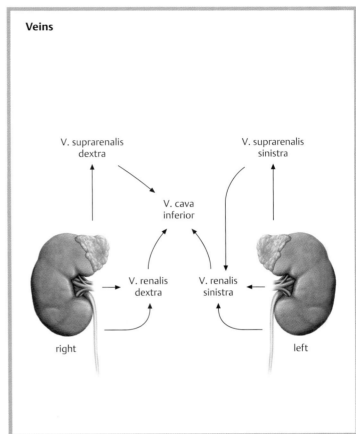

Lymph nodes

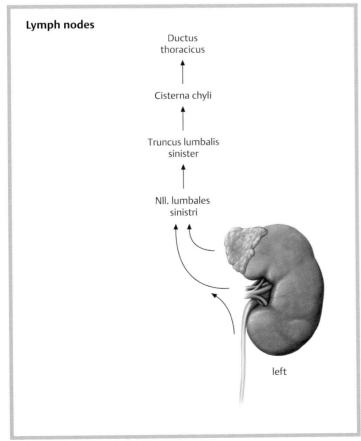

Innervation

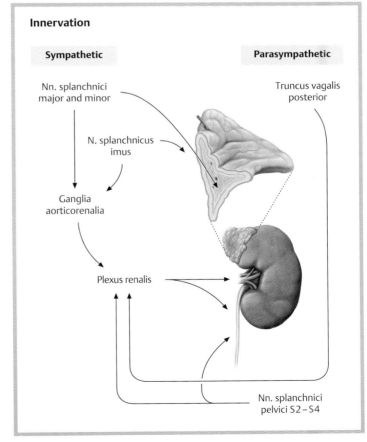

1.15 Vesica Urinaria, Prostata, and Glandula Vesiculosa

Arteries

Aorta abdominalis
↓
A. iliaca communis
↓
A. iliaca interna

A. umbilicalis

Aa. vesicales
superiores

Rr. ureterici

A. vesicalis
inferior

Rr. prostatici

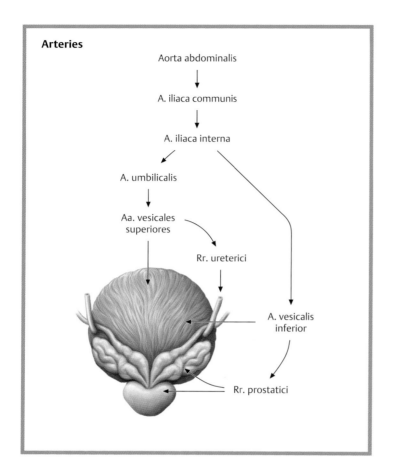

Veins

V. cava superior   V. cava inferior

V. azygos/
hemiazygos

Vv. lumbales
ascendentes

V. iliaca
communis

V. iliaca interna

Plexus venosus
vertebralis

Vv. vesicales

Plexus venosus
vesicalis

Plexus venosus
prostaticus

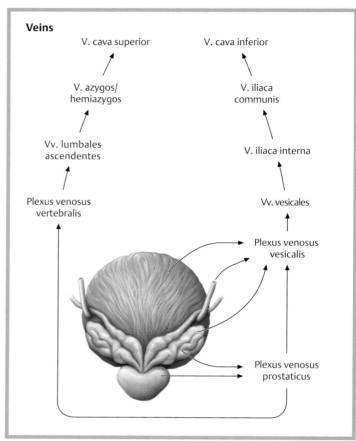

Lymph nodes

Ductus thoracicus
↑
Cisterna chyli

Truncus lumbalis
dexter and sinister

Nll. lumbales dextri/
intermedii/sinistri

Nll. iliaci communes

Nll. iliaci externi/interni

Nll. vesicales
laterales

Nll. prevesicales/
retrovesicales

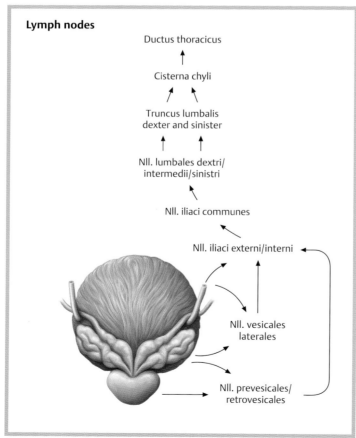

Innervation

Sympathetic	Parasympathetic

Nn. splanchnici
lumbales

Ganglion mesen-
tericum inferius

Plexus hypogastricus
superior

Plexus hypo-
gastricus inferior

Plexus
vesicalis

Plexus
prostaticus

Nn. splanchnici
pelvici S2–S4

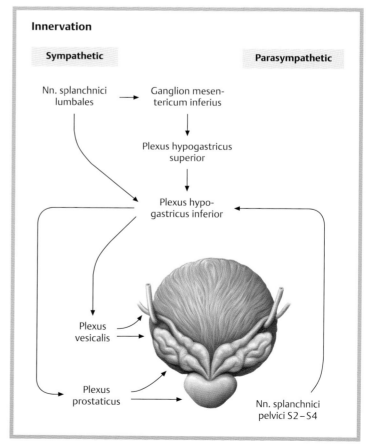

1.16 Testis, Epididymis, and Ductus Deferens

Arteries

Aorta abdominalis

A. iliaca communis

A. testicularis

A. iliaca interna

A. umbilicalis

A. ductus deferentis

A. vesicalis inferior (variant)

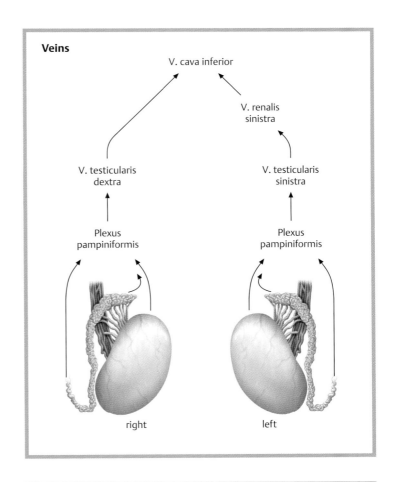

Veins

V. cava inferior

V. renalis sinistra

V. testicularis dextra

V. testicularis sinistra

Plexus pampiniformis

Plexus pampiniformis

right

left

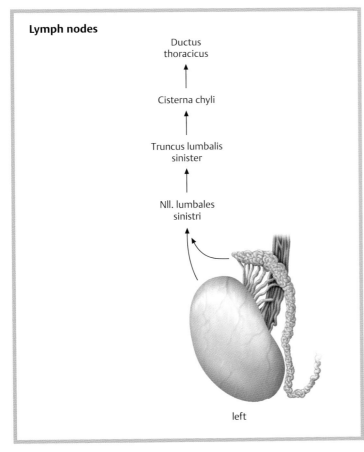

Lymph nodes

Ductus thoracicus

Cisterna chyli

Truncus lumbalis sinister

Nll. lumbales sinistri

left

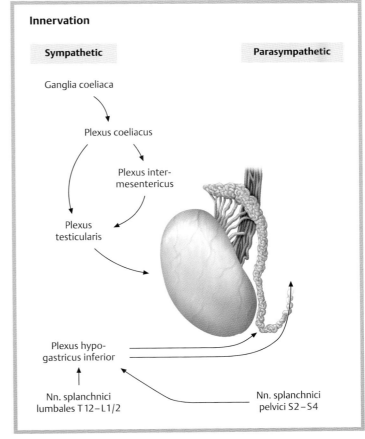

Innervation

Sympathetic		Parasympathetic

Ganglia coeliaca

Plexus coeliacus

Plexus inter-mesentericus

Plexus testicularis

Plexus hypo-gastricus inferior

Nn. splanchnici lumbales T 12–L1/2

Nn. splanchnici pelvici S2–S4

1.17 Uterus, Tuba Uterina, and Vagina

Arteries

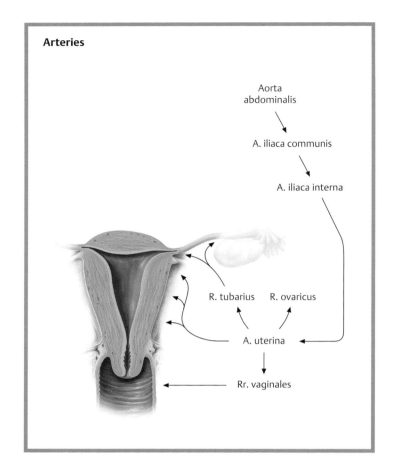

Aorta abdominalis

A. iliaca communis

A. iliaca interna

R. tubarius   R. ovaricus

A. uterina

Rr. vaginales

Veins

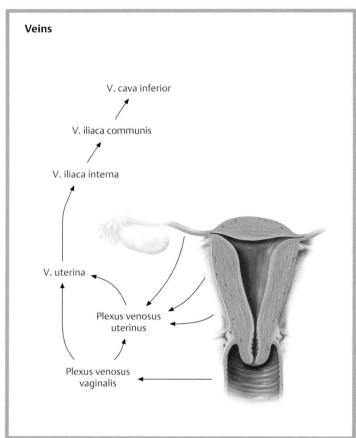

V. cava inferior

V. iliaca communis

V. iliaca interna

V. uterina

Plexus venosus uterinus

Plexus venosus vaginalis

Lymph nodes

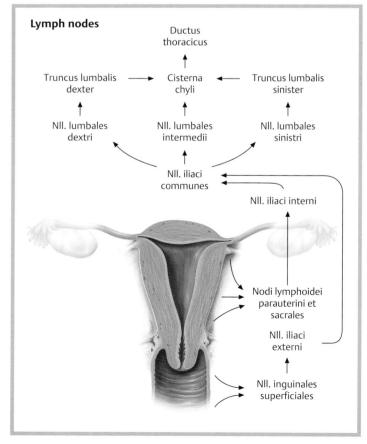

Ductus thoracicus

Truncus lumbalis dexter → Cisterna chyli ← Truncus lumbalis sinister

Nll. lumbales dextri   Nll. lumbales intermedii   Nll. lumbales sinistri

Nll. iliaci communes

Nll. iliaci interni

Nodi lymphoidei parauterini et sacrales

Nll. iliaci externi

Nll. inguinales superficiales

Innervation

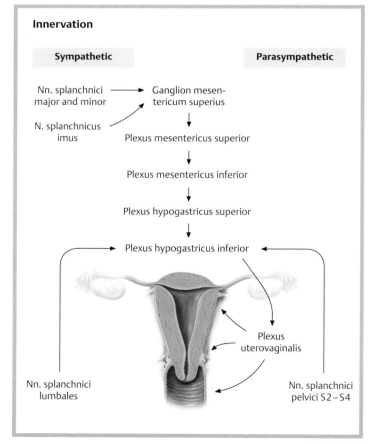

Sympathetic	**Parasympathetic**

Nn. splanchnici major and minor → Ganglion mesentericum superius

N. splanchnicus imus

Plexus mesentericus superior

Plexus mesentericus inferior

Plexus hypogastricus superior

Plexus hypogastricus inferior

Plexus uterovaginalis

Nn. splanchnici lumbales

Nn. splanchnici pelvici S2–S4

1.18 Tuba Uterina and Ovarium

Arteries

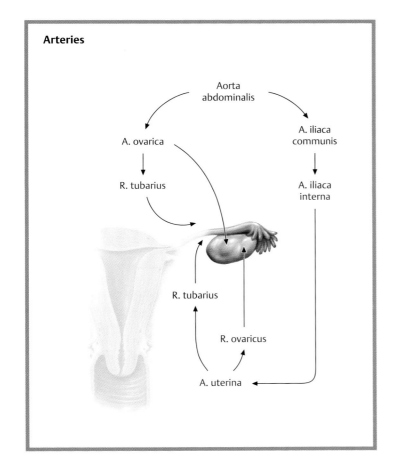

Aorta
abdominalis

A. ovarica

R. tubarius

A. iliaca
communis

A. iliaca
interna

R. tubarius

R. ovaricus

A. uterina

Veins

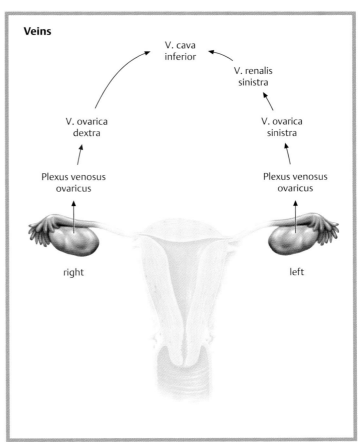

V. cava
inferior

V. renalis
sinistra

V. ovarica
dextra

V. ovarica
sinistra

Plexus venosus
ovaricus

Plexus venosus
ovaricus

right

left

Lymph nodes

Ductus
thoracicus

Cisterna chyli

Truncus lumbalis

Nll. lumbales

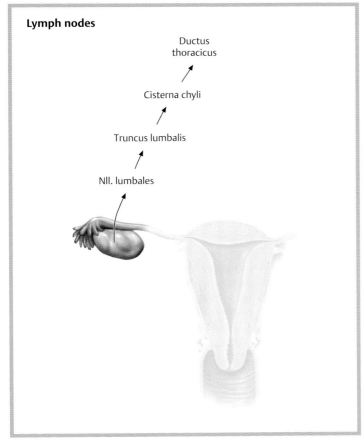

Innervation

Sympathetic	Parasympathetic

Nn. splanchnici
major and minor

Ganglion
mesentericum
superius

Truncus
vagalis posterior

N. splanchnicus
imus

Plexus renalis

Plexus
mesentericus
superior

Plexus ovaricus

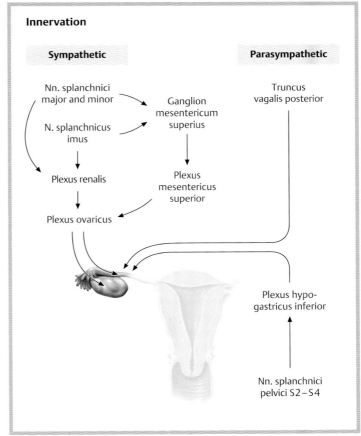

Plexus hypo-
gastricus inferior

Nn. splanchnici
pelvici S2–S4

E   Organ Fact Sheets

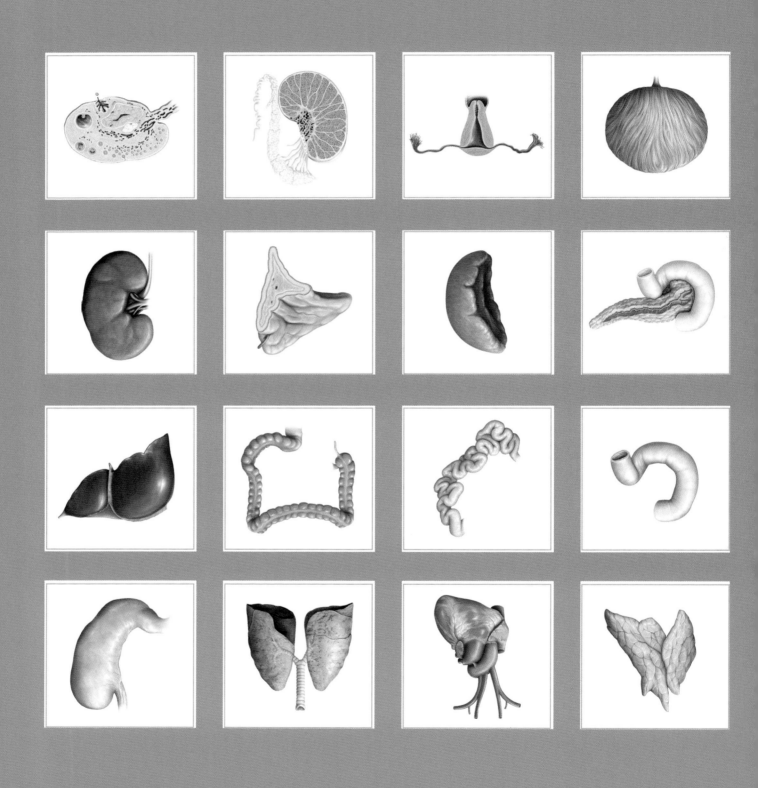

1.1   Thymus

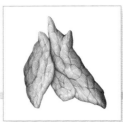

Location	• Situated in the mediastinum superius posterior to the sternum, and anterior to the pericardium and major vessels at the basis cordis	• Projection on the thorax is referred to as the thymic triangle.
Shape and structure	• Lymphoepithelial organ, usually consists of two lobi (left and right lobes). • Delicate connective tissue capsule, and trabeculae that extend into the parenchyma subdividing the thymus into lobuli • Each lobulus is divided into a (darker) cortex and (lighter) medulla. Epithelial cells form a densely packed subcap-	sular layer around the fibrous trabeculae (blood–thymus barrier) and join together inside the thymus to form a three-dimensional network that encloses the lymphocytes. Epithelial cells in the medulla aggregate to form Hassall's corpuscles. • Other cell types: macrophages, myoid cells, dendritic cells
Neurovascular structures (see also p. 408)	Mediastinal circulation. Owing to its location in the mediastinum superius, the thymus is supplied by the neurovascular structures of the mediastinum (entering and exiting the head). • *Arteries:* rr. thymici arising from the a. thoracica interna (proximity to sternum); • *Veins:* vv. thymicae drain into the vv. brachiocephalicae.	• *Lymphatic drainage:* through the nll. brachiocephalici into the trunci bronchomediastinales • *Autonomic innervation:* – parasympathetic through both nn. vagi, especially the nn. laryngei recurrentes – sympathetic through branches of the ganglia cervicalia (nn. cardiaci cervicales)
Function	• Maturation and differentiation (conferring immunological competence) of T-cells • Induction of programmed cell death (apoptosis) in T-cells that respond to antigens: approximately 90% of immature T-cells die in the thymus. • Production of immune-modulating hormones (thymosin, thymopoietin, thymulin) • Primary lymphatic organ	*Note:* The thymus is an organ "of childhood and adolescence." It reaches its maximum size during puberty (approximately 30 grams). The degree of atrophy of thymic tissue in adults varies.
Embryonic development	• The thymic epithelium is derived from the epithelium of the saccus pharyngeus tertius (endodermal origin). • The epithelial primordium is populated with lymphocytes (mesodermal origin).	
Major diseases	• Disorders of the thymus are very rare • Absence of the thymus may be life-threatening (thymic aplasia), resulting in lack of cellular immunity • Lymphatic diseases (e.g., certain types of leukemia) may affect the thymus	• Thymomas: tumors that originate from the epithelial cells of the thymus, and because of the immunologic function of the thymus are often accompanied by autoimmune diseases: myasthenia gravis (muscle weakness).

1.2   Pericardium

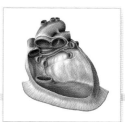

Location	Situated in the thorax (mediastinum medium)

Shape and structure	Fibrous sac that surrounds the cor consisting of • Pericardium fibrosum (outermost layer composed of dense connective tissue; extends to the roots of the great vessels at the basis cordis); • Pericardium serosum (serous membrane) with – lamina *parietalis* (adhered to the pericardium fibrosum), – lamina *visceralis* (epicardium, attached to the myocardium);	• Between laminae parietalis and visceralis: cavitas pericardiaca (narrow space); • At the location where the lamina visceralis is folded back onto the lamina parietalis near the basis cordis, two sinuses are formed: – *sinus transversus pericardii* (between the arteries and veins) – *sinus obliquus pericardii* (between the vv. pulmonales sinistrae and dextrae).

Openings	• One for the aorta ascendens • One for the truncus pulmonalis • Two for both vv. cavae • Four for the four vv. pulmonales.

Neurovascular structures (see also p. 411)	• Mediastinal circulation • *Arteries:* a. pericardiacophrenica (from the a. thoracica interna) • *Veins:* v. pericardiacophrenica (to the v. brachiocephalica) • *Lymphatic drainage:* nll. prepericardiaci, nll. pericardiaci laterales (also nll. phrenici superiores and nll. tracheobronchiales into the truncus bronchomediastinalis)	• *Autonomic innervation:* negligible • *Somatosensory innervation:* n. phrenicus (from the plexus cervicalis)

Function	Provides sliding-surface for the heart, however the pericardium is not essential for life.

Embryonic development	Derived from mesoderma laminae lateralis: • Visceral parts derived from mesenchyma splanchnopleurale • Parietal parts derived from mesenchyma somatopleurale

Major diseases	• Pericarditis: inflammation usually caused by viral or bacterial infection. • Tuberculous pericarditis, which is rare nowadays, can lead to pericardial calcium deposits. As a result, the	heart can no longer expand; it is constricted (also known as constrictive pericarditis).

1.3   Cor (Heart)

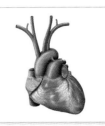

Location	• Located in the thorax within the pericardium. • The basis cordis is directed upward, backward, and to the right. The basis cordis is the location of the venous entry and arterial exit points (vv. cavae inferior and superior, vv. pulmonales, aorta ascendens and truncus pulmonalis).

• The apex cordis is directed downward, forward and to the left.
• The longitudinal axis of the cor (from the base to the apex, the anatomical axis of the cor) is at a 45-degree angle to all body planes.

Shape and structure

• Hollow organ, shaped like a cone: measures 12–14 cm in length, 9 cm in width at its broadest part.

• Weight: up to 300 g.

External structures of the cor

• **Surfaces:**
 – facies sternocostalis (facies anterior)
 – facies pulmonales dextra and sinistra
 – facies diaphragmatica (facies inferior)

• **Grooves on the outside of the cor:**
 – sulci interventriculares anterior/posterior
 – sulcus coronarius

• **Auriculae atrii:** (auricula sinistra/dextra): protrusions attached to the atria (analogous to the primitive atria; potential site for thrombus formation) produce atrial natriuretic peptide (ANP) for regulation of blood pressure.

Internal structures of the cor

Chambers and openings of the cor

• **Four contractile chambers:**
 – two atria: atria sinistrum and dextrum separated by the septum interatriale (muscle);
 – two ventriculi: ventriculi sinister and dexter, separated by the septum interventriculare (pars muscularis and pars membranacea, thus part muscle and part connective tissue); both ventriculi have an inflow tract (with trabeculae carneae) and an outflow tract (smooth-walled) following the direction of blood flow.

• **Four openings** that connect the atria and ventriculi, the ventriculus dexter and truncus pulmonalis, and the ventriculus sinister and aorta ascendens:

 – two openings in the right side of the cor: ostium atrioventriculare dextrum and ostium trunci pulmonalis;
 – two openings in the left side of the cor: ostium atrioventriculare sinistrum and ostium aortae.

• Additionally, **openings for the two vv. cavae** (in the atrium dextrum) and the four vv. pulmonales (in the atrium sinistrum, see flow of blood below) as well as the ostium sinus coronarii (in the atrium dextrum: opening of sinus coronarius with the valvula sinus coronarii).

Flow of blood through the heart chambers

• Generally: from the right cor to the lungs (oxygen absorption), from there to the left cor and then to the aorta (oxygen is released to serially connected organs)
• More specifically: from the vv. cavae superior and inferior into the atrium dextrum, from there through the ostium atrioventriculare dextrum to the ventriculus dexter and through the ostium trunci pulmonalis to the truncus pulmonalis, through both of the aa. pulmonales, and into the lungs; from there to the four vv. pulmonales, then to the atrium sinistrum and through the ostium atrioventriculare sinistrum to the ventriculus sinister and finally through the ostium aortae to the aorta.

Cardiac valves

• By closing and opening (mm. papillares, see below) **four valves** ensure that blood flows in only one direction through the cor:

 – two valvae atrioventriculares;
 – two semilunar valves (valva trunci pulmonalis and valva aortae).

During ventricular contraction, the valvae atrioventriculares prevent backflow of blood from the ventriculi into the atria; when the ventriculi relax, the semilunar valves prevent the return of blood from the truncus pulmonalis and aorta ascendens back into the ventricles.

• **Valves of the right side of the cor:**
 – valva atrioventricularis dextra at the ostium atrioventriculare dextrum = cuspid valve with three cusps: cuspides septalis/anterior/posterior = tricuspid valve;
 – valva trunci pulmonalis at the ostium trunci pulmonalis in the outflow tract of the ventriculus dexter = semilunar valve with three cusps: valvula semilunares anterior/sinistra/dextra;

• **Valves of the left side of the cor:**
 – valva atrioventricularis sinistra at the ostium atrioventriculare sinistrum = cuspid valve with two cusps = bicuspid valve: cuspides anterior/posterior = valva mitralis;
 – valva aortae at the ostium aortae in the outflow tract of the ventriculus sinister = semilunar valve also with three cusps: valvulae semilunares posterior/sinistra/dextra.

Grooves and crests on the inner walls of the chambers of the cor

Grooves (only in the atria):

- Right: fossa ovalis in the septum interatriale is the embryonic remnant of the foramen ovale.
- Left: valvula foraminis ovalis is the counterpart of the fossa ovalis on the right side.

Crests (in atria and ventriculi):

- *Atria* dextrum and sinistrum: mm. pectinati: ridge-like muscle protrusions in the auricula, see above, correspond to the primitive atrium of the embryonic cor.
- *Ventriculi* dexter and sinister:
  - trabeculae carneae (muscular columns that line the ventriculi; more prominent in the ventriculus dexter than in the ventriculus sinister)
  - mm. papillares: specialized extensions of the trabeculae carneae that project into the lumen of the ventriculus; prevent the inversion or prolapse of valves during ventricular contraction
  - in the ventriculus dexter: *three* mm. papillares for the *three* cusps of the valva tricuspidalis, see above, (anterior, posterior, and septalis)

- in the ventriculus sinister: *two* mm. papillares for the *two* cusps of the bicuspid valve (valva mitralis), see above (mm. papillares anterior and posterior)

Skeleton of the cor

The heart valves all lie in one plane (valve plane) and are covered by endocardium. The valve rings are composed of dense connective tissue. All anuli fibrosi, together with the collagenous bands through which they are connected, form the cardiac skeleton.

Layers of the heart wall

The wall of the cor consists of three layers. From the inside to the outside they are

- endocardium (simple squamous epithelium): lines the cavities of the cor and covers the heart valves;
- myocardium (muscle, the fibers of which are arranged in different directions): muscle fibers roughly arranged in three layers;
- epicardium (tunica serosa of the pericardium, simple squamous epithelium): strictly speaking, it is part of the pericardium, although it is often referred to as part of the cor.

Neurovascular structures (see also p. 410)	<ul><li>Mediastinal circulation</li><li>*Arteries:* a. coronaria sinistra (with r. interventricularis anterior and r. circumflexus) and a. coronaria dextra (with r. interventricularis posterior), both arise from the aorta ascendens where it exits the ventriculus sinister.</li><li>*Veins:* vv. cardiacae (magna, media, parva), like the v. ventriculi sinistri posterior, the vv. cardiacae return blood to the atrium dextrum through the sinus coronarius.</li></ul> • *Lymphatic drainage:* through the nll. brachiocephalici and the nll. tracheobronchiales into the truncus bronchomediastinalis • *Autonomic innervation:* parasympathetic through the two nn. vagi (rr. cardiaci cervicales and thoracici). The neuronal cell bodies are in the nuclei posteriores nervorum vagorum; sympathetic through branches of ganglia thoracica 2–5 (nn. cardiaci cervicales superior, medius and inferior) and rr. cardiaci thoracici.

Function	The cor functions as a suction-pressure pump to distribute blood around the body (heart volume approximately 780 ml, ventricular stroke volume 70 ml). • The heartbeat can be felt as pulse (resting heart rate ~ 1 Hz). • Cardiac activity is divided into two phases: systole (contraction of the myocardium) and diastole (relaxation of the myocardium). • Contraction of the ventricular myocardium (closure of the AV valves) and closure of the valvae aortae and trunci pulmonalis are audible as the first and second heart sounds. • Cardiac excitation conduction system composed of specialized myocardial cells: impulses are generated by the nodus sinuatrialis (SA node) in the atrium dextrum adjacent to the opening of the v. cava superior. Excitation is spread to the ventriculi through the nodus atrioventricularis (AV node), at the junction of atrium dextrum and ventriculus dexter, and then through the fasciculus atrioventricularis (bundle of His) with its crura dextrum and sinistrum, which terminate in the Purkinje fibers. *Note:* Because of its autonomous excitation, the cor can trigger the impulse that generates the heartbeat. Even an isolated heart beats. The autonomic innervation (see above) modifies only the activities of the autonomous excitation and conduction system. The parasympathetic nervous system reduces the heart rate and atrioventricular conduction. The sympathetic nervous system increases both as well as the stroke volume.

Embryonic Development	Of mesodermal origin, derived from the primitive cor tubulare and subsequently formed ansa cordis.

Major diseases	<ul><li>Heart diseases are important and are the leading cause of death in the industrialized world: *myocardial infarction* = occluded aa. coronariae that lead to inadequate blood flow to distinct parts of the myocardium, which results in myocardial necrosis</li><li>*Arrhythmia* and dysfunction of the conduction system</li><li>*Valve defects* (congenital or caused by inflammation of the endocardium) = incomplete opening of the valve (valve stenosis) or incomplete valve closure (valve insufficiency)</li></ul> • With *myocardial injuries* without damage to the pericardium, the cor continues to pump blood into the cavitas pericardiaca until cardiac arrest occurs (*cardiac tamponade*). • Generally: formation of pathological blood clots (thromboses) in the cor, which may travel through the blood stream, for example, to the encephalon.

1.4 Trachea, Bronchi, and Lungs

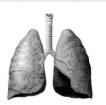

Location	• Pars cervicalis of the trachea situated in the neck • Pars thoracica of the trachea and bronchi principales situated in the mediastinum • Bronchi lobares and all segments inferior: intrapulmonary location • Lungs: situated on either side of the mediastinum	• Surface of the lung covered by pleura visceralis (pleura pulmonalis). On the facies mediastinalis at the lig. pulmonale the pleura parietalis is folded back onto the pleura visceralis.
External structure of the lung	• Apex pulmonis • Basis pulmonis • Lobi pulmonis. Three lobi in the right lung: lobus superior, lobus medius, and lobus inferior; two in the left lung: lobus superior and lobus inferior • Fissures, two in the right lung: fissura horizontalis below the lobus superior; fissura obliqua between the lobus medius and lobus inferior. In the left lung one fissura obliqua between the lobi superior and inferior • Two margines: margines anterior and inferior	• Four surfaces: facies costalis (adjacent to the ribs), facies diaphragmatica (at the basis pulmonis, adjacent to the diaphragma), facies mediastinalis (adjacent to the mediastinum), facies interlobaris (in the fissurae between lobi) *Note:* A term for the posterior margin of the lung (where the facies costalis and mediastinalis meet) is not listed in the official Terminologia Anatomica.
Shape and structure of the airways	• Generally: tubes that divide by dichotomous branching with decreasing caliber • The intrapulmonary airways, connective tissue, and neurovascular structures form a spongy organ—the paired pulmones. **Structure of the trachea and arbor bronchialis:** • Trachea to bronchioli terminales = conducting (carrying air) portion. • Bronchioli terminales to alveoli = respiratory (gas exchange) portion. **Components of the conducting portion:** • Pars cervicalis of the trachea: first tracheal ring, see below, to apertura thoracis superior • Pars thoracica of the trachea: apertura thoracis superior to bifurcatio tracheae • At the bifurcatio tracheae: division of the trachea into the bronchi principales dexter and bronchi principales dexter	• Division of the bronchus principalis dexter into three bronchi lobares: bronchi lobares superior dexter, medius and inferior dexter • Division of the bronchus principalis sinister into two bronchi lobares: bronchi lobares superior sinister and inferior sinister • Division of the bronchi lobares into bronchi segmentales: ten bronchi segmentales in the right lung and nine bronchi segmentales in the left lung • Division of the bronchi segmentales into bronchi intrasegmentales **Components of the respiratory portion:** • Bronchioli respiratorii: first to third order (where alveoli begin to appear) • Ductuli alveolares • Sacculi alveolares
Structure of the airway wall	**Trachea:** • Hollow, tubular organ with 16–20 horseshoe-shaped cartilage rings • Tracheal rings joined together by collagen and elastic fibers (ligg. anularia) • Tunica mucosa of the trachea covered with respiratory epithelium, contains multiple glands (gll. tracheales). • Posterior tracheal wall: non-cartilaginous, composed of connective tissue (membranous wall of trachea), permeated by smooth-muscle cells (m. trachealis). **Bronchi principales, lobares, segmentales and intrasegmentales:** • Generally similar in structure to the trachea.	• Concentric or spiral sheets of smooth-muscle cells in all bronchi (active changes in caliber) • In bronchi segmentales and intrasegmentales cartilaginous plates instead of cartilage rings • Pseudostratified respiratory epithelium like tracheal mucosa **Starting from the bronchioli respiratorii:** • Non-cartilaginous walls • Ciliated epithelium with type I and type II pneumocytes (in the alveoli)
Internal structure of the lungs	Structure of the airways determines the structure of the pulmones: • Both lungs aerated by trachea. • Bronchi principales (sinister and dexter, respectively) each aerate one lung (sinister and dexter, respectively). • Bronchi lobales each aerate one lobus.	• Bronchi segmentales each aerate one segmentum bronchopulmonale. • Bronchioli terminales each aerate one lobulus (pulmonary lobule). • Bronchioli respiratorii each aerate one acinus; a group of acini forms a lobulus.

Neurovascular structures (see also p. 412)	Mediastinal circulation

Neurovascular structures (see also p. 412)

Mediastinal circulation

- The intrapulmonary neurovascular structures in the lung either run along the divisions of the arbor bronchialis or within the connective tissue framework.
- Characteristic feature of the lungs: two circulation systems: rr. bronchiales (aortae) and vv. bronchiales to supply the lung itself, and aa. and vv. pulmonales for gas exchange through the entire body.

Bronchial arteries and veins:
- *Arteries:* rr. bronchiales directly from the aorta thoracica or indirectly from aa. intercostales posteriores
- *Veins:* on the right, vv. bronchiales to the v. azygos, on the left to the v. hemiazygos or v. hemiazygos accessoria

Arteriae and venae pulmonales:
- *Arteries:* the aa. pulmonales (sinistra, dextra) carry deoxygenated blood from the truncus pulmonalis. Segmental branches (aa. segmentales) of the aa. pulmonales follow the bronchi segmentales into the center of one of the 10 or 9 segmenta bronchopulmonalia.
- *Veins:* drainage of oxygenated blood usually through four vv. pulmonales into the atrium sinistrum of the cor
- *Lymphatic drainage:* through the nll. intrapulmonales, bronchopulmonales, tracheobronchiales, and paratracheales into the trunci bronchomediastinales
- *Autonomic innervation:*
  - parasympathetic through the two nn. vagi to the plexus pulmonalis,
  - sympathetic through branches mainly from ganglia thoracica 2 or 3–4 (varies), also to the plexus pulmonalis

Function

Generally, the exchange of oxygen and carbon dioxide between the atmosphere and blood circulation, more specifically:

- Trachea and bronchi as well as their divisions (arbor bronchialis) except for the finest terminal portions: air conduction
- Final divisions of the arbor bronchialis (alveoli): gas exchange between atmosphere and blood; thus the important role of the lungs for
  - energy production: oxygen is extracted from the atmosphere for oxidation processes.
  - regulation of acid-base balance (release of carbon dioxide in the air when exhaling and thus influencing bicarbonate levels in the blood)
- Following changes in the thoracic volume through the pleural layers (capillary forces cause the pleura visceralis, which is attached to the lungs, to adhere to the pleura parietalis, which is attached to the inner surface of the thoracic wall); a change in lung volume leads to a change in intrapulmonary pressure resulting in drawing in or expelling air from the lungs.

Embryonic development

Of endodermal origin, derived from the cranial praeenteron:

- Gemma respiratoria or diverticulum laryngotracheale develops from a small outpouching on the ventral surface of the embryonic oesophagus.
- Gemma respiratoria undergoes repeated dichotomous branching (total of 22) to give rise to the trachea along with the arbor bronchialis including the alveoli.

Note: The lungs are fully matured at approximately the age of 10.

Major diseases

The arbor bronchialis and lungs are the parts of the body most commonly affected by diseases (entry points for infectious pathogens):

- Acute inflammation of the arbor bronchialis (bronchitis, bronchial catarrh, cold) is usually caused by viral infections and is generally harmless.
- Chronic inflammation (chronic bronchitis) is much more common in smokers.
- Bronchial asthma (often triggered by allergies) is a result of insufficient expansion of small bronchi and bronchioli during expiration.
- Lung overexpansion and rupture of the alveoli (pulmonary emphysema)
- Chronic obstructive pulmonary disease (COPD): endstage of the three previously mentioned diseases, with destruction of gas exchange tissue
- Malignant tumors (bronchial carcinoma) is among the leading causes of death for smokers.
- Pulmonary embolism: Acute occlusion of an a. pulmonalis (or one of its branches) is caused by a blood clot that most commonly was formed in a vein and carried from the right cor to the lung. In that case it is crucial that the pulmones possess a double circulation. Blood from the bronchial branches is sufficient to supply the tissue. Hence, blockage of the a. pulmonalis does not result in tissue undersupply and subsequent destruction.

1.5 Oesophagus

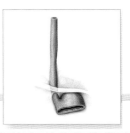

Location	Situated in the neck and thorax (mediastinum) between the trachea and columna vertebralis, as well as in the abdomen

Shape, size and segments	• Tubular organ, measures about 23–27 cm in length from the entrance of the oesophagus to its terminal portion. • Measures about 20 mm in width (but see constrictions of the oesophagus). Divided into three parts corresponding to the regions of the body they are located in (see above)	• Pars cervicalis (C6–T1): to the apertura thoracis superior • Pars thoracica (T1–T11): to the hiatus oesophageus (site where the oesophagus passes through the diaphragma) • Pars abdominalis: to the ostium cardiacum of the gaster (shortest segment, measures only 2–3 cm in length, lies intraperitoneally).

Esophageal constrictions (maximum width of 14 mm instead of the usual 20 mm)	• Upper constriction: constrictio pharyngooesophagealis at the C6 level; 14–16 cm from the dentes incisivi • Middle constriction: constrictio partis thoracicae at the T4/T5 level; 25–27 cm from the dentes incisivi, oesophagus passes to the right of the aorta thoracica.	• Lower constriction: constrictio phrenica at the T10/T11 level; 36–38 cm from the dentes incisivi, site where the oesophagus pierces the diaphragma; functional closure of the esophagus by muscles and venous cushions of the oesophageal wall, and muscles of the diaphragma

Wall structure	• Basically the same as in the gastrointestinal tract: tunica mucosa, tela submucosa, tunica muscularis, and tunica adventitia, or in the lower part in proximity to the gaster: tela subserosa and tunica serosa. • Tunica mucosa with stratified non-keratinized squamous epithelium (has no digestive function but provides mechanical protection against passing food, lubricated by gll. oesophageae) • Musculature in the upper oesophagus (variable degree of expansion), striated (like the mm. pharyngis), in the	middle and lower part smooth muscle (like the gaster), the lower part contains numerous veins. • Muscles also contain fibers that wind obliquely around the oesophagus. • Combination of circular and longitudinal muscle fibers allows for the expansion and constriction of the oesophageal inlet and outlet (swallowing).

Neurovascular structures (see also p. 409)	• Primarily mediastinal circulation (pars thoracica); to a lesser extent also cervical (pars cervicalis) and upper abdominal circulation (pars abdominalis)
	• *Arteries:* numerous rr. oesophageales of the a. thyroidea inferior (pars cervicalis), aorta thoracica (pars thoracica), and a. gastrica sinistra (pars abdominalis)
	• *Veins:* numerous vv. oesophageales to the v. thyroidea inferior (pars cervicalis), vv. azygos and hemiazygos (pars thoracica), and v. gastrica sinistra (pars abdominalis)
	• *Lymphatic drainage* through the nll. juxtaoesophageales into the nll. cervicales profundi (pars cervicalis), trunci bronchomediastinales (pars thoracica) and nll. gastrici sinistri (pars abdominalis)
		• *Autonomic innervation:*
		  – parasympathetic through the two nn. vagi (trunci vagales), in the neck region specifically through the nn. laryngei recurrentes. Neurons for the smooth esophageal muscles in the nucleus posterior nervi vagi, neurons for the striated muscles in nucleus ambiguus
		  – sympathetic through branches of ganglia thoracica 2–5.
		
		The autonomic fibers form the plexus oesophageus on the oesophagus.

Function	During swallowing, active transport of solids and liquids from the pharynx to the gaster; when vomiting, transport	of gaster contents from the gaster to the pharynx

Embryonic development	• Derived from the endoderm of the cranial praeenteron. • Lower part of the mesoesophagus may remain in the form of the lig. hepatoesophageale (connects hepar to pars abdominalis of oesophagus).	*Note:* As a result of the rotation of the gaster in the embryo, the oesophagus also shifts slightly. Thus, the longitudinal layer of the smooth esophageal muscles is arranged in a rightward spiral pattern.

Major diseases	Diseases of the oesophagus itself (rare except for esophageal reflux): • Diverticulum (outpouchings of the wall), most common at the junction between the hypopharynx (pars laryngea pharyngis) and oesophagus (also known as Zenker's diverticulum, which is not an esophageal but a hypopharyngeal diverticulum). • Malignant tumors (esophageal carcinoma; relatively rare) • Inflammation of the tunica mucosa oesophagi as a result of chronic alcohol consumption • Esophageal reflux: inflammation of the esophageal epithelium caused by reflux of stomach acid; caused by	insufficient closing mechanisms at the junction of the oesophagus and gaster. • Barrett's oesophagus: as a result of chronic esophageal reflux, the columnar epithelium of the gaster may replace the squamous epithelium of the oesophagus: increased risk of cancer. In the case of liver cirrhosis, abnormally enlarged esophageal veins (esophageal varices: hemorrhagic risk) serve as a portacaval detour (drainage into the azygos system!).

1.6   Gaster (Stomach)

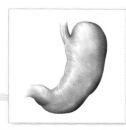

Location	*Lies intraperitoneally in the left upper quadrant (=epigastrium).*

Shape and segments	• Sac-like hollow organ with parietes anterior and posterior; different shapes may be encountered (hook-shaped gaster, bull-horn-shaped gaster, long gaster).
	• Four parts of the gaster in cranial to caudal direction:
	  – top right: cardia = ostium cardiacum = esophageal inlet
	  – fundus gastricus (base or dome of the gaster; appears on radiographs as an air-filled space above a fluid level)
	  – corpus gastricum
	  – bottom right: pars pylorica of gaster = pylorus with antrum pyloricum and canalis pyloricus; stomach terminates at the pylorus, which closes the ostium pyloricum (exit from the gaster into the duodenum)
		• The corpus gastricum has two curvaturae:
		  – *curvatura minor,* faces right and upward, omentum minus (connects the hepar to the gaster) extends from it.
		  – *curvatura major,* faces left and downward, omentum majus extends from it.
		• The gaster has two notches:
		  – the incisura cardialis at the junction between the cardia and the corpus gastricum
		  – the incisura angularis at the junction between the corpus gastricum and the pylorus

Wall structure	• Basically the same wall structure as the entire gastrointestinal tract: tunica mucosa, tela submucosa, tunica muscularis, and tela subserosa and tunica serosa. • Exception: tunica muscularis consists of three layers: fibrae obliquae, stratum circulare and stratum longitudinale (important for peristaltic motion).	• Tunica mucosa contains specialized glandular cells that produce HCl and intrinsic factor (parietal cells), pepsinogen (chief cells; protein digestion) and mucus (surface epithelial cells and accessory cells, mucin-producing; protection against self-digestion).

Neurovascular structures
(see also p. 415)
	Upper abdominal circulation.
	
	• *Arteries*: owing to the location in the upper abdomen, all aa. gastricae arise directly (a. gastrica sinistra) or indirectly (through the a. hepatica communis or a. splenica) from the truncus coeliacus: aa. gastricae sinistra and dextra supply the curvatura minor, aa. gastroomentales sinistra and dextra supply the curvatura major; variably an a. gastrica posterior for the paries posterior of the gaster.
	• *Veins:* vv. gastricae sinistra and dextra, vv. gastroomentales sinistra and dextra, v. prepylorica and vv. gastricae breves directly or indirectly (v. splenica or v. mesenterica
		superior) into the v. portae hepatis
		• *Lymphatic drainage:* through groups of nodi lymphoidei at the curvatura minor (nll. gastrici sinistri and dextri), curvatura major (nll. gastroomentales sinistri and dextri), and at the pylorus (nll. pylorici) into the nll. coeliaci and from there into the cisterna chyli
		• *Autonomic innervation:*
		  – parasympathetic through the two nn. vagi (trunci vagales)
		  – sympathetic, primarily through the n. splanchnicus major and partially through the nn. splanchnici minores (through the ganglia coeliaca)

Function	• Temporary reservoir for food, hence its large volume (1.2–1.8 L) and high elasticity.
	• Start of digestive process requirements:
	  – production of gastric juice containing HCl (approximately 2 L per day, responsible for protein denaturation and sterilizing food, HCl concentration 5 M/L) and protein-digesting enzymes (pepsin)
		– liquefaction and mechanical grinding (through peristaltic motion of the paries gastricus) of food into chyme which is passed in small amounts through the pylorus to the duodenum. Peristaltic transport of chyme
		  – secretion of intrinsic factor for the intestinal resorption of vitamin B_{12}

Embryonic development	• Of endodermal origin, derived from the praeenteron. • The gaster has a mesogastrium dorsale and a mesogastrium ventrale that develop into the omentum majus and minus, respectively.	• As the gaster and the mesogastrium rotate, the hepar and splen shift to the right and left upper quadrants and the duodenum comes to lie retroperitoneally.

Major diseases	• Acute and chronic inflammation (gastritis) • Ulcer (often caused by a type of bacteria called *Helicobacter pylori*)	• Malignant gastric tumor (gastric carcinoma)

1.7   Intestinum Tenue: Duodenum

Location	• Largely secondarily retroperitoneal in the right upper quadrant just below the hepar, with approximately 2 cm of the superior part in proximity to the gaster remaining intraperitoneal. • As a result of the tilt and rotation of the gaster during embryonic development the duodenum shifts to	the right, superior and posterior.

Shape and parts of the duodenum	• Hollow, tubular organ, in anterior view: c-shaped • Shortest segment of the intestinum tenue and has a length of approximately 12 finger-widths • 4 parts from top to bottom: – pars superior	– pars descendens – pars inferior or horizontalis – pars ascendens

Wall structure	• Basically the same wall structure as the entire gastro-intestinal tract: tunica mucosa, tela submucosa, tunica muscularis (with strata circulare and longitudinale), tela subserosa, and tunica serosa or adventitia, with the pli-cae longitudinales duodeni being the most distinct and diminishing in size toward the end of the intestinum tenue.	• Tunica mucosa with specialized circular folds (also known as Kerckring's folds). Gll. duodenales (also known as Brunner's glands) open into the intestinal lumen.

Neurovascular structures
(see also p. 416)
	Upper abdominal circulation and superior mesenteric circulation
	
	• *Arteries:* indirect branches of the truncus coeliacus (rr. duodenales of the a. gastroduodenalis with aa. pan-creaticoduodenales superiores anterior and posterior) and the a. mesenterica superior (small branches of the a. pancreaticoduodenalis inferior)
	• *Veins:* drainage via the vv. pancreaticoduodenales into the v. portae hepatis
		• *Lymphatic drainage:* indirectly through the nll. pancreati-coduodenales and pancreatici to the nll. coeliaci or into the truncus intestinalis
		• *Autonomic innervation:*
		  – parasympathetic primarily through the right n. vagus (truncus vagalis posterior)
		  – sympathetic through the nn. splanchnici majores (ganglia coeliaca)

Function	• Digestion of food through enzymatic breakdown of car-bohydrates, fat, and proteins. The enzymes are pro-duced by the duodenal epithelium or are secreted by the pancreas and released through the papilla duodeni major (opening of the joined ductus choledochus and ductus pancreaticus) and papilla duodeni minor (open-ing of the ductus pancreaticus accessorius) into the duo-denal lumen. The addition of the ductus choledochus serves to supply bile for emulsifying fat.	• Transport of absorbed nutrients in the bloodstream directly to the hepar (with the exception of fats) • Peristaltic transport of chyme *Note:* Gallstones may obstruct the common opening for the ductus choledochus and pancreaticus, and reflux of pancre-atic juice that contains highly active enzymes may cause an acute inflammation of the pancreas (pancreatitis).

Embryonic development	• Of endodermal origin, derived from the praeenteron • Mesoduodenum dorsale and a smaller mesoduodenum ventrale	*Note:* The duodenal epithelium gives rise to the primordia for the hepar, vesica biliaris, and pancreas.

Major diseases	• Duodenal ulcer • Acute and chronic inflammation (duodenitis) • Malignant tumors (very rare)

1.8 Intestinum Tenue: Jejunum and Ileum

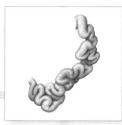

Location	• Lies *intraperitoneally* between the mesocolon transversum and the level of the apertura pelvis superior in the upper part of the cavitas peritonealis. • Defining their location by reference to skeletal landmarks is not useful because the small bowel loops are	very mobile, generally-surrounded and framed by the intestinum crassum.
Shape and parts	• Hollow, tubular organ with numerous loops • Longest single organ (measures up to 5 m), ensures long transit time of food: *jejunum* (longest single segment) accounts for approximately ⅔ of the entire length; *ileum* accounts for approximately ⅓.	*Note:* The ileum is connected in an end-to-side fashion to the caecum.
Wall structure	• Basically the same wall structure as the entire gastrointestinal tract: tunica mucosa, submucosa, tunica muscularis (with strata circulare and longitudinale), tela subserosa, and tunica serosa. • Tunica mucosa with numerous plicae and villi. Plica height decreases from proximal to distal, thus from jejunum to ileum.	• Tela submucosa (particularly in the pars terminalis ilei) with distinct collections of lymphoid follicles for immune response to antigens present in intestinal contents (noduli lymphoidei aggregati = Peyer's patches). Effect of oral inoculation is based on the stimulation of Peyer's patches.

Neurovascular structures (see also p. 417)	Superior mesenteric circulation.
	
	• *Arteries:* numerous aa. jejunales and ileales (branches of the a. mesenterica superior). Additionally, in the pars terminalis ilei the a. ileocolica. Arteries extend in the mesenterium to the intestinal segments and form arcades close to the bowel, thus forming anastomoses, hence impaired circulation in the intestinum is very rare.
	• *Veins:* vv. jejunales and ileales into the v. mesenterica superior and from there into the v. portae hepatis. The pars terminalis ilei is also drained by the v. ileocolica.
		• *Lymphatic drainage:* through nodi lymphoidei located in the mesenterium (nodi juxtaintestinales) into the nll. mesenterici superiores
		• *Autonomic innervation:*
		  – parasympathetic primarily through the right n. vagus (truncus vagalis posterior)
		  – sympathetic through the nn. splanchnici major and minor (partially ganglia coeliaca, but mainly ganglia mesenterica superiora)

Function	• Enzymatic breakdown and digestion of carbohydrates, proteins, and fats as well as absorption of their components; additionally, absorption of vitamins, trace elements and minerals • Slow (transit time 8–16 h) peristaltic transport of chyme through the jejunum and ileum, with mucosal lining in close contact with food	• Absorbed nutrients are carried off in the bloodstream directly to the liver (via the v. portae hepatis) (with the exception of lipids: they are transported via vasa lymphocapillaria to the cisterna chyli).
Embryonic development	• Of endodermal origin, derived from the mesenteron • Jejunum and ileum with mesenterium dorsale	
Major diseases	• Acute and chronic inflammation (enteritis) • Ulcers primarily in the presence of chronic inflammation (Crohn's disease); malignant tumors (very rare) • At the three constrictions (ostium pyloricum, flexura duodenojejunalis, and ostium ileale) foreign bodies that	have been swallowed may get stuck (risk of life-threatening *mechanical ileus*).

1.9   Intestinum Crassum: Caecum with Appendix Vermiformis and Colon

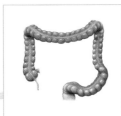

Location	Frame-like, primarily in the lower abdomen, transverse and lateral segments: <ul><li>Cola ascendens and descendens secondarily retroperitoneal</li><li>Cola transversum and sigmoideum intraperitoneal</li><li>Caecum intraperitoneal or more or less fully secondarily retroperitoneal</li></ul>

- Appendix vermiformis remains intraperitoneal.

Note: Only the intraperitoneal segments of the mature organism have a mesenterium dorsale.

Shape and parts

Hollow, tubular organ, shaped like a frame that is partially open at its inferior aspect, with caecum and appendix vermiformis; and cola ascendens, transversum, descendens, and sigmoideum

---

Wall structure

- Basically the same wall structure as the entire gastrointestinal tract
- Deep mucosal depressions (crypts), but, unlike the small intestine, no plicae circulares or villi
- Numerous lymphoid follicles in the tela submucosa (recognize enteric antigens), unlike the sterile intestinum tenue, the intestinum crassum is always populated by bacteria.

Note: The strata longitudinalia of the tunica muscularis of the colon are in the form of three discontinuous longitudinal bands of muscle (taeniae libera, mesocolica, omentalis).

- The circular layers of the muscularis form constrictions (visible internally as plicae semilunares) with sacculations located between the folds (haustra = haustrations of colon). Tunica serosa with fat deposition (appendices omentales).
- Taeniae, haustra, and appendices omentales are distinctive morphological features of the colon and caecum, which are helpful in distinguishing the intestinum crassum from the intestinum tenue during surgery. Taeniae are not present in the rectum where the longitudinal muscle fibers again form a continuous layer. (The junction between the colon and rectum is visible externally.)

Neurovascular structures
(see also p. 418f)

Proximal to the flexura coli sinistra **superior mesenteric circulation:**
- *Arteries:* aa. colicae dextra and media and a. ileocolica (from the a. mesenterica superior) with aa. caecales anterior and posterior and a. appendicularis
- *Veins:* vv. colicae dextra and media and v. ileocolica with v. appendicularis into the v. mesenterica superior and from there into the v. portae hepatis
- *Lymphatic drainage:* through the nll. precaecales and retrocaecales and nodi appendiculares, and nll. colici dextri and medii, into the nll. mesenterici superiores
- *Autonomic innervation:*
  - parasympathetic primarily through the right n. vagus (trruncus vagalis posterior)
  - sympathetic through the nn. splanchnici major and minor (ganglia mesenterica superiora)

Distal to the flexura coli sinistra, **inferior mesenteric circulation:**
- *Arteries:* a. colica sinistra and aa. sigmoideae arising from the a. mesenterica inferior

- *Veins:* v. colica sinistra and vv. sigmoideae into the v. mesenterica inferior and from there into the v. portae hepatis
- *Lymphatic drainage:* through mesenteric lymph nodes (left colic lymph nodes and sigmoid lymph nodes) into the inferior mesenteric lymph nodes and from there into the trunci lumbales or via the nodi lymphoidei lumbales sinistri into the cisterna chyli
- *Autonomic innervation:*
  - parasympathetic through the nn. splanchnici pelvici (from S 2–S 4) via the plexus hypogastricus inferior,
  - sympathetic through the nn. splanchnici lumbales (via the plexus hypogastricus inferior), partially through the nn. splanchnici major and minor (ganglia mesenterica superiora).

Note: Close to the flexura coli sinistra distinct anastomoses between the a. colica media and a. colica sinistra (Riolan anastomosis) and convergence of autonomic fibers (Cannon-Böhm point) mark the boundary between the mesenteron and metenteron.

Function

- To some extent resorption of food components broken down by enzymes
- Primarily thickening of the chyme through salt and water absorption (colon), hence slow peristaltic transport of the chyme

- Immune recognition of antigens in the food (mainly caecum and appendix vermiformis = "tonsil" of the gastrointestinal tract).

Embryonic development

Of endodermal origin, derived from the mesenteron and metenteron.

Major diseases

- Acute and chronic inflammation (enteritis)
- Benign tumors (polyps), which often become malignant (Large intestine carcinomas are one of the most common malignant tumors in the industrialized world.)
- Acute inflammation (mostly bacterial) of the appendix vermiformis is very common (acute appendicitis,

mistakenly referred to as typhlitis). Spreading of the inflammation to the peritoneum can lead to life-threatening peritonitis. Therapy: surgical removal of the appendix (appendectomy).

1.10 Intestinum Crassum: Rectum

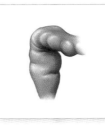

Location	Situated in the pelvis minor, extends anterior to the os sacrum to the diaphragma pelvis, largely in the spatium extraperitoneale in the pelvis. The proximal end may be	intraperitoneal, and the rest lies in the spatium extraperitoneale (retroperitoneal and subperitoneal).
Shape and parts	Hollow, tubular organ with • Ampulla recti (ampulla = circumscribed dilation) that serves as a stool reservoir and • Canalis analis.	*Note:* The rectum (straight) is by no means straight but has curves proximal to the os sacrum (flexura sacralis) and above the diaphragma pelvis (flexura perinealis).
Wall structure	Basically the same wall structure as the gastrointestinal tract with tunica mucosa, tela submucosa, tunica muscularis (with strata circulare and longitudinale), tela subserosa, and tunica serosa or adventitia.	*Note* the following characteristics in which the rectum differs from the rest of the intestinum crassum: absence of taeniae and haustra, no appendices omentales; three plicae transversae instead of plicae semilunares.

Neurovascular structures
(see also p. 420)
	Blood and lymphatic vessels (not the autonomic innervation) originate from **two sources:**
	
	Metenteron derivatives of the rectum, primarily the ampulla recti, **inferior mesenteric circulation:**
	• *Arteries:* unpaired a. rectalis superior from the a. mesenterica inferior
	• *Veins:* v. rectalis superior into the v. mesenterica inferior and from there into the v. portae hepatis to the hepar
	• *Lymphatic drainage:* 2 ways:
	  – through nll. rectales superiores into the nll. mesenterici inferiores
	  – through nll. sacrales and pararectales into the nodi iliaci interni
	
	Diaphragma pelvis derivatives, the canalis analis and anus, **pelvic circulation** (iliac circulation)**:**
	• *Arteries:* paired aa. rectales mediae (not always present) from the aa. iliacae internae, and aa. rectales inferiores from the aa. pudendae internae
		• *Veins:* (paired) vv. rectales mediae directly and (paired) vv. rectales inferiores via vv. pudendae internae into the vv. iliacae internae
		• *Lymphatic drainage:* through the nodi pararectales and nodi inguinales superficiales into the nodi iliaci interni
		
		Autonomic innervation (the same for both parts):
		• Parasympathetic through the nn. splanchnici pelvici (S 2–S 4)
		• Sympathetic through the nn. splanchnici lumbales and (to a lesser extent) sacrales (via plexus rectales superior, medius, and inferior)

Function	As part of the intestinum crassum, temporary and controlled storage of fecal matter (continence) and its controlled elimination (defecation). *Note:* Functional continence is ensured by gas-tight closure of the rectum. The rectal cavernous plexus (hemorrhoidal	plexus), which is supplied by the a. rectalis superior, remains filled up as part of the permanent contraction of the muscular sphincter apparatus.
Embryonic development	• Largely (mainly the ampulla recti) derived from the metenteron with an endodermal lining. • The distal part of the rectum, the canalis analis, develops from the ectodermal cells of the diaphragma pelvis.	*Note:* Terminologically, the canalis analis is considered either part of the rectum (with the ampulla recti as the part derived from the endoderm) or as a separate part of the intestine.
Major diseases	• Malignant tumors (rectal cancers) are one of the most common malignant tumors in industrialized nations. • Hemorrhoidal disease (dilation of the hemorrhoidal plexus; when bleeding occurs: bright red arterial blood)	• Anal fistulas and anal abscesses

1.11 Hepar (Liver)

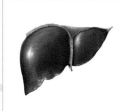

Location	• Lies intraperitoneally in the right upper quadrant. • As a result of the rotation of the gaster and the mesogastrium ventrale in the embryo, the hepar moves under surface of the diaphragma where it becomes partially attached (the area of the liver devoid of peritoneum = area nuda), moves with respiration.
Shape and parts	• Heaviest human parenchymal organ (weighs approximately 1.5 kg), in anterior view almost triangular in shape • Morphologically divided into lobi hepatici dexter and sinister, with lobi caudatus and quadratus included on the facies visceralis. • Based on vascular structures it is functionally and clinically divided into 8 segmenta; one segmentum = area supplied by one a. segmenti branch of the a. hepatica propria. **Models to describe the microstructure of the hepatic parenchyma:** • *(central venous) lobulus hepatis*: lobuli measuring 1-2 mm in size. In their midst lies the v. centralis. Cube-shaped hepatocytes are arranged around the v. centralis in a star-like pattern. Venous drainage is of primary importance to this concept of liver organization. • *(peri-) portal lobuli*: where multiple lobuli touch, they are connected through periportal areas (connective tissue with a. interlobularis, v. interlobularis, and ductus bilifer interlobularis = trias hepatica). At the center of the periportal lobulus is the periportal area or trias hepatica; this structural organization of the hepar is based on bile secretion (hepar as exocrine gland), however this model is no longer used. • *Hepatic acinus*: in the shape of a rhombus, the outer angles of which are formed by two opposite periportal areas and two opposite vv. centrales. This concept is based on arterial supply as the structural organization, most recent concept, important for pathophysiology.

Neurovascular structures
(see also p. 414)
	Upper abdominal circulation.
	
	• *Arteries:* a. hepatica propria from the a. hepatica communis (branch of the truncus coeliacus)
	• *Portal vein:* venous inflow from most of the entire gastrointestinal tract via the v. portae hepatis
	• *Veins:* vv. hepaticae (usually three) open into the v. cava inferior.
	• *Lymphatic drainage:* primarily through the nll. hepatici into the nll. coeliaci, but also through the diaphragma into the nll. mediastinales
	• *Autonomic innervation:*
	  – parasympathetic through the nn. vagi (trunci vagales)
	  – sympathetic primarily through the nn. splanchnici majores, but also partially through the nn. splanchnici minores (ganglia coeliaca)
	
	Note: The hepar has two sources of vascular inflow: the a. hepatica propria and the v. portae hepatis. Blood supplied by the a. hepatica propria is sufficient to sustain hepar function. The vv. hepaticae transverse the area nuda and open into the v. cava inferior. Segmenta hepatis can be resected individually, as the remaining parts of the hepar have high regenerative potential.

Function	• Largest "metabolic laboratory" of the human body. The v. portae hepatis carries the nutrient-rich blood from the gastrointestinal tract to the hepar. • *Exocrine* gland: via intra- and extrahepatic bile ducts, bile is secreted into the duodenum discontinuously and as needed. In the duodenum, bile emulsifies dietary fat. Emulsified fat particles have enlarged surface areas making it easier for duodenal enzymes to further break them down. • *Endocrine* gland: produces most of the blood proteins including coagulation factors and the prohormone angiotensinogen. The proteins are released into the vv. hepaticae. • Detoxification (metabolism) of numerous pharmaceuticals. They become water-soluble through metabolism and can thus be excreted through bile or blood (kidney).
Embryonic development	Of endodermal origin, derived from the gemma hepatopancreatica, sprouting of duodenal epithelium into the mesogastrium ventrale and the very small mesoduodenum ventrale.
Major diseases	• Acute and chronic inflammation (hepatitis), usually caused by alcohol or viral infection (hepatitis A, B or C). • Primary liver cell carcinoma is very rare in Europe, however, the hepar is often the site of metastases of carcinoma of the intestinum crassum (metastatic migration of tumor cells through the venous bloodstream via the v. portae hepatis).

1.12   Vesica Biliaris (Gallbladder) and Bile Ducts

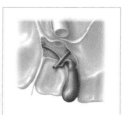

Location	• Vesica biliaris: lies *intraperitoneally* at the facies visceralis of the hepar. The collum of the vesica biliaris (exit point of the vesica biliaris) is oriented toward the fissura portalis principalis. The fundus of the vesica biliaris is just visible below the sharp margo inferior of the hepar along the mid-clavicular line beneath the arcus costalis. (When the vesica biliaris is inflamed, tenderness to pressure may be noted at this location.) • Extrahepatic bile ducts: lie *intraperitoneally* mainly in the lig. hepatoduodenale (part of the omentum minus). The terminal portion of the ductus choledochus that	traverses the pancreas and approaches the duodenum is secondarily *retroperitoneal*. *Note:* By definition the vesica biliaris is part of the bile duct system. In order to provide a better overview and because it is a blind sac connecting to the duodenum, it is listed separately. The intrahepatic bile ducts (canaliculi biliferi and ductus biliferi interlobulares), as intrinsic components of the hepar structure (see hepar), are not mentioned separately.
Shape, parts, and wall structure	• Vesica biliaris: small, pear-shaped pouch, measures up to 12 cm in length. • Extrahepatic bile ducts are divided into – ductus hepatici dexter and sinister – ductus hepaticus communis – ductus cysticus – ductus choledochus (formed by the merger of the ductus hepaticus communis and ductus cysticus) opens into the duodenum.	*Note:* Right before opening into the duodenum, the ductus choledochus and the ductus pancreaticus join. The walls of the vesica biliaris and the extrahepatic bile ducts include a tunica mucosa and a strong tunica muscularis for transporting bile.
Neurovascular structures (see also p. 414)	• *Arteries:* because of its proximity to the hepar, the arterial supply (a. cystica) is provided by the a. hepatica propria (from the r. dexter). • *Veins:* v. cystica into the v. portae hepatis • *Lymphatic drainage* (through the nll. hepatici and cystici) primarily into the nll. coeliaci	• *Autonomic innervation* same as for the liver: – parasympathetic through the nn. vagi (trunci vagales) – sympathetic through the n. splanchnicus major (ganglia coeliaca)
Function	• Storage and thickening of the bile produced by the hepatic cells, and the controlled release of bile through the ductus cysticus and ductus choledochus into the duodenum (through contraction of the muscular wall)	• Reservoir function: the vesica biliaris can store up to 50 mL of bile.
Embryonic development	Of endodermal origin. All parts of the bile ducts develop from the gemma hepatopancreatica, from a sprouting of the duodenal epithelium into the mesogastrium ventrale and the very small mesuoduodenum ventrale.	
Major diseases	• Gallbladder stones (concrements, crystal-like, hard substances in the liquid bile) not painful per se, painful only when the vesica biliaris tries to push out the stones through rhythmic muscle contractions, causing sudden onset of severe pain (colic); Fat digestion is possible even after surgical removal of the vesica biliaris because	the liver continues to produce bile; however, due to the absence of the bile reservoir, large amounts of fat can no longer be digested. • Inflammation of the vesica biliaris (cholecystitis) and malignant tumors are rare.

1.13 **Pancreas**

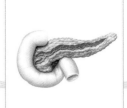

Location	Lies obliquely in the upper abdomen along the posterior wall of the bursa omentalis. Most of the corpus pancreatis lies at the L1 level, the caput pancreatis extends to the L2 level.
Shape and parts	Elongated gland with little connective tissue composed of • Caput pancreatis • Corpus pancreatis • Processus uncinatus (pancreatis) • Cauda pancreatis
Structure	Histologically and functionally the pancreas can be divided into • *Exocrine pancreas*: numerous small glands that secrete through an outflow duct (ductus pancreaticus)—mostly together with the ductus choledochus—into the duodenum. Often, there is a second pancreatic duct (ductus pancreaticus accessorius) present. • *Endocrine pancreas*: islets of epithelial cells (insulae pancreaticae) scattered throughout the exocrine pancreas. The islet cells release hormones directly into the bloodstream.

Neurovascular structures
(see also p. 416)
	Upper abdominal and mediastinal circulation:
	
	• *Arteries:* the arterial supply is from two directions via the pancreatic arcade:
	  – superiorly from branches of the truncus coeliacus (branches of the a. splenica: a. pancreatica magna; rr. pancreatici; a. pancreatica inferior. Branches of the a. hepatica communis: a. gastroduodenalis with aa. pancreaticoduodenales superiores anterior and posterior)
	  – inferiorly from a branch of the a. mesenterica superior: the a. pancreaticoduodenalis inferior
	• *Veins:* vv. pancreaticae (via v. splenicae) or vv. pancreaticoduodenales (via v. mesenterica superior) or directly into the v. portae hepatis
	
	• *Lymphatic drainage:* through nll. pancreatici superiores and inferiores and nll. pancreaticoduodenales into the nll. coeliaci and nll. mesenterici superiores
	• *Autonomic innervation:*
	  – parasympathetic through nn. vagi (primarily right n. vagus as truncus vagalis posterior)
	  – sympathetic through nn. splanchnici major and minor (ganglia coeliaca and ganglia mesenterica superiora)

Function	• *Endocrine part* (insulae pancreaticae): predominantly production of insulin and glucagon (two antagonistic hormones of glucose metabolism) • *Exocrine part:* production of numerous enzymes for the digestion of carbohydrates, fats, proteins and nucleic acids in the small intestine
Embryonic development	• Exocrine pancreas of endodermal origin, derived from two epithelial buds of the duodenum (gemmae pancreaticae ventralis and dorsalis) that later merge • Endocrine pancreas from endoderm derived insulae pancreaticae initiales
Major diseases	• Inflammation of the pancreas (pancreatitis) can be caused by bile reflux due to blockage of the ductus choledochus from a gallstone, or from chronic alcohol consumption. Insufficient secretion from the exocrine pancreas leads to lack of digestive enzymes and maldigestion. • The most common disease of the endocrine pancreas (and the pancreas in general) is insufficient insulin production from the islet cells that leads to type 1 diabetes. *Note:* The a. and v. mesentericae superiores pass adjacent to the pancreatic tissue in the area between caput and corpus pancreatis. Pancreatic tumors can lead to possible occlusion of these vessels. Cancer of the caput pancreatis can lead to occlusion of the ductus choledochus.

1.14   Splen (Spleen)

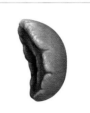

Location	Lies intraperitoneally in the left upper quadrant directly above the flexura coli sinister. Its longitudinal axis is oriented parallel to the 10th rib. Because of its location just below the diaphragma its position varies considerably with respiration.
Shape and parts	"Coffee bean shaped" with • The hilum splenicum, the entry and exit route for neurovascular structures, directed toward the gaster • One pole directed forward and downward (extremitas anterior) and one pole directed backward and upward (extremitas posterior) as well as a margo inferior and a margo superior • The facies diaphragmatica of the splen is directed toward the diaphragm and ribs. The facies gastrica, colica, and renalis are directed toward the corresponding organs. • Thickness by width by length approximately 4 x 7 x 11 cm (4711 rule), and reddish-brown color because of its abundance of red blood cells
Microstructure	• Blood from vessels located in strands of connective tissue (trabeculae splenicae) flows into the reticular meshwork through profusely branching vessels that are surrounded by aggregations of lymphocytes (lymphoreticular organ). • The blood vessels empty into the meshwork (sinus splenici) with low flow velocity (allowing for age verification of erythrocytes) and into the connective tissue itself (open circulation, a distinctive feature of the splen). The blood then flows back from the sinus splenici into the trabecular veins.
Neurovascular structures (see also p. 414)	Upper abdominal circulation: • *Arteries:* a. splenica from truncus coeliacus • *Veins:* through the v. splenica to the v. portae hepatis • *Lymphatic drainage:* through the nll. splenici (some through the nll. coeliaci) into the truncus intestinalis • *Autonomic innervation:* – parasympathetic: primarily through the right n. vagus (truncus vagalis posterior) – sympathetic through n. splanchnicus major and partly through the n. splanchnicus minor (ganglia coeliaca).
Function	• Largest lymphoid organ • Monitors the blood immunologically. • Destroys aged (80–100 days old) erythrocytes.
Embryonic development	• Derived from mesodermal tissue that sprouts into the mesogastrium dorsale • As the gaster rotates, the splen moves to the left upper quadrant. *Note:* During physical exercise (running), blood flow to the splen increases, and as a result the splen swells. Stretching of the peritoneal connection between the splen and colon (lig. splenocolicum) is believed to be the cause of "side stitch" (a piercing sensation felt below the rib cage).
Major diseases	• Affected by dysfunction of the hemolymphatic system (e.g., leukemia) • Painful swelling of the splen resulting from mononucleosis (a common viral infection) • Until recently, in cases of more severe upper abdominal injuries, a damaged splen was often removed because it is very difficult to repair due to its soft consistency.	Today, because the immune function of the splen is very important, surgical procedures where the splen is preserved are increasingly common (using fibrin glue). 5% of patients who have undergone splenectomy are affected by overwhelming post-splenectomy infection (OPSI) syndrome, a condition in which encapsulated bacteria often cause fatal sepsis.

1.15 Glandulae Suprarenales (Suprarenal or Adrenal Glands)

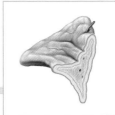

Location	• Primarily retroperitoneal (extraperitoneal) in the spatium retroperitoneale in the cavitas abdominis, each of the glands lies on the superior pole of the associated ren	• Located together with the renes in the capsulae adiposae
Shape and structure	• Triangular-shaped (cocked hat of Napoleon; facies renalis, anterior and posterior) • Larger (three-layered) outer cortex (with zona glomerulosa, zona fasciculata, and zona reticularis), the epithelial cells of the cortex form columns and conglomerates.	• Smaller inner medulla consists of sympathetic neurons that secrete into the blood: sympathetic paraneurons. • Suprarenal endothelial cells are active in phagocytosis—part of Aschoff's reticuloendothelial system.

Neurovascular structures (see also p. 421)	Retroperitoneal abdominal circulation:
	
	• *Arteries:* arterial supply provided by three tiers of arteries:
	  – aa. suprarenales superiores from the aa. phrenicae inferiores
	  – aa. suprarenales mediae from the aorta abdominalis
	  – aa. suprarenales inferiores from the aa. renales
	• *Veins:* drainage through the aa. suprarenales, on the right side (a. suprarenalis dextra) into the v. cava inferior and on the left side (v. suprarenalis sinistra) into the v. renalis
	• *Lymphatic drainage:* directly into the nll. lumbales
	• *Autonomic innervation:*
	  – parasympathetic: unclear.
		– sympathetic: preganglionic sympathetic fibers from the nn. splanchnici majores supply innervation to the medulla.
		
		Note: The preganglionic sympathetic nerve fibers synapse with the postganglionic cells directly in the medulla glandulae suprarenalis and not in the truncus sympathicus as is often the case in the pars sympathica of the nervous system. Thus, the preganglionic transmitter of the first sympathetic neuron is acetylcholine as is generally the case in the pars sympathica, whereas the second paraneuron secretes mainly epinephrine and some norepinephrine (10 %).

Function	Each of the paired gll. suprarenales consists of two endocrine parts, which have different embryonic origins: • *Cortex:* production of steroid hormones (glucocorticoids, mineralocorticoids, and male sex hormones) affecting glucose, fat and protein metabolism, and mineral balance	• *Medulla:* release of epinephrine and norepinephrine directly into the blood; functional component of the pars sympathica of the nervous system ("two glands one organ") *Note:* Blood flows from the cortex to the medulla (downstream).
Embryonic development	• Cortex: cells originate from the steroidogenic zone (mesodermal). • Medulla: cells migrate from the crista neuralis (ectodermal).	
Major diseases	Dysfunction of the cortex • Loss of cortex glandulae suprarenalis (suprarenal hypofunction, Addison's disease; without hormone replacement it is life-threatening), for example, resulting from destruction of the gl. suprarenalis through tuberculosis or metastatic involvement (malignant melanoma) or	• Hyperfunction of the cortex glandulae suprarenalis (Cushing's syndrome), which may occur as a result of ACTH producing tumors.

1.16   Renes (Kidneys)

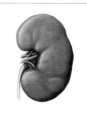

Location	• Lies primarily retroperitoneally (extraperitoneally) in the spatium retroperitoneale of the cavitas abdominis at the L1/L2 level, together with the gll. suprarenales within the capsula adiposa.	• Right ren lower than the left ren because it is pushed down by the larger hepar.
Shape and structure	• Bean-shaped, measuring 12 x 6 x 3cm (length x width x thickness) • The hilum renalis, directed medially, is the site of entry and exit for neurovascular structures and the ureter. • Extremitates (poli) superior and inferior, and facies anterior and posterior	• Margines lateralis and medialis • The entire renal tissue mass is enveloped by a tough capsula fibrosa.
Microstructure	• The outer cortex renalis contains numerous corpuscula renalia for formation of primary urine by ultrafiltration. • Toward the medulla renalis are microscopically fine tubular systems (pars convoluta of tubuli proximales and	pars convoluta and pars recta of tubuli distales with ansa nephroni) for concentration of primary urine. • Urine is discharged via calices renales into the pelvis renalis adjacent to the hilum renale, and then into the ureter.
Neurovascular structures (see also p. 421)	Retroperitoneal abdominal circulation • *Arteries:* left and right aa. renales directly from the aorta abdominalis • *Veins:* left and right vv. renales directly into the v. cava inferior • *Lymphatic drainage:* directly into the nll. lumbales • *Autonomic innervation:* – parasympathetic primarily through the nn. vagi (truncus vagalis posterior), and partially through nn. splanchnici pelvici from S2–S4 (mainly to the pelvis renalis)	– sympathetic primarily through the nn. splanchnici minor and imus (ganglia coeliaca and aorticorenalis), and partially through the plexus hypogastricus inferior (mainly to the pelvis renalis) *Note:* On the left side the left v. renalis receives the v. testicularis/ovarica sinistra and the v. suprarenalis sinister. The left v. renalis runs between the aorta abdominalis and a. mesenterica superior and can become compressed ("nutcracker syndrome") as it courses right into the v. cava inferior.
Function	• Regulation of water-, acid-base- and sodium-balance • Excretion of substances normally discharged with urine • Regulation of blood pressure • Stimulation of red blood cell production	• Influences metabolism of Vitamin D for regulation of calcium.
Embryonic development	Of mesodermal (intermediate mesoderm) origin, derived from the primitive metanephros (blastema metanephrogenicum). The primitive metanephros develops in the	pelvis and migrates upward until it is just inferior to the diaphragma (renal ascent).
Major diseases	• *Kidney stones:* when the solubility of compounds in the urine is exceeded, dissolved components may form crystallization nuclei. They may develop anywhere in the ren (e.g., staghorn calculi in the pelvis renalis). If they become lodged in the ureter, they may stimulate muscular contractions causing severe pain (colic). • Inflammation of the ren (*nephritis*) is possibly caused by bacterial involvement of the pelvis renalis (*pyelonephritis*), or autoimmunological involvement of the corpuscula renalia (glomerulonephritis).	• *Renal artery constriction* caused by atherosclerosis (with a drop in blood pressure) may lead to an increase in systemic blood pressure due to the ren's compensatory ability in blood pressure regulation. • Chronically elevated blood sugar (*diabetes*) may lead to renal dysfunction and increased blood pressure as a result of damage to the small renal arteries (microangiopathy).

1.17 **Ureter**

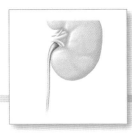

Location	Lies primarily retroperitoneal (extraperitoneal) in the abdomen and pelvis.
Shape and parts	Hollow tubular organ (pipeline) with narrow lumen; measures 24–31 cm in length, three parts: • Pars abdominalis: in the spatium retroperitoneale of the cavitas abdominis adjacent to the columna vertebralis, it runs from pelvis renalis to linea terminalis of bony pelvis. • Pars pelvica: in front of the os sacrum in the spatium retroperitoneale and subperitoneal pelvis; runs from linea terminalis to vesica urinaria wall.	• Pars intramuralis: in the vesica wall. *Note:* In the female, the ureter passes through the lig. latum uteri and crosses below the a. uterina (risk of injury during surgery!).
Structure	• Tunica mucosa with specialized urothelium (protection against hyperosmotic urine) • Submucosa • Tunica muscularis with strong muscle fibers (active transport)	• Tunica adventitia for integration into the connective tissue of the spatium extraperitoneale of the abdomen and pelvis

Neurovascular structures (see also p 421f)	Retroperitoneal abdominal circulation and pelvic circulation (iliac circulation):
	
	• *Arteries:* depending on which part of the ureter, rr. ureterici of the neighboring arteries of abdomen (a. renales) and pelvis (aa. vesicales superiores: possibly aa. iliacae internae)
	• *Veins:* depending on which part of the ureter, into the neighboring abdominal veins (vv. renales) and pelvic veins (plexus venosus vesicalis: possibly vv. iliacae internae)
		• *Lymphatic drainage:* depending on which part of the ureter directly into the nll. lumbales, vesicales or nll. iliaci
		• *Autonomic innervation:*
		  – parasympathetic through nn. splanchnici pelvici primarily from S2–S4
		  – sympathetic through nn. splanchnici minores or imi via the ganglia coeliaca and aorticorenalia, as well as nn. splanchnici lumbales via the plexus hypogastricus inferior

Function	• Active peristaltic transport of urine in quanta from pelvis renalis to vesica urinaria • Preventing reflux of urine and thus ascending infection in cases of vesica urinaria infection	
Embryonic development	Of mesodermal origin, in both the male and female the ureter is derived from the ductus mesonephricus. The ureter develops in the pelvis and moves upward with renal ascent.	
Distinctive features	Clinically significant constrictions (3 ureteral constrictions) due to • Proximity of the ureter to the extremitas inferior of the ren • The ureter being crossed by vessels (a. iliaca communis) at the level of the linea terminalis, as well as	• Passage of the ureter through the muscular vesica urinaria wall • An additional fourth constriction may occur where the ureter crosses below the testicular or ovarian vessels. The constrictions are potential sites where stones from the renes may lodge (ureteral stones).
Major diseases	• Ureteral stones, which may lodge at ureteral constrictions, may cause severe pain when the ureter contracts in order to push the stones toward the vesica urinaria (*ureteral colic*)	• Bacterial inflammation of the vesica urinaria may cause pathogens to pass through the ureters to the ren, resulting in ureteral inflammation (*ureteritis*).

1.18   Vesica Urinaria (Urinary Bladder)

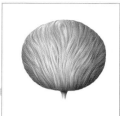

Location	Situated in the spatium extraperitoneale of the pelvis minor posterior to the symphysis pubica; the vesica urinaria sits on top of the diaphragma pelvis.
Peritoneal relations	The superior surface of the vesica urinaria is covered by peritoneum urogenitale (viscerale). The peritoneum is reflected onto the anterior abdominal wall and behind the vesica urinaria onto the anterior wall of the adjacent organ located posteriorly (uterus or rectum) where it is continuous with the peritoneum parietale.	*Note:* A well-distended vesica urinaria pushes the peritoneum superiorly. When it rises above the symphysis pubica this provides an access route for puncture of the anterior wall of the vesica urinaria that is devoid of peritoneum (suprapubic bladder aspiration).
Shape	Hollow organ shaped like a tureen or ball depending on the degree of distention, can hold up to 500–1000 mL. Corpus vesicae with apex vesicae (upper portion) and fundus vesicae, and cervix vesicae (toward the diaphragma pelvis).	The ostia ureterum and the ostium urethrae internum (with uvula vesicae) form a triangle (trigonum vesicae) on the inside wall of the fundus vesicae.
Wall structure	• Tunica ucosa with specialized urothelium (protection against osmotic effects of urine) • Tela submucosa • Distinct multilayered tunica muscularis, responsible for closing (continence) and opening (micturition) the bladder	• Adventitial layer (fascia pelvis visceralis), integrates the vesica urinaria into the surrounding connective tissue. The superior surface of the vesica urinaria is covered by peritoneum urogenitale, a serosa.
Neurovascular structures (see also p. 422)	Pelvic circulation (iliac circulation). • *Arteries:* via the visceral branches of the aa. iliacae internae: Aa. vesicales superiores and inferiores • *Veins:* drainage into the visceral branches of the vv. iliacae internae via the vv. vesicales • *Lymphatic drainage:* into the nll. iliaci interni	• *Autonomic innervation:* – *parasympathetic* through the nn. splanchnici pelvici from S 2–S 4 – *sympathetic* through the nn. splanchnici lumbales and sacrales (via the plexus hypogastricus inferior)
Function	Temporary and controlled storage of final urine (continence) and controlled discharge of urine (micturition)	
Embryonic development	Largely of endodermal origin, derived from the sinus urogenitalis, part of the cloaca; a small part (a portion of the posterior wall) of mesodermal origin, derived from both of the ductus mesonephrici that are integrated into the vesica urinaria. *Note:* An enlarged uterus, located posterior to the vesica urinaria (during pregnancy or resulting from muscular | tumors in the wall of the uterus [myoma]), reduces the bladder capacity resulting in frequent urination. Descent of the muscular diaphragma pelvis due to structural weakness caused by multiple vaginal deliveries may lead to failure of the closure mechanism and thus to urinary incontinence.
Major diseases	• Bacterial inflammation (cystitis) caused by germs that enter through the urethra, and is much more common in the female than the male due to the short urethra in the female. • Bladder carcinoma as a malignant tumor • Urinary incontinence resulting from diaphragma pelvis descent (mechanical insufficiency of the pelvic floor, | which may develop if the diaphragma pelvis slackens and descends after multiple vaginal deliveries). • Trabeculated bladder: obstruction of the outlet of the vesica urinaria with hypertrophied muscle bundles due to benign prostatic hyperplasia (BPH)

1.19 Urethra

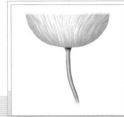

Note: Owing to gender differences regarding shape and function, the urethra is differentiated into

- Urethra feminina
- Urethra masculina

Location	In both the male and the female the urethra is directly below the vesica urinaria in the spatium extraperitoneale of the cavitas pelvis. In the male it is also in the corpus spongiosum penis. A portion of the urethra masculina below the bladder is surrounded by the prostata.
Shape	Hollow tubular organ with two orifices: • Ostium urethrae internum at the vesica urinaria outlet (in both the male and female) • Ostium urethrae externum on the body surface: in the female into the vestibulum vaginae, in the male on the glans penis

Parts	**Urethra feminina** (straight and approximately 3–5 cm long) divided into two parts:
	• Pars intramuralis (very short, in the vesica urinaria wall)
	• Spongy part (longer portion, opens into the vestibulum vaginae)
	
	Urethra masculina (20 cm long, has two curves) divided into four parts:
	• Pars intramuralis (very short, in the bladder wall, only for urine passage; with m. sphincter urethrae internus)
	• Pars prostatica (3 cm long, urinary and seminal passage, surrounded by prostata; with crista urethralis and colliculus seminalis)
	• Pars membranacea (1–2 cm long, passes through the hiatus urogenitalis in the diaphragma pelvis, distal portion with expandable urethral ampulla)
	• Pars spongiosa (15 cm long; in the corpus spongiosum penis, the dilated part known as the fossa navicularis is right before the ostium urethrae externum; the proximal portion of the pars spongiosa is attached to the diaphragma pelvis; the distal portion is suspended).
	
	• *Two curves of the urethra masculina:*
	  – infrapubic curve: at the junction between the partes membranacea and spongiosa
	  – prepubic curve: at the junction between the proximal and distal portions of the pars spongiosa
	• *Three constrictions of the urethra masculina:*
	  – pars intramuralis
	  – pars membranacea (proximal portion)
	  – ostium urethrae externum
	• *Three dilated parts of the urethra masculina:*
	  – pars prostatica
	  – urethral ampulla
	  – fossa navicularis

Wall structure	Tunica mucosa (urothelium in proximal portion, stratified non-keratinized squamous epithelium in distal portion) with gll. urethrales, tunica muscularis and adventitial coat

Neurovascular structures	Pelvic circulation.
	
	• *Arteries:* a. urethralis from the a. pudenda interna and smaller branches (in the male from the rr. prostatici; in the female from the a. vesicalis inferior and a. rectalis media)
	• *Veins:* drainage to the plexus venosus vesicalis (in the female) or plexus vesicalis, plexus venosus prostaticus, and veins of the penis (in the male)
	
	• *Lymphatic drainage:* nll. lumbales (via nll. iliaci interni or nodi inguinales)
	• *Autonomic innervation* (sparse):
	  – parasympathetic through the nn. splanchnici pelvici (S2–S4)
	  – sympathetic through the nn. splanchnici sacrales or plexus hypogastricus inferior
	  – somatic sensory innervation through the n. pudendus

Function	Discharge of urine from the body (in both the male and the female); transport of semen during ejaculation (in the male)
Embryonic development	Derived from the sinus urogenitalis (males and females), and an ingrowth of ectodermal cells from the glans penis (males)
Major diseases	• Acute or chronic inflammation (urethritis, very common!) caused by bacteria (in most cases) or fungus (less common). Burning sensation while urinating. Women are much more frequently affected than men. • Deformities during fetal development include urethrovaginal fistulas in young girls, or an atypical opening on the penis (mostly on the underside of the penis, known as hypospadias) in young boys.

1.20   Vagina

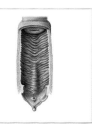

Location	Lies extraperitoneally in the spatium extraperitoneale of the pelvis. The vagina traverses the diaphragma pelvis posterior to the urethra in the hiatus urogenitalis and opens into the vestibulum vaginae between the labia minora.
Shape	Hollow, elongated tubular organ (measuring 8–10 cm in length)

Wall structure

- Specialized mucosa composed of stratified epithelium (mechanically resilient) where bacteria convert glycogen into lactic acid (acidic pH protects against ascending infections)
- Strong tunica muscularis

- Adventitia integrates the vagina into the surrounding pelvic connective tissue.

Note: There are no glands in the parietes vaginae. The wall is moistened by transudation.

Neurovascular structures
(see also p. 424)

Pelvic circulation (iliac circulation)

- *Arteries:* aa. vaginales (not always present) as distinct branches of the aa. iliacae internae, or rr. vaginales of the aa. uterinae
- *Veins:* plexus venosus vaginalis directly into the vv. uterinae or via the plexus venosus uterinus
- *Lymphatic drainage:* partially (only the superior portion) into the nll. parauterini, mostly into the nll. inguinales

superficiales (given that the vagina is a derivative of the diaphragma pelvis) and then into the nll. iliaci externi
- *Autonomic innervation:*
  - parasympathetic through the nn. splanchnici pelvici (S2–S4)
  - sympathetic through the nn. splanchnici lumbales and sacrales (via the plexus hypogastricus inferior)
- additional *somatosensory* innervation through the n. pudendus

Function	Copulatory organ, birth canal
Embryonic development	Derived from epithelial evaginations in the diaphragma pelvis (bulbi sinovaginales that fuse to form the lamina vaginae). The lamina vaginae develops initially as a solid structure that later undergoes secondary canalization.

Major diseases

- Infections caused by bacteria or fungi because of disruption of the normal vaginal milieu
- Malignant tumors (vaginal carcinoma) are rather rare.
- Rare, but explainable with regard to fetal development, are congenital fistulas to the urethra or rectum resulting in urine or feces being passed through the vagina (bacterial infections).

- Atrophy of the vaginal epithelium after menopause: strictly speaking this is not a disease given that menopause is a physiological process. It may however lead to subjective symptoms (vaginal dryness).

1.21 Uterus and Tubae Uterinae (Uterine Tubes)

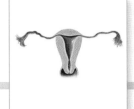

Location	Lies intraperitoneally in the pelvis minor (covered by peritoneum viscerale urogenitale). Only a small portion of the cervix uteri lies extraperitoneally. **Uterus:** • Between the vesica urinaria and rectum • The lig. latum uteri attaches the uterus to the lateral pelvic walls; the uterus is tilted anteriorly (anteverted); the corpus uteri forms an angle with cervix uteri and is bent forward (anteflexed).	*Note:* The lig. latum uteri is a sheet of connective tissue in which courses the neurovascular structures to the uterus and tubae uterinae, and partially also to the ovaria. That is why it is considered as "meso" (mesometrium/mesosalpinx/mesovarium = mesentery component of the uterus/tuba uterina/ovarium). **Tubae uterinae:** situated in the upper margin of the lig. latum uteri
Shape and parts	• Hollow, muscular, pear-shaped organ (uterus) • On the left and right sides arise a 7–10 cm long hollow tubular organ (right and left tubae uterinae). • The end of the tuba uterina (ampulla tubae uterinae) curves over a plum-sized and shaped organ (ovarium) in order to receive the ovulated egg (see ovarium). **Parts of the uterus:** • Corpus uteri (⅔) with facies posterior and anterior, and the blind-ended fundus uteri • Cervix uteri (⅓) with isthmus uteri and canalis cervicis uteri, portiones vaginalis and supravaginalis cervicis • Ostium uteri (opening in the vagina)	*Note:* A cervical mucus plug seals off the cervix uteri from the vagina and guards against the passage of bacteria ascending from the vagina. **Parts of the tubae uterinae** from lateral to medial: • Ostium abdominale tubae uterinae (fimbriated funnel-shaped end) • Infundibulum tubae uterinae • Ampulla tubae uterinae • Isthmus tubae uterinae • Pars uterina (very narrow, passes through the wall of the uterus) with ostium uterinum tubae uterinae
Wall structure	**Uterus:** • Tunica mucosa (endometrium with basal and functional layers), specialized to receive zygote. In sexually mature woman the endometrium undergoes cyclic changes with menstruation. • Tunica muscularis (myometrium): during pregnancy maintains uterine closure (cervical closure); expulsion of the fetus • Tunica serosa (perimetrium): allows for growth of the uterus in the cavitas peritonealis during pregnancy. *Note:* Contraction of the muscles in the uterine wall is controlled not only by nerves but also by hormones (oxytocin).	**Tubae uterinae:** • Tunica mucosa specialized to generate fluid flow (kinocilia) toward uterus, helps to transport the immobile zygote and to move mobile sperm in the required direction (positive rheotaxis). • Tunica muscularis: responsible for movement of tubae uterinae when sweeping the surface of the ovaria. • Tunica serosa (peritoneal covering) of the tuba uterina is continuous with the mesosalpinx (see "location" above).

Neurovascular structures (see also p. 424f)	Pelvic circulation (iliac circulation)
	
	Uterus:
	• *Arteries:* aa. uterinae from the aa. iliacae internae
	• *Veins:* drainage to the plexus venosus uterinus and to the vv. iliacae internae
	• *Lymphatic drainage:* via nodi lymphoidei parauterini et sacrales to internal and common iliac lymph nodes (mainly from the body of the uterus) and inguinal lymph nodes (cervix, drainage same as external genitals)
	• *Autonomic innervation:*
	  – parasympathetic: nn. splanchnici pelvici (S2–S4)
	  – sympathetic: mainly nn. splanchnici lumbales and partly nn. splanchnici sacrales (via plexus hypogastricus inferior)
		Uterine tubes:
		• *Arteries:* rr. tubarii from the aa. uterinae and aa. ovarici
		• *Veins:* drainage to plexus venosus uterinus or v. ovarica
		• *Lymphatic drainage:* directly or indirectly (via nll. parauterini) into nll. lumbales
		• *Autonomic innervation:* see uterus
		
		Note the uterus–tuba uterina angle: In the female, the lig. teres uteri traverses through the canalis inguinalis along with vasa lymphatica. Thus, metastatic tumor cells from the uterus–tuba uterina angle may settle within the nll. inguinales.

Function	**Uterus:** • Nurturing and sheltering of fetus during pregnancy • Expulsion of fetus	**Tubae uterinae:** • Collection of ovulated egg • Passage-way for ascending sperm • Site for fertilization • Transport of zygote to uterus
Embryonic development	**The uterus and tubae uterinae** are of mesodermal origin, derived from the ductus paramesonephrici: • Uterus derived from the fused ducts • Tubae uterinae derived from parts of the ducts that remain unfused	
Major diseases	**Uterus:** • Benign muscle tumors (myomas or fibroids), the growth of which may be influenced by sex hormones. They may put pressure on surrounding organs (vesica urinaria, rectum) or the tunica mucosa uteri (possible disruption of menstrual cycle). • Malignant tumors may develop in the tunica mucosa of the corpus uteri (endometrial carcinoma) or the cervix uteri (cervical carcinoma). • Descent of the diaphragma pelvis may lead to descent of the uterus.	**Tubae uterinae:** • Bacterial inflammation (adnexitis) generally ascends from the uterus. • Chronic inflammation may lead to occlusion of the tubal lumen (may inhibit conception). • Infections may spread from the ostium abdominale tubae uterinae to the cavitas peritonealis.

1.22 **Prostata and Glandula Vesiculosa (Seminal Vesicle)**

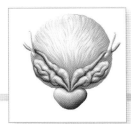

Location	**Prostata:** lies extraperitoneally just inferior to the vesica urinaria in the subperitoneal space of the cavitas pelvis; lies upon the m. levator ani, surrounds the proximal portion of the urethra (pars prostatica urethrae). **Gl. vesiculosa:** lies largely extraperitoneally directly adjacent to the posterior vesica urinaria wall (the most
	posterosuperior tip is the only portion covered by peritoneum).

Shape and structure	**Prostata:** • Unpaired gland that is enveloped by a fibrous capsula prostatae • Numerous branched epithelial ducts that empty into the urethra by small ductuli • The ductus excretorius of each gl. vesiculosa merges with the adjacent ductus deferens to form the ductus ejaculatorius that passes through the prostata.	**Gl. vesiculosa:** • Paired, elongated (5cm long) organs consisting of a tube that is coiled upon itself • The glands are surrounded by a fine capsule. *Note:* The histological division of the prostata into zones is done for clinical purposes. The term "seminal vesicle" is misleading: the gl. vesiculosa does not store semen. Their secretions constitute approximately 70% of the ejaculate.

Neurovascular structures
 (see also p. 422)
	Pelvic circulation (iliac circulation) for both organs
	
	 • *Arteries:* rr. prostatici mainly from the aa. vesicales inferiores
	 • *Veins:* plexus venosus prostaticus with drainage into the plexus venosus vesicalis (often described together as the vesicoprostatic venous plexus)
	 • *Lymphatic drainage:* partially into nll. prevesicales/retro-vesicales and then into the nll. iliaci interni, sacrales and lumbales
		• *Autonomic innervation:*
		   – parasympathetic through the nn. splanchnici pelvici (S2–S4)
		   – sympathetic through the nn. splanchnici lumbales and (to a lesser extent) the nn. splanchnici sacrales (via the plexus hypogastricus inferior)

Function	Produce secretions that, as components of the ejaculate, contains substances of functional importance for sperm motility. Secretions are alkaline and (particularly for the gll. vesiculosae) rich in fructose (energy source for sperm).

Embryonic development	**Prostata:** outgrowths of the urethral epithelium **Gl. vesiculosa:** outgrowths of the mesonephric epithelium (ductus mesonephrici)

Major diseases	**Prostata:** benign and malignant tumors: • Benign hyperplasia of the epithelium and stroma with urethral stricture and urinary retention is particularly common in the transition zone of older men. As the prostata enlarges it causes the vesica urinaria wall to thicken (known as trabeculated bladder) as the vesica urinaria tries to force urine out. Treatment consists of urethral dilation. • Prostatic carcinoma: develops in the peripheral zone in the epithelium below the capsula prostatica. Prostatic carcinoma is one of the most common malignant	tumors in older men. Often, tumor cells spread to the bones, particularly to the columna vertebralis, because the veins between the plexus venosus prostaticus and the plexus venosi vertebrales lack valves (pain in the lower region of the columna vertebralis in older men). **Gl. vesiculosa:** rare cases of inflammation caused by genital infections

1.23 Epididymis and Ductus Deferens

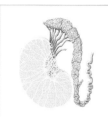

Location	**Epididymis:** lies extraperitoneally (not in the tunica vaginalis surrounding the testis) in the scrotum on the posterolateral aspect of the testis. **Ductus deferens:** (continuous with epididymis) passes through the canalis inguinalis and runs along the superior and posterior surface of the vesica urinaria to the prostata. The part that is situated on the superior surface of the vesica urinaria is covered by peritoneum urogenitale ("subperitoneal location").

Shape and structure	**Epididymis:** up to 12 m long, highly convoluted duct (ductus epididymidis), that is divided into the caput, corpus, and cauda epididymidis. The cauda epididymidis is continuous with the ductus deferens. **Ductus deferens:** approximately 40 cm in length with strong muscle fibers that spiral around the very narrow lumen (often appears three-layered in histological section). The epithelium bears stereocilia. At the prostata the duct widens out to form the ampulla ductus deferentis where it then continues as the ductus ejaculatorius (after joining with the ductus excretorius of the gl. vesiculosa) through the prostata. *Note:* Owing to its strong muscle fibers, the ductus deferens has the thickness of a pencil and is palpable in the canalis inguinalis.

Neurovascular structures
(see also p. 423)
	Epididymis: retroperitoneal abdominal circulation (with testicular vessels). Partially pelvic circulation as well (iliac circulation). Some of the epididymal neurovascular structures join the neurovascular structures of the testis.
	
	• *Arteries:* branches (rr. epididymales) of the aa. testiculares
	• *Veins:* drainage to the plexus pampiniformis into the vv. testiculares
	• *Lymphatic drainage:* nll. lumbales
	• *Autonomic innervation:*
	  – parasympathetic through nn. splanchnici pelvici (S2–S4)
	  – sympathetic through nn. splanchnici lumbales and via the plexus hypogastricus inferior
	Ductus deferens: pelvic circulation (iliac circulation)
	
	• *Arteries:* a. ductus deferentis from the a. umbilicalis
	• *Veins:* drainage partially to plexus pampiniformis, partially to plexus venosus vesicalis
	• *Lymphatic drainage:* nll. lumbales
	• *Autonomic innervation:*
	  – parasympathetic through nn. splanchnici pelvici (S2–S4)
	  – sympathetic through nn. splanchnici lumbales and via the plexus hypogastricus inferior

Function	**Epididymis:** storage and maturation of sperm produced in the testes **Ductus deferens:** rapid transport of sperm into the urethra during ejaculation *Note:* The formation and maturation of sperm in the testis and epididymis, the migration of sperm in the epididymis, and their final storage in the caudal part of the ductus epididymidis takes approximately 80 days.

Embryonic development	Both organs are of mesodermal origin, derived from the caudal portion of the ductus mesonephricus.

Major diseases	Inflammation of the epididymis (epididymitis) or ductus deferens is rare.

1.24 **Testis**

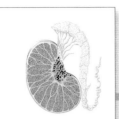

Location	Extracorporeal in the scrotum; largely surrounded by a closed peritoneal sac (tunica vaginalis testis). The position in the scrotum is the result of fetal testicular descent.
Shape and structure	Paired organ with the approximate size and shape of a plum, divided by fibrous septula testis into approximately 350 lobuli testis. Each lobulus testis contains 2–4 tubuli seminiferi contorti lined by specialized epithelium where the spermatocytes develop (spermatogenesis). The tissue between the tubuli contains Leydig cells, which produce testosterone.

Neurovascular structures (see also p. 423)	Retroperitoneal abdominal circulation (despite extracorporeal location)
	During development, the testis together with its neurovascular structures descend from the upper abdomen into the scrotum. Thus, the neurovascular structures do not arise from structures in the pelvis (analogous to the ovarium).
	
	• *Arteries:* aa. testiculares from the upper portion of the aorta abdominalis
	• *Veins:* drainage to the plexus pampiniformis and then through the vv. testiculares on the right side directly into the v. cava inferior, and on the left side into the left v. renalis
	• *Lymphatic drainage:* nll. lumbales
	• *Autonomic innervation:*
	  – from nn. sacrales S2–S4 (nn. splanchnici pelvici)
	  – sympathetic primarily through the nn. splanchnici minor and imus via the ganglia mesenterica superiora and aorticorenalia (via the plexus testicularis)

Function	Produce gametes (sperm) and male sex hormones (testosterone).
Embryonic development	Of mesodermal origin, derived from the initially undifferentiated gonadal primordia in the crista mesonephrica in the area of the upper vertebrae lumbales. Sperm precursor cells migrate secondarily from the wall of the saccus vitellinus. *Note:* The testes are located in the scrotum (extracorporeal location) because the higher temperature within the cavitas abdominalis would inhibit spermatogenesis.
Major diseases	• Failure of normal testicular descent leads to abdominal testes (testis remains in the cavitas abdominis or pelvis) or inguinal testes (testis remains in the canalis inguinalis). The higher temperature within the cavitas abdominis or pelvis (as the testis is located closer to the core) inhibits the production of sperm and may lead to male infertility (with normal hormone production). • Dilations of the plexus pampiniformis (varicoceles, mainly left sided) may lead to overheating of the testis (due to the increased amount of warm blood) and reduced fertility. • Malignant testicular carcinoma is one of the most common cancers in young men. The risk of malignant testicular cancer (seminoma, teratoma) increases with cryptorchidism (an undescended testis located within a body cavity).

1.25 Ovarium

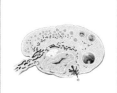

Location	Lies intraperitoneally in the pelvis minor in the fossa iliaca (after descent). *Note:* The peritoneal covering of the ovarium has mistakenly been referred to as germinal epithelium although it does not participate in egg production. The "germinal epithelium" of the testis, however, does not describe a peritoneal covering but rather the epithelium that produces sperm.

Shape and structure	• Paired organ with the approximate size and shape of a plum, presenting an extremitas tubaria (vascular pole) and an extremitas uterina (uterine pole)
	• Divided into
	  – connective tissue capsule (tunica albuginea),
	  – cortex ovarii and medulla ovarii.
		The cortex ovarii consists of folliculi ovarici at various stages of development. Each folliculus contains a single oocyte surrounded by follicular epithelial cells and an envelope of connective tissue (theca folliculi).
		Note: Female sex hormones are not produced by the ovum but by cells of the connective tissue surrounding it.

Neurovascular structures
(see also p. 425)
	Primarily retroperitoneal abdominal circulation, pelvic circulation (iliac circulation) plays a minor role.
	
	• *Arteries:* aa. ovaricae from the aorta abdominalis, and rr. ovarici of the aa. uterinae (together they form the ovarian arcade)
	Note: When surgically removing the ovarium two vascular systems need to be ligated due to the ovarium's dual blood supply.
	• *Veins:* on the right side the v. ovarica dextra into the v. cava inferior, on the left side the v. ovarica sinistra into
		the left v. renalis; also ovarian venous plexus to plexus venosus uterinus
		• *Lymphatic drainage:* into the nll. lumbales
		• *Autonomic innervation:*
		  – parasympathetic primarily through the nn. vagi
		  – sympathetic primarily through the nn. splanchnici minor and imus (via ganglia mesenterica superiora and aorticorenalia)

Function	• Production of female gametes (eggs) • Cyclic production of female sex hormones	
Embryonic development	Derived from the gonadal primordia in the intermediate mesoderm of the crista mesonephrica in the area of the upper vertebrae lumbales. From there, the ovarium descends into the pelvis minor (ovarian descent). *Note:* The embryonic ovarium is initially retroperitoneal in location, and moves intraperitoneal as the cristae	mesonephricae fuse. As the ovarium descends from the upper abdomen into the pelvis, it drags its neurovascular structures with it. Thus, the neurovascular structures course within a fold of the peritoneum (the lig. suspensorium ovarii).
Major diseases	• Ovarian cancer: particularly malignant because the tumor cells can easily spread within the entire cavitas abdominalis.	• Dysfunction of follicular development leading to reduced fertility or menstrual cycle disorder.

Appendix

References

Agur AMR. Grants Anatomie. Lehrbuch und Atlas. Stuttgart: Enke; 1999

Anschütz F. Die körperliche Untersuchung. 3. Aufl. Heidelberg: Springer; 1978

Aumüller G, Aust G, Doll A et al. Anatomie. Duale Reihe. Stuttgart: Thieme; 2007

Bähr M, Frotscher M. Duus' Neurologisch-topische Diagnostik. 8. Aufl. Stuttgart: Thieme; 2003

Becker C. CT-Diagnostik der koronaren Herzkrankheit. Teil I: Indikation, Durchführung und Normalbefundung der CT-Koronarographie. Radiologie up2date 2008; 1: 55-67; DOI 10.1055/s-2007-995498

Block B, Meier PN, Manns MP. Lehratlas der Gastroskopie. Stuttgart: Thieme; 1997

Block B, Schachschal G, Schmidt H. Der Gastroskopie-Trainer. Stuttgart: Thieme; 2003

Brambs H-J. Pareto-Reihe Radiologie. Gastrointestinales System. Stuttgart: Thieme; 2007

Claussen CD, Miller S, Fenchel M et al. Pareto-Reihe Radiologie. Herz. Stuttgart: Thieme; 2007

Dauber, W. Feneis' Bild-Lexikon der Anatomie. 9. Aufl. Stuttgart: Thieme; 2005

Dietrich Ch, Hrsg. Endosonographie. Lehrbuch und Atlas des endoskop-ischen Ultraschalls. Stuttgart: Thieme; 2007

Dorschner W, Stolzenburg J-U, Neuhaus J. Structure and Function of the Bladder Neck. Advances in Anatomy, Embryology and Cell Biology Vol. 159. Berlin: Springer; 2001

Drews U. Taschenatlas der Embryologie. 2. Aufl. Stuttgart: Thieme; 2006

Faller A, Schünke M. Der Körper des Menschen—Einführung in Bau und Funktion. 15. Aufl. Stuttgart: Thieme; 2008

Fanghänel J, Pera F, Anderhuber F, Nitsch R, Hrsg. Waldeyer - Anatomie des Menschen. Berlin: De Gruyter; 2003

Flachskampf F. Kursbuch Echokardiografie. 4. Aufl. Stuttgart: Thieme; 2008

Földi M, Kubik S. Lehrbuch der Lymphologie. 3. Aufl. Stuttgart: Gustav Fischer; 1993

Frick H, Leonhardt H, Starck D. Allgemeine und spezielle Anatomie. Taschenlehrbuch der gesamten Anatomie, Bd. 1 u. 2. 4. Aufl. Stuttgart: Thieme; 1992

Fritsch H, Kühnel W. Taschenatlas der Anatomie. Bd. 2. 7. Aufl. Stuttgart: Thieme; 2001

Graumann W, v. Keyserlingk D, Sasse D. Taschenbuch der Anatomie. Stuttgart: Gustav Fischer; 1994

Greten H, Hrsg. Innere Medizin. 12. Aufl. Stuttgart: Thieme; 2005

Hamm B, Krestin GP, Laniado M, Paul G, Volkmar N, Taupitz M, Hrsg. MRT von Abdomen und Becken. 2. Aufl. Stuttgart: Thieme; 2006

Hegglin J. Chirurgische Untersuchung. Stuttgart: Thieme; 1976

Heinecker R. EKG in Klinik und Praxis. Stuttgart: Thieme; 1975

Ignjatovic D et al. Can the gastrocolic trunk of Henle serve as an anatomical landmark in laparoscopic right colectomy? A postmortem anatomical study. The American Journal of Surgery 2010; 199: 249–254

Jin G, Tuo H, Sugiyama M et. al. Anatomic study of the superior right colic vein: its relevance to pancreatic and colonic surgery. The American Journal of Surgery 2006; 191: 100–103

Kahle W, Frotscher M. Taschenatlas der Anatomie. Bd. 1. Stuttgart: Thieme; 2001

Klinke R, Silbernagl S. Lehrbuch der Physiologie. 3. Aufl. Stuttgart: Thieme; 2001

Lange S. Radiologische Diagnostik der Thoraxerkrankungen. 3. Aufl. Stuttgart: Thieme; 2005

von Lanz T, Wachsmuth W. Praktische Anatomie. Bd. II/6 Bauch. Berlin: Springer; 1993

Lippert H, Pabst R. Arterial Variations in Man. München: Bergmann; 1985

Loeweneck H. Diagnostische Anatomie. Berlin: Springer; 1981

Lüllmann-Rauch R. Histologie. 2. Aufl. Stuttgart: Thieme; 2006

Masuhr KF, Neumann M. Neurologie. Duale Reihe. 5. Aufl. Stuttgart: Thieme; 2005

McNeal JE. Regional morphology and pathology of the prostate. Am J Clin Pathol 1968; 49: 347–357

Möller TB, Reif E. Taschenatlas der Röntgenanatomie. 3. Aufl. Stuttgart: Thieme; 2006

Möller TB, Reif E. Taschenatlas der Schnittbildanatomie. Bd. 2: Thorax, Abdomen, Becken. 2. Aufl. Stuttgart: Thieme; 2000

Moore KL, Persaud TVN. Embryologie. 5. Aufl. München: Urban & Fischer bei Elsevier; 2007

Nauth HF. Gynäkologische Zytodiagnostik. Stuttgart: Thieme; 2002

Netter FH. Farbatlanten der Medizin. Stuttgart: Thieme; 2000

Platzer W. Taschenatlas der Anatomie. Bd. 1. Stuttgart: Thieme; 1999

Platzer W. Atlas der topographischen Anatomie. Stuttgart: Thieme; 1982

Rauber A, Kopsch F. Anatomie des Menschen. Bd. 1 -4. Stuttgart: Thieme; Bd 1. 2. Aufl. 1997; Bde. 2 u. 3 1987; Bd. 4 1988

Reiser M, Kuhn FP, Debus J. Radiologie. Duale Reihe. 2. Aufl. Stuttgart: Thieme; 2006

Rohde H. Lehratlas der Proktologie. Stuttgart: Thieme; 2006

Rohen JW. Topographische Anatomie. 10. Aufl. Stuttgart: Schattauer; 2000

Romer AS, Parson TS. Vergleichende Anatomie der Wirbeltiere. 5. Aufl. Hamburg und Berlin: Parey; 1983

Sadler ThW. Medizinische Embryologie. 11. Aufl. Stuttgart: Thieme; 2008

Schneider H, Ince H, Kische S, Rehders TC et al. Management der Aortenisthmusstenose im Erwachsenenalter: Diagnostik, Prognose und Behandlung. Kardiologie up2date 2008; 4: 85–99; DOI: 10.1055/s-2007-995625

Schünke M. Funktionelle Anatomie - Topographie und Funktion des Bewegungssystems. Stuttgart: Thieme; 2000

Schumacher GH, Aumüller G. Topographische Anatomie des Menschen. 6. Aufl. Stuttgart: Gustav Fischer; 1994

Schumpelick V, Bleese N, Mommsen U. Chirurgie. 4. Aufl. Stuttgart: Enke; 1999

Schwalenberg T, Neuhaus J, Dartsch M et al. Funktionelle Anatomie des männlichen Kontinenzmechanismus. Der Urologe 2010; 49: 472–480

Silbernagl S, Despopoulos A. Taschenatlas der Physiologie. 6. Aufl. Stuttgart: Thieme; 2003

Silbernagl S, Despopoulos A. Taschenatlas der Physiologie. 6. Aufl. Stuttgart: Thieme; 2003

Stelzner F. Chirurgie an viszeralen Abschlußsystemen. Stuttgart: Thieme; 1998. Unter Benutzung der Ergebnisse von Widmer O. Die Rektalarterien des Menschen. Z Anat Entwickl-Gesch 1955; 118

Stelzner F. Der Verschluß der terminalen Speiseröhre. Deutsch Med Wochensch 1968; 93: 1679 -1685

Strohmeyer G, Dölle W. Ösophagusvarizen: Bedeutung, Ursachen und Behandlung. Med Klein 1963; 58: 1649 -1653 Thelen M, Erbel R, Kreitner KF, Barkhausen J, Hrsg. Bildgebende Kardiodiagnostik. Stuttgart: Thieme; 2007

Tillmann B. Farbatlas der Anatomie. Zahnmedizin—Humanmedizin. Stuttgart: Thieme; 1997

Thurn P, Bücheler E. Einführung in die Röntgendiagnostik. 6. Aufl. Stuttgart: Thieme; 1979

Wallner C, Dabhoiwala NF, DeRuiter MC et al. The Anatomical Components of Urinary Continence. European Urology 2009; 55/4: 932–944

Wedel T. Funktionelle Anatomie—Voraussetzung zum Verständnis von Defäkationsstörungen. In: Chir Gastroenterol 2007; 23: 220–227

Wedel T, Stelzner S. Persönliche Mitteilung

Subject Index